EMERGING THEORIES IN HEALTH PROMOTION PRACTICE AND RESEARCH

In the world of theory there strode three giants:
Albert Bandura, Martin Fishbein,
Everett Rogers

Many have stood on their broad shoulders and
benefited from their seminal research. To them the
field owes a great debt of gratitude.

EMERGING THEORIES IN HEALTH PROMOTION PRACTICE AND RESEARCH

Second Edition

RALPH J. DICLEMENTE
RICHARD A. CROSBY
MICHELLE C. KEGLER

Editors

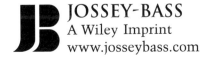

JOSSEY-BASS
A Wiley Imprint
www.josseybass.com

Published by Jossey-Bass
A Wiley Imprint
989 Market Street, San Francisco, CA 94103-1741—www.josseybass.com

Jossey-Bass books and products are available through most bookstores. To contact Jossey-Bass directly call our Customer Care Department within the U.S. at 800-956-7739, outside the U.S. at 317-572-3986, or fax 317-572-4002.

Jossey-Bass also publishes its books in a variety of electronic formats. Some content that appears in print may not be available in electronic books.

Library of Congress Cataloging-in-Publication Data

Emerging theories in health promotion practice and research / Ralph J. DiClemente, Richard A. Crosby, Michelle C. Kegler, editors ; foreword by Ross Brownson.—2nd ed.
    p.   cm.
  Includes bibliographical references and index.
    ISBN 978-0-470-17913-0 (cloth)
      1. Health promotion--United States. 2.   Health promotion—Research--United States.
  3. Community health services—United States.   4. Public health—United States.
  I. DiClemente, Ralph J.   II. Crosby, Richard A., 1959-   III. Kegler, Michelle C., 1961-
  [DNLM: 1. Health Promotion. 2.   Community Health Services.   3. Health Behavior.
  4. Models, Organizational. WA 590 E53 2010]
  RA427.8.E447 2010
  613.0973—dc22
                                                                            2009032202

Printed in the United States of America
SECOND EDITION

PB Printing   10 9 8 7 6 5 4 3 2 1

CONTENTS

TABLES AND FIGURES

TABLES

FIGURES

FOREWORD

As illustrated in this volume, we are learning more about the important role of existing and new theories in promoting health. A theory is a set of interrelated concepts, definitions, and propositions that presents a systematic view of events by specifying relations among variables to explain and predict the events. Theories help to explain behavior and

In theory there is no difference between theory and practice. In practice there is.
—Yogi Berra

suggest ways to achieve behavior change, and are created after observation and testing. They are designed to rationally and clearly explain a phenomenon. As noted by Bandura,[1] in some scientific disciplines (for instance, mathematics), theories integrate laws, whereas in newer fields (for example, public health, behavioral science), theories describe or specify the determinants governing the phenomena of interest. Moreover, when planning programs, theory can point to important intervention and evaluation strategies. For example, if perceptions are considered important in maintaining behavior, then it will be crucial to include some strategies to alter perceptions, whereas if skills are considered important to change behavior, then some strategy to alter skills must be included in the intervention. Does theory matter when developing and implementing interventions to improve public health? The verdict is in on this question, and the answer is a resounding "Yes." It is now established that the effectiveness of public health interventions can be enhanced by use of theory-based planning frameworks such as those described in the second edition of *Emerging Theories in Health Promotion Practice and Research*.

Knowing the importance of theory, we are beginning to document the use of theory in behavior-change interventions, thus identifying gaps needing attention. Painter and colleagues recently reviewed articles in ten leading public health, medicine, and psychology journals.[2] They found that 36 percent of studies mentioned theory. The most commonly used theories were those focusing on either individual-level behavior change (for example, the health belief model) or at the interpersonal level (for example, the social cognitive theory). Articles using theory most often were informed by theory (68 percent), whereas a smaller proportion sought to build theory (9 percent) or tested theory (4 percent). This suggests a significant gap the literature that is filled by this volume—that is, the development and testing of theories for specific populations, settings, and approaches to intervention. The chapters in *Emerging Theories in Health Promotion* lie at the nexus between what we have learned from past theory-driven research, the challenges that we face in continuing to build the evidence base, and the application of theory in "real-world" settings. As theories have evolved, it is likely that the earliest individually focused theories were developed in less complex systems compared to many of the theories described in this volume, which are applied in complex and multidisciplinary systems and often to underserved populations. Three particularly important themes are woven through various chapters in the current volume: a priority on eliminating health disparities, the need for an "upstream" focus, and an improved understanding of how to apply theory in practice settings.

Theory can play a crucial role in addressing health disparities. The elimination of health disparities is one of the two overarching goals of the Healthy People 2010 national health agenda. Recent data show large and growing differences in disease burden and health outcomes between high- and low-income groups.[3] The health disparities also persist in other population subgroups, such as African Americans, Hispanic/Mexican Americans, and American Indians/Alaskan Natives. As noted in several chapters in this book, health disparities are often associated with poverty and social fragmentation. Theory-based approaches show promise in addressing these health disparities. For example, diverse community coalitions with active participation can lead to more effective intermediate outcomes. Much of the evidence on the use and effectiveness of theory has developed in Western, European-American settings. This book makes an important contribution by exploring how theory can be applied in other cultures. Often these are populations with significant health disparities.

While interventions are often organized around ecological frameworks, the existing health behavior change literature has lacked sufficient focus on "upstream" intervention levels of such frameworks. The upstream, sociopolitical public health actions (for example, raising the price of tobacco) are likely to be more cost-effective and save more lives than downstream interventions (for example, conducting smoking cessation classes).[4] Thus, we know that public health policy, in the form of laws, guidelines, and regulations, can have a profound effect on health status. In a review of behavioral research articles,[2] only 2 percent of studies were policy-focused. Policy, in the form of laws, regulations, and organizational guidelines, has a profound effect on our daily lives and health status. Policy interventions have the potential to equalize the environment in a way that may significantly reduce the growing disparities. However, upstream approaches can be subject to the "inverse evidence" law, in which there is less evidence on social and policy determinants of health than on individual-level interventions, due in part to the difficulty in studying these issues with "gold standard" research designs (for example, randomized trials).[5] Therefore, we often have the right answers to the wrong questions.

As noted in this volume, the challenges in putting theory to work in public health practice are not trivial. It is very likely that the capacity of an organization has a direct bearing on its ability to implement theory-driven interventions. The lack of trained staff, facilities, and external funding, along with a lack of appropriate infrastructure for adoption, can often inhibit implementation and maintenance of even the most effective interventions. Implementation research seeks to understand the processes and factors that are associated with successful integration of evidence-based interventions within a particular setting (for example, a worksite or school).[6] Implementation of theory-based programs often results in a tension between fidelity (maintaining the original program design) and reinvention (changes needed for replication in a new setting). As noted in this text, participatory processes are increasingly being used with evidence-based efforts to understand local context while maintaining some degree of fidelity. In addition, when practice settings seek out appropriate and adequate resources (for example, training, technical assistance), the likelihood of success in adopting and maintaining theory-driven interventions is increased.

This timely and well-conceived second edition of *Emerging Theories in Health Promotion* covers these issues and a wide range of others, forging new ground on numerous topics. This text will become treasured reading for researchers or practitioners interested in having the most up-to-date set of tools in their health promotion toolbox.

Ross C. Brownson, PhD

REFERENCES

1. Bandura A. *Social foundations of thought and action: A social cognitive theory.* Englewood Cliffs, NJ: Prentice Hall, 1986.

2. Painter, J. E., Borba, C. P., Hynes, M., Mays, D., and Glanz, K. (2008). The use of theory in health behavior research from 2000 to 2005: A systematic review. *Annals of Behavioral Medicine.*

3. Ezzati, M., Friedman, A. B., Kulkarni, S. C., and Murray, C. J. (2008). The reversal of fortunes: Trends in county mortality and cross-county mortality disparities in the United States. *PLoS Medicine, 5*(4), e66.

4. McKinlay, J. B., and Marceau, L. D. (2000). Upstream healthy public policy: Lessons from the battle of tobacco. *International Journal of Health Services, 30*(1), 49–69.

5. Nutbeam, D. (2003). How does evidence influence public health policy? Tackling health inequalities in England. *Health Promotion Journal of Australia, 14*, 154–158.

6. Rabin, B. A., Brownson, R. C., Haire-Joshu, D., Kreuter, M. W., and Weaver, N. L. (2008). A glossary for dissemination and implementation research in health. *Journal of Public Health Management Practice, 14*(2), 117–123.

ACKNOWLEDGMENTS

We wish to acknowledge all our wonderful and talented contributors for their time, effort, and dedication. Their research, practice, and advocacy make life better for all people. We thank Andrew Pasternack, our editor, for his encouragement, steadfast support, and valuable feedback, Seth Schwartz, whose acumen and assistance have been instrumental to creating this volume, and Seth Miller and Merrill Peterson at Matrix Productions, for their diligence in producing it.

THE EDITORS

Ralph J. DiClemente, PhD, is Charles Howard Candler Professor at the Rollins School of Public Health, Emory University. He holds concurrent appointments in the School of Medicine, Department of Medicine, Division of Infectious Diseases, and the Department of Pediatrics, Division of Infectious Diseases, Epidemiology, and Immunology. He is also associate director, Center for AIDS Research. His research focuses on identifying the determinants of adolescent/young adults' HIV/STD-associated sexual behavior and designing interventions to reduce sexual risk behaviors and their adverse health consequences. He has authored or edited fourteen books and written over three hundred scientific articles.

Richard A. Crosby, PhD, is an endowed professor and chair of the Department of Health Behavior in the College of Public Health at the University of Kentucky. He was previously an assistant professor at the Rollins School of Public Health and served as a Fellow of the Association of Teachers for Preventive Medicine at CDC. He has published numerous journal articles addressing empirical questions related to safer sex practices among persons at high risk of acquiring sexually transmitted infections. Dr. Crosby is also an author of a textbook devoted to research methods (*Research Methods for Health Promotion*) and coeditor of a textbook devoted to the promotion of adolescent health (*Adolescent Health: Understanding and Preventing Risk*). As a dedicated teacher, Dr. Crosby has shared in the training of countless numbers of students earning their Masters in Public Health degree.

Michelle C. Kegler, DrPH, MPH, is an associate professor and director of Graduate Studies in the Department of Behavioral Sciences and Health Education in the Rollins School of Public Health at Emory University. She is also deputy director of the Emory Prevention Research Center. Dr. Kegler received her BA degree (1983) in psychology from the University of Minnesota, her MPH (1985) in health behavior and health education from the University of Michigan, and her DrPH (1995) in the same field from University of North Carolina at Chapel Hill. Her research interests include community-based approaches to chronic disease prevention, with an emphasis on community coalitions and program evaluation. She has published numerous articles on community coalitions, community capacity, and evaluation results from community-based programs. She is also interested in environmental approaches to health promotion, with recent work focusing on the home environment as a setting for obesity prevention and reduction of exposure to secondhand smoke. Dr. Kegler teaches program evaluation and health promotion interventions.

THE CONTRIBUTORS

Marc A. Adams, MPH, is a doctoral candidate in the Joint Doctoral Program in Public Health (Health Behavior) between San Diego State University and the University of California, San Diego. He is also a research associate at the Center for Behavioral Epidemiology and Community Health (CBEACH) and at the Center for Wireless and Population Health Systems. His research interests include theory development and promotion of physical activity and healthy diets; tobacco control, and sun protection behavior.

Angie Alaniz is the Brazos Valley Regional Director for the Center for Community Health Development at the Texas A&M Health Science Center, School of Rural Public Health, one of CDC's thirty-three designated Prevention Research Centers. Her work focuses on building capacity of rural communities through leadership development, training, and technical assistance. She has extensive expertise in community health development and partnership facilitation.

Moya L. Alfonso, PhD, MSPH, is a research assistant professor with the Florida Prevention Research Center at the University of South Florida. She is also senior research coordinator for the Center for Social Marketing at the University of South Florida. She has a decade of experience in community-based participatory research and evaluation. Her research interests include community youth development and adolescent health, with an emphasis on the prevention of alcohol use.

Julie A. Baldwin, PhD, is professor and chair of the Department of Community and Family Health, College of Public Health, University of South Florida, Tampa. She has collaborated with the Florida Prevention Research Center for four years and has an extensive publication record and a history of federally funded, community-based projects. Dr. Baldwin has also served on several NIH review panels, including two standing committees: the Behavioral and Social Consequences of HIV/AIDS, and the Community Influences on Health Behavior.

Jamie Barden has been an assistant professor in the Department of Psychology at Howard University since receiving his doctorate from Ohio State University in 2005. Much of his research is focused on the processes that produce evaluative judgments, from less thoughtful automatic processes to more thoughtful meta-cognitive processes. A second line of inquiry explores the processes and biases that result from placing the self and others into social categories including race, gender, and political party.

Carol Bryant, PhD, is a Distinguished USF Health Professor and codirector of the Florida Prevention Research in the College of Public Health at the University of South Florida. For the past twenty years, she has directed marketing research to design public health interventions on a wide variety of topics. With her colleagues at USF, she is developing and evaluating the community-based prevention marketing framework described in Chapter Twelve.

James N. Burdine, DrPH, serves as director and co-principal investigator of the Center for Community Health Development, a CDC-designated Prevention Research Center, and as a professor in the Department of Social and Behavioral Health at the School of Rural Public Health, Texas A&M Health Science Center in College Station. Dr. Burdine is an internationally recognized expert in population health status assessment and community health development. Over the course of his career, Dr. Burdine has coauthored more than two hundred papers presented at national professional meetings, and has been awarded more than $15 million in grants and contracts for community health improvement related research, demonstration, and evaluation projects.

Frances Dunn Butterfoss, PhD, MSEd, is president of *Coalitions Work,* a consulting group that trains coalitions to build, sustain, and evaluate themselves. Dr. Butterfoss is a professor at Eastern Virginia Medical School and Old Dominion University. She has provided technical assistance on improving coalition effectiveness to federal agencies, foundations, health departments, and community-based organizations. Her research and practice focus on promoting access to insurance, health care and immunizations, managing asthma, and preventing obesity and injury.

Christina M. Camp, PhD, is currently a director of research in Emory University's Rollins School of Public Health, Department of Behavioral Science and Health Education. Her research interests lie in the areas of bio-behavioral processes, ethnocultural issues in mental health, and the development of culturally appropriate interventions to reduce sexual risk behaviors and the spread of HIV/AIDS.

Hannah Cooper, ScD, MPH, is an assistant professor in the Department of Behavioral Sciences and Health Education at the Emory University Rollins School of Public Health. Her research focuses on the social determinants of health, including the social determinants of substance use and related harms.

Rita DiGioacchino DeBate, PhD, MPH, CHES, is an associate professor in the Department of Community and Family Health, College of Public Health at the University of South Florida. She has a background in health behavior/health education and public health. Her research interests include obesity and eating disorders. She has authored numerous articles on body image, physical activity, and secondary prevention of eating disorders. She has also developed a training program for oral health professionals on secondary prevention of eating disorders.

David L. DuBois, PhD, is a professor in the Division of Community Health Sciences within the School of Public Health at the University of Illinois at Chicago. He has authored numerous peer-reviewed studies addressing factors that may contribute to youth resilience, particularly self-esteem and mentoring relationships. He is the lead editor of the award-winning *Handbook of Youth Mentoring* and of special issues of the *Journal of Early Adolescence* and the *Journal of Community Psychology*.

Kristin Dunkle is an assistant professor of Behavioral Sciences and Health Education at Emory Rollins School of Public Health. She works both domestically and internationally on gender, power, poverty, violence and HIV, and has an emerging interest in men as both survivors and perpetrators of violence. She has worked with inner-city sex workers in Johannesburg, pregnant women in South African townships, rural South African youth, heterosexual couples in Zambia and Rwanda, and women and men in the United States; her research and publications focus on understanding HIV risk and developing evidence-based interventions.

Eugenia Eng, DrPH, MPH, is a professor of Health Behavior and Health Education and director of the Kellogg Health Scholars Postdoctoral Program at the University of North Carolina at Chapel Hill, Gillings School of Global Public Health. Dr. Eng's body of work examines the lay health advisor intervention model, the concepts of community competence and natural helping, and the community assessment procedure, Action-Oriented Community Diagnosis. She has more than twenty-five years of community-based participatory research experience, including field studies conducted with rural communities of the southern United States, West Africa, and Southeast Asia to address socially stigmatizing health problems such as pesticide poisoning, breast and prostate cancer, and STDs.

Craig Ewart, PhD, is professor of psychology and senior scientist in the Center for Health and Behavior at Syracuse University, and senior associate in the Department of Environmental Health Sciences, Bloomberg School of Public Health, at Johns Hopkins University. He developed Social Action Theory as a foundation for his Project Heart studies of emotional stress and resilience in urban youth, which he has conducted in Baltimore and Syracuse for the past twenty-five years. This community- and laboratory-based research program investigates how personal goal strivings, emotion regulation skills, and neighborhood environments combine to raise or lower cardiovascular disease risk in adolescents and young adults.

Michael C. Fagen, PhD, MPH, is a clinical assistant professor of community health sciences at the University of Illinois-Chicago School of Public Health. His research focuses on systemic approaches to school-based health promotion. He was recently appointed as an associate editor of *Health Promotion Practice*.

Michael R. J. Felix, of Community Health Development Specialists in Allentown, Pennsylvania, works with states and local communities across the United States applying the Partnership Approach to health networks for population health improvement. His recent work is focused on the strategic integration of mental health, substance abuse, oral health, and wrap-around services in primary care settings as Patient-Centered Health Homes.

Jeffrey D. Fisher is a professor of Psychology at the University of Connecticut. He is the founder and director of its Center for Health, Intervention, and Prevention (CHIP). He received his Master's degree and PhD from Purdue University. Professor Fisher has been awarded seven major NIMH grants since 1989 on HIV risk reduction and medical adherence, totaling over $28 million as PI. Most of his work has involved theory and empirical work on the dynamics of unhealthy behavior and on social psychological factors that can affect the success of interventions to change such behavior. He has lectured internationally and published extensively on factors associated with HIV risk behavior, and has done a great deal of conceptual and empirical work in the area of interventions to increase HIV preventive behavior. His work also focuses on designing theoretically based interventions to increase adherence to antiretroviral therapy, and on health behavior change in general. New work focuses on dissemination of effective health behavior change interventions.

William Fisher is Distinguished University Professor in the Department of Psychology and the Department of Obstetrics and Gynaecology at the University of Western Ontario and Research Affiliate at the Center for Health, Intervention, and Prevention at the University of Connecticut. Dr. William Fisher is codeveloper with Dr. Jeffrey Fisher of the Information-Motivation-Behavioral Skills model of health behavior, he has held a National Health Scientist award from Health Canada, and his research has been supported by the U.S. National Institute of Mental Health for the past two decades.

Martin Fishbein, PhD, is the Harry C. Coles Jr. Distinguished Professor of Communication at the Annenberg School for Communication, and director of the Health Communications Area in the Annenberg Public Policy Center. Developer of the Theory of Reasoned Action and the Integrative Model of Behavioral Prediction, his current research interests are focused on understanding the role of the media as an influence on adolescent and adult behavior.

Brian R. Flay, PhD, is professor of public health at Oregon State University. He has a long history in prevention research, including school-based randomized trials, methodological developments, and the development of health behavior theory. Most of his past work has concerned the development and evaluation of programs for the prevention of substance abuse, violence, and AIDS. Recent studies focus on positive youth development, including social and character education. Dr. Flay is currently conducting several studies of the *Positive Action* program, which addresses most of the distal and proximal influences on youth development, and so is likely to influence a broad array of both positive and negative behaviors as well as school performance.

Michelle Fortier, PhD, is a physical activity psychology researcher and a professor at the School of Human Kinetics at the University of Ottawa. Her research program aims to understand and promote physical activity behavior change with an emphasis on motivation. She has extensive research experience examining the determinants of physical activity adoption and maintenance in different healthy and clinical populations, and has been involved in the development and evaluation of physical activity promotion interventions.

David Groulx is the acting policy and planning specialist in the Resources, Research, Evaluation, and Development Division at the Sudbury and District Health Unit. He received his BScN from Laurentian University and his MPH from Lakehead University. He has spent the last decade working as a public health nurse, with a particular focus in health promotion.

Denise Haynie, PhD, MPH, is a staff scientist in the Prevention Research Branch, Division of Epidemiology, Statistics and Prevention Research, Eunice Kennedy Shriver National Institute of Child Health and Human Development, National Institutes of Health. Her training is in developmental psychology and maternal and child health. Dr. Haynie's research interest focus is on adolescent health behavior, including peer and parent influences.

Stevan E. Hobfoll, PhD, is the Judd and Marjorie Weinberg Presidential Professor and Chair of the Department of Behavioral Sciences at Rush Medical College. His Conservation of Resources (COR) theory has become one of two most widely cited theories of stress and has been related to the full spectrum of stress from burnout to mass casualty. His most recent work focuses on the lifetime impact of trauma in women's lives and on the impact of war and terrorism.

Everold Hosein, PhD, born in Trinidad and Tobago, is the senior communication advisor-consultant, World Health Organization (WHO), Geneva and is an international communication expert with more than thirty years of experience in strategic communication, integrated marketing communication, advocacy, and public relations, health education, and IEC (information-education-communication) related to social development issues and behavioral impact/behavior change/behavioral development.

Mel Hovell, PhD, is an Al Johnson Distinguished Professor of Public Health and director of the Center for Behavioral Epidemiology and Community Health, San Diego State University, San Diego. His areas of expertise include behavioral epidemiology, individual and population experimental trials, and theory development. He has published more than 250 coauthored peer-reviewed articles in national and international journals. Dr. Hovell has an established record of NIH funding, including current research concerning HIV/TB epidemiology, tobacco prevention, and promotion of diet and activity in youth and young adults. He is coprincipal investigator for the National Children's Study, a twenty-one year analysis of healthy development and disease processes in children and families.

Barbara Kahan is a principal of Kael Consulting, and editor of the Web site IDM Best Practices (www.idmbestpractices.ca). She received her MHSc in health promotion from the University of Toronto. For the last twelve years she has focused on developing and applying a comprehensive, situation-sensitive health promotion best practices approach.

Kelli McCormack Brown, PhD, CHES, is a professor of health education and behavior at the University of Florida. She was the director of the first community-based prevention marketing project conducted in Sarasota, Florida. She has been able to blend her health education experience with community-based prevention marketing and through these efforts has written numerous peer-reviewed articles on how health educators and communities can use social marketing to develop behavior change interventions.

Robert J. McDermott received his BS, MS, and PhD degrees from the University of Wisconsin-Madison. He was a faculty member in the Department of Health Education, at Southern Illinois University, Carbondale, from 1981 to 1986. Dr. McDermott came to the University of South Florida College of Public Health in 1986. He headed an effort that successfully led to its being designated a Prevention Research Center by the U.S. Centers for Disease Control and Prevention (CDC) in 1998. He continues to serve as co-director of this Center, which has created and field-tested a new model for health behavior change in communities—community-based prevention marketing (CBPM). In addition to more than 220 scientific articles, he has written 56 book chapters, and three books, each of which appeared in multiple editions.

Kenneth R. McLeroy, PhD, is professor of Social and Behavioral Health at the Texas A&M Health Science Center. He has written extensively about community-based programs and interventions and currently serves as principal investigator on the

CDC-funded Prevention Research Center for Community Health Development and the National Center on Minority Health and Health Disparities–funded Program for Rural and Minority Health Disparities Research.

Paul Monaghan, PhD, MA, is an assistant professor in the Department of Agricultural Education and Communication at the University of Florida. His research focuses on community participation in behavior change on topics such as farmworker health safety, homeowner water conservation, and environmental protection in the state of Florida.

Elizabeth Noelcke is a project assistant, focusing on Medicaid and state policy issues, at the Center for Health Transformation in Washington. Prior to that, she was a post-baccalaureate research fellow in the Prevention Research Branch, Division of Epidemiology, Statistics, and Prevention Research, Eunice Kennedy Shriver National Institute of Child Health and Human Development, National Institutes of Health. She is a graduate of the University of North Carolina at Chapel Hill.

Barbara L. Norton is an assistant professor of research at the University of Oklahoma, College of Public Health, and in 2008 served as managing associate for the Association for the Study and Development of Community in Gaithersburg, Maryland. She received her DrPH from the University of Oklahoma, conducting research on the relationship between community connectedness and health behaviors in an environmentally stressed community.

Edith A. Parker, DrPH, is an associate professor of Health Behavior and Health Education and the Associate Dean for Academic Affairs at the University of Michigan at Ann Arbor, School of Public Health. Dr. Parker's research focuses on development, implementation, and evaluation of community-based participatory interventions to improve health status and reduce racial disparities in health, with a special interest in both epidemiological research on environmental causes of disease and research on public health and policy interventions to address environmental causes of disease.

Will Parks, PhD, is an internationally recognized specialist in social policy, public health, medical anthropology, health promotion, and participatory appraisal, monitoring, and evaluation. For the past seventeen years, he has contributed to the planning, management, and evaluation of international and national social policies and public health programs, as well as conducted training and research for the prevention and control of communicable and noncommunicable diseases in close collaboration with ministries of health and nongovernment organizations throughout the world. Based in Fiji, Parks is currently Chief of Policy, Advocacy, Planning, and Evaluation with UNICEF Pacific covering child-focused programs in fourteen Pacific Island countries.

Dr. Heather Patrick is a Research Assistant Professor at the University of Rochester working with Dr. Geoffrey C. Williams on a large tobacco-cessation induction trial and developing translational projects for nutrition, physical activity, and diabetes prevention. She earned her PhD in Social Psychology from the University of Houston in 2003. She completed a post-doctoral fellowship in Behavioral Nutrition at the Children's Nutrition Research Center (CNRC) at Baylor College of Medicine. While at the CNRC, Dr. Patrick received funding from the US National Cancer Institute to pilot a self-determination theory-based intervention utilizing computerized personal trainers.

John Petraitis, PhD, is a professor of psychology at the University of Alaska Anchorage. His research focuses on risk factors for adolescent substance use—an area in which he has coauthored numerous articles and book chapters—and potential evolutionary explanations for sex and age differences in risky behaviors.

Richard E. Petty is Distinguished University Professor and chair of the Department of Psychology at Ohio State University. He received his BA from the University of Virginia and his PhD from Ohio State. Petty's research focuses on the factors (both conscious and unconscious) that are responsible for changes in beliefs, attitudes, and behaviors.

Leah M. Phillips, MPH, is the coordinator for the Florida Prevention Research Center at the University of South Florida. Her interests include community-based participatory research, social marketing, research methods and evaluation, and project administration.

Scott D. Rhodes, MD, MPH, CHES, is an associate professor in the Departments of Social Sciences and Health Policy and Internal Medicine at Wake Forest University, School of Medicine. His research explores sexual health, HIV and sexually transmitted disease (STD) prevention, obesity prevention, and other health disparities among vulnerable communities. Committed to partnership approaches to blend research and practice, Dr. Rhodes has extensive experience working with Latino communities, urban African American adolescents, persons living with HIV and AIDS, men of color, self-identifying gay and bisexual men, and men who have sex with men.

Renata Schiavo, PhD, MA, is the founder and principal of Strategic Communication Resources, which provides health communication and strategic planning counseling and training to leading U.S. and international organizations in the public health field. She has almost two decades of U.S. and global health experience. Select experience includes the National Association of Pediatric Nurse Practitioners (NAPNAP); National Ministry of Health (Angola); Solving Kids' Cancer; UNICEF; and the World Bank. In addition to her consulting practice, she is also an adjunct assistant professor of public health at New York University, Steinhardt School, where she is on the faculty of the Community Public Health and Global Public Health MPH programs. She is the author of *Health Communication: From Theory to Practice* (San Francisco: Jossey Bass, 2007) and several peer-reviewed publications.

Jeremiah A. Schumm, PhD, formerly at Harvard Medical School and the VA Boston Healthcare System, is now assistant professor of clinical psychiatry at the University of Cincinnati and staff psychologist at the Cincinnati VA Medical Center's PTSD and Anxiety Disorders Division. His work focuses on the impact of stress and substance abuse on PTSD and individual and family-focused interventions.

Paul A. Shuper, PhD, is an Independent Scientist at the Centre for Addiction and Mental Health and an assistant professor in the Department of Psychology at the University of Toronto in Toronto, Canada. His research focuses on behavioral and psychological factors associated with health outcomes, particularly in the area of HIV prevention. Dr. Shuper's work has ranged from controlled laboratory research assessing the impact of sexual arousal and sexual partner characteristics on HIV+ MSM's condom use intentions, to the development, implementation, and evaluation of theory-based adherence-promotion and risk-reduction interventions for people living with HIV/AIDS.

Bruce Simons-Morton, ED, MPH, is chief of the Prevention Research Branch, Division of Epidemiology, Statistics, and Prevention Research, Eunice Kennedy Shriver National Institute of Child Health and Human Development, National Institutes of Health. Dr. Simons-Morton directs an intramural research group that conducts research on adolescent health behavior, with an emphasis on social influences. He is the author of the textbook, *Introduction to Health Education and Promotion,* second edition, and 2006 Research Laureate of the American Academy of Health Behavior.

Shane Sweet is a doctoral student at the School of Psychology at the University of Ottawa. His doctoral research focuses on understanding physical activity behavior change using theoretical-based motivational constructs. His research experience centers on motivation and confidence towards physical activity across healthy and clinical populations. He was the principal research assistant in Dr. Michelle Fortier's

Physical Activity Counseling Randomized Controlled Trial (2004–2006) which was a theoretically-based motivational trial investigating the effect of adding a physical activity counselor to the primary health care team. He is also the project coordinator for Dr Fortier's Social Science and Humanities Research Council grant (SSHRC; 2008–2011) entitled: *Understanding Physical Activity Adoption and Maintenance in Cardiac Rehabilitation.* He was awarded a SSHRC doctoral fellowship (2006–2010). He has published in *Psychology, Health & Medicine*, and coauthored in manuscripts appearing in *Psychology of Sport and Exercise and Annals of Behavioral Medicine.*

Dennis R. Wahlgren, MA, is a research associate with the Center for Behavioral Epidemiology and Community Health, Graduate School of Public Health, San Diego State University. His work has included pediatric tobacco control (for example, secondhand smoke exposure), low back pain, and theory development.

Monica L. Wendel, MA, MPH, is the associate director of the Center for Community Health Development at the Texas A&M Health Science Center School of Rural Public Health, one of CDC's thirty-three designated Prevention Research Centers. Her research focuses on community health development and capacity building, specifically in rural and underserved communities. She also has extensive experience in community assessment, program development, and program evaluation.

S. Christian Wheeler's research comprises three interrelated streams on attitudes and persuasion, automaticity, and the self. His research has been published in outlets such as *Journal of Consumer Research, Journal of Marketing Research, Journal of Personality and Social Psychology, Personality and Social Psychology Review, Proceedings of the National Academy of Science, and Psychological Bulletin.* He is an associate professor of marketing at Stanford University. He holds a BA in psychology from the University of Northern Iowa and MA and PhD degrees in psychology from the Ohio State University.

Geoffrey C. Williams received his MD from Wayne State University in 1983. He completed training in Internal Medicine and completed fellowships in biopsychosocial medicine and in general internal medicine, at the University of Rochester Medical Center. He then received his PhD in health psychology from the University of Rochester, supervised by Prof. Edward L. Deci. He was awarded an Individual NRSA postdoctoral fellowship from the National Cancer Institute study smoking cessation. Dr. Williams is associate professor of medicine, psychiatry, and psychology at the University of Rochester, and is a staff physician in the Department of Medicine at the University's Strong Memorial Hospital. He has done several research projects on the relation of motivation to medication adherence, health behavior change, and health status.

Gina M. Wingood, ScD, MPH is professor in the Department of Behavioral Sciences and Health Education and the Agnes Moore Endowed Faculty in HIV/AIDS Research at Emory University, Rollins School of Public Health. She also serves as director, of the Social and Behavioral Science Core, Emory Center for AIDS Research. Dr. Wingood received her doctoral degree from the Harvard University School of Public Health. Dr. Wingood's research examines gender and social factors (for example stigma, discrimination, partner abuse) that affect the sexual health of African American women. Dr. Wingood has served as the principal investigator on several NIH randomized controlled behavioral intervention to reduce HIV risk among women. The Center's for Disease Control and Prevention (CDC) is currently disseminating a suite of three evidence-based HIV prevention programs for African American women (the SiSTA study), African American female adolescents (the SiHLE study) and HIV positive African American women (the WiLLOW study) developed by Dr. Wingood. CDC refers to this suite of programs as the "Continuum of HIV prevention services for African American women."

Josephine Pui-Hing Wong is a nurse with extensive experience in critical health promotion and community-based action research. She is a doctoral candidate in the Dalla Lana School of Public Health (Social Science and Health Program) at the University of Toronto. Her research focuses on sexuality, mental health, and marginalization. She currently holds a CIHR-Institute of Gender and Health doctoral fellowship and an appointment as associate professor at Ryerson University.

EMERGING THEORIES IN HEALTH PROMOTION PRACTICE AND RESEARCH

CHAPTER

1

THEORY IN HEALTH PROMOTION PRACTICE AND RESEARCH

Richard A. Crosby
Michelle C. Kegler
Ralph J. DiClemente

PROMOTING HEALTHY BEHAVIOR

One commonly used definition of public health is "the science and art of protecting and improving community health through health education, promotion, research, and disease prevention strategies" (Association of Schools of Public Health, 2006). Notably important in this definition is that "public health" is not synonymous with "health care." Indeed, the lion's share of any health care system's resources is dedicated to providing clinical and diagnostic services. For example, in the United States, our health care budget exceeds $1 trillion annually; however, only about 1 percent is allocated to population-based prevention. A landmark report in the 1970s noted that health is based largely on human biology, environment, and lifestyle, with health care playing a much smaller role in preventing mortality (Lalonde, 1974). Although adequate health care services remain critical, equally critical are efforts to "move upstream" and prevent the causes of morbidity. Thus, public health adopts a proactive approach that is based solidly on the premise that health is a product of lifestyle, shaped heavily by social and physical environments. As such, diverse strategies can be employed to substantially alter risk behaviors and environments and, in so doing, markedly change the disease trajectory and reduce morbidity. The mission of public health is to fulfill "society's interest in assuring conditions in which people can be healthy" (IOM, 1998, page 7). This mission is based on the premise that multiple aspects of the environment (physical, economic, legal, political, cultural, and so on) act as powerful determinants of health as well as health-related behaviors. The differences between treating disease, as exemplified in the health care approach, versus modifying lifestyle and environments, as exemplified in a public health approach, have been eloquently described in a recent text entitled, *Prescription for a Healthy Nation* (Farley and Cohen, 2005).

The practice of public health, then, can be viewed as a diverse array of strategies, methods, and efforts that are designed to protect people by mitigating risk factors associated with morbidity and premature mortality and by creating environments that are conducive to healthy practices. Given that the basic purpose of public health practice is to prevent morbidity and premature mortality, it is important to have an understanding of the causes of disease, disability, and death. In a classic article, McGinnis and Foege (1993) articulated actual causes of death in the United States. A recent update of this work provides a foundation for understanding how changing health behavior can lead to improvements in the health of the public (Mokdad et al. 2004). The top ten "offenders" are shown below in descending order of importance.

- Tobacco use
- Poor diet and physical inactivity
- Alcohol use
- Infection with microbes
- Toxins
- Motor vehicle crashes

- Firearm trauma
- Sexual risk behaviors
- Illicit drug use

Consider just the first two actual causes of death. Collectively, tobacco use, poor diet, and physical inactivity account for about 35 percent of all premature deaths in the United States. The implications for public health are simple and obvious, yet the solutions are elusive and complex. It is obvious that the health of the public would be greatly improved if people would stop smoking and overeating and begin exercising on a routine basis. But identifying solutions to these health problems is "elusive and complex." Smoking, overeating, and sedentary lifestyles are culturally ingrained for many Americans. Moreover, private sector forces with vested fiscal interests have supported, reinforced, and promoted behaviors that are clearly deleterious to the health of Americans. The obvious question then is: Where does one even begin the seemingly insurmountable task of reversing this trend?

Even relatively "small" changes in health behavior may yield substantial benefits to public health.

Looking at the remainder of the items representing actual causes of death, it becomes apparent that changing health behavior is the likely turning point for protecting the public from harm. Even relatively "small" changes in health behavior may yield substantial benefits to public health.

For example, the simple elimination of table salt could result in a 20 percent nationwide decrease of stroke (Law et al., 1991). Of course, removing salt-shakers from all eating tables in the United States is a formidable challenge. Meeting this challenge involves providing health education about the health hazard of adding salt to foods and is contingent upon people's willingness to comply with this health-protective information, a type of "medical advice," when they feel perfectly healthy and, as important, have cultivated a taste for salt in their food. The question then becomes, are health promotion efforts always at the mercy of public acceptance? To answer this question, a second example is needed.

Tobacco use illustrates how even a seemingly small change in health behavior can yield substantive rewards in public health. In 1989, the state of California imposed a tax on the sale of cigarettes (25 cents per pack). Estimates suggest that this tax led to at least a 5 percent decline in tobacco use (Flewelling et al., 1992), to which, in the ensuing decade, the 20 percent decline in heart disease-related mortality was partly attributable (Fichtenberg et al., 2003). In this example, the change in health behavior was related to a carefully calibrated change in policy (increasing cigarette tax) as a means of discouraging use. The additional financial pressure exerted through the tax acted as a catalyst by providing a tangible, and important, incentive to reduce smoking.

Although vastly different from each other, the aforementioned examples regarding table salt elimination (a lifestyle change) and taxation of cigarettes (a change to the environment) illustrate that changes in health behavior can markedly effect reductions in morbidity and mortality. In fact, a nearly infinite number of health-protective behaviors could be listed. Many of these may be simple, one-time acts, such as testing your home for radon or being vaccinated for diseases like tetanus or measles. Others may require periodic repetition, such as semi-annual dental cleanings, Pap testing, or screening for high cholesterol. However, the majority of health-protective behaviors require constant (often daily) repetition. Examples include: eating high-fiber, low-fat foods; drinking clean water; engaging in aerobic exercise, and maintaining musculoskeletal health through stretching and weight-bearing exercises. Many of the behaviors requiring constant repetition are avoidance behaviors, such as avoiding toxins in the environment (including environmental tobacco smoke); abstaining from the use of illicit drugs and the use of more than moderate amounts of alcohol; not using tobacco; not consuming foods associated with an increased risk of heart disease, cancer, or diabetes; and not engaging in unprotected sex that could lead to infection with sexually transmitted pathogens, including HIV. Still other repetitive behaviors entail daily habits such as safe driving practices and the intentional practice of home and workplace safety.

The profound role of **social determinants** in shaping health behavior is becoming increasingly apparent. The influence of social capital, for example, is well-documented. Culturally ingrained health-risk behaviors are common in every nation of the world and serve to remind us that social norms are powerful antecedents of health behavior. Entire epidemics can rightfully be said to proliferate as a consequence of unyielding adherence to socially accepted practices, as happened with the AIDS epidemic in that millions of people resisted advice to use condoms to prevent acquisition and transmission of HIV. With respect to chronic disease, two extremely critical health behaviors, diet and physical activity, are largely products of social customs, traditions, and norms. Given the strength of social determinants in shaping health behavior, the expanding role of macro-level theory in fostering the long-term adoption of health-protective behaviors is clearly a valuable asset to public health practice.

Regardless of the exact approach used, public health is achieved through carefully designed efforts to foster health-protective behavior, not through surgery or medicine. In the words of former Surgeon General C. Everett Koop, "Health care is vital to all of us some of the time, but public health is vital to all of us all of the time." Thus, the mandate of public health is deeply rooted in the process of influencing people to adopt healthy behaviors. Herein lies the ultimate challenge to public health: "how can such change be achieved?" The answers to this fundamental question are nearly as infinite as the number of health behaviors; however, they all share one common thread—theory! Although theory is not a panacea, it has been embraced by the public health profession as a means of guiding investigation (research) and informing the content of health education and health promotion efforts.

THE ROLE OF THEORY IN HEALTH BEHAVIOR

Understanding the application of theory to changing health behavior requires mastery of a few fundamental concepts. This section of the chapter will begin by briefly addressing these.

Fundamental Concept 1: Theory Is Dynamic

Theories are seldom static; instead they change and evolve to better serve public health (Crosby, Kegler, and DiClemente, 2002). The evolution of theory refers generically to the discipline of health promotion rather than focusing on the improvements made within existing theories. For example, the concept of natural helper models is a relatively new method of effectively leveraging change in health behaviors. Rather than being an improvement over a previous version of a single theory, natural helper models represent a true innovation in the paradigm used to change behavior. Indeed, innovative paradigms are the seed of this evolutionary process. The evolutionary process is vital because the challenges in public health change, as do the populations served. As practice needs change, research is conducted to help identify new solutions in the form of health promotion strategies, methods, techniques, and policy. Theories are utilized to inform these solutions. Solutions are tested using rigorous evaluation methodologies designed to isolate and quantify the effect of the solution on health behavior. By identifying efficacious "solutions" and assessing the link between the underlying theory and behavior change, we strengthen the empirical evidence in support of theory. Theory, however, must also be able to accommodate new and emergent challenges to public health. Thus, theory must be capable of adapting to the needs imposed by established or emergent threats to public health.

> Theory must be capable of adapting to the needs imposed by established or emergent threats to public health.

Theory cannot be rigid, simply because people and public health issues are diverse and continually evolve. This concept is illustrated in Figure 1.1.

Fundamental Concept 2: Theories Have Different Paradigms

A paradigm may or may not be something that is a recognized part of thinking and problem solving. Frequently, however, scholars may fail to recognize that their

FIGURE 1.1 *Relationship Between Theory, Research, and Practice in Public Health*

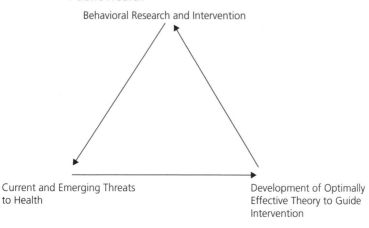

thinking is restricted by a given paradigm. In fact, paradigms can sometimes act as blinders, precluding alternative views. Consider, for example, the relatively common problem of hospital-acquired infections. One way to reduce the incidence of these infections is to ensure that all clinical staff thoroughly wash their hands between seeing patients. In an "education paradigm" the solution to this problem would be constantly reminding clinical staff about the problem of hospital-acquired infections and the benefits of thorough hand-washing. Unfortunately, this **education-based** paradigm often fails to solve the problem, and it offers no other solution beyond intensifying education efforts. Now, consider an **ecological approach** as an alternative paradigm. Ecological approaches to health behavior change go beyond education by actions such as influencing social norms, building community infrastructures, providing skills and resources that people need to practice healthy behaviors, and by making changes to the physical, economic, legal, political, and cultural environment. Actions that may result from this paradigm might then lead to the discovery that clinical staff members are frequently "pressed for time," to the point that traversing a long hospital hallway to wash their hands is inconvenient. One potential solution would be installing large hand-washing stations along the hallway to reduce the distance staff have to travel, thus enhancing convenience and, as a direct outcome, hand-washing behavior.

The two examples reflect different perspectives on how best to catalyze behavior change and represent opposing ends on a continuum of theory, as illustrated in Figure 1.2.

Health promotion is exciting because it is dynamic. For example, rather than implementing a staff educational campaign alone or modifying the hospital environment alone, a more effective approach may involve both a change in hospital environment and concomitant staff education regarding the benefits of hand-washing. Together, modification of the hospital environment and staff education may be more effective at promoting the desired behavior change than either strategy alone. Creatively designing "solutions" to enhance health implies the necessity of understanding the barriers to adopting health-protective behaviors. It also means developing new strategies to inform and motivate individuals and manipulate social/environmental contingencies to catalyze the long-term adoption of health-protective behaviors.

FIGURE 1.2   *A Continuum of Theory*

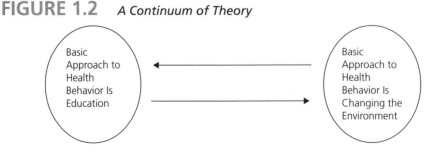

Fundamental Concept 3: Theories Have Multiple Functions

Students of behavioral theory have often raised inquiries such as "Why couldn't there be just one theory that does it all?" or "Would it be possible to know just one or two theories really well and still serve the goals of public health?" Unfortunately, the answer to both questions would be "no," simply because theory aids public health intervention efforts in multiple ways, depending on the specified objectives to be achieved.

A convenient way to think about any intervention effort is to view the process as occurring in three sequential phases. The first phase would be to ask and empirically answer two fundamentally discrete, though related, questions: (1) Why do people engage in behaviors that increase their risk for adverse health outcomes; and (2) What factors predict adoption of health-protective behaviors? For convenience, we can refer to the first phase as the "why" phase. In this phase of the overall effort to develop an effective health promotion program, the program objectives will be developed based on theory-guided investigation.

The next phase involves understanding how people go about the somewhat cumbersome process of actually adopting, performing, and possibly repeating the health-protective behavior in question. For convenience, we can refer to this as the "how" phase. In this phase the content of the health promotion program will be developed. Content refers to the strategies, techniques, and methods that will be employed to achieve the objectives. Stated differently, the content is the specific "action plan" to help people adopt and maintain health-protective behavior. Development of the specific action plan or program content is, of course, critically important, loosely analogous to a "drug" in medicine. For all intents and purposes, the program content is the "active ingredient" that catalyzes behavior change. Thus, substantial time and resources are dedicated to developing program content. The end product of this stage is usually an action plan or intervention manual that spells out in great detail the program content in a step-by-step plan for achieving the objectives identified in the "why" phase.

Fundamental Concept 4: Theory Guided Planning

Health promotion programs generally follow a well-established and sequential process that is generically known as program planning. This process begins with a needs assessment of individuals and their community. Broadly speaking, these assessments seek to understand the "why" phase previously described. Community assessments include extensive identification of physical, social, legal, cultural, economic, and policy-related factors that may be related to the health behaviors in question. **Theory-based planning frameworks** can be used to guide these assessments, which in turn can be used to plan the action steps of the health promotion program.

One example of a planning model is PRECEDE-PROCEED (Green and Kreuter, 2005). In this approach to planning, assessment of the social context and general quality-of-life indicators in a community is considered a first and paramount step.

Assessment at multiple levels leads to identification of important and "changeable" behaviors and environments, as well as identification of predisposing, reinforcing, and enabling factors related to the priority health behaviors. The planning process then shifts focus to examine the relevant policy, regulation, and organizational factors that can be changed or used in any way to influence the predisposing, reinforcing, or enabling factors. Moreover, the planning framework provides for the use of behavioral theory to guide the process of changing these factors. Different theories may be used in combination to target the full range of factors that affect the health behavior. In essence, theory-guided planning frameworks, such as PRECEDE-PROCEED, provide a "blueprint" for health promotion specialists to follow.

Ultimately, the blueprint created through the process of theory-guided program planning yields a set of criteria that can be used to evaluate the effectiveness of both the process and the targeted outcomes. Indeed, evaluation is the mainstay of planning, as it is the only mechanism that provides corrective feedback to the health promotion program and the various objectives specified by the blueprint.

Theory and evaluation are inexorably linked; the choice of theory-guided planning models then has direct implications for what to measure in an evaluation. For example, if a community-needs assessment finds that elderly residents of an urban area are largely sedentary because they feel threatened by crime when they leave their homes, then one objective of the planned program may be to construct designated and secure recreational areas for these elderly residents. Process objectives tied to this larger objective can readily become the target of evaluation efforts. One process objective might be the formation and maintenance of a community coalition that advocates for public funding to build secure recreational areas. The formation, functionality, and ongoing level of effort from this coalition can each be measured, and can serve as a part of a larger evaluation process. Theories can also help to identify a program's model of change, as well as specific outcome objectives that can be measured in an evaluation, such as increased self-efficacy or increased behavioral intention to exercise.

Fundamental Concept 5: Theory Is a Tool

Much like biostatistics, theory is a necessary system of thinking needed to efficiently understand and address public health problems. It is a means to an end, with the "end" being some form of tangible benefit to public health. As a tool, then, this volume may be viewed as a repository of the emerging theories and models used in the trade of health promotion. The selection of a single "tool" is rarely, if ever, adequate. Thus, the wise professional will be dedicated to a working knowledge of multiple tools to better meet the diversity of prevention opportunities in health promotion practice. Theories, as a set of tools, have the potential to facilitate or streamline the planning process. Indeed, nearly every prevention opportunity will have a corresponding theory (or theories) that can greatly aid the task of intervention development and dissemination.

Theory, research, and practice are interrelated. As theory-guided practice and research unfold, empirical findings subsequently suggest needed refinements in the theory that was applied (Jenson, 1999).

As theory-guided practice and research unfold, empirical findings subsequently suggest needed refinements in the theory that was applied.

Although the evolution of theory is an expected and desirable consequence of research and practice, one inherent difficulty is conveying the substance of these emerging theories to health-promotion professionals. The purpose of this volume is to provide the reader with an understanding of new developments in the field of behavioral and social science theory as applied to health promotion practice and research. Because the discipline of health promotion is newly emerging and transdisciplinary, it does not have a long legacy of scientific theory, principles, and axioms to provide a foundation for informing research relative to other social and behavioral sciences. The range of theoretical approaches in health promotion practice is a reflection of the discipline itself, eclectic and diverse. Theoretical approaches from a broad spectrum of disciplines have been utilized. Indeed, health promotion is currently a highly diverse and interdisciplinary field of practice and research. This diversity is important because advances in health promotion are most readily made through the use of interdisciplinary approaches. In a sense, theory can be viewed as a focal point that brings this diversity into a unified set of propositions about people and their health behaviors.

Although theory is not a panacea, it does provide a conceptual framework for selecting key constructs hypothesized to influence health behavior and, as such, provides a foundation for empirical investigations, intervention development, implementation, and evaluation. Theory also facilitates the complex process of organizing and understanding information obtained from these efforts. In addition, theory provides a useful reference point to help keep research and implementation activities clearly focused.

With increasing recognition that morbidity and mortality, for both adolescents and adults, are predominantly linked to behavioral and social factors (Smedley and Syme, 2000), the role of behavioral and social science theory in public health becomes paramount. In the coming years, noncommunicable disease (for example, tobacco-associated coronary heart and pulmonary disease and malignancies) will account for an increasingly larger proportion of the global disease burden. Fortunately, these diseases are typically amenable to behavioral and social interventions. Communicable diseases (for example, HIV and tuberculosis) and emerging communicable diseases (for example, Lyme disease and pulmonary hantavirus) may also require solutions that include modification of behavioral and social factors; the HIV epidemic is a primary example. Thus, there is a continual need to expand and refine theories that may ultimately prove valuable in informing and guiding the design and implementation of health promotion programs. As described in this volume, theory expansion and refinement is occurring in response to accumulating empirical evidence obtained through research and evaluation, in combination with the iterative process of theory development and testing.

A TRAJECTORY OF THEORY DEVELOPMENT

Theory development is a dynamic process. Systematic and consistent use of theory across a range of behaviors, populations, and settings is necessary to advance the science of health promotion.

Robust theories are flexible, accommodating a wide range of populations with different cultural perspectives. Constantly reevaluating the explanatory and predictive capacity of theory allows the discipline of health promotion to grow and mature. By definition, any maturational process involves change. Thus, as theories become less useful (that is, they explain an insufficient amount of variance, particularly in risk behaviors) or are found wanting as a foundation for guiding the design and implementation of behavior change interventions, they are modified or even discarded in favor of potentially more useful theories. This process of development, evaluation, elimination/refinement, and replacement is incremental. As new theories are synthesized and embraced, they too are subject to empirical validation and, if found lacking, are similarly discarded.

> Systematic and consistent use of theory across a range of behaviors, populations, and settings is necessary to advance the science of health promotion.

Individual-Level Approaches

Traditionally, behavioral and social science theories tended to focus on identifying, quantifying, and understanding the impact of individual-level determinants of specific health behaviors. For example, the health belief model, the theory of reasoned action, and the theory of planned behavior have been widely applied to health issues such as vaccine acceptance (Armstrong, Berlin, Schwartz, et al. 2001; Liau and Zimet 2000; Zimet, Blythe, and Fortenberry, 2000), understanding why people do not adopt HIV-protective behaviors (see Fisher and Fisher, 2000 for a review), and what psychosocial factors predict mammography use (Michels et al., 1995; Montano, Kasprzyk, and Taplin, 1997). Theories have also been developed to guide intervention programs that target individual-level determinants of health behavior (for example, the Transtheoretical Model).

In many respects, **individual-level theories** have dominated health promotion efforts. For example, Waldo and Coates (2000) noted, that "Virtually all of the psychological theories that have been applied to explain HIV risk behavior locate it at the individual level" (page S24). Possible reasons for the widespread use of individual-level theories may be that: (1) they tacitly posit the individual as the key decision-maker responsible for his or her health and, as a corollary, individuals can implement changes to enhance their health; (2) they assume that people value good health and will make the necessary changes to reduce behaviors associated with adverse health outcomes; (3) they assume that behavior is under volitional control; (4) they assume that cognitive predisposition (that is, beliefs, attitudes, and perceptions) drives health behavior; (5) they entail relatively manageable study designs and data analytic procedures (for example, the randomized, controlled clinical trial design can be used to test the efficacy of interventions delivered to individuals and small groups); (6) a substantial proportion of health promotion researchers are trained in psychology, a discipline that traditionally focuses on cognitive processes as a cornerstone of individual-level change; and (7) the accumulating empirical evidence suggests that theory-based, individual-level approaches to changing health behaviors can be effective. Given the popularity of this approach and the wealth of associated theories, researchers have

Although many well-established individual-level theories have been refined, others have been newly created, based largely on the lessons learned from application of the established theories.

continued the quest to develop and improve individual-level behavioral theories. One such example is the information-motivation-behavioral skills model (**Chapter Two** of this volume) that represents an eloquent synthesis of many of the individual-level theories that preceded this model.

Although many well-established individual-level theories have been refined, others have been newly created, based largely on the lessons learned from application of the established theories. An example of this is social influence theory, found in **Chapter Three** of this volume. Self-esteem enhancement theory (**Chapter Four**) and conservation of resources theory (**Chapter Five**) are two important innovations on traditional individual-level approaches that have great potential for application in health promotion research and practice. The former aims to build resilience in people, thereby conferring protection against health-compromising behaviors; the latter is designed for application with populations experiencing extreme stress or trauma. Yet another example is self-determination theory (**Chapter Six**), which is predicated on the humanistic perspective that people are inherently seeking growth and health. The next chapter in this first section provides insight into how people change their attitudes toward given health behaviors as a product of exposure to messages promulgated through mass media (**Chapter Seven**). The final chapter in this section provides an example of a theory (the theory of reasoned action) that has effectively changed to better predict health-related behaviors: The integrative model for behavioral prediction (**Chapter Eight**) includes the extremely important construct of self-efficacy in addition to the previous constructs of attitude toward the behavioral and subjective norms.

While the repertoire of individual-level theories has been expanding, researchers have questioned the wisdom of relying exclusively on individual-level approaches to achieve substantive changes in health behavior and, as important, sustain these changes over time in the face of countervailing social influences and pressures (McLeroy, Bibeau, Steckler, and Glanz, 1988; Rutten 1995; Salis and Owen, 1997; Smedley and Syme, 2000). Thus, **community-based approaches** are an important complement or alternative to individual-level approaches.

Community-Based Approaches

Community-based approaches and associated theories that transcend the individual level have been much more difficult to develop, refine, make operational, and evaluate. Yet they hold great potential to promote and support health behavior change and the long-term maintenance of newly adopted health behaviors necessary to achieve reductions in morbidity and mortality. It is important to realize that theories applied at this level seek to utilize the strength of local leaders and the "will" of the public (or key sectors in a community) to leverage changes in social norms, local policy, and community practices that will ultimately lead to changes in health behavior. The principles of these approaches are often used without formal recognition of an underlying theory or model. One of the best examples is the global work conducted by the Carter Center to eradicate dracunculiasis (Guinea worm). The prevention challenge with this disease was that all community residents needed to filter their drinking water through finely woven cloth. A second, and equally daunting, challenge was to keep people with Guinea worms from wading in the waters that others would eventually drink. Yet another challenge was to convince local residents that treating water supplies with a commercially produced pesticide would avert future cases of Guinea worm infection. Each of these challenges was met—in communities across countries such as Kenya, India, Senegal, Yemen, Cameroon, and Chad—through skilled negotiation with community leaders combined with the assistance of local volunteers to educate community residents about preventive measures and to distribute needed supplies (Carter, 2007).

The principles used by the Carter Center in this and many of their other disease prevention efforts are covered in the section of this volume delineating various community-based approaches to health promotion. Paramount among these are coalition theory (**Chapter Nine**), and the concept of developing community capacity (**Chapter Ten**). Natural helper models (**Chapter Eleven**) are then described as a method of enhancing the implementation of prevention plans created through community efforts. The final chapter of this section (**Chapter Twelve**) provides a framework for using the principles of community-based health promotion in conjunction with the individual-level theories described in the previous section and in conjunction with principles from the field of marketing. Given the mandate of health promotion to effect behavioral and environmental changes in the United States and globally, these emerging community-based approaches have substantial implications for public health practice.

Ecological Approaches

Some theories shift the intervention emphasis from the individual to the environment. In this paradigm, behavior is viewed as a product of society's rules and regulations. These theories typically seek to change policy- and social-level determinants of health. Although the obstacles to achieving these changes are often formidable, the potential for influencing large numbers of people is substantial. Examples of this type of approach include mandatory installation of car air bags (Loo, Siegel, Dischinger, et al., 1996), tax levies on tobacco and alcohol that have resulted in lower consumption (Chaloupka, Grossman, and Saffer, 2002; Cook and Tauchen, 1982; Lee, 2007; Meier and Licari, 1997), and the widespread success of bans on smoking in public places (Sargent, Shepard, and Glantz, 2004; Siegel, Albers, Cheng, Biener, and Rigotti, 2005).

In the third section of this volume several emerging ecological approaches to health promotion are described. This adaptation aptly illustrates the principle that ecological approaches can embody principles from community-based approaches, as well as principles from individual-level approaches. For example, Ewart's social action theory (**Chapter Thirteen**) provides an eloquent synthesis of all three approaches to changing health behaviors. Next, the theory of gender and power is described (**Chapter Fourteen**) as an ecological approach to disease prevention with global implications, given the widespread prevalence of patriarchal societies and the continued repression of women. Although the changes in culture and policy necessitated by this theory are immense, the potential for long-term payoffs in public health is tremendous. The behavioral ecological model (**Chapter Fifteen**) provides an equally important theory that functions at a super-structural level to shape behavior using principles from operant learning. Next, the theory of triadic influence (**Chapter Sixteen**) is presented. This theory draws on the academic disciplines of health education, social psychology, developmental psychology, sociology, and education, as well as general systems theories. The theory considers influence on behaviors emanating from intrapersonal, interpersonal, and sociocultural levels (again illustrating that ecological approaches do not necessarily preclude a focus on the individual level or the community level). In **Chapter Seventeen**, the interactive domain model is presented. This model posits that several domains and subdomains interact in the context of the sociopolitical, economic, psychological, and physical environments. Finally, **Chapter Eighteen** describes a planning model developed and used by the World Health Organization in more than fifty countries. The approach—known as communication for behavioral impact—is predicated on social mobilization, combined with principles from the disciplines of communication and social marketing.

THE UTILITY OF EMERGING THEORIES AND APPROACHES

The brief description of theory development suggests that the range of theories available for application in health promotion is rapidly expanding. We view this expansion as a positive development. Indeed, increasing the range of theories (that is, "tools") can lead to more options for practitioners and researchers alike, which may culminate in better theory selection. In turn, improved selection can optimize the ability of any program to mitigate health risk behaviors and subsequently promote protective behaviors.

Every level of theory (individual, community, and ecological) has utility and no one level is inherently "better" than another. Instead, the "best theory" is a function of how well it serves the objectives that must be met to achieve sustainable protective behaviors among a specified population. In essence, the range of behavioral and social science theories available for both health promotion practice and research affords the practitioner and researcher an opportunity to select the theories that are the most appropriate, feasible, and practical for a particular setting or population. Because global populations are extremely diverse in almost every conceivable respect, theory must be flexible and capable of adaptation.

Although this volume is not an exhaustive review of emerging theories, we believe it represents a well-rounded picture of new thinking and new applications of theory for health promotion practice and research. Given the rapid escalation of health care costs in many industrialized nations, and the nearly complete lack of health care in many other economically disadvantaged nations, prioritization of "prevention" over "treatment" may be an economic imperative. Consequently, this volume represents one step forward in the progress of public health toward the goal of preserving quality and quantity of life.

Every level of theory (individual, community, and ecological) has utility and no one level is inherently "better" than another.

SUMMARY

The rapidly changing landscapes of public health practice necessitate continued refinement of theory-based approaches to prevention. To serve public health effectively, theories need to be flexible, and capable of accommodating new ideas. Moreover, the evolution of theory should be passionately embraced by professionals, as doing so will greatly contribute to the overall effectiveness of health promotion efforts. Finally, it is vital to understand that theory can be an effective tool at multiple levels of influence, including the individual level, the community level, and the much broader ecological level.

REFERENCES

Armstrong, K., Berlin, M., Sanford-Swartz, J., Propert, K., and Ubel, P. A. (2001). Barriers to influenza immunization in a low-income urban population. *The American Journal of Preventive Medicine*, *20*, 2–25.

Association of Schools of Public Health (2006). What is public health? Available online at: http://www.whatispublichealth.org/what/index.html. Accessed 2/15/08.

Carter, J. (2007). *Beyond the White House: Waging peace, fighting disease, building hope*. New York, NY: Simon and Schuster.

Chaloupka, F. J., Grossman, M., and Saffer, H. (2002). The effects of price on alcohol consumption and alcohol-related problems. *Alcohol Research and Health*, 26.

Cook, P. J., and Tauchen G. (1982). The effect of liquor taxes on heavy drinking. *The Bell Journal of Economics*, *13*(2), 379–390.

Crosby, R. A., Kegler, M. C., and DiClemente, R. J. (2002). Understanding and Applying Theory in Health Promotion Practice and Research. In, DiClemente, R. J., Crosby, R. A., and Kegler, M. (eds.) *Emerging theories in health promotion practice and research* (pp. 1–15). San Francisco: Jossey-Bass.

Farley, T., and Cohen D. A. (2005). *Prescription for a Health Nation: A new approach to improving our lives by fixing our everyday world*. Boston, MA: Beacon Press.

Fichtenberg, C. M., and Glantz, S. A. (2000). Association of the California tobacco control program with declines in cigarette consumption and mortality from heart disease. *New England Journal of Medicine*; *343*:1772–1777.

Fisher, J. D., and Fisher, W. A. (2000). Theoretical approaches to individual-level change in HIV-risk. In J. L. Peterson and R. J. DiClemente (eds.), *Handbook of HIV prevention* (pp. 3–56). New York: Plenum Press.

Flewelling, R. L., et al. (1992). First-year impact of the 1989 California cigarette tax increase on cigarette consumption. *American Journal of Public Health*; *82*:867–869.

Jenson, P. S. (1999). Links among theory, research, and practice: Cornerstones of clinical scientific progress. *Journal of Clinical Child Psychology*, *28*, 553–557.

Institute of Medicine. (1988). *The future of public health*. Washington DC: National Academy Press.

Lalonde, M. (1974). *A new perspective on the health of Canadians*. National Health and Welfare, Government of Canada. Ottawa, Canada.

Law, M. R., et al. (1991). How much does dietary salt reduction lower blood pressure: III-analysis of data from trials of salt reduction. *British Medical Journal*; *302*:819–824.

Lee, J. (2007). The synergistic effect of cigarette taxes on the consumption of cigarettes, alcohol and betel nuts. *BMC Public Health*, *7*, 121.

Liau, A., and Zimet, G. D. (2000). Undergraduates' perception of HIV immunization: attitudes and behaviours as determining factors. *International Journal of STD and AIDS*, *11*, 445–50.

Loo, G. T., Siegel, J. H., Dischinger, P. C., Rixen, D., Burgess, A. R., Addis, M. D., O'Quinn, T., et al. (1996). Airbag protection versus compartment intrusion effect determines the pattern of injuries in multiple trauma motor vehicle crashes. *Journal of Trauma-Injury and Critical Care, 41*(6), 935–951.

McGinnis, J. M., and Foege, W. H. (1993). Actual causes of death in the United States. *Journal of the American Medical Association, 270*; 2207–2212.

McLeroy, K. R., Steckler, A. B., Simons-Morton, B., Goodman, R. M., Gottlieb, N., and Burdine, J. N. (1993). Social science theory in health education: time for a new model? *Health Education Research, Theory, and Practice, 9*, 305–312.

Meier, K. J., and Licari, M. J. (1997). The effect of cigarette taxes on cigarette consumption, 1955 through 1994. *American Journal of Public Health, 87*(7), 1126–1130.

Michels, T. C., Taplin, S. M., Carter, W. B., and Kugler, J. P. (1995). Barriers to screening: the theory of reasoned action applied to mammography use in a military beneficiary population. *Military Medicine, 160*, 431–437.

Mokdad, A. S., et al. (2004). Actual causes of death in the United States, 2000. *Journal of the American Medical Association, 291*; 1238–1245.

Montano, D. E., Kasprzyk, D., and Taplin, S. H. (1997). The theory of reasoned action and the theory of planned behavior. In K. Glanz, F. M. Lewis, and B. K. Rimer (eds.), *Health behavior and health education: Theory research, and practice* (2nd ed., pp. 85–112). San Francisco: Jossey-Bass.

Rutten, A. (1995). The implementation of health promotion: A new structural perspective. *Social Science in Medicine, 41*, 1627–1637.

Salis, J. F., and Owen, N. (1997). Ecological models. In K. Glanz, F. M. Lewis, and B. K. Rimer (eds.), *Health behavior and health education: Theory research, and practice* (2nd ed., pp.403–424). San Francisco: Jossey-Bass.

Sargent, R. P., Shepard, R. M., and Glantz, S. A. (2004). Reduced incidence of admissions for myocardial infarction associated with public smoking ban: before and after study. *British Medical Journal, 328*(7446), 977–980.

Siegel, M., Albers, A. B., Cheng, D. M., Biener, L., and Rigotti, N. A. (2005). Effect of local restaurant smoking regulations on progression to established smoking among youths. *Tobacco Control, 14*(5), 300–306.

Smedley, B. D., and Syme, S. L. (Eds.) (2000). *Promoting health: Intervention strategies from social and behavioral research*. Washington, DC: National Academy Press.

Waldo, R., and Coates, T. J. (2000). Multiple levels of analysis and intervention in HIV prevention science: exemplars and directions for new research. *AIDS, 14* (Suppl. 2), S18–S26.

Zimet, G. D, Blythe, M. J., and Fortenberry, J. D. (2000). Vaccine characteristics and acceptability of HIV immunization among adolescents. *International Journal of STD and AIDS, 11*,143–149.

PART

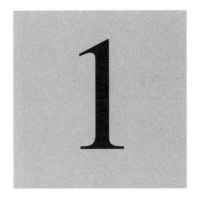

1

INDIVIDUAL-LEVEL APPROACHES

THE INFORMATION-MOTIVATION-BEHAVIORAL SKILLS MODEL OF HIV PREVENTIVE BEHAVIOR

Jeffrey D. Fisher
William A. Fisher
Paul A. Shuper

STUDYING HIV RISK BEHAVIOR WITH THE INFORMATION-MOTIVATION-BEHAVIORAL SKILLS MODEL

The Information-Motivation-Behavioral Skills (IMB) Model (J. Fisher and Fisher, 1992; W. Fisher and Fisher, 1993) has been used as a basis for understanding HIV risk behavior and for constructing theoretically and empirically based interventions to change this behavior across a wide range of populations of interest. The IMB model has been applied as a conceptual framework for studying—or intervening to alter—HIV risk behavior among adolescents (Arnowitz and Munzert, 2006; Arnowitz, Rennells, and Todd, 2005; Fisher, Fisher, Bryan, and Misovich, 2002; Fisher, Fisher, Misovich, Kimble, and Malloy, 1996; Rotheran-Borus, Gwadz, Fernandez, and Srinivasan, 1998; St. Lawrence et al., 1995; St. Lawrence, Crosby, Brasfield, and O'Bannon, 2002; Walter and Vaughn, 1993), individuals in close relationships (Misovich, Fisher, and Fisher, 1997), homosexual men (deWit, Stroebe, DeVroome, Sandfort, and van Griensven, 2000), military personnel (Boyer et al., 2001, 2005), injection drug users (Avants, Margolin, Usubiaga, and Doebrick, 2004; Avants, Warbuton, Hawkins, and Margolin, 2000; Bryan, Fisher, Fisher, and Murray, 2000), severely mentally ill individuals (Carey, Carey, and Kalichman, 1997; Carey, Carey, and Weinhardt, 1997; Kalichman, Malow, Dévieux, Stein, and Piedman, 2005; Otto-Salaj, Kelly, Stevenson, Hoffmann, and Kalichman, 2001; Weinhardt, Carey, Carey, and Verdecias, 1998), and HIV infected persons (Fisher, Kimble, Misovich, and Weinstein, 1998; Fisher, Fisher, Cornman, et al., 2006), among others. The model has also been used as a basis for understanding and promoting adolescent contraception (Byrne, Kelley, and Fisher, 1993), abstinence from sexual activity (Bazargan and West, 2006), sexually transmitted infection (STI) risk reduction (Fisher, 1997), and as a conceptual and empirical basis for reproductive health promotion education efforts (Barak and Fisher, 2003; Connecticut Department of Public Health, 1997; Health Canada, 2003; Fisher and Fisher, 1999). More recently, the IMB model has been articulated as a general model of health behavior change (Fisher, Fisher, and Harman, 2003) and has received support in that context (Fisher, Fisher, and Harman, 2003; Misovich, Martinez, Fisher, and Bryan, 2003; Murray, 2000). Standardized measures of the IMB model's constructs have been developed and validated for use with a number of populations and health behaviors of interest (Fisher and Fisher, 1996; Fisher, Fisher, Cornman, et al., 2006; Fisher, Fisher, Williams, and Malloy, 1994; Fisher and Fisher, 1993; Misovich, Fisher, and Fisher, 1996; Misovich, Fisher, and Fisher, 1998; Murray, 2000; Williams et al., 1998), and the IMB model may be systematically applied to create theoretically and empirically based health risk reduction interventions (J. Fisher and Fisher, 1992, W. Fisher and Fisher, 1993, 1999). A discussion of its widespread use appears later in this chapter. Although the IMB model now has broad application in health promotion practice, it was originally developed in response to the HIV epidemic (Fisher, Cornman, Norton, and Fisher, 2006; J. Fisher and Fisher, 1992; W. Fisher and Fisher, 1993). Consequently, we examine the utility of the IMB model with special reference to HIV.

EPIDEMIOLOGY OF HIV

The HIV epidemic has had a devastating global impact. Since 1981, it is estimated that 65 million people worldwide have been infected with HIV, and that 25 million have died as a result of AIDS (UNAIDS, 2006b). Recent data estimate 2.5 million new HIV infections globally in 2007, contributing to a total of 33.2 million people worldwide currently living with HIV (UNAIDS, 2007). In 2007 alone there were 2.1 million deaths attributable to AIDS-related illnesses (UNAIDS, 2007). Sub-Saharan Africa, where more than two-thirds (68 percent) of all HIV infections are found (UNAIDS, 2007), continues to be especially affected by the HIV epidemic.

In the United States, approximately 55,000 people become infected with HIV each year (Hall et al., 2008). From the beginning of the epidemic through 2005, there have been 550,394 AIDS-related deaths (CDC, 2007), and data suggest that at the end of 2003 there were 1,039,000 to 1,185,000 people living with HIV in the United States (Glynn and Rhodes, 2005). The effects of HIV/AIDS in the United States have been felt disproportionately among minorities, injection drug users, and men who have sex with men (CDC, 2007).

LIMITATIONS OF HIV PREVENTION APPROACHES

Over the course of the HIV epidemic, large numbers of HIV prevention interventions have been implemented in a broad array of settings. Unfortunately, there has typically been an enormous gap between the state of the science with respect to HIV prevention interventions and HIV prevention practice as typically implemented (Auerbach and Coates, 2000; Fenton and Valdiserri, 2006; Fisher and Fisher, 2000; Gluck and Rosenthal, 1995; Kegeles, Rebchook, and Tebbetts, 2005; Kelly et al., 2000; Rebchook, Kegeles, Huebner, et al., 2006; Ruiz et al., 2001). To date, as with other public health interventions, many of those targeting groups which practice HIV risk behavior are implemented directly by state or federal health departments, or funded by them and administered by community-based organizations (CBOs). All too often, neither behavioral scientists nor well-tested theories of behavior change are incorporated into the intervention design process (Fisher, Cornman, et al., 2006; Fisher and Fisher, 2000; Holtgrave et al., 1995; Kelly, Murphy, Sikkema, and Kalichman, 1993). In addition, rigorous evaluations of the efficacy of these programs are all too rare. A large number of HIV prevention interventions have also been undertaken by public schools (Health Canada, 2003; Kirby and DiClemente, 1994), and in many jurisdictions there are laws mandating that HIV education be provided, but without stipulations concerning *how* this should be done. Primary and secondary educational institutions have generally fielded weak, atheoretical interventions, with content that is often irrelevant to the practice of specific HIV/AIDS preventive actions and highly unlikely to effectively change HIV risk behavior. Until relatively recently, of the entire "portfolio" of HIV prevention interventions that have been implemented, too many have focused primarily—and in some cases *solely*—on providing **information** about HIV. Such information has consistently been shown to be unrelated to HIV risk behavior change (see, for example, Brunswick and Banaszak-Hol, 1996; Exner, Seal, and Ehrhardt, 1997; J. Fisher and Fisher, 1992, 2000; Helweg-Larsen and Collins, 1997; Kalichman, Cain, et al., 2005; Kalichman and Cherry, 1999; St. Lawrence et al., 1995; St. Lawrence et al., 2002).

In the past several years, a greater level of sophistication than that described above has begun to emerge in public health sector HIV prevention programs, especially in the United States since the U.S. Centers for Disease Control mandated that behavioral scientists become involved in intervention design, implementation, and evaluation, and that evidence-based programs be utilized (for example, Collins, Harshbarger, Sawyer, and Hamdallah, 2006; U.S. Department of Health and Human Services et al., 1993). Greater sophistication can also be found in some school-based programs (Fisher et al., 2002). Over the course of the entire HIV epidemic, most "cutting-edge" HIV prevention research has involved interventions designed, implemented, and evaluated by behavioral scientists—generally based at academic institutions—with funding from government agencies. This work has been much more theoretically elegant, and much more likely to have been rigorously evaluated and proven to be effective than other interventions. Unfortunately, such interventions make up a relatively small percentage of those that have been undertaken, and only a small proportion of the total HIV prevention intervention funds spent. Further, relatively few of these interventions have been broadly disseminated beyond the research setting (Ruiz et al., 2001).

When one reviews the body of HIV prevention intervention work conducted to date, a number of limitations that curtail intervention impact become clear (Coates, 1990; Fisher, Cornman, et al., 2006; J. Fisher and Fisher, 1992, 2000; Gluck and Rosenthal, 1995; Kelly et al., 1993). First, while relevant conceptual frameworks for HIV-risk behavior change have been proposed (for example, the health belief model, Rosenstock et al., 1994; the HIV risk-reduction model, Catania et al., 1990; the theory of reasoned action, Fishbein, Middlestadt, and Hitchcock, 1994; social cognitive theory, Bandura, 1994; the information-motivation-behavioral skills model of HIV risk behavior change, J. Fisher and Fisher, 1992, 2000; the transtheoretical model, Prochaska et al., 1994), many interventions have been intuitively and not theoretically based, and have failed to benefit from the substantial theoretical literature that is available to provide guidance for them (see Coates, 1990; deWit, 1996; J. Fisher and Fisher, 1992, 2000; W. Fisher and Fisher, 1993; Gluck and Rosenthal, 1995; Holtgrave et al., 1995, and Wingood and DiClemente, 1996 for discussion of this issue). This trend does appear to be changing, however, with the development of an increasing number of theory-based HIV risk-reduction interventions over recent years (Noar, 2008).

Second, relatively few interventions have systematically assessed target group members' *preintervention* HIV prevention **information** base, their HIV risk reduction **motivation**, and their **behavioral skills** with respect to HIV prevention, in order to tailor interventions to target group needs. Consequently, many interventions have involved empirically untargeted "shooting in the dark" (see J. Fisher and Fisher, 1992, 2000, and W. Fisher and Fisher, 1993, 1999) for discussion of this issue).

Third, interventions often focus on efforts to change *general* patterns of behavior (for example, encouraging people to practice "safer sex") as opposed to focusing on increasing individuals' inclination and ability to practice specific risk-reduction acts, even though a great deal of social psychological research suggests that it is more effective to focus on specific acts than on general patterns of behavior (see Ajzen and Fishbein, 1980; Fishbein and Ajzen, 1975; and Fishbein et al., 1994 for discussion of this issue).

Fourth, as noted earlier, a number of interventions implemented outside of research settings—in "real world" intervention contexts—have focused solely on providing information about HIV. Even *within* this narrow focus, the information that they provide is often relatively irrelevant to preventive behavior (for example, information about "modes of infection" is not directly relevant to enacting *specific* behaviors that are instrumental to HIV prevention), or the information which is offered is difficult to comprehend, unnecessarily frightening, sexist, or overtly risk-provoking (see W. Fisher and Fisher, 1993 for discussion of this issue).

Fifth, a number of HIV risk-reduction interventions that have been implemented have failed to motivate individuals to change their risky behavior or to provide training to help them acquire, rehearse, and refine the requisite behavioral skills for HIV risk behavior change (Bandura, 1994; J. Fisher and Fisher, 1992, 2000; W. Fisher and Fisher, 1993; Kelly, 1995).

Sixth, the majority of HIV prevention interventions have focused on individuals who are *not* likely to be HIV infected, and have generally not addressed the need for behavior change (for example, safer sex or injection drug use) in HIV-infected individuals, who are directly capable of spreading the virus to others (Crepaz et al., 2006; Kelly and Kalichman, 2002). For HIV-infected individuals, moreover, antiretroviral medication adherence promotion interventions (to increase consistent adherence to combination therapies) are also critical to maintain patient health and to avoid development and transmission of treatment-resistant strains of HIV (for example, Amico et al., 2009; Amico, Toro-Alfonso, and Fisher, 2005; Fisher, Fisher, Amico, and Harman, 2006; Fisher, Fisher, and Amico, 2001; Fisher, 2000, 2001; Kalichman et al., 2001; Starace, Massa, Amico, and Fisher, 2006).

Finally, many existing interventions have not been evaluated with sufficient rigor to determine whether intended changes in mediating factors (for example, knowledge, motivation, behavioral skills) and in HIV preventive behavior have actually occurred in the short- or long-term and in relation to both direct and indirect and nonreactive indicators of intervention outcome (see Exner et al., 1997; Gluck and Rosenthal, 1995; Johnson, Ostrow, and Joseph, 1990; Kelly et al., 1993; Leviton and Valdiserri, 1990; Oakley, Fullerton, and Holland, 1995; and Wingood and DiClemente, 1996 for discussion of this issue).

ORIGINS OF THE IMB MODEL

The IMB model was created in an attempt to apply social psychological conceptualizations, methodologies, and measurement techniques to address the critical need for a strong theoretical basis for HIV/AIDS prevention efforts that also addresses the problems with existing work cited above. The model is rooted in an analysis and integration of theory and research in the HIV prevention and social psychological literatures (J. Fisher and Fisher, 1992, 2000; Fisher and Fisher, 1993; Fisher, Fisher, and Harman, 2003). It was influenced by earlier work by J. Fisher (1988), and Fisher and Misovich (1990) on the effects of social influence on HIV preventive behavior, and on the conditions under which behavior change is likely and unlikely (Fisher, Silver, Chinsky, Goff, Klar, and Zagieboylo, 1989). The model was further influenced by earlier conceptual and empirical work by W. Fisher on affective determinants of sexual and reproductive health behavior (Fisher, Fisher, and Byrne, 1977; Fisher, Byrne, Kelly, and White, 1988; Fisher and Fisher, 1999), on the Sexual Behavior Sequence theory of the determinants of sexual behavior (Byrne, 1977; Fisher 1986) and work on changing risky sexual behavior (Fisher, Byrne, and White, 1983). Since its initial publication in *Psychological Bulletin* in 1992, the IMB model has been widely cited and tested in the context of HIV prevention with diverse populations, and has received support both in correlational and experimental intervention research in the context of HIV prevention and other health behaviors (for example, Albarracín et al., 2005; J. Fisher and Fisher, 1992, 2000; Fisher, Fisher, and Harman, 2003; Johnson, Carey, Chaudoir, and Reid, 2006; Johnson, Carey, Marsh, Levin, and Scott-Sheldon, 2003).

THE IMB MODEL OF HIV PREVENTIVE BEHAVIOR

The IMB model conceptualizes the psychological determinants of HIV preventive behavior and provides a general framework for understanding and promoting prevention across populations and preventive behaviors of interest (J. Fisher and Fisher, 1992, 2000; Fisher and Fisher, 1993; Fisher, Fisher and Harmon, 2003). The model focuses comprehensively on the set of informational (for example, U.S. Department of Health and Human Services, 1988), motivational (for example, Fishbein and Middlestadt, 1989), and behavioral skills (for example, Kelly and St. Lawrence, 1988) factors which are conceptually and empirically associated with HIV prevention but which are often dealt with in isolation (J. Fisher and Fisher, 1992, 2000). It specifies a set of causal relationships among these constructs, and a set of operations to be utilized in translating this approach into conceptually-based and empirically-targeted HIV prevention interventions (J. Fisher and Fisher, 1992, 2000; W. Fisher and Fisher, 1993, 1999).

Fundamental Assumptions

The IMB model asserts that HIV prevention information, HIV prevention motivation, and HIV prevention behavioral skills are the **fundamental determinants** of HIV preventive behavior (J. Fisher and Fisher, 1992, 2000; J. Fisher et al., 1996; W. Fisher and Fisher, 1993). To the extent that individuals are well-informed, motivated to act, and possess the behavioral skills required to act effectively, they will be likely to initiate and maintain patterns of HIV preventive behavior.

According to the IMB model, HIV prevention *information* that is directly relevant to preventive behavior, and that can be enacted easily in the social ecology of the individual, is a prerequisite of HIV preventive behavior (J. Fisher and Fisher, 1992, 2000; Kelly and St. Lawrence, 1988). HIV prevention information that is closely related to preventive behavior enactment can include specific facts about *HIV transmission* (for example, "Oral sex is a safer alternative to vaginal intercourse"), as well as facts relevant to *HIV prevention* (for example, "Consistent condom use can prevent HIV"), that serve as guides for personal preventive actions.

In addition to facts that are easy to translate into behavior, the IMB model recognizes additional cognitive processes and content categories that significantly influence performance of preventive behavior. Individuals often rely heavily on ***HIV prevention heuristics***—simple decision rules which permit automatic and cognitively effortless (but often incorrect) decisions about whether or not to engage in HIV preventive behavior. Endorsement of such heuristics appears to be strongly related to HIV preventive practices (Hammer, Fisher, and Fitzgerald, 1996; Misovich et al., 1996; Offir, Fisher, and Williams, 1993). For example, reliance on HIV prevention heuristics such as "monogamous sex is safe sex" and "known partners are safe partners" is ubiquitous and substantially interferes with performance of objectively effective preventive behaviors (Hammer et al., 1996; Misovich et al., 1996). Individuals also operate on the basis of *implicit theories of HIV risk* that (again incorrectly) hold that it is possible to detect and avoid HIV risk on the basis of assessment of a partner's externally visible characteristics such as dress, demeanor, personality, or social associations. Based upon estimates of HIV risk made by assessing a partner's overtly accessible profile of supposed risk cues, people often decide that the partner poses little risk and that preventive behaviors are not warranted (Hammer et al., 1996; Misovich et al., 1996, 1997; Offir et al., 1993; Shuper and Fisher, 2008; Williams et al., 1992).

Motivation to engage in HIV preventive acts is an additional determinant of preventive behavior and influences whether even well-informed individuals will be inclined to act on what they know about prevention. According to the IMB model (J. Fisher and Fisher, 1992, 2000; Fisher and Fisher, 1993; Fisher, Fisher, and Harman, 2003), HIV prevention motivation includes personal motivation to practice preventive behaviors (attitudes towards practicing specific preventive acts) and social motivation to engage in prevention (perceptions of social support for performing such acts) (Fishbein and Ajzen, 1975).

Behavioral skills for performing HIV preventive acts are an additional prerequisite of HIV preventive behavior, and determine whether even well-informed and well-motivated individuals will be capable of practicing prevention effectively. The behavioral skills component of the IMB model is composed of an individual's objective ability and his or her perceived self-efficacy in performing the sequence of HIV preventive behaviors that are involved in the practice of prevention (Bandura, 1989, 1994; J. Fisher and Fisher, 1992, 2000; W. Fisher, 1990; Kelly and St. Lawrence, 1988). Behavioral skills involved in HIV prevention can include objective and perceived abilities to purchase and to put on condoms; to negotiate consistent condom use before, or during, sexual contact; to negotiate HIV testing and monogamy; and the ability to reinforce the self and the partner for maintaining patterns of preventive behaviors across time, among many other such behaviors.

The IMB model (see Figure 2.1) specifies that HIV prevention information and HIV prevention motivation work primarily through HIV prevention behavioral skills to influence HIV preventive behavior.

The effects of prevention information and prevention motivation are a result of the development and deployment of prevention behavioral skills directly applied to the initiation and maintenance of preventive behavior. The IMB model also specifies that prevention information and prevention motivation may have direct effects on preventive behavior, in cases in which complicated or novel behavioral skills are not necessary to effect prevention. For example, HIV prevention information may have a direct effect on preventive behavior when a pregnant woman learns of the benefits of prenatal HIV antibody testing and simply agrees with her physician's suggestion that she undergo such testing. Motivation may have a direct effect on behavior, as when a motivated couple who have both been tested for HIV status maintain a sexually monogamous pattern of behavior as opposed to multiple partnering, with attendant behavioral skills demands for using condoms, including condom acquisition, discussion, negotiation, and consistent use. Finally, from the perspective of the IMB model, information and motivation are regarded as generally independent constructs, in that well-informed individuals are not necessarily well-motivated to practice prevention, and well-motivated individuals are not always well-informed about prevention (J. Fisher and Fisher, 1992, 2000; Fisher et al., 1994). The model's basic constructs and the relationships among them are depicted in Figure 2.1.

The IMB model's information, motivation, and behavioral skills constructs are regarded as highly generalizable determinants of HIV preventive behavior across populations and preventive behaviors of interest (J. Fisher and Fisher, 1992, 1996, 2000; W. Fisher and Fisher, 1993). At the same time, however, these constructs should have specific content that is most relevant to the prevention needs of particular populations and particular preventive practices. Thus, within the IMB model, it is presumed that *specific* HIV prevention information, motivation, and behavioral skills may be especially relevant to understanding and promoting prevention among males (as compared to females),

FIGURE 2.1 *The Information-Motivation-Behavioral Skills Model of HIV Prevention Health Behavior*

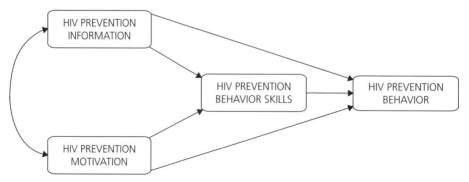

Source: Fisher, J.D., & Fisher, W.A. "Changing AIDS Risk Behavior." *Psychological Bulletin,* 111(3), 455-474, 1992, APA Reprinted with permission.

among African Americans (as compared to whites), and among members of particular ethnic groups and persons of particular sexual orientation, chemical dependency status, and the like. Similarly, specific HIV prevention information, motivation, and behavioral skills content will be especially relevant to specific HIV preventive practices, such as abstinence, condom use, and HIV antibody testing, within specific populations of interest. Also following this logic, the IMB model proposes that particular constructs of the model, and particular causal pathways among them, will emerge as more or less powerful determinants of HIV preventive practices for specific populations and specific preventive behaviors (J. Fisher and Fisher, 1992, 1996, 2000; W. Fisher and Fisher, 1993). Such differences should be informative with respect to understanding and promoting the practice of specific preventive behaviors in specific populations of interest.

The IMB approach specifies measurement and statistical procedures for eliciting information, motivation, and behavioral skills content that is relevant to HIV prevention for particular populations and behaviors of interest. These procedures may then be used to identify specific causal elements and paths in the model that are especially influential in determining a given population's practice of a particular preventive behavior (J. Fisher and Fisher, 1992, 2000; Fisher et al., 1996; W. Fisher and Fisher, 1993). According to the IMB model, specification of the information, motivation, and behavioral skills content most relevant to a population's practice of a particular preventive behavior, and identification of IMB model constructs that most powerfully influence the population's practice of the preventive behavior, are crucial to the design of effective conceptually-based and empirically-targeted prevention interventions for the population and preventive behavior of interest (J. Fisher and Fisher, 1992, 2000; Fisher et al., 1996; W. Fisher and Fisher, 1993).

The IMB approach to understanding and promoting HIV preventive behavior specifies a set of generalizable operations for constructing, implementing, and evaluating HIV prevention interventions for particular target populations and behaviors (J. Fisher and Fisher, 1992, 1996, 2000; W. Fisher and Fisher, 1993; Fisher, Cornman, et al., 2006). (Figure 2.2.)

On the basis of the model, the first step in the process of changing HIV preventive behavior involves *elicitation research* conducted with a subsample of a population of interest, to empirically identify population-specific deficits and assets in HIV prevention information, motivation, behavioral skills, and HIV risk and preventive behavior. The use of open-ended data collection techniques such as focus groups and open-ended questionnaires to avoid providing occasions for prompted responses is advocated, in addition to the use of close-ended techniques that lend themselves to quantitative analyses (W. Fisher and Fisher, 1993). The second step in this process of changing HIV risk behavior involves the design and implementation of *conceptually-based, empirically-targeted, population-specific* interventions, constructed on the basis of elicitation research findings. These targeted interventions address identified deficits in HIV prevention information, motivation, behavioral skills, and behavior, and capitalize on assets that may characterize a population. The third step in the process of HIV risk behavior change involves methodologically rigorous *evaluation research* conducted to determine whether an intervention has had significant and sustained

FIGURE 2.2 *Elicitation, Intervention, and Evaluation*

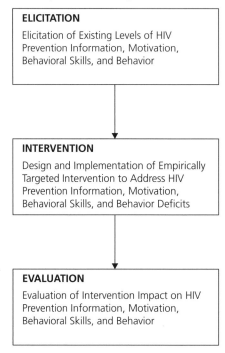

Source: J. Fisher and Fisher (1992) and W. Fisher and Fisher (1993), *Psychological Bulletin, 111*, 455-474. Copyright by APA. Reprinted with permission.

effects on the information, motivation, and behavioral skills determinants of HIV preventive behavior, and on HIV preventive behavior *per se*. The IMB approach advocates evaluation research that relies upon multiple convergent sources of data, at least some of which are relatively nonreactive, and at least some of which are collected in a context that appears to participants to be unrelated to the intervention *per se* (J. Fisher and Fisher, 1992, 1996, 2000; W. Fisher and Fisher, 1993).

EMPIRICAL SUPPORT FOR THE IMB MODEL

Considerable empirical support for the fundamental assumptions of the IMB model has been accumulated in multivariate correlational research concerning informational, motivational, and behavioral skills determinants of HIV preventive behavior across populations and preventive behaviors of interest (see Table 2.1 for IMB model tests in the context of HIV risk and preventive behavior).

Confirming evidence concerning the IMB model's HIV risk-reduction behavior change implications has also been accumulated in model-based experimental intervention research, in which interventions have resulted in significant and sustained increases in HIV risk-reduction information, motivation, behavioral skills, and preventive behavior over time and across diverse populations at risk for HIV (see Table 2.2 for successful

TABLE 2.1 Tests of the Information-Motivation-Behavioral Skills Model with Respect to Sexual Risk Behavior: Summary of Reported Associations Among IMB Components.

Location/Sample	Information-motivation	Information-behavioral skills	Motivation-behavioral skills	Behavioral skills-behavior	Information-behavior	Motivation-behavior	Percent variance
Urban housing developments in NY, OH, VA, WA, and WI N = 557 low income women (76% African American) (1)			✓	✓		✓	50%
Methadone maintenance program in Hartford, CT N = 156 heroin-addicted adults receiving methadone treatment (2)			✓		✓	✓	35%
Chennai, India N = 300 male truck drivers (3)				✓	✓	✓	40–51%[1]
University in Storrs, CT N = 259 university students (4)		✓	✓	✓		✓	10%
Hartford and New Haven, CT N = 126 gay men (5)		✓	✓	✓		✓	35%

(Continued)

TABLE 2.1 (Continued)

Miami, FL N=87 male high school students (6)			✓	✓	75%
Miami, FL N=61 female high school students (7)		✓	✓	✓	45%
Inner-city areas of Miami-Dade County, FL N=320 substance abusing severely mentally ill adults (8)	✓	✓	✓	✓	not stated
STI clinic in Cape Town, South Africa N=191 STI clinic patients (9)	✓		✓	✓	not stated
"Juvenile detention center in a Southern U.S. city" N=195 female incarcerated juvenile offenders (10)	✓		✓	✓	not stated
Juvenile detention center in a southern U.S. city N=328 male incarcerated juvenile offenders (11)	✓	✓		✓	not stated

[1]Findings from Bryan et al. (2001) represent tests of relationships of information, motivation, behavioral skills with behavior, and percent of variance accounted for in condom use with wives and with commercial sex workers.

Sources: (1) Anderson et al. (2006); (2) Bryan et al. (2000); (3) Bryan et al. (2001); (4) Fisher et al. (1994); (5) Fisher et al. (1994); (6) Fisher et al. (1999); (7) Fisher et al. (1999); (8) Kalichman, Malow, et al. (2005); (9) Kalichman et al. (2006) ; (10) Robertson et al. (2006) ; (11) Robertson et al. (2006).

TABLE 2.2 Effective Sexual Risk-Reduction Interventions Using the Information-Motivation-Behavioral Skills (IMB Model)[1].

Location/Sample	IMB Model-Based Intervention
Urban housing developments in NY, OH, VA, WA, and WI N = 557 low income women (76% African American) (1)	Five 90-minute group workshops emphasizing HIV-related information, positive attitudes, and condom use and negotiation skills. The intervention also included community-based activities and the formation of a community-based Women's Health Council.
Methadone maintenance program in New Haven, CT N = 220 Injection drug users (2)	Twelve-session harm reduction group intervention emphasizing AIDS education, the development of a personalized risk-reduction plan, and skills development.
Low-income, inner city community in Atlanta, GA N = 74 women (95% African American) (3)	Single-session HIV prevention intervention focusing on HIV-related education, problem solving, communication skills, self-efficacy, assertiveness training, and development of action plans.
U.S. Marines in the Western Pacific N = 619 male U.S. Marines (4)	Four 2-hour interactive group sessions focusing on STI/HIV risk-related knowledge, alcohol use, and skills training.
U.S. Marines stationed in the U.S. and abroad N = 2,157 female U.S. Marine recruits (5)	Four 2-hour group sessions addressing HIV-risk-related IMB factors through didactic teaching, interactive group activities, and videos.
Syracuse, NY N = 102 women (76% African American) (6)	Four 90-minute group sessions involving motivational interviewing techniques, HIV-related knowledge enhancement, and interpersonal skills building.

(Continued)

TABLE 2.2 *(Continued)*

CBO in Syracuse, NY N = 102 women (88% African American) (7)	Four 90-minute group sessions involving motivational interviewing techniques, HIV-related knowledge enhancement, and interpersonal skills building.
Cohen (2000) University in Austin, TX N=88 university students	Two-session intervention emphasizing HIV/AIDS information, condom demonstrations, and self-management techniques.
Urban HIV-care clinic in KwaZulu-Natal, South Africa N = 152 HIV+ patients on ARVs receiving clinical care (9)	Multiple 15-minute intervention sessions delivered by counselors during routine care aimed at increasing HIV-related knowledge, changing negative attitudes, building skills, and setting goals.
Chennai, India N = 250 male truck drivers (10)	Single-session group interactive workshop that focused on addressing information deficits, decreasing negative condom attitudes, and rehearsing condom use skills.
University in Storrs, CT N = 744 undergraduate dormitory residents (11)	Three 2-hour sessions involving a slide show to present HIV-related information; group discussions to enhance attitudes; and video-based and in-vivo skills training.
Four inner-city high schools in CT N = 1577 High school students (12)	Five-session classroom-based intervention providing HIV-related information, attitudinal change videos, and video-based and hands-on skills training.
Two of the largest HIV clinics in CT N = 497 HIV+ patients receiving clinical care (13)	Multiple 5–10 minute intervention sessions delivered by clinicians during routine care addressing IMB barriers, ambivalence to behavior change, and risk-reduction goals.
University in Syracuse, NY N = 78 University students	Single-session intervention emphasizing STI information, advantages of risk-reduction, and skills training.

STI Clinic in Milwaukee, WI N = 612 STI Clinic patients (15)	Single 90-minute counseling session emphasizing HIV-related information and personal responsibility and providing personalized feedback and skills training.
STI Clinic in Atlanta, GA N = 106 male STI Clinic patients (100% African American) (16)	Single 3-hour group-based session providing HIV-related information along with motivational and skills training (for either latex or polyurethane condoms).
STI Clinic in Atlanta, GA N = 117 male STI Clinic patients (100% African American) (17)	Two 3-hour video-based intervention sessions involving HIV-related information, motivational training, and skills acquisition and practice.
STI Clinic in Atlanta, GA N = 81 female STI Clinic patients (100% African American) (18)	Single 2.5-hour workshop emphasizing HIV-related information, female condom use and skills, and communication skills.
University in Storrs, CT N = 157 university students (19)	Two-session computer-based intervention emphasizing HIV-related information, advantages of using condoms, normative support, behavioral skills, and goal setting.
Methadone maintenance program in New Haven, CT N = 90 HIV+ Injection drug users (20)	Twice-weekly, 2-hour HIV harm-reduction sessions involving skills training, cognitive remediation strategies, and behavioral games.
Public Health STI Clinics in Oregon N = 339 adolescents (21)	Five 60-90 minute individual counselor-participant sessions emphasizing goal setting; assertiveness training, social skills training, and behavioral self-management.
Community mental health clinics in Milwaukee, WI N = 189 men and women from outpatient programs (22)	Seven-session small group intervention (+2 booster sessions) emphasizing HIV/AIDS risk, self-efficacy, condom use skills, and safer-sex role plays.
University in Pullman, WA N = 386 university students (23)	15-session interventions (self-management and peer norm) emphasizing HIV-related information, condom use skills, role-playing, self-management skills training, and enhancement of positive peer norms.

(Continued)

TABLE 2.2 (Continued)

University in Storrs, CT N = 701 university students (24)	Three-session intervention emphasizing AIDS information, attitudes, social norms, and skills training.
Social service agency in New York, NY N = 151 adolescents (25)	Seven 1.5-hour intervention sessions emphasizing HIV knowledge, perceived risk, self-efficacy, negotiation and condom use skills, and goal setting.
Southern U.S. City N = 246 Adolescents (100% African American) (26)	Eight weekly group sessions of 1.5 to 2 hours emphasizing HIV-related information, values, empowerment, perceived vulnerability, and communication and condom use skills.
Residential drug treatment programs in MS N = 161 substance-dependent adolescents (27)	Twelve 90-minute group sessions emphasizing HIV risk-related knowledge, personal responsibility, condom and negotiation skills, and personal vulnerability.
STI Clinic in Cape Town, South Africa N = 228 STI Clinic patients (28)	Single 60-minute counseling session emphasizing HIV-related knowledge, motivation and commitment to change, and behavioral self-management and communication skills.
High schools in New York, NY N = 1201 9th and 11th grade students (29)	Six in-class sessions emphasizing AIDS transmission and prevention information, appraisal of perceived risk, personal values, condom skills, and negotiation skills.
Public psychiatric hospital in upstate NY N = 22 female outpatients living with mental illness (30)	Ten daily 75-minute treatment sessions focusing on HIV-related information, vulnerability, negotiation skills, and sexual assertiveness training.

[1]Due to space limitations, information presented in Table 2.2 provides only very brief descriptions of studies and interventions. Please refer to the cited studies for complete descriptions of samples, IMB model-based interventions, and sexual risk-reduction outcomes.

Source: (1) Anderson et al. (2006); (2) Avants et al. (2004); (3) Belcher et al. (1998); (4) Boyer et al. (2001); (5) Boyer et al. (2005); (6) Carey, Maisto, et al. (1997); (7) Carey et al. (2000); (8) Cohen (2000); (9) Cornman et al. (2008) ; (10) Cornman et al. (2007); (11) Fisher et al. (1996); (12) Fisher et al. (2002); (13) Fisher et al. (2006); (14) Jaworski et al. (2001); (15) Kalichman, Cain et al. (2005); (16) Kalichman and Cherry (1999); (17) Kalichman, Cherry et al. (1999); (18) Kalichman, Williams, et al. (1999); (19) Kiene and Barta (2006); (20) Margolin et al. (2003); (21) Metzler et al. (2000); (22) Otto-Salaj et al. (2001); (23) Peeler (2000); (24) Rosengard (1992); (25) Rotheram-Borus et al. (1998); (26) St. Lawrence et al. (1995); (27) St. Lawrence et al. (2002); (28) Simbayi et al. (2004); (29) Walter and Vaughn (1993); (30) Weinhardt et al. (1998);

HIV risk-reduction IMB-model based intervention studies). Finally, a number of systematic reviews and meta-analyses of HIV risk-reduction interventions provide support for the underlying assumptions of the IMB model (for example, Albarracín et al., 2005; Albarracín, Durantini, and Earl, 2006; Copenhaver et al., 2006; Crepaz et al., 2006, 2007; Herbst et al., 2005; Herbst, Beeker, et al., 2007; Herbst, Kay, et al., 2007; Johnson et al., 2003, 2006; Johnson et al., 2002; Noar, 2008).

Multivariate correlational evidence consistently supports the IMB model's assumptions concerning the determinants of HIV preventive behavior. In an initial study in this research line, J. Fisher et al. (1994) used a structural equation modeling approach to empirically test the IMB model's assumptions concerning the determinants of HIV preventive behavior within a heterosexual university student sample. In this sample, HIV prevention information and HIV prevention motivation were statistically independent factors; each was related to HIV prevention behavioral skills; and HIV prevention behavioral skills were related to HIV preventive behavior per se: Each of these relationships was precisely as predicted by the IMB model. In an additional study in this series, J. Fisher et al. (1994) examined HIV preventive behavior from the perspective of the IMB model within a community sample of adult homosexual men. Once again, it was found that information and motivation were independent constructs; that they were each associated with behavioral skills; and that behavioral skills were associated with preventive behavior, as predicted by the model. A direct link between HIV prevention motivation and HIV preventive behavior was observed as well, also in accord with the model's assumptions. Subsequent research has confirmed the IMB model's propositions concerning the determinants of HIV preventive behavior in populations of sexually active minority high school students (Fisher, Williams, Fisher, and Malloy, 1999), low-income women (Anderson et al., 2006), heroin users on methadone treatment (Bryan et al., 2000), male Indian truck drivers (Bryan, Fisher, and Benziger, 2001), substance-abusing adults with serious mental illness (Kalichman, Malow, et al., 2005), STI clinic patients in South Africa (Kalichman et al., 2006), and incarcerated juvenile offenders (Robertson, Stein, and Baird-Thomas, 2006).

The findings observed across multiple empirical tests of the IMB model's relationships are summarized in Table 2.1. It is evident that the general propositions of the IMB model are supported and that the data are in accord with the assertion that HIV prevention information and HIV prevention motivation stimulate the application of HIV prevention behavioral skills to effect HIV preventive behavior. It is also clear that there is often a direct link between HIV prevention motivation and HIV preventive behavior, in accord with the model's supposition that motivation may directly influence the practice of preventive behaviors that are not complicated or novel. Finally, in these model tests, the constructs of the IMB model generally account for a substantial proportion of the variance in HIV preventive behavior.

With respect to HIV risk-reduction behavior change, IMB model-based experimental intervention research has demonstrated the utility of the approach in producing significant and sustained changes in HIV prevention information, motivation, behavioral skills, and behavior (Table 2.2).

In research reported by J. Fisher et al. (1996), samples of primarily heterosexual university students participated in elicitation studies to identify deficits in their HIV prevention information, motivation, and behavioral skills, and to determine their most significant HIV risk behaviors. Based on elicitation findings, an IMB model-based, empirically-targeted HIV risk-reduction intervention was designed to address HIV prevention information gaps, motivational obstacles, and behavioral skills deficits related to this population's primary HIV risk behaviors. The intervention comprised a field experiment in which paired male and female dormitory floors received an IMB model-based intervention—consisting of information, motivation, and behavioral skills–focused slide shows, videos, group discussions, and role plays, delivered by a health educator and peer educators—or were assigned to a control condition. Evaluation research showed that the intervention had significant effects on multiple measures of HIV prevention information, motivation, and behavioral skills at four weeks post-intervention, and significant effects on discussing condom use with sexual partners, keeping condoms accessible, and using condoms during sexual intercourse at this interval. Results of a follow-up assessment indicated that the intervention had significant and sustained effects on condom accessibility and condom use, and on HIV antibody testing, two to four months post-intervention.

Anderson and her colleagues (2006) developed and tested an IMB model–based intervention aimed at increasing condom use among women living in a number of low-income urban housing developments. Women in housing developments that were randomly assigned to the IMB model–based intervention condition took part in five 90-minute small group workshops that emphasized HIV prevention-related information, motivation (positive attitudes and beliefs about HIV risk-reduction behaviors), and behavioral skills (for negotiating condom use and using condoms correctly). In each of the housing developments in which the IMB model intervention was implemented, a Women's Health Council was formed to conduct community-based activities corresponding with the small group workshops and to reinforce the IMB–model related HIV risk-reduction messages that workshop participants had received. Women in the IMB model–based intervention were also sent coupons for free condoms and AIDS-related information. In contrast, women residing in the control condition developments received only coupons for free condoms and AIDS-related information. Results demonstrated that at follow-up, whereas women who had received the IMB model–based intervention significantly increased their use of condoms, women in the control condition showed a slight decrease in condom use. Furthermore, women receiving the IMB model–based intervention demonstrated significant increases in HIV risk-related information, perceived pro-prevention social norms, and condom use intentions, and reported engaging in significantly higher rates of condom procurement and condom-related discussions with partners. Finally, providing further support for the IMB model, structural analysis of the outcome data demonstrated that increases in reported condom use resulted from women's increases in motivation and behavioral skills. Results from Anderson et al. (2006) and J. Fisher et al. (1996), along with findings from a substantial number of other successful IMB model–based intervention outcome studies (for example, Belcher et al., 1998; Boyer et al., 2001, 2005; Carey, Braaten, et al., 2000; Carey, Maisto, et al., 1997; Cohen, 2000; Fisher et al., 2002; Fisher, Fisher, Cornman, et al., 2006; Jaworski and Carey, 2001; Kalichman and Cherry, 1999; Kalichman, Cherry, and Browne-Sperling, 1999; Kalichman, Williams, and Nachimson, 1999; Kalichman, Cain, et al., 2005; Kiene and Barta, 2006; Metzler, Biglan, Noell, Ary, and Ochs, 2000; Peeler, 2000; Rosengard, 1992; Rotheram-Borus et al., 1998; St Lawrence et al., 1995; Walter and Vaughn, 1993), demonstrate the efficacy of IMB model–based interventions in reducing HIV transmission risk behavior among a variety of heterosexual, MSM, and noninjection drug–using populations.

Several IMB model–based interventions have also been specifically developed to reduce risky sexual and drug use behavior among samples of injection drug users (for example, Avants et al., 2004; Margolin, Avants, Warburton, Hawkins, and Shi, 2003). Margolin et al. (2003), for example, developed and tested through a randomized controlled trial an IMB model–based intervention aimed at reducing needle sharing and unprotected sexual behavior among HIV+ injection drug users entering a methadone maintenance program. Posttreatment results demonstrated that participants receiving the IMB model–based intervention were significantly less likely to have reported sharing needles and were three times less likely to have reported engaging in unprotected sex than participants in the control condition. Overall, these findings provide support for the use of the IMB model in developing risk-reduction interventions for traditionally difficult-to-treat populations.

Rates of HIV among individuals living with a severe mental illness are significantly higher than rates of HIV among the general population, with reported HIV prevalence rates ranging from 3.1 percent (Rosenberg et al., 2001) to 22.9 percent (Silberstein, Galanter, Marmor, Lifshutz, and Krasinski, 1994) among individuals with mental illness (see Cournos and McKinnon, 1997, for a review). Several IMB model–based interventions targeting individuals with severe mental illness have been developed, and these interventions have been shown to have a significant impact on HIV risk behavior among members of this population (for example, Carey, Carey, and Kalichman, 1997; Carey, Carey, and Weinhardt, 1997; Kalichman, Malow, et al., 2005; Otto-Salaj et al., 2001; Weinhardt et al., 1997, 1998). Weinhardt and his colleagues (1998) developed a ten-session, two-week IMB model–based intervention for female psychiatric outpatients. The IMB model–based intervention provided participants with HIV-related information and, to enhance participants' motivation to enact safer behaviors, participants were also provided with a personalized risk summary aimed at increasing awareness of their susceptibility to HIV infections. Behavioral skills were addressed in a sexual assertiveness training component that emphasized negotiating condom use, dealing with partners who resisted safer behavior, and refusing to engage in unsafe sexual behavior. Two months after completing the intervention, results showed that compared to those in a wait-list control condition, participants receiving the IMB model–based intervention reported significantly higher levels of protected sexual intercourse, significantly stronger sexual assertiveness skills, and significantly higher levels of HIV-related knowledge. Overall, these findings, along with the findings from a number of other IMB model–based research studies involving individuals with severe mental illness (for example, Carey, Carey, and Kalichman, 1997; Carey, Carey, and Weinhardt, 1997; Kalichman et al., 2005; Otto-Salaj et al., 2001; Weinhardt et al., 1997), suggest that IMB model–based interventions can effectively reduce HIV risk behavior among individuals with severe cognitive, affective, and behavioral difficulties who are particularly at risk for acquiring HIV.

In addition to a large number of IMB model–based interventions that have been successfully tested in the Unites States, IMB model–based interventions aimed at reducing HIV risk behavior have recently been shown to be effective in international settings (for example, Cornman et al., 2008; Cornman et al., 2007; Simbayi et al., 2004). In South Africa, HIV prevalence rates are among the highest in the world, with an estimated 5.5 million people currently living with HIV (UNAIDS, 2006a). Within this epidemic context, Simbayi and his colleagues developed an IMB model–based intervention designed to reduce HIV risk behavior among a sample of high-risk individuals—patients who had been seen for repeat STIs at an STI clinic in Cape Town, South Africa. The IMB model framework was used to create a brief (sixty-minute) culturally appropriate intervention designed for the South African clinical care context and clinical population. Specifically, with respect to HIV-related information, the intervention focused on correcting local misinformation about HIV (for example, having sex with a virgin can rid a person of HIV), providing information about local HIV prevalence, and discussing community-based HIV resources available locally. With respect to motivation, emphasis was placed on personal responsibility, feedback was provided regarding participants' own risk behavior, and participants engaged in a risk-reduction goal-setting exercise. Finally, participants were taught a number of risk-reduction skills that included identifying social and environmental triggers associated with potentially risky situations, managing these triggers for risk, and choosing safer alternatives over risky sexual behavior. Results indicated that compared to participants receiving a control condition intervention consisting only of HIV information/education, STI clinic patients who received the culturally tailored IMB model–based intervention reported engaging in significantly lower levels of unprotected sex, and reported a lower proportion of unprotected intercourse occasions. Those receiving the IMB model–based intervention also showed higher levels of HIV-related knowledge and greater confidence in their ability to reduce their risk for HIV compared to participants receiving the HIV education/information only intervention. These findings, along with additional intervention research conducted in South Africa (Cornman et al., 2008) and in other international settings (for example, Cornman et al., 2007), provide support for the use of the IMB framework in the development of effective, culturally appropriate, HIV risk-reduction interventions in very high HIV prevalence areas of the world.

Strong support for the general propositions of the IMB model with respect to HIV prevention has also been demonstrated in a series of meta-analytic and systematic reviews of studies involving HIV risk-reduction interventions (for example, Albarracín et al., 2005; Albarracín, et al., 2006; Copenhaver et al., 2006; Crepaz et al., 2006, 2007; Herbst et al., 2005; Herbst, Beeker, et al., 2007; Herbst, Kay, et al., 2007; Johnson et al., 2006; 2003; 2002; Noar, 2008). First, a number of these reviews have found that interventions grounded in behavioral theory are more effective than interventions that are not theoretically based (for example, Albarracín et al., 2005; 2006; Crepaz et al., 2006, 2007; Herbst et al., 2005; Noar, 2008). It should be noted, however, that not all behavioral theories have been shown to be equally efficacious when it comes to using them as the basis for HIV risk-reduction interventions. Specifically, upon examining risk-reduction interventions based on different behavioral theories, Albarracín and her colleagues (2005, 2006) found that whereas interventions based on the IMB model, the theory of reasoned action (Fishbein and Ajzen, 1975; Ajzen and Fishbein, 1980), the theory of planned behavior (Ajzen, 1985), and self-efficacy/social cognitive theory (for example, Bandura, 1989, 1992) were effective, interventions based on theories emphasizing fear appeals were not. In fact, and providing strong support for the IMB model approach, Albarracín and her colleagues (2005) found in a comprehensive review of HIV prevention interventions conducted between 1985 and 2003 that HIV risk-reduction interventions were most effective when they included HIV-related information, motivational components, and behavioral skills training. In addition, in a meta-analytic examination of theory-specific components of HIV risk-reduction interventions, Noar (2008) has shown that, consistent with the IMB model, interventions that include behavioral skills training components were significantly more effective than interventions not including such components. This meta-analytic effect for behavioral skills training was found in a number of different populations, including injection drug users (Copenhaver et al., 2006), Black and Hispanic STI clinic patients (Crepaz et al., 2007), individuals living with HIV (Crepaz et al., 2006; Johnson et al., 2006), Hispanics in the United States and Puerto Rico (Herbst, Kay, et al., 2007), men who have sex with men (Herbst et al., 2005; Johnson et al., 2002), and adolescents (Johnson et al., 2003). Also in accord with the IMB model, meta-analytic support has been shown for informational and motivational aspects of behavior change, indicating increased intervention impact for interventions providing condom-related information (Johnson et al., 2003) and interventions emphasizing motivational aspects (Johnson et al., 2006), including peer norms (Herbst, Kay, et al., 2007). Across meta-analytic and individual studies, then, a substantial amount of empirical support has clearly been demonstrated for the IMB model in the domain of HIV intervention and prevention.

CASE APPLICATION OF THE IMB MODEL

A key factor in sustaining the HIV epidemic is the continued risky sexual behavior of some individuals who are living with HIV. Over 70 percent of HIV+ individuals remain sexually active after learning their HIV status (Crepaz and Marks, 2002), and approximately one-third of all HIV+ individuals continue to engage in unsafe sexual behaviors (Kalichman, 2000), with some reports demonstrating as many as 84 percent of HIV+ individuals engaging in unprotected sex (Halkitis and Parsons, 2003). In many instances, these unprotected acts occur with partners who are HIV-negative or who are of unknown HIV status (van Kesteren, Hospers, and Kok, 2007). Despite the high level of HIV transmission risk behavior in which HIV+ individuals may continue to engage, and despite the fact that the number of people living with HIV is increasing (in part due to reduced AIDS-related mortality resulting from ARV treatment availability [UNAIDS, 2007]), HIV risk-reduction interventions have traditionally been focused on HIV–, not HIV+ persons (Crepaz et al., 2006; Kelly and Kalichman, 2002). Recognizing the need to help support HIV+ individuals practice of safer sex, Fisher and his colleagues (Fisher, Fisher, Cornman, et al., 2006) utilized the IMB model to design, implement, and evaluate the Options intervention; an HIV clinic–based, collaborative, clinician-initiated safer sex intervention aimed at reducing the HIV transmission risk behavior of HIV-infected clinical care patients.

Phase I: Elicitation Research

Following the IMB model approach, the first phase in developing the Options intervention involved conducting open-ended elicitation research with HIV+ patients and with HIV care providers to identify patients' information, motivation, and behavioral skills deficits associated with HIV transmission risk behavior, and to determine the most effective and acceptable manner for integrating the intervention into routine clinical care (Fisher et al., 2004). Elicitation work consisted of patient and health care provider focus groups at the Nathan Smith Clinic at Yale-New Haven Hospital in New Haven, Connecticut. Patient focus groups discussed a wide variety of information, motivation, and behavioral skills barriers associated with risky behavior among people living with HIV. Similarly, focus groups composed of HIV health care providers discussed their own information, motivation, and behavioral skills assets and limitations in providing intervention support for safer sexual behavior for their HIV+ patients, and discussed as well their perceptions of patients' risk behavior and barriers to safer behavior.

Findings from these focus groups indicated that with respect to HIV prevention-related informational deficits, although HIV+ patients were knowledgeable about HIV transmission and prevention, many had difficulty in applying or acting on that knowledge. Furthermore, a number of faulty HIV-related heuristics were reported by patients. For example, one heuristic prevalent among the patients was the belief that having an undetectable viral load indicated that one could not transmit one's HIV to a noninfected individual. Additionally, providers reported that a number of their HIV+ patients believed that having unprotected sex or sharing needles with another HIV+ individual posed little or no risk for either partner. Some HIV+ patients perceived that there was very low or no risk of HIV transmission associated with oral sex, and some believed that it was difficult for an HIV+ woman to transmit her HIV to a noninfected man through unprotected sex. Finally, some participants discussed the use of heuristics or implicit theories when trying to determine a partner's HIV serostatus, indicating that a partner could be perceived as being HIV+ solely based on the venue where the partner was met or on the partner's willingness to have sex without a condom (Fisher et al., 2004).

With respect to motivational factors associated with risky behavior, HIV+ patients and HIV health care providers reported that because of the perceived lack of intimacy associated with using condoms, patients were at times not motivated to use condoms with their long-term or committed relationship partners. This desire for intimacy was shown to extend to casual relationships, with some individuals reporting having engaged in sex without a condom in their search for emotional closeness. In other instances, HIV+ patients reluctantly engaged in sex without condoms, and this may have resulted from a fear of being abused by their partner had they insisted on a condom being used. Additionally, negative attitudes toward condoms were reported as reasons for engaging in unprotected sex.

Finally, barriers to safer sex associated with deficits in behavioral skills were reported by HIV-positive patients and by HIV health care providers. Many patients reported that they lacked the skills to effectively negotiate condom use with their partners, and this finding was mirrored by their health care providers' reports. Patients and providers also indicated that using condoms was particularly difficult for patients when under the influence of alcohol or drugs.

Focus groups also discussed the feasibility of implementing an HIV risk-reduction intervention in the clinical care setting (Fisher et al., 2004). HIV+ patients were open to the idea of discussing risk-reduction strategies with their providers but had concerns about such discussions occurring within the context of a traditional patient-provider interaction that tended to be hierarchical in nature. Some HIV+ patients also had reservations about divulging unsafe sexual and injection drug use practices to their provider. From the providers' perspective, although providers recognized the importance of discussing risk-reduction counseling with their patients, concern was expressed with regard to their self-perceived ability to change their patients' behavior. Additionally, some providers indicated that they would feel uncomfortable discussing sexual and drug use behavior with their patients. Other difficulties associated with implementing a risk-reduction intervention that were reported by providers included cultural barriers, a lack of training to conduct risk-reduction counseling, and a lack of knowledge about sex and drug use. Both HIV+ patients and HIV health care providers were also concerned that there would not be sufficient time to incorporate a risk-reduction intervention into a routine clinical care visit.

Phase II: Intervention

Findings from the elicitation research phase were used to guide the development of an IMB model–based HIV risk-reduction intervention, to be initiated by HIV clinical care providers to support HIV+ patients' practice of safer sexual behavior. The intervention was designed to be delivered in the context of routine HIV clinical care visits and as such to capitalize on the repeated regular contact and often positive relationship existing between clinician and patient.

Based on formative research, it was decided that motivational interviewing techniques (Rollnick, Mason, and Butler, 1999) would be used as a delivery mechanism for the IMB model–based intervention. Motivational interviewing (MI) uses empirically tested counseling techniques for very brief one-on-one interventions and serves as an effective delivery system for clinicians to convey appropriate HIV prevention information, motivation and behavioral skills content to HIV+ patients in support of HIV risk-reduction behavior change. MI was originally created as a method to increase substance abusers' motivation to change their unhealthy behavior and as a means to provide the information, motivation, and skills needed to make such changes (Miller and Rollnick, 1991; Rollnick, Heather, and Bell, 1992). As such, MI strategies are conceptually and operationally ideal for the delivery of IMB model–based content in the clinical care context. Additionally, MI also provides a specific structure for delivering interventions, ensuring the structural uniformity of an intervention across clinicians and patients and relative ease of teaching intervention techniques to providers. MI techniques also place patients and providers on an equal footing during risk-reduction intervention sessions, and this was seen as a significant benefit of using MI, particularly for patients who did not feel comfortable discussing sex- and drug-related behaviors with their providers through interactions that were traditionally hierarchical in nature. Finally, MI techniques also enable clinicians to quickly identify a patient's information, motivation, and behavioral skills barriers to safer behavior, and, through a brief discussion with the patient, to work collaboratively to develop strategies for overcoming such barriers. Therefore, an intervention employing MI techniques was seen as an ideal mechanism that could be used to implement an IMB model–based HIV risk-reduction intervention into the existing ecology of a high-volume inner city HIV clinical care setting.

Through collaborative efforts among behavioral scientists, HIV health care providers, and HIV+ patients, the IMB model–based intervention using MI techniques was developed, piloted, and further refined to create a final version of the Options intervention as a mechanism for providing information, motivation, and behavioral skills inputs to support safer sexual behavior among HIV infected individuals. The Options intervention was designed as a clinician-delivered intervention to be administered through brief, five- to ten-minute clinician-patient interactions occurring during routine clinical care visits.

Each Options intervention session follows a specific protocol in which HIV+ patients and providers engage in a semi-structured conversation regarding HIV risk. A flowchart outlining the general Options intervention protocol can be found in Figure 2.3.

As seen in the figure, Step 1 of the intervention involves the clinician asking the patient in an open, nonconfrontational manner for permission to discuss HIV risk behavior. For example, the provider could say:

"I now talk with all of my patients about their sexual behavior. I know that it can be uncomfortable to talk about sex, but I think it's important to do so because of how it can affect your health and the health of others. So I would like to spend a few minutes talking about this. Is that okay with you?"

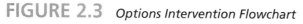

FIGURE 2.3   *Options Intervention Flowchart*

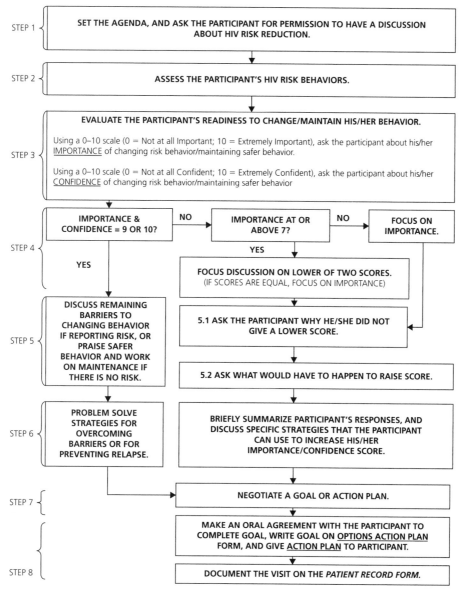

Through this introduction, participants experience a sense of control over what was happening and believe that their wishes are being respected, minimizing their defensiveness and increasing the likelihood for subsequent cooperation for behavior change.

Step 2 of the Options intervention involves an assessment of the participant's risk behavior. Here, participants are made to feel comfortable disclosing risky behavior with their clinician. Clinicians therefore set the stage by first telling the participant that many patients have a difficult time always practicing safer behavior, and that it would not be surprising if the participant also had a difficult time staying safe. The goal of this exercise is to obtain a general assessment of the nature of risk behavior in which the participant is engaging.

Step 3 focuses on identifying participants' readiness to change their HIV risk behavior. On a 0–10 scale, participants are asked how *important* it would be for them to change from risky to safer behavior. Similarly, participants are also asked to indicate on a scale of 0–10 how *confident* they are that they could change their risky behavior (participants who are not engaging in risk behavior are asked how important it is for them to maintain safer behavior and how confident they are that they can do so). Whereas low importance ratings are generally indicative of deficits in information (for example, believing that having an undetectable viral load means that one cannot transmit HIV) and motivation (for example, possessing negative attitudes toward condoms), low confidence ratings are generally indicative of deficits in behavioral skills (for example, low self-efficacy with respect to negotiating condom use with one's partner). Based on the participant's responses to these questions, clinicians use algorithm-based decision rules (see Figure 2.3) to determine whether importance or confidence becomes an initial focus during the Options intervention session (Step 4).

Focusing initially on either importance or confidence, the clinician first asks the participant why he or she did not give a *lower* score on the importance/confidence scale (Step 5). By asking the participant why a *lower* score was not given, participants are tasked with presenting self-motivating reasons supporting a change toward safer behavior. After participants verbally express their supporting reasons for safer behavior, clinicians ask participants to indicate what it would take for their importance/confidence score to increase. Here, it is the participant, who is truly the foremost expert on his or her own behavior and situation, that is tasked with coming up with his or her own set of risk-reduction strategies.

In Step 6, the clinician briefly summarizes the participant's responses and discusses the risk-reduction strategies that the participant had proposed. If a participant is unable to come up with any of his or her own strategies, the clinician presents a number of different risk-reduction strategies tailored to the specific IMB barriers to safer behavior that the participant has reported experiencing. Subsequently, the clinician and participant negotiate a goal and decide on an action plan for the participant to enact before his or her next clinic visit (Step 7). Finally, in Step 8, an oral agreement is made between the clinician and patient, and the participant is given a "Prevention Prescription" which not only serves as a written reminder of the goal that was set, but also serves as a type of contract clearly stating the participant's commitment to complete the goal.

Phase III: Evaluation

The efficacy of the Options intervention (Fisher, Fisher, Cornman, et al., 2006) was assessed through an eighteen-month clinical trial that was conducted at two of the largest HIV care clinics in Connecticut. One clinic was randomly assigned to receive the intervention and the other to serve as the standard-of-care control. At the intervention clinic, prior to initiating the intervention trial, HIV clinical care providers received extensive intervention-related training. This involved (1) a four-hour didactic and interactive session that focused on the IMB model–based Options intervention protocol and MI techniques; (2) a two-hour workshop that focused on risky sexual and drug use behaviors, along with risk-reduction strategies; and (3) a one-hour session in which clinicians practiced the Options intervention protocol through role plays (Fisher et al., 2004). All participating clinicians at the intervention site were required to meet intervention-related performance requirements to ensure that the intervention would be delivered consistently and with sufficient fidelity.

During the eighteen-month trial at the intervention clinic, the Options intervention was built into participants' routine clinical care visits with their HIV care clinician. Specifically, HIV care clinicians spent approximately five to ten minutes of each clinical care visit going through the Options intervention protocol with each of their HIV+ participants, assessing HIV+ participants' risk behavior, determining participants' importance and confidence with respect to enacting safer behavior, developing risk-reduction strategies, and setting risk-reduction goals. During all follow-up visits, clinicians also discussed the goals that participants had set in their previous sessions and, if there were reported difficulties in achieving these goals, possible barriers to goal completion and how they might be addressed were also discussed. At the standard-of-care control clinic, HIV+ participants continued to meet with clinicians for regularly scheduled routine care visits, but visits did not involve structured, theory-based discussions on HIV risk reduction. Risk-reduction discussions taking place during these visits occurred only on an ad-hoc basis. As part of the eighteen-month clinical trial, at both the intervention clinic and the standard-of-care control clinic, HIV+ participants completed measures at baseline, six months, twelve months, and eighteen months that assessed their risky and safer behavior along with their levels of HIV risk reduction–related information, motivation, and behavioral skills.

Results from the clinical trial provided support for the effectiveness of the Options intervention (Fisher, Fisher, Cornman, et al., 2006). Overall, the intervention was well accepted and was delivered with fidelity (Fisher et al., 2004). The vast majority (73 percent) of the 1,455 possible intervention medical visits over the course of the eighteen-month study period included the Options intervention, and HIV+ participants responded quite positively to it, rating their clinicians as very helpful ($M=9.08$ on a 10-point scale) and very understanding ($M=9.30$ on a 10 point scale) (Fisher et al., 2004).

Importantly, the Options intervention was shown to have a significant impact on HIV risk behavior. Whereas HIV+ participants who received the Options intervention showed a significant decrease in unprotected vaginal, anal, or insertive oral sex events over time, HIV+ participants in the standard-of-care control condition showed a significant increase in these behaviors over time, reflecting a behavioral pattern of safer sex fatigue. Similarly, when focusing only on unprotected vaginal or anal sex events, HIV+

participants receiving the Options intervention showed a marginally significant decrease in these events, while control condition participants showed a significant increase.

Overall, results from this clinical trial demonstrate that a brief, clinician-delivered IMB model–based intervention presented during routine clinical care can effectively and efficiently reduce risk behavior among individuals living with HIV. Furthermore, this test of the Options intervention not only demonstrates a high level of acceptability to HIV+ patients and their clinicians, but also suggests that the intervention can be feasibly integrated into the existing ecology of a busy, and at times overburdened, HIV clinical care setting.

FUTURE DIRECTIONS: THE IMB MODEL AS A GENERAL HEALTH BEHAVIOR CHANGE CONCEPTUALIZATION

Beyond its established strength in predicting, understanding, and intervening to change HIV risk behavior, the IMB model is viewed as a generalizable approach to understanding and promoting heath behavior more broadly defined (Fisher and Fisher, 1999; Fisher, Fisher, and Harman, 2003). A review of correlational research literature concerning psychological factors linked to performance of diverse health behaviors demonstrated that information, motivation, and behavioral skills elements are consistently related with health behavior performance across diverse areas including exercise behavior, smoking cessation, breast and cardiovascular health, and other domains. In effect, correlational evidence supports the IMB model's assertion that the three factors in the model are critical determinants of health behavior outside the domain of HIV prevention (for further details, see Fisher, Fisher, and Harman, 2003). Similarly, a review of experimental intervention research across the same health domains demonstrated that interventions that contain information, motivation, and behavioral skills elements were more effective in promoting health behavior change than interventions that lacked one or more of these elements. Further, when comparing the intensity of the information, motivation, and behavioral skills content of interventions that had strong behavior change effects, versus those with weak effects, it appears that the former have greater information, motivation, and behavioral skills–related content than the latter (for further details, see Fisher, Fisher, and Harman, 2003). Overall, these findings provide support for IMB model elements as determinants of health behavior change intervention efficacy across health behavior change domains.

TESTS OF THE IMB MODEL IN OTHER HEALTH DOMAINS

Breast Self-Examination (BSE)

Although BSE was regarded as effective in the early detection and subsequent cure of breast cancer, it was practiced by relatively few women (W. Fisher, Dervatis, Bryan, Silcox, and Kohn, 2000; Misovich, Martinez, Fisher, and Bryan, 2003). (Note that in the past few years, there has been some controversy over the relative role and importance of BSE in cancer detection; see, for example, Hackshaw and Paul, 2003.)

During the time when BSE was more clearly viewed as advantageous, Misovich et al. (2003) conducted a research study in which women in workplace settings were recruited to complete questionnaires measuring levels of BSE-relevant information, motivation, behavioral skills, and behavior. In addition to identifying critical deficits in BSE-relevant information, motivation, behavioral skills and behavior among women in the sample (see Misovich et al., 2003 for specifics), the investigators tested the hypothesized interrelations among the IMB model constructs (depicted in Figure 2.4 for the context of BSE) using structural equation modeling procedures.

Results showed that each of the relationships specified by the IMB model was confirmed, and that the model provided an acceptable fit to the data (CFI = 96, RMSEA = 07). As can be seen in Figure 2.4, BSE information and motivation are statistically independent constructs; each is significantly linked with BSE behavioral skills; and behavioral skills are significantly associated with performance of BSE-related behaviors, all as specified by the IMB model. In addition, and also predicted by the model, there is an independent link between BSE motivation and BSE-related behavioral performance. The three components of the IMB model account for 70 percent of the variance in BSE-related behaviors, which is regarded as a large effect size for a prediction model in the behavioral sciences (Cohen, 1988).

Motorcycle Safety

Murray (2000) conducted an IMB model test to assess the psychological determinants of another preventive health behavior—motorcycle safety gear utilization. Motorcycle accidents and associated injury and death are very common occurrences (U.S. Department of Transportation, 2005). Although motorcycle safety gear use has been demonstrated

FIGURE 2.4 *Empirical Test of the Information-Motivation-Behavioral Skills Model of the Determinants of Breast Self-Examination Behavior*

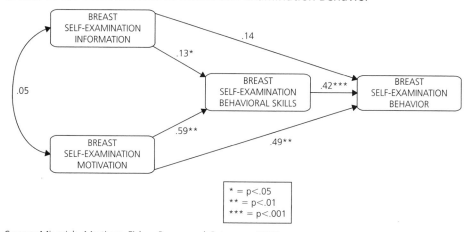

Source: Misovich, Martinez, Fisher, Bryan, and Catapano, 2001

to save hundreds of lives annually (U.S. Department of Transportation, 2005), such equipment is used inconsistently by motorcycle riders at risk. In her investigation, Murray first created elicitation research–based sets of information, motivation, behavioral skills, and behavior items relating to motorcycle safety gear use. Data collection for the research to test the IMB model in the context of motorcycle safety then took place with "in person" samples of motorcycle riders recruited at a "Super Sunday" biker event, at motorcycle shops, and via flyers posted on a university campus (N = 180). An additional sample (N = 701) was recruited through Internet motorcycle-related Web sites and Web-based mailing lists, and questionnaires which were completed on the Internet were returned via email.

Findings from this cross-sectional study revealed that motorcycle riders had significant information, motivation, behavioral skills, and behavior deficits with respect to motorcycle safety gear use (for specific findings see Murray, 2000). With respect to behavior, for example, motorcycle helmets, which are particularly critical for saving lives, were reportedly used only 58 percent of the time. Concerning the IMB model, results of structural equation modeling analyses again showed that the relationships specified by the IMB approach were confirmed, and that the model provided an acceptable fit to the data (CFI = 97, RMSEA = 07). As can be seen in Figure 2.5, information and motivation concerning motorcycle safety gear use were statistically related constructs (note that while the IMB model suggests that information and motivation are often independent constructs, because well-informed persons are not necessarily well motivated to practice health behaviors, the model does not require the statistical independence of the information and motivation constructs).

FIGURE 2.5 *Empirical Test of the Information-Motivation-Behavioral Skills Model of the Determinants of Complex Motorcycle Safety Gear Utilization*

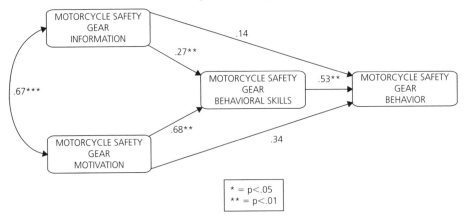

Source: Murray, 2000.

Further, and as predicted by the IMB model, for complex tasks (that is, wearing helmets, jackets, and pants, which can be challenging to put on because they involve snaps, velcro, zippers, and so on and more important, which can impair one's sense of control and mobility while riding), both information and motivation were linked to behavioral skills for motorcycle safety gear use. In addition, behavioral skills were significantly associated with reported complex motorcycle safety gear use behavior as such. Thus, the IMB model was supported in the context of a complex preventive health behavior performance—motorcycle safety gear utilization.

Adherence to antiretroviral medications

Understanding and promoting adherence to antiretroviral medications (ARVs) in HIV+ individuals is of enormous individual and public health significance. On the one hand, ARVs have proven dramatically effective in reducing the viral load and associated morbidity of persons living with HIV, and have contributed directly to dramatic declines in HIV-related mortality (Greenberg et al., 1999; Montaner et al., 1998). On the other hand, adherence to ARVs must be highly consistent, generally in the range of 90–95 percent (Bartlett, 2002; Patterson et al., 2000); but among individuals on ARVs, adherence to ARV regimens, which may be complicated and side-effect laden, is generally much lower (Bangsberg and Deeks, 2002). When ARV adherence is suboptimal, treatment failure, viral mutation, and development of multidrug-resistant HIV can take place (for example, Bangsberg et al., 2006; Hogg, Yip, Chan, O'Shaughnessy, and Montaner, 2000; Ickovics and Chesney, 1997; Knobel et al, 2002; Spire et al., 2002; Walsh et al., 2001). HIV+ individuals who are inconsistently adherent are therefore at significant personal health risk, and may pose a substantial public health challenge involving the development and transmission of multidrug-resistant HIV to others as well (Hecht et al., 1998).

From the perspective of the IMB model, adherence to medical regimen shares much in common with other critical health behaviors (Fisher, Fisher, and Harman, 2003; Fisher, Fisher, Amico, et al., 2006). Therefore, ARV adherence is conceptualized to occur as a function of the presence of a specific set of relevant information, motivation, and behavioral skills factors. All else being equal, to the extent that an HIV+ individual is well informed about ARVs, motivated to act, and possesses the requisite behavioral skills to act effectively, he or she will be likely to adhere to ARV regimens, and to reap substantial health benefits. To the extent that an HIV+ individual is poorly informed, unmotivated to act, and lacks the requisite behavioral skills for effective adherence, the individual will be nonadherent to ARVs and will fail to realize their health benefits. An IMB model–based conceptualization of ARV adherence is presented in Figure 2.6. It describes specific information, motivation, behavioral skills, and adherence behavior parameters, and the relationships among them, as well as a set of moderating and feedback factors regarded as relevant in the context of ARV adherence.

According to the IMB model articulated to adherence, *information* that is directly relevant to antiretroviral therapy is an initial prerequisite for ARV adherence. *Motivation* and *behavioral skills* are also critical for adherence (see Figure 2.6 for the

FIGURE 2.6 *An Information-Motivation-Behavioral Skills Model Analysis of Adherence to Antiretroviral Medication*

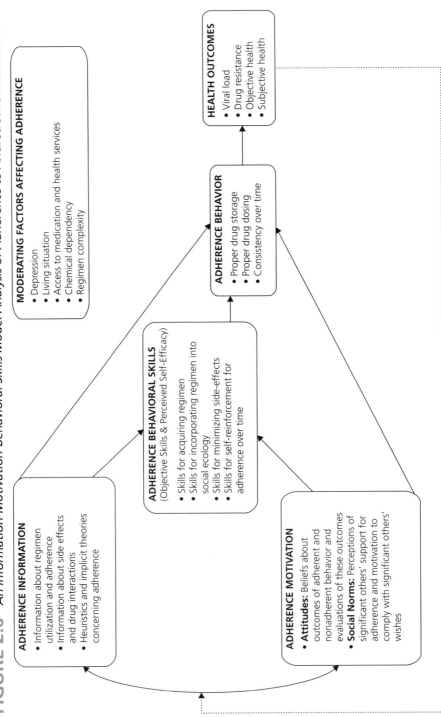

Source: J. Fisher, Fisher, Amico, and Harman, 2006)

specific types of information, motivation, and behavioral skills that may be most essential). Consistent with other health behaviors, the IMB model of adherence specifies that adherence information and motivation are often statistically independent factors that work primarily through behavioral skills to affect adherence behavior *per se* (Figure 2.6). Adherence information and motivation may also have direct effects on adherence behavior, in situations in which novel or complicated behavioral skills may not be required for ARV adherence. The IMB approach described in Figure 2.6 involves some critical additional elements including moderating factors and feedback loops (see Fisher, Fisher, Amico, et al., 2006, and Fisher, Fisher, and Harman, 2003, for details), suggesting that factors such as homelessness, and increased or decreased subjective and objective health resulting from adherence or nonadherence, may, for example, lead to changes in one's motivation to adhere (in the case of subjective health) or in one's ability to mobilize information, motivation, and behavioral skills in the service of adherence (in the case of homelessness).

The IMB model of ARV adherence has been supported in a number of investigations. Starace et al. (2006), for example, conducted a test of the model that was based on measures of ARV-related information, motivation, and behavioral skills completed by a sample of 100 HIV clinical care patients in Italy. As can be seen in Figure 2.7, the results show that both adherence-related information and adherence-related motivation are significantly associated with adherence-related behavioral skills. Additionally, adherence-related behavioral skills were shown to be significantly associated with adherence behavior. The model demonstrates good fit (CFI = .996, RMSEA = .028), accounting for approximately 52 percent of the variability in adherence. Similar tests of the IMB model of ARV adherence have demonstrated comparable patterns of results in other populations, including women living with HIV (Kalichman et al., 2001), HIV+ patients in clinical care in Puerto Rico (Amico et al., 2005), and HIV+ patients in clinical care

FIGURE 2.7   *Empirical Test of the Information-Motivation-Behavioral Skills Model ARV Adherence (Restricted [Mediated] Model)*

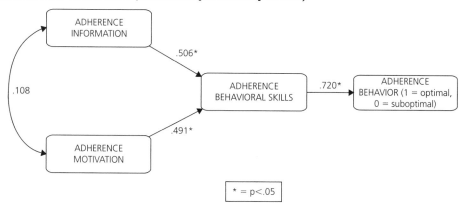

Source: Starace et al., 2006.

in the Deep South (Amico et al., 2009). Overall, this research provides supportive evidence for IMB model constructs as they relate to adherence behavior.

CRITIQUE OF THE IMB MODEL

Empirical tests of the IMB model have suggested criticisms of the IMB approach to understanding and promoting health behavior change which need to be addressed in future conceptual and empirical work. On a conceptual level, our review raises questions about the role of the IMB model's information construct, which across studies continues to be a relatively inconsistent contributor to the prediction of preventive behavior. Although the IMB model has specified situations in which information is expected to be a substantial contributor to health behavior (for example, early in epidemics such as the HIV epidemic) and when it will not (for example, later on in epidemics, J. Fisher and Fisher, 1992, 2000), further empirical study of the IMB model's conceptualization of the role of information is necessary. Most but not all extant tests of the IMB model have taken place with samples that may be assumed to have above-threshold levels of information and which may have blunted the contribution of this construct in research tests. Our review also raises questions concerning the relationship of the information and motivation constructs, which are sometimes independent and sometimes not. The model's logic—which holds that well-informed people are not necessarily well motivated to practice prevention, and vice versa (J. Fisher and Fisher, 1992, 2000)—permits the possibility of a relationship between informational and motivational factors, but it would appear to be important to establish conceptually when such a relationship may or may not be anticipated by the theory. Other questions remaining for future conceptual and empirical consideration involve specification of when—in terms of populations at risk and preventive behaviors of interest—specific model constructs concerning information, motivation, and behavioral skills may prove to be most important.

SUMMARY

The IMB model's assumptions concerning the determinants of HIV prevention and other health behaviors have been consistently confirmed in multivariate correlational research and in experimental intervention research conducted across a diversity of populations and behaviors, and its constructs account for a substantial proportion of the variance in HIV prevention and other health behaviors. The IMB model's approach to HIV risk and other health behavior change has been supported as well in elicitation, experimental intervention, and outcome evaluation research which have established the model's ability to promote sustained risk-reduction behavior change across diverse populations. Results of this research are consistent with the IMB model's focus on identifying and addressing weaknesses in HIV and health-relevant information, motivation, and behavioral skills as an effective means for promoting health behavior change. Overall, the IMB model provides a comprehensive conceptual approach to understanding the determi-nants of HIV prevention and other health behaviors, and may constitute a general-izable methodology for intervening to promote such behavior.

REFERENCES

Ajzen, I. (1985). From intentions to actions: A theory of planned behavior. In J. Kuhi and J. Beckmann (Eds.), *Action-control: From cognition to behavior* (pp. 11–39). Heildelberg, Germany: Springer.

Ajzen, I., and Fishbein, M. (1980). *Understanding attitudes and predicting social behavior.* New Jersey: Prentice Hall.

Albarracín, D., Durantini, M. R., and Earl, A. (2006). Empirical and theoretical conclusions of an analysis of outcomes of HIV-prevention interventions. *Current Directions in Psychological Science, 15,* 73–78.

Albarracín, D., Gillette, J. C., Earl, A. N., Glasman, L. R., Durantini, M. R., and Ho, M. (2005). A test of the major assumptions about behavior change: A comprehensive look at the effects of passive and active HIV-prevention interventions since the beginning of the epidemic. *Psychological Bulletin, 131,* 856–897.

Amico, K. R., Barta, W., Konkle-Parker, D. J., Fisher, J. D., Cornman, D. H., Shuper, P. A., et al. (2009). The information-motivation-behavioral skills model of ART adherence in a Deep South HIV+ clinic sample. *AIDS and Behavior, 13,* 66–75.

Amico, K. R., Toro-Alfonso, J., and Fisher, J. D. (2005). An empirical test of the information, motivation, and behavioral skills model of antiretroviral therapy adherence. *AIDS Care, 17,* 661–673.

Anderson, E. S., Wagstaff, D. A., Heckman, T. G., Winett, R. A., Roffman, R. A., Solomon, L. J., et al. (2006). Information-motivation-behavioral skills (IMB) model: Testing direct and mediated treatment effects on con-dom use among women in low-income housing. *Annals of Behavioral Medicine, 31,* 70–79.

Arnowitz, T., and Munzert, T. (2006). An expansion and modification of the information, motivation, and behav-ioral skills model: Implications from a study with African American girls and their mothers. *Issues in Comprehensive Pediatric Nursing, 29,* 89–101.

Arnowitz, T., Rennells, R. E., and Todd, E. (2005). Heterosocial behaviors in early adolescent African American girls: The role of mother-daughter relationships. *Journal of Family Nursing, 11,* 122–139.

Auerbach, J. A., and Coates, T. J. (2000). HIV prevention research: Accomplishments and challenges for the third decade of AIDS. *American Journal of Public Health, 90,* 1029–1032.

Avants, S. K., Margolin, A., Usubiaga, M. H., and Doebrick, C. (2004). Targeting HIV-related outcomes with intraveneous drug users maintained on methadone: A randomized clinical trial of a harm reduction group ther-apy. *Journal of Substance Abuse Treatment, 26,* 67–78.

Avants, S. K., Warburton, L. A., Hawkins, K. A., and Margolin, A. (2000). Continuation of high-risk behavior by HIV-positive drug users. Treatment implications. *Journal of Substance Abuse Treatment, 19,* 15–22.

Bandura, A. (1989). Perceived self-efficacy in the exercise of control over AIDS infection. In V. M. Mays and G. W. Albee and S. M. Schneider (eds.), *Primary Prevention of AIDS* (pp. 128–141). Newbury Park, CA: Sage.

Bandura, A. (1992). Social-cognitive approach of thought to the exercise of control over AIDS infection. In J. R. DiClemente (Ed.), *Adolescents and AIDS: A generation in jeopardy.* Newbury Park, CA: Sage.

Bandura, A. (1994). Social cognitive theory and exercise control of HIV infection. In R. J. DiClemente and J. L. Peterson (eds.), *Preventing AIDS: Theories and methods of behavioral interventions.* (pp. 25–59). New York: Plenum.

Note: Work on this chapter was supported by grants from the National Institutes of Health (1 R01 MH066684; R01 MH077524–01)

Bangsberg, D. R., Acosta, E. P., Gupta, R., Guzman, D., Riley, E. D., Harrogan, P. R., et al. (2006). Adherence-resistance relationships for protease and non-nucleoside reverse transcriptase inhibitors explained by virological fitness. *AIDS*, *20*, 223–231.

Bangsberg, D. R., and Deeks, S. G. (2002). Is average adherence to HIV antiretroviral therapy enough? *Journal of General Internal Medicine*, *17*, 812–813.

Barak, A., and Fisher, W. A. (2003). Experience with an internet-based theoretically grounded educational resource for promotion of sexual and reproductive health. *Sexual and Relationship Therapy*, *18*, 293–308.

Bartlett, J. A. (2002). Addressing the challenges of adherence. *Journal of Acquired Immune Deficiency Syndromes*, *29*, S2–S10.

Bazargan, M., and West, K. (2006). Correlates of the intention to remain sexually inactive among underserved Hispanic and African American high school students. *Journal of School Health*, *76*, 25–32.

Belcher, L., Kalichman, S., Topping, M., Smith, S., Emshoff, J., Norris, F., et al., (1998). A randomized trial of a brief HIV risk reduction counseling intervention for women. *Journal of Consulting and Clinical Psychology*, *66*, 856–861.

Boyer, C. B., Shafer, M. B., Shaffer, R. A., Brodine, S. K., Ito, S. I., Ynigues, D. L., et al. (2001). Prevention of sexually transmitted diseases and HIV in young military men: Evaluation of a cognitive-behavioral skills-building intervention. *Sexually Transmitted Diseases*, *28*, 349–355.

Boyer, C. B., Shafer, M., Shaffer, R. A., Brodine, S. K., Pollack, L. M., Betsinger, K., et al. (2005). Evaluation of a cognitive-behavioral, group, randomized controlled intervention trial to prevent sexually transmitted infections and unintended pregnancies in young women. *Preventive Medicine*, *40*, 420–431.

Brunswick, A. F., and Banaszak-Hol, J. (1996). HIV risk behavior and the health belief model: An empirical test in an African American community sample. *Journal of Community Psychology*, *24*, 44–65.

Bryan, A. D., Fisher, J. D., and Benziger, T. J. (2000). HIV prevention information, motivation, behavioral skills among Indian truck drivers in Chennai, India. *AIDS*, *14*, 756–758.

Bryan, A. D., Fisher, J. D., and Benziger, T. J. (2001). Determinants of HIV risks among Indian truck drivers: An information, motivation, behavioral skills approach. *Social Science and Medicine*, *53*, 1413–1426.

Bryan, A. D., Fisher, J. D., Fisher, W. A., and Murray, D. M. (2000). Understanding condom use among heroin addicts in methadone maintenance using the information, motivation, behavioral skills model. *Substance Use and Misuse*, *35*, 451–471.

Byrne, D. (1977). Social psychology and the study of sexual behavior. *Personality and Social Psychology Bulletin*, *3*, 3–30.

Byrne, D., Kelley, K., and Fisher, W. A. (1993). Unwanted teenage pregnancies: Incidence, interpretation, intervention. *Applied Preventive Psychology*, *2*, 101–113.

Carey, M. P., Braaten, L. S., Maisto, S. A., Gleason, J. R., Forsyth, A. D., Durant, L. E., et al. (2000). Using information, motivational enhancement, and skills training to reduce the risk of HIV infection for low-income urban women: A second randomized clinical trial. *Health Psychology*, *19*, 3–11.

Carey, M. P., Carey, K. B., and Kalichman, S. C. (1997). Risk for human immunodeficiency virus (HIV) infection among persons with severe mental illnesses. *Clinical Psychological Review*, *17*, 271–291.

Carey, M. P., Carey, K. B., and Weinhardt, L. S. (1997). Behavioral risk for HIV infection among adults with a severe and persistent mental illness: Patterns and psychological antecedents. *Journal of Community Mental Health*, *33*, 133–142.

Carey, M. P., Maisto, S. A., Kalichman, S. C., Forsyth, A.D., Wright, E.M., and Johnson, B.T. (1997). Enhancing motivation to reduce the risk of HIV infection for economically disadvantaged urban women. *Journal of Consulting Clinical Psychology*, *65*, 531–541.

Catania, J. A., Gibson, D. R., Chitwood, D. D., et al. (1990). Methodological problems in AIDS behavioral research: Influences on measurement error and participation bias in studies of sexual behavior. *Psychological Bulletin*, *108*, 339–362.

CDC (2007). *HIV/AIDS surveillance report, 2005*, Vol. 17 (Revised Edition). Atlanta, GA: U.S. Department of Health and Human Services, Centers for Disease Control and Prevention.

Coates, T. J. (1990). Strategies for modifying sexual behavior patterns for primary and secondary prevention of HIV disease. *Journal of Consulting and Clinical Psychology*, *58*, 57–69.

Cohen, J. (1988). *Statistical power analysis for the behavioral sciences* (2nd ed). Hillsdale, NJ: Erlbaum.

Cohen, E. S. (2000). *High-risk sexual behavior in the context of alcohol use: An intervention for college students*. Unpublished doctoral dissertation, University of Texas at Austin.

Collins, C., Harshbarger, C., and Sawyer, R. (2006). The diffusion of effective behavioral interventions project. Development, implementation, and lessons learned. *AIDS Education and Prevention*, *18*, 5–20.

Connecticut Department of Public Health. (1997). *Program goals: AIDS prevention education services*. Hartford, CT.

Copenhaver, M. M., Johnson, B. T., Lee, I., Harman, J. J., and Carey, M. P. (2006). Behavioral HIV risk reduction among people who inject drugs: Meta-analytic evidence of efficacy. *Journal of Substance Abuse Treatment*, *31*, 163–171.

Cornman, D. H., Kiene, S. M., Fisher, W. A., Shuper, P. A., Pillay, S., Friedland, G. H., et al. (2008). Clinic-based intervention reduces unprotected sexual behavior among HIV-infected patients in KwaZulu-Natal, South Africa: Results of a pilot study. *Journal of Acquired Immune Deficiency Syndromes*, *48*, 553–560.

Cornman, D. H., Schmiege, S. J., Bryan, A., Benziger, T. J., and Fisher, J. D. (2007). An information-motivation-behavioral skills (IMB) model-based HIV prevention intervention for truck drivers in India. *Social Science and Medicine*, *64*, 1572–1584.

Cournos, F., and McKinnon, K. (1997). HIV seroprevalence among people with severe mental illness in the Unites States: A critical review. *Clinical Psychology Review*, *17*, 259–269.

Crepaz, N., Horn, A. K., Rama, S. M., Griffin, T., DeLuca, J. B., Mullins, M. M., et al. (2007). The efficacy of behavioral interventions in reducing HIV risk sex behaviors and incident sexually transmitted disease in Black and Hispanic sexually transmitted disease clinic patients in the United States: A meta-analytic review. *Sexually Transmitted Diseases*, *34*, 319–332.

Crepaz, N., Lyles, C. M., Wolitski, R. J., Passin W. F., Rama, S. M., Herbst, J. H., et al. (2006). Do prevention interventions reduce HIV risk behaviours among people living with HIV? A meta-analytic review of controlled trials. *AIDS*, *20*, 143–157.

Crepaz, N., and Marks, G. (2002). Towards an understanding of sexual risk behavior in people living with HIV: A review of social, psychological, and medical findings. *AIDS*, *16*, 135–149.

deWit, J. B., Stroebe, W., DeVroome, E.M.M., Sandfort, T.G.M., and van Griensven, G.J.P. (2000). Understanding AIDS preventive behavior with casual and primary partners in homosexual men: The theory of planned behavior and the information-motivation-behavioral-skills model. *Psychology and Health*, *15*, 325–340.

deWit, J. B. (1996). The epidemic of HIV among young homosexual men. *AIDS*, *10*, 21–25.

Exner, T. M., Seal, D. W., and Ehrhardt, A. A. (1997). A review of HIV interventions for at-risk women. *AIDS and Behavior*, *1*, 93–124.

Fenton, K. A., and Valdiserri, R. O. (2006). Twenty-five years of HIV/AIDS—United States, 1981–2006. *Morbidity and Mortality Report Weekly*, *55*, 585–589.

Fishbein, M., and Ajzen, I. (1975). *Belief, attitude, intention and behavior: An introduction to theory and research*. Reading, MA: Addison-Wesley.

Fishbein, M., and Middlestadt, S. E. (1989). Using the theory of reasoned action as a framework for understanding and changing AIDS-related behaviors. In V. M. Mays and G. W. Albee and S. M. Schneider (eds.), *Primary prevention of psychopathology* (pp. 93–110). Newbury Park, CA: Sage.

Fishbein, M., Middlestadt, S. E., and Hitchcock, P. J. (1994). Using information to change sexually transmitted disease-related behaviors. In R. J. DiClemente and J. L. Peterson (eds.), *Preventing AIDS: Theories and methods of behavioral interventions*. (pp. 61–78). New York: Plenum.

Fisher, J. D. (1988). Possible effects of reference group-based social influence on AIDS-risk behavior and AIDS-prevention [Special issue on AIDS]. *American Psychologist, 43*, 914–920.

Fisher, J. D. (2000). The IMB model of adherence. Invited presentation at the 1st International Workshop on the Information-Motivation-Behavioral Skills Model, Hotel Continental, Naples, Italy, June 1–2, 2000.

Fisher, J. D. (2001). Physician-Delivered Interventions: The Options Project. Presented at the HIV Prevention in Treatment Settings: U.S. and International Priorities conference, sponsored by the Center for Mental Health Research on AIDS, and NIMH, Washington, D.C., August 3, 2001.

Fisher, J. D., Cornman, D. H., Norton, W. E., and Fisher. W. A. (2006). Involving behavioral scientists, health care providers, and HIV-infected patients as collaborators in theory-based HIV prevention and antiretroviral adherence interventions. *Journal of Acquired Immune Deficiency Syndromes*, *43*, S10–S17.

Fisher, J. D., Cornman, D. H., Osborn, C. Y., Amico, K. R., Fisher, W. A., and Friedland, G. H. (2004). Clinician-initiated HIV-risk reduction intervention for HIV+ persons: Formative research, acceptability, and fidelity of the Options project. *Journal of Acquired Immune Deficiency Syndromes*, *37*, S78–S87.

Fisher, J. D., and Fisher, W. A. (1992). Changing AIDS risk behavior. *Psychological Bulletin*, *111*, 455–474.

Fisher, J. D., and Fisher, W. A. (1996). The information-motivation-behavioral skills model of AIDS risk behavior change: Empirical support and application. In S. Oskamp and S. Thompson (eds.), *Understanding and preventing HIV risk behavior: Safer sex and drug use* (pp. 100–127). Thousand Oaks, CA: Sage.

Fisher, J. D., and Fisher, W. A. (2000). Theoretical approaches to individual-level change. In Peterson, J. and DiClemente, R. (eds.), *HIV Prevention Handbook*. (pp. 3–55). New York: Kluwer Academic/Plenum Press.

Fisher, J. D., Fisher, W. A., and Amico, R. (2001). An information-motivation-behavior skills model of adherence to highly active antiretroviral therapy. Paper presented at AIDS Impact: Biopsychosocial Aspects of HIV Infection, Fifth International Conference, Brighton, UK, July 8–11, 2001.

Fisher, J. D., Fisher, W. A., Amico, K. R., and Harman, J. J. (2006). An information-motivation-behavioral skills model of adherence to antiretroviral therapy. *Health Psychology*, *25*, 462–473.

Fisher, J.D., Fisher, W.A., Bryan, A.D., Misovich, S.J. (2002). Information-motivation-behavioral skills model-based HIV risk behavior change intervention for inner-city high school youth. *Health Psychology*, *21*, 177–186.

Fisher, J. D., Fisher, W. A., Cornman, D. H., Amico, K. R., Bryan, A., and Friedland, G. H. (2006). Clinician-delivered intervention during routine clinical care reduces unprotected sexual behavior among HIV-infected patients. *Journal of Acquired Immune Deficiency Syndromes*, *41*, 44–52.

Fisher, J. D., Fisher, W. A., Misovich, S. J., Kimble, D. L., and Malloy, T. E. (1996). Changing AIDS risk behavior: Effects of an intervention emphasizing AIDS risk reduction information, motivation, and behavioral skills in a college student population. *Health Psychology*, *15*, 114–123.

Fisher, J. D., Fisher, W. A., Williams, S. S., and Malloy, T. E. (1994). Empirical tests of an information-motivation-behavioral skills model of AIDS preventive behavior in gay men and heterosexual university students. *Health Psychology*, *13*(3), 238–250.

Fisher, J. D., Kimble, D. L., Misovich, S. J., and Weinstein, B. (1998). Dynamic of sexual risk behavior in HIV-infected men who have sex with men. *AIDS and Behavior*, *2*, 101–113.

Fisher, J. D. and Misovich, S. (1990). Evolution of College Students' AIDS-Related Behavioral Responses, Attitudes, Knowledge, and Fear. *AIDS Education and Prevention*, *2*, 322–337.

Fisher, J. D., Silver, R., Chinksy, J., Goff, B., Klar, Y. and Zagieboylo, C. (1989). Psychological effects of participation in a large group awareness training. *Journal of Consulting and Clinical Psychology*, *57*, 747–755.

Fisher, W. A. (1986). A psychological approach to human sexuality: The sexual behavior sequence. In D. Byrne and K. Kelley (eds.), *Approaches to Human Sexuality*. Hillsdale, NJ: Erlbaum.

Fisher, W. A. (1990). Understanding and preventing adolescent pregnancy and sexually transmissible disease/ AIDS. In J. Edwards and R. S. Tindale and L. Health and E. J. Posavac (eds.), *Social influence processes and prevention* (pp. 71–101). New York: Plenum Press.

Fisher, W. A. (1997). A theory-based framework for intervention and evaluation in STD/HIV prevention. *Canadian Journal of Human Sexuality*, *6*, 105–111.

Fisher, W. A., Byrne, D., Kelley, K., and White, L. A. (1988). Erotophobia—erotophilia as a dimension of personality. *Journal of Sex Research*, *25*, 123–151.

Fisher, W. A., Byrne, D., and White, L. A. (1983). Emotional barriers to contraception. In D. Byrne and W. A. Fisher (eds.), *Adolescents, sex, and contraception*. Hillsdale, NJ: Erlbaum.

Fisher, W. A., Dervatis, K. A., Bryan, A. D., Silcox, J., and Kohn, H. (2000). Sexual health, reproductive health, sexual coercion, and partner abuse indicators in a Canadian obstetrics and gynaecology outpatient population. *Journal of the Society of Obstetricians and Gynaecologists of Canada, 22,* 714–724.

Fisher, W. A., and Fisher, J. D. (1993). A general social psychological model for changing AIDS risk behavior. In L. Pryor and G. Reeder (eds.), *The social psychology of HIV infection* (pp. 127–153). Hillsdale, NJ: Erlbaum.

Fisher, W. A., and Fisher, J. D. (1999) Understanding and promoting sexual and reproductive health behavior: Theory and method. In Rosen, R. C., Davis, C. M., Ruppel, H. J., Jr. *Annual review of sex research, Vol. 9.* (pp. 39–76). Lake Mills, IA: Society of Scientific Study of Sex.

Fisher, W. A., Fisher, J. D., and Byrne, D. (1977). Consumer reactions to contraception purchasing. *Personality and Social Psychology Bulletin, 3,* 293–296.

Fisher, W. A., Fisher, J. D., and Harman, J. (2003). The Information-Motivation-Behavioral Skills model: A general social psychological approach to understanding and promoting health behavior. In J. Suls and K. A. Wallston (eds.), *Social psychological foundations of health and illness.* (pp. 82–106). Malden, MA: Blackwell.

Fisher, W. A., Williams, S. S., Fisher, J. D., and Malloy, T. E. (1999). Understanding AIDS risk behavior among sexually active urban adolescents. An empirical test of the Information-Motivation-Behavioral Skills model. *AIDS and Behavior, 3,* 13–23.

Gluck, M., and Rosenthal, E. (1995). *OTA Report: The effectiveness of AIDS prevention efforts.* American Psychological Association, Washington, DC.

Glynn, M., and Rhodes, P. (2005). Estimated HIV prevalence in the United States at the end of 2003. National HIV Prevention Conference; June 2005; Atlanta, GA. Abstract T1-B1101. Available at http://www.aegis.com/conferences/NHIVPC/2005/T1-B1101.html. Accessed December 1, 2007.

Greenberg, B., Berkman, A., Thomas, R., Hoos, D., Finkelstein, R., Astemborski, J., and Vlahov, D. (1999). Evaluating supervised HAART in late-stage HIV among drug users: A preliminary report. *Journal of Urban Health, 76,* 468–480.

Hackshaw, A. K., and Paul, E. A. (2003). Breast self-examination and death from breast cancer: A meta-analysis. *British Journal of Cancer, 88,* 1047–1053.

Halkitis, P. N., and Parsons, J. T. (2003). Intentional unsafe sex (barebacking) among HIV-positive gay men who seek sexual partners on the internet. *AIDS Care, 15,* 367–378.

Hall, H. I., Song, R., Rhodes, P., Prejean, J., An, Q., Lee, L. M., et al. (2008). Estimation of HIV incidence in the United States. *Journal of the American Medical Association, 300,* 520–529.

Hammer, J. C., Fisher, J. D., and Fitzgerald, P. (1996). When two heads aren't better than one: AIDS risk behavior in college-age couples. *Journal of Applied Social Psychology, 26,* 375–397.

Health Canada. (2003). *Canadian guidelines for sexual health education.* Ottawa, Canada. http://pubs.cpha.ca/PDF/P6/20652.pdf.

Hecht, F. M., Grant, R. M., Petropoulos, C. J., Chesney, M. A., Tian, H., Hellmann, N. S., et al. (1998). Sexual transmission of an HIV-1 variant resistant to multiple reverse-transcriptase and protease inhibitors. *New England Journal of Medicine, 339,* 307–311.

Helweg-Larsen, M., and Collins, B. E. (1997). A social psychological perspective on the role of knowledge about AIDS in AIDS prevention. *Current Directions in Psychological Science, 6,* 23–53.

Herbst, J. H., Beeker, C., Mathew, A., McNally, T., Passin, W. F., Kay, L. S., et al. (2007). The effectiveness of individual-, group-, and community-level HIV behavioral risk-reduction interventions for adult men who have sex with men: A systematic review. *American Journal of Preventive Medicine, 32,* S38–S67.

Herbst, J. H., Kay, L. S., Passin, W. F., Lyles, C. M., Crepaz, N., and Marín, B. V. (2007). A systematic review and meta-analysis of behavioral interventions to reduce HIV risk behaviors of Hispanics in the United States and Puerto Rico. *AIDS and Behavior, 11,* 25–47.

Herbst, J. H., Sherba. R. T., Crepaz. N., DeLuca, J. B., Zohrabyan, L., Stall. R. D., et al. (2005). A meta-analytic review of HIV behavioral interventions for reducing sexual risk behavior of men who have sex with men. *Journal of Acquired Immune Deficiency Syndromes, 39,* 228–241.

Hogg, R. S., Yip, B., K., C., O'Shaughnessy, M. V., and Montaner, S. G. (2000). *Nonadherence to triple combination therapy is predictive of AIDS progression and death in HIV-positive men and women.* Program and abstracts of 7th Conference on Retroviruses and Opportunistic Infections. San Francisco, California January 30 to February 2, 2000.

Holtgrave, D. R., Qualls, N. L., Curran, J. W., et al. (1995). An overview of the effectiveness and efficiency of HIV prevention programs. *Public Health Reports, 110,* 134–146.

Ickovics, J., and Chesney, M. (1997). Issues regarding antiretroviral treatment for patients with HIV-1 infection. *Journal of the American Medical Association, 278,* 1233–1234.

Jaworski, B. C., and Carey, M. C. (2001). Effects of a brief, theory-based STD-prevention program for female college students. *Journal of Adolescent Health, 29,* 417–425.

Johnson, B. T., Carey, M. P., Chaudoir, S. R., and Reid, A. (2006). Sexual risk reduction for persons living with HIV: Research synthesis of randomized controlled trials, 1993 to 2004. *Journal of Acquired Immune Deficiency Syndromes, 41,* 642–650.

Johnson, B. T., Carey, M. P., Marsh, K. L., Levin, K. D., and Scott-Sheldon, L.A.J. (2003). Interventions to reduce sexual risk for the Human Immunodeficiency Virus in Adolescents, 1985–2000. *Archives of Pediatrics and Adolescent Medicine, 157,* 381–388.

Johnson, R. W., Ostrow, D. G., and Joseph, J. G. (1990). Educational strategies for prevention of sexual transmission of HIV. In D. G. Ostrow (Ed.), *Behavioral aspects of AIDS* (pp. 43–73). New York: Plenum.

Johnson, W. D., Hedges, L. V., Ramirez, G., Semaan, S., Norman, L. R., Sogolow, E., Sweat, M. D., and Diaz, R. M. (2002). HIV prevention research for men who have sex with men: A systematic review and meta analysis. *Journal of Acquired Immune Deficiency Syndromes, 30,* S118–S129.

Kalichman, S. C. (2000). HIV transmission risk behaviors of men and women living with HIV-AIDS: Prevalence, predictors, and emerging clinical interventions. *Clinical Psychology: Science and Practice, 7,* 32–47.

Kalichman, S. C., Cain, D., Weinhardt, L., Benotsch, E., Presser, K., Zweben, A., et al. (2005). Experimental components analysis of brief theory-based HIV/AIDS risk-reduction counseling for sexually transmitted infection patients. *Health Psychology, 24,* 198–208.

Kalichman, S. C., and Cherry, C. (1999). Male polyurethane condoms do not enhance brief HIV-STD risk reduction interventions for heterosexually active men: Results from a randomized test of concept. *International Journal of STD and AIDS, 10,* 548–553.

Kalichman, S.C., Cherry, C., and Browne-Sperling, F. (1999). Effectiveness of a video-based motivational skills-building HIV risk-reduction intervention for inner-city African American men. *Journal of Consulting and Clinical Psychology, 67,* 959–966.

Kalichman, S. C., Malow, R., Dévieux, J., Stein, J. A., and Piedman, F. (2005). HIV risk reduction for substance using seriously mentally ill adults: Test of the information-motivation-behavioral skills (IMB) model. *Community Mental Health Journal, 41,* 277–290.

Kalichman, S.C., Rompa, D., DiFonzo, K., Simpson, D., Austin, J., Luke, W., et al. (2001). HIV treatment adherence in women living with HIV/AIDS: Research based on the information-motivation-behavioral skills model of health behavior. *Journal of the Association of Nurses in AIDS Care, 12,* 58–67.

Kalichman, S. C., Simbayi, L. C., Cain, D., Jooste, S., Skinner, D., and Cherry, C. (2006). Generalizing a model of health behaviour change and AIDS stigma for use with sexually transmitted infection clinic patients in Cape Town, South Africa. *AIDS Care, 18,* 178–182.

Kalichman, S. C., Williams, E., and Nachimson, D. (1999). Brief behavioral skills building intervention for female controlled methods of STD-HIV prevention: Outcomes of a randomized clinical field trial. *International Journal of STD and AIDS, 10,* 174–181.

Kegeles, S. M., Rebchook, G. M., and Tebbetts, S. (2005). Challenges and facilitators to building program evaluation capacity among community-based organizations. *AIDS Education and Prevention, 17,* 284–299.

Kelly, J. A. (1995). *Changing HIV risk behavior: Practical strategies.* New York: The Guilford Press.

Kelly, J. A., and Kalichman, S. C. (2002). Behavioral research in HIV/AIDS primary and secondary prevention: Recent advances and future directions. *Journal of Consulting and Clinical Psychology, 70,* 626–639.

Kelly, J. A., Murphy, D. A., Sikkema, K. L., and Kalichman, S. C. (1993). Psychological interventions to prevent HIV infection are urgently needed: New priorities for behavioral research in the second decade of AIDS. *American Psychologist*, *48*, 1023–1034.

Kelly, J. A., and St. Lawrence, J. S. (1988). *The AIDS health crisis: Psychological and social interventions.* New York: Plenum Press. Kirby, D. (1999). Reflections on two decades of research on teen sexual behavior and pregnancy. *Journal of School Health*, *69*, 89–94.

Kelly, J. A., Somlai, A. M., DiFranceisco, W. J., Otto-Salaj, L. L., McAuliffe, T. L., Hackl, K. L., et al. (2000). Bridging the gap between the science and service of HIV prevention: Transferring effective research-based HIV prevention interventions to community AIDS service providers. *American Journal of Public Health*, *90*, 1082–1088.

Kiene, S. M., and Barta, W. D. (2006). A brief individualized computer-delivered sexual risk reduction intervention increases HIV/AIDS preventive behavior. *Journal of Adolescent Health*, *39*, 404–410.

Kirby, D., and DiClemente, R. J. (1994). School-based interventions to prevent unprotected sex and HIV among adolescents. In R. J. DiClemente and J. L. Peterson (eds.), *Preventing AIDS: Theories and methods of behavioral interventions*. (pp. 117–139). New York: Plenum Press.

Knobel, H., Alonso, J., Casado, J. L., Collazos, J., Gonzales, J., Ruiz, I., et al. (2002). Validation of a simplified medication adherence questionnaire in a large cohort of HIV-infected patients: The GEEMA Study. *AIDS*, *16*, 605–613.

Leviton, L. C., and Valdiserri, R. O. (1990). Evaluating AIDS prevention: Outcome, implementation, and mediating variables. *Evaluation and Program Planning*, *13*, 55–66.

Margolin, A., Avants, S. K., Warburton, L. A., Hawkins, K. A., and Shi, J. (2003). A randomized clinical trial of a manual-guided risk-reduction intervention for HIV-positive injection drug users. *Health Psychology*, *22*, 223–228.

Metzler, C. W., Biglan, A., Noell, J., Ary, D. V., and Ochs, L. (2000). A randomized controlled trial of a behavioral intervention to reduce high-risk sexual behavior among adolescents in STD clinics. *Behavior Therapy*, *31*, 27–54.

Miller, W. R., and Rollnick, S. (1991). *Motivational interviewing: Preparing people to change addictive behavior.* New York: Guilford Press.

Misovich, S. J., Fisher, J. D., and Fisher, W. A. (1996). The perceived AIDS-preventive utility of knowing one's partner well: A public health dictum and individual's risky sexual behavior. *Canadian Journal of Human Sexuality*, *5*, 83–90.

Misovich, S. J., Fisher, J. D., and Fisher, W. A. (1997). Close relationships and HIV risk behavior: Evidence and possible underlying psychological processes. *General Psychology Review*, *1*, 72–107.

Misovich, S. J., Fisher, W. A., and Fisher, J. D. (1998). A measure of AIDS prevention information, motivation and behavioral skills. In C. M. Davis and R. Yarber and G. Bauserman and G. Schreer and S. L. Davis (eds.), *Sexuality related measures: A compendium*. Newbury Park CA: Sage.

Misovich, S. J., Martinez, T., Fisher, J. D., Bryan, A. D., and Catapano, N. (2003). Breast self-examination: A test of the information, motivation, and behavioral skills model. *Journal of Applied Social Psychology*, *33*, 775–790.

Montaner, J. D., Reiss, P., Cooper, D., Vella, S., Harris, M., Conway, B., Weinberg, M.A., Smith, et al. (1998). A randomized, double-blind trial comparing combinations of nevirapine, didanosine, and zidovudine for HIV-infected patients. *Journal of the American Medical Association*, *279*, 930–937.

Murray, D. M. (2000). Exploring motorcycle safety gear use: A theoretical approach. Unpublished doctoral thesis, University of Connecticut.

Noar, S. M. (2008). Behavioral interventions to reduce HIV-related sexual risk behavior: Review and synthesis of meta-analytic evidence. *AIDS and Behavior, 12*, 335–353.

Oakley, A., Fullerton, D., and Holland, J. (1995). Behavioral interventions for HIV/AIDS prevention. *AIDS*, *9*, 479–486.

Offir, J. T., Fisher, J. D., and Williams, S. S. (1993). Possible reasons for inconsistent AIDS prevention behaviors among gay men. *Journal of Sex Research*, *30*, 62–69.

Otto-Salaj, L. L., Kelly, J. A., Stevenson, L. Y., Hoffmann, R., and Kalichman, S. C. (2001). Outcomes of a randomized small-group HIV prevention intervention trial for people with serious mental illness. *Community Mental Health Journal, 37*, 123–144.

Patterson, D. L., Swindells, S., Mohr, J., Brester, M., Vergis, E. N., Aquier, C., et al. (2000). Adherence to protease inhibitor therapy and outcomes in patients with HIV infection. *Annals of Internal Medicine, 133*, 21–30.

Peeler, C.M. (2000). An analysis of the effects of a course designed to reduce frequency of high-risk sexual behavior and heavy drinking. Unpublished doctoral thesis, Washington State University.

Prochaska, J. O., Redding, C. A., Harlow, L. L., et al. (1994). The transtheoretical model of change and HIV prevention: A review. *Health Education Quarterly, 21*, 471–486.

Rebchook, G. M., Kegeles, S. M., Huebner, D., and the TRIP Research Team. (2006). Translating research into practice: The dissemination and initial implementation of an evidence-based HIV prevention program. *AIDS Education and Prevention, 18*, 119–136.

Robertson, A. A., Stein, J. A., and Baird-Thomas, C. (2006). Gender differences in the prediction of condom use among incarcerated juvenile offenders: testing the information-motivation-behavior skills (IMB) model. *Journal of Adolescent Health, 38*, 18–25.

Rollnick, S., Heather, N., and Bell, A. (1992). Negotiating behaviour change in medical settings: The development of brief motivational interviewing. *Journal of Mental Health, 1*, 25–37.

Rollnick, S., Mason, P. and Butler, C. (1999). *Health behavior change: A guide for practitioners*. Edinburgh: Churchill Livingstone.

Rosenberg, S. D., Goodman, L. A., Osher, F. C., Swartz, M. S., Essock, S. M., Butterfield, M. I., et al. (2001). Prevalence of HIV, hepatitis B, and hepatitis C in people with severe mental illness. *American Journal of Public Health, 91*, 31–37.

Rosengard, C. (1992). Safer sex behavior change in college students: Exploration of a stage of behavior change model. Unpublished master's thesis, University of Connecticut.

Rosenstock, I. M., Stretcher, V. J., and Becker, M. H. (1994). The health belief model and HIV risk behavior change. In R. J. DiClemente and J. L. Peterson (eds.), *Preventing AIDS: Theories and methods of behavioral interventions*. (pp. 5–25). New York: Plenum Press.

Rotheram-Borus, M. J., Gwadz, M., Fernandez, M. I., and Srinivasan, S. (1998). Timing of HIV interventions on reductions in sexual risk among adolescents. *American Journal of Community Psychology, 26*, 73–96.

Ruiz, M. S., Gable, A. R., Kaplan, E. H., Stoto, M. A., Fineberg, H. V., and Trussell, J. (eds.) (2001). *No time to lose: Getting more from HIV prevention*. Washington, DC: National Academy Press.

St. Lawrence, J. S., Brasfield, T. L., and Jefferson, K. W., Alleyne, E., O'Bannon, R.E., and Shirley, A. (1995). Cognitive-behavioral intervention to reduce African American adolescents' risk for HIV infection. *Journal of Consulting Clinical Psychology, 63*, 221–237.

St. Lawrence, J. S., Crosby, R. A., Brasfield, T. L., and O'Bannon III, R. E. (2002). Reducing STD and HIV risk behavior of substance-dependent adolescents: A randomized controlled trial. *Journal of Consulting and Clinical Psychology, 4*, 1010–1021.

Shuper, P. A., and Fisher, W. A. (2008). The role of sexual arousal and sexual partner characteristics in HIV + MSM's intentions to engage in unprotected sexual intercourse. *Health Psychology, 27*, 445–454.

Silberstein, C., Galanter, M., Marmor, M., Lifshutz, H., and Krasinski, K. (1994). HIV-1 among inner city dually diagnosed inpatients. *American Journal of Drug and Alcohol Abuse, 20*, 101–131.

Simbayi, L. C., Kalichman, S. C., Skinner, D., Jooste, S., Cain, D., Cherry, C., et al. (2004). Theory-based HIV risk reduction counseling for sexually transmitted infection clinic patients in Cape Town, South Africa. *Sexually Transmitted Diseases, 31*, 727–733.

Spire, B., Duran, S., Souville, M., Leport, C., Raffi, F., Moatti, J. P., et al. (2002). Adherence to highly active antiretroviral therapies (HAART) in HIV-infected patients: From a predictive to dynamic approach. *Social Science and Medicine, 54*, 1481–1496.

Starace, F., Massa, A., Amico, K. R., and Fisher, J. D. (2006). Adherence to antiretroviral therapy: An empirical test of the information-motivation-behavioral skills model. *Health Psychology, 25*, 153–162.

U.S. Department of Health and Human Services (1988). *Understanding AIDS*. Rockville, MD: Centers for Disease Control.

U.S. Department of Health and Human Services (1993). *Planning and evaluating HIV/AIDS prevention programs in State and local health departments: A companion to program announcement 300*. Public Health Service; Atlanta, GA: Centers for Disease Control.

U.S. Department of Transportation. (2005). *Traffic safety facts: Motorcycles*. http://www-nrd.nhtsa.dot.gov/pdf/nrd-30/NCSA/TSF2005/2005TSF/810_620/images/810620.pdf

UNAIDS. (2006a). AIDS epidemic update. Switzerland: Joint United Nations Programme on HIV/AIDS (UNAIDS) and World Health Organization (WHO).

UNAIDS. (2006b). UNAIDS annual report: Making the money work. Switzerland: Joint United Nations Programme on HIV/AIDS (UNAIDS).

UNAIDS. (2007). AIDS epidemic update. Switzerland: Joint United Nations Programme on HIV/AIDS (UNAIDS) and World Health Organization (WHO).

van Kesteren, N.M.C., Hospers, H. J., and Kok, G. (2007). Sexual risk behavior among HIV-positive men who have sex with men: A literature review. *Patient Education and Counseling, 65,* 5–20.

Walsh, J. C., Horne, R., Dalton, M., Burgess, A. P., and Gazzard, B. G. (2001). Reasons for nonadherence to antiretroviral therapy: Patients' perspectives provide evidence of multiple causes. *AIDS Care, 16,* 269–277.

Walter, H., and Vaughn, R. D. (1993). AIDS risk reduction among a multi-ethnic sample of urban high school students. *Journal of the American Medical Association, 270,* 725–730.

Weinhardt, L. S., Carey, M. P., and Carey, K. B. (1997). HIV risk reduction for the seriously mentally ill: Pilot investigation and call for research. *Journal of Behavior Therapy and Experimental Psychiatry, 28,* 1–8.

Weinhardt, L. S., Carey, M. P., and Carey, K. B., and Verdecias, R. N. (1998). Increasing assertiveness skills to reduce HIV risk among women living with a severe and persistent mental illness. *Journal of Consulting and Clinical Psychology, 66,* 680–684.

Williams, S. S., Doyle, T. M., Pittman, L. D., Weiss, L. H., Fisher, J. D., and Fisher, W. A. (1998). Roleplayed safer sex skills of heterosexual college students influenced by both personal and partner factors. *AIDS and Behavior, 2*(3), 177–187.

Williams, S. S., Kimble, D. L., Covell, N. H., Weiss, L. H., Newton, K. S., Fisher, J. D., and Fisher, W. A. (1992). College students use implicit personality theory instead of safer sex. *Journal of Applied Social Psychology, 22,* 921–933.

Wingood, G. M., and DiClemente, R. J. (1996). HIV sexual risk reduction interventions for women: A review. *American Journal of Preventive Medicine, 12*(3), 209–217.

CHAPTER

3

SOCIAL INFLUENCES: THE EFFECTS OF SOCIALIZATION, SELECTION, AND SOCIAL NORMATIVE PROCESSES ON HEALTH BEHAVIOR

Bruce G. Simons-Morton
Denise Haynie
Elizabeth Noelcke

SOCIAL INFLUENCES ON HEALTH BEHAVIOR

Compared with older, more experienced drivers, novice young drivers tend to drive faster and follow the vehicle ahead of them more closely. This may reflect inexperience or a tendency of young drivers to take greater risks than others. Curiously, the presence of teenage passengers alters risky driving behavior decidedly. In the presence of a male teenage passenger, teenage males drive much faster and follow more closely than do teenage males driving without passengers. Similarly, teenage females drive faster and closer to the car in front of them when a teenage male passenger is present, but not when a teenage female passenger is present. With a teenage female passenger, teenage male drivers tend to drive about the same speed and follow at the same distance as older drivers. It seems that teenage passengers provide a social influence that alters teenage risky driving behavior (Simons-Morton, Lerner, and Singer, 2005).

The presence of passengers increases crash risk among teenage drivers, but not among adult drivers (Chen, Baker, Braver, and Li, 2000). As noted, crash data have been corroborated by observational behavior showing that the presence of teenage passengers, particularly males, increases speed and reduces following distance, two measures of risky driving behavior (Simons-Morton, Lerner, et al., 2005). However, it is unclear why teenagers engage in risky driving behavior in the presence of other teenagers. While inexperience and distraction may provide partial explanations, the variability among teenage males and females of the effect of teenage passengers on driving performance suggests that social influences are a major contributor.

The effect of teenage passengers on teenage driving performance is hardly an isolated example of social influences on health behavior. Indeed, social influence occurs among virtually all population groups in association with a wide range of behaviors and social outcomes (Forgas and Williams, 2001; Berkman and Kawachi, 2000). Although there is a great deal of theory and research about social influences, these processes are not fully understood.

Social influence can best be appreciated within expansive social contexts, including social norms and networks. Viewed broadly, social influences occur at multiple levels and include policies, programs, and media, as well as more proximal interpersonal influences such as friends and family (Glass and McAfee, 2006).

Many authors have noted that health behavior is largely contextual and only partly volitional (Buchanan, 2000). Population and environmental determinants explain more of the variation in diet, physical activity, and smoking, for example, than personal characteristics (McKinlay and Marceau, 2000). In large part, social context shapes not just the interpretation of information, but also the types of sources used and frequency with which it is sought.

The broad social context provides both direct effects on individual behavior and indirect effects through other societal levels. In general, direct interpersonal influences, particularly those of close others such as family and friends, are thought to be primary, while personal observation

Social context shapes not just the interpretation of information, but also the types of sources used and frequency with which it is sought.

and macro-level effects such as media and policy are thought to be secondary. However, **macro-level influences** also operate indirectly on the behavior of an individual or group by affecting the social norms of their proximal influences (Glass and McAfee, 2006).

Within the social context, several social influence processes are important. The first of these is **socialization**, which is the effect of interactions with others on one's thoughts, feelings, and behavior. For example, an adolescent may be persuaded to stop playing soccer or basketball because his or her current friends do not favor it. A second social influence process is **selection**, which is the process of befriending or associating with people who share common perspectives and behaviors. For example, an early adolescent who wishes to experiment with cigarettes would tend to associate with other youth who are already experimenting with cigarettes. A third social influence process involves **social norms**. This is not discrete from selection or socialization, but may be one of the ways that socialization and selection exert influence. The interesting thing about social norms is they do not have to be accurate to be influential (Berkowitz, 2004).

Social influence processes are relevant to a wide range of health behaviors. The creation of effective health promotion programs can be improved through a better understanding of the nature of social influences on health behavior. In this chapter, we provide a conceptual model describing the relationships between social influences and health behavior. We use the example of adolescent health behavior because it is well studied and illustrates the range of social influences.

GENESIS OF THE MODEL

Health behavior researchers and health promotion professionals are interested in social influences because they are among the most pervasive and substantial predictors of health behavior. There are many examples of health behaviors known to be greatly influenced by both broad, long-term social support and more proximal and immediate social influence. In general, there is remarkable consistency in thought, feeling, and behavior within social groups with respect to many health behaviors. For example, dietary behavior is highly associated with family eating experiences (Larson, Neumark-Sztainer, Hannan, and Story, 2007) and social context (Sorensen et al., 2007). Obesity is a social phenomenon, as well as an energy intake-expenditure issue (Christakis and Fowler, 2007). Patients with good social support are more likely to seek health care when warranted and follow medical advice than those without good social support (Berkman, 2000). People who exercise tend to have friends who exercise and make additional friends who exercise (McNeill, Kreuter, and Subramanian, 2006). Having friends who smoke increases the likelihood that an adolescent will take up smoking in the future (Simons-Morton, Chen, Abroms, and Haynie, 2004).

Social influence is an integral part of many prominent theories of development and behavior. Perhaps because social influence involves a complex set of processes, there is no unifying social influence theory, although aspects of social influence are emphasized or recognized by many theories commonly employed in health behavior research, as shown in Table 3.1. Basically, all of these theories agree that social

TABLE 3.1 **Theory and Social Influences.**

Theory	Concepts
Social Network Theory: SNT posits that the relationship of the individual within a social system influences dispositions and behavior (Berkman, 2000)	Social networks: • Provide context for social interaction, communication channels, reference points for decision making • An individual's location/status within the system matters with respect to influence • May be narrow or widespread, dynamic or static, homogeneous or heterogeneous, transient or stable
Primary Socialization (and peer cluster theory): theory posits that norms and behaviors are learned in social contexts (Oetting, 1999)	Norms and behavior are influenced by bonding with primary socialization sources: • Family, school, peer groups are primary sources • Media and other macro sources are secondary, indirect sources of influence • Weak social bonds increase likelihood and influence of affiliation with antisocial peers • Personal traits may have direct or indirect effects or may interact with socialization source influences
Social Cognitive Theory: SCT posits that learning is socially and cognitively mediated (Bandura, 1986)	Learning and self-control occur through reciprocal determinism, the dynamic interaction of person, environment, and behavior • Direct experience provides feedback and reinforcement • Vicarious experience through observation and modeling also provides feedback and reinforcement • Cognitive processing of information: • Outcome and efficacy expectations and expectancies • Behavioral capability • Parent and peers are primary social factors • Media is secondary social factor

Theory of Reasoned Action: TRA posits that intent is influenced by attitudes about the behavior and the relevant subjective norms (Fishbein and Ajzen, 1975)	<ul><li>Attitudes predict intent, but action depends on opportunity and other contextual factors</li><li>Attitudes are made up of beliefs</li><li>Attitudes about the relative advantages of the behavior predict behavior</li><li>Attitudes about the subjective norms predict behavior</li><li>Personality and other factors can mediate relationship between attitudes and intent</li></ul>
Social Norms Theory: SNT suggests that behavior is influenced by perceptions of social norms (Berkowitz, 2004)	<ul><li>Norms are contextual and cultural</li><li>Individuals are not always aware of their perceptions of norms</li><li>Salience of norms varies by group</li><li>Perceptions are influential, even if they are not accurate</li><li>Perceived norms are real in their consequences</li><li>There are many sources of misinformation about norms, including false consensus and pluralistic ignorance</li></ul>

influence is the product of information obtained from social interactions. This information is processed and interpreted variously by the recipient and often by the other parties involved. Many theories relate to social influences, including a number of information processing and developmental psychology theories, but space allows brief description of only a few theories that are both prominent and representative. These include social network theory, primary socialization theory, social cognitive theory, theory of reasoned action, and social norms theory.

SOCIAL NETWORK THEORY

Social network theory posits that the position of the individual within a social system influences dispositions (perceptions and attitudes) and behavior. **Social networks** refer to the structure of relationships that provide information on how an individual is integrated with others (Institute of Medicine, 2001). Social networks are definable, but often have amorphous boundaries. One can be part of multiple social networks. Networks can include close others, casual friends, people and groups known only by reputation, media, and other vicarious sources. **Proximal social influences** stemming from interactions with family and friends are embedded within other levels of social influence that act both directly and indirectly through proximal others to reinforce social norms. Social networks provide context for social interactions and for gaining and determining the value of information. Social networks not only channel information, but also determine the value and importance of it. Of course, information does not need to be based on fact to be influential. Indeed, not everyone values fact-based information or is as exposed to accurate and impartial sources of information as they are to other highly influential sources that may or may not be credible, reliable, or unbiased.

Within a social network, members offer social support, typically provided by close others, but sometimes through groups organized for this purpose (Cohen and Syme, 1985; House, Landis, and Umberson, 1988). Social support involves the provision of resources by other persons, which can include emotional, instrumental, informational, and appraisal support (House et al., 1988). Social support is typically purposeful, with the support person intending to be helpful. However, some attempts at social support may not be helpful or may even be harmful, even if unintended. Nevertheless, there is substantial evidence that social support can be important in a variety of areas of health and behavior and is essential in areas such as adherence to medical regimen (Berkman, 2000). Social support can be provided with respect to any topic or behavior, but it is most often studied as an essential helping process provided mainly by family members and close friends of individuals coping with a health problem. However, it is also an element in health promotion and disease prevention. Lack of social support is associated with negative health outcomes, and the presence of social support and its quality are associated with positive outcomes (Berkman, 2000). However, there are benefits from less tangible forms of social relations. All other things being equal, social integration—that is, being part of a social network—seems to contribute positively to health outcomes (Berkman and Glass, 2000).

Some individuals may have limited social networks, while others have extensive social networks. Social networks can be quite widespread and unstructured, existing mainly through vicarious sources such as the Internet, television, or radio. Moreover, social networks can be mixed, in that they include both overt contacts and vicarious information sources. Social networks can also be dynamic, change over time, and be complex. Social networks can exist among people who do not know each other, but share common interests in dress, music, or activities. Social networks can also be tightly knit and coherent, as in a family, a gang, or among close friends. People often use their social networks as a reference point, seeing how others react to thoughts and ideas. By doing so, they gain useful feedback about social norms and the credibility and importance of the idea. Also, the influence of social networks can vary by topic. Individuals may obtain and rely on information about specific topics from different networks. For example, youth may rely on their parents for information about topics like politics, but rely mainly on their peers for information about sex and drugs (Ennett and Bauman, 1994). A person with a health problem may rely solely on a health care provider for information, or may solicit information from a broader network of friends, social contacts, and others so afflicted. The Internet has allowed for the development of instant networks in which anyone with an interest can become involved.

PRIMARY SOCIALIZATION THEORY

Primary socialization theory (Oetting and Donnermeyer, 1998) applies the theories of Durkeim (1897) to adolescent development. The theory shares much in common with social bonding theory (Hirshi, 1969) and social development theory (Hawkins and Weiss, 1985; Hawkins, Catalano, and Miller, 1992). Accordingly, norms and behaviors are learned within social contexts, particularly within the primary contexts of family, peers, and school. In particular, the relationship bonds between the adolescent and the primary social-ization contexts serve as channels through which information and val-ues about norms and behaviors are transmitted. Strong bonds with family, school, and prosocial peers should be protective against prob-lem behavior. However, weak bonds with family and school are likely to increase affiliation with antisocial youth and heighten the influence of the peer cluster. Individual personality traits, particularly low self-evaluation, lack of self-control, and/or propensity for sensation-seeking, may negatively interact with family and school bonds and foster bonds with peers who engage in antisocial or deviant behavior.

Weak bonds with family and school are likely to increase affiliation with antisocial youth and heighten the influence of the peer cluster.

SOCIAL COGNITIVE THEORY

Bandura (1986) introduced the concept of reciprocal determinism, which is the dynamic interaction of the person, behavior, and the environment. Social cognitive theory (SCT) posits, among other things, that people learn through experience. Experiences, which can be direct or vicarious through observation, provide feedback that is cognitively processed by the individual. This cognitive processing provides information about reinforcement. A principal premise of SCT is operant condition-ing, which is largely concerned with how reinforcement influences behavior. Behaviors that are reinforced, more or less, tend to be sustained, while those that are not reinforced tend to decrease, all other things being equal. However, as tidy as rein-forcement theory might be, reinforcement itself has turned out to be quite complex, because it is subjective to cognitive interpretation and varies according to context. To demonstrate, food is not reinforcing to a satiated rat and, of course, people are greatly more complicated than rats. Personal attention is known to be a powerful source of reinforcement (Kazdin, 2001). However, in some instances, any attention can be rein-forcing, while in others, no amount of attention is sufficiently powerful to alter behav-ior. Moreover, not all attention is equal, so the effect of attention on behavior is variable. For example, an adolescent may crave and respond to attention from one particular parent or teacher. Nonetheless, social reinforcement, particularly from fam-ily and friends in the form of praise or recognition, is both a powerful and prevalent source of influence on human behavior.

Social cognitive theory is uniquely concerned with how individuals cognitively process the reinforcement potential of a behavior based on information gathered from experience. Some behaviors, such as eating, smoking, drugs, and physical activity, are largely self-reinforcing because the behavior triggers positive feedback that reinforces the behavior. These and other behaviors are often reinforced indirectly through social interaction rather than materially. For example, an adolescent may study more or less because of recognition and praise for doing so (or possibly punishment or disapproval for not doing so) from a parent or teacher. Thus, motivation to act is based on the cognitive processing of information from direct or vicarious experience about the reinforcing properties of the behavior. Accordingly, people are motivated to engage in a particular behavior (for example, smoking, drinking, exercising, or meditating) when they perceive it as providing positive outcomes, consider it within their ability (behavioral capability), are reasonably confident they can implement it (self-efficacy), and assume the outcomes are both likely (expectations) and valued (expectancies). Individuals may also be motivated to engage in a behavior if they observe someone successfully engage in the behavior and be rewarded for it (vicarious reinforcement). For example, upon observing a peer smoking and seeming to achieve positive outcomes as a result, an adolescent may become motivated to try smoking as well. Moreover, an adolescent's initial experiences with smoking may provide a great deal of information about norms and future outcome expectations by way of the reactions of the adolescent to the experience, including the act of smoking, the real or perceived reactions of other youth, and possibly the expected or perceived perceptions of parents or other adult role models. Adolescents may also judge their own behavior in terms of their perceptions of the values of vicarious role models such as movie stars, musicians, or other media figures.

THEORY OF REASONED ACTION

According to the theory of reasoned action (TRA) and its more recent incarnation as the theory of planned behavior (TPB), intent predicts behavior, except that environmental influences sometimes get in the way. Intent is largely the product of several categories of perceptions: (1) perceptions about the relative advantages of engaging in the behavior in question; (2) perceptions about norms (**subjective norms**) with respect to how relevant others would view the individual if they knew the individual engaged in the behavior; and (3) perceptions about social pressure to engage or not engage in the behavior (Fishbein and Ajzen, 1975; Ajzen, 1988). For example, an adolescent might evaluate the relative advantages of going to a party by considering not only his or her expectations with respect to the direct outcomes of attending the party, such as having a good time and being with those in attendance, but also perceptions about what others, such as party attendees, close friends, peer referents and parents, would think about his or her going. Of course, personality may moderate the relationships between beliefs and behavior. The essential contribution of TRA to the discussion of social influence is the central emphasis it places on perceptions about norms.

SOCIAL NORMS THEORY

Social norms theory (SNT) suggests that the extent of social influence is due largely to perceptions about social norms (Berkowitz, 2004). While TRA is primarily concerned with subjective norms (perceptions about others' expectations and values with respect to the behavior and the individual), SNT is largely concerned with norms with respect to perceived acceptability and prevalence. SNT has been studied primarily within the context of adolescent alcohol use and sexual behavior. This theory suggests that adolescents will be more or less predisposed to engage in these behaviors to the extent they perceive that they are acceptable and popular with their peer group. A central feature of the theory is that *perceptions* about the prevalence and acceptability of a behavior, rather than *actual* prevalence and acceptance, influence behavior. According to the theory, perceptions are often erroneous. **False consensus** is the incorrect belief that one's attitudes and behaviors represent that of the majority when one is actually a minority (for example, because I smoke or my friends smoke, most adolescents must smoke or think it is okay to smoke). Conversely, **pluralistic ignorance,** the incorrect belief that one's perceptions are unique, tends to discourage the expression of opinions or actions perceived to be nonconforming, contributing to false consensus.

Social norms, actual or perceived, are complicated because they may vary in the groups for which they are salient and are highly dependent on specific social and cultural contexts. Both perceived and actual social norms of adolescents regarding sex, drugs, school, and other topics may vary greatly among members of different groups, such as church groups or sports teams, and among those who identify with certain types of music, such as rap, country, or alternative. Furthermore, norms exist not only for the proximal peer group, but also at broader social levels, for example, by ethnicity, religion, or geographic region.

> Social norms, actual or perceived, are complicated because they may vary in the groups for which they are salient and are highly dependent on specific social and cultural contexts.

THEORY SUMMARY

Each of these theories provides useful perspectives on aspects of social influences on behavior. Each theory emphasizes how individuals process and interpret information. Except for social network theory, the theories focus primarily on proximal social influences and take into account only indirectly the substantial influence exerted by the larger and more distal social context. The point of introducing these theories, however briefly, is not to suggest that any of them fully describes social influences or that other theories do not offer useful perspectives on social influences, but more to suggest that social influence is a recognized concern in many popular psychosocial theories. It should be noted that due to space limitations, we did not describe how social influence fits into information processing and social marketing theories and approaches, which are generally concerned with social influences from various perspectives, including influences of information on perceived social norms and the indirect effects of information transmitted to influential sources and not the primary target (Andreasen, 1994;

Gass, and Seiter, 2003). While many psychosocial theories provide insight into social influence processes, there remains a need to better integrate social-psychological theory with a broader understanding of social networks and contexts.

DESCRIPTION AND EMPIRICAL EVIDENCE

Social influence is a complicated and dynamic process that is best understood within social contexts and by considering the nature of information as it is obtained from various sources and interpreted by the individual. Figure 3.1 provides a conceptualization of the relationships between key information sources, influence processes, and health behavior. Accordingly, the two major sources of information are sociocultural and interpersonal. Sociocultural context, which is composed of mass media, politics, policies and programs, religion, national and regional factors, and other aspects of culture and society, conveys information about norms and values. In addition, social interactions, such as conversations with friends and family and messages delivered by teachers, coworkers, or even complete strangers, provide additional information about values and norms. These various sources provide information that is cognitively processed based on the receiver's past experiences and cultural context. Accordingly, the receiver interprets the information so that it is personally relevant (or not). The information is stored as perceptions and values that become major contributors to the three key social influence processes: **socialization**, or overt social influence; **selection**, the tendency to befriend others with common values and behavior; and **social norms**, which are the actual and perceived norms about a particular behavior. These social influence processes directly affect health behavior. Of course, behavior also affects these processes because it provides feedback about social influences. The following paragraphs describe the importance of social context, the relative importance of various sources of information, and the primary social influences processes.

FIGURE 3.1 *Social Influences Model*

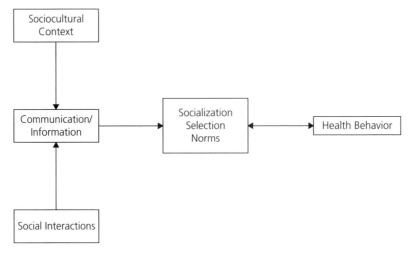

SOCIAL CONTEXT

Proximal social influence cannot be understood without an appreciation of social context. Values and norms are inculcated throughout the lifespan and maintained by broad social influences. Given the need for people to work together and contribute to common goals in modern society, laws, policies, and programs (for example, public education) are largely designed to transmit and enforce social values and encourage individuals to conform and adhere to generally accepted behaviors. Hence, each individual grows up with substantial cultural expectations and tremendous social pressures to accept normative perspectives and conform to socially prescribed perceptions and practices. However, despite increases in homogenizing social influences such as national media, the social contexts of individuals and groups can vary considerably, and not all groups in society have the same opportunities, constraints, experiences, and perceptions of their experiences. Socioeconomic status (SES) matters in terms of health, with higher SES groups, relative to lower SES groups, less likely to engage in health-damaging practices such as smoking or overeating, more likely to engage in health-promoting activities such as exercising, and better able to change to improve both health-promoting and health-damaging behaviors (Institute of Medicine, 2003).

In general, lifetime social experience and contemporary social contexts are thought to influence interpretation of social interactions. Social context can be dynamic, as people come into contact over time with new institutions (for example, churches, schools, or businesses), ideas, and individuals. In general, owing to numerous factors associated with development (for example, increased independence or reliance on peers), adolescents can experience quite different social contexts than they did as preadolescents. Notably, the transition from high school to college is associated with increases in risk-taking behavior that appears to be associated with social context (Read, Wood, Davidoff, McLacken, and Campbell, 2002; Arnett, 2000).

Culture is a dominant yet subtle influence on behavior; people may not always be aware of it or the power of its influence on their behavior.

Culture is a dominant yet subtle influence on behavior; people may not always be aware of it or the power of its influence on their behavior. Glass and McAfee (2006) conceptualized nested hierarchies of social context, including global, national, work/school/community, and social group and family. These embedded hierarchies reinforce conventional norms and values and largely determine the kinds of opportunities and constraints experienced by the population and therefore their motivation and behavior. Socioeconomic status and other social factors such as race and religion provide social contexts that have pervasive and lasting influences on motivation and behavior (Harding, 2003).

While macro-level social factors provide context, family is the primary social unit for the transmission of values and norms (Oetting, 1999). The great influence of family and close others is due to proximity and longevity. For example, an adolescent's response to specific parenting behavior may depend not only on the entire past history of the parent-teen relationship, but also on the particular teen behavior, the context of the parenting behavior, and other factors (Darling and Steinberg, 1993). Additionally, the effect of a spouse encouraging a mate to follow a prescribed medical regimen may depend in part on the history of the couple's relationship, as well as the proximal dynamics of communication about adherence, what the prescribing medical provider said to the patient, and what the patient and spouse understood of these instructions (Berkman and Kawachi, 2000). Ultimately, long-term social context effects can contribute to proximal social influences.

Moreover, while some social influence may be entirely intentional, for example, parents' efforts to encourage school performance and discourage smoking, much of it may be unwitting. A parent's attitudes about school performance, alcohol, or safety, for instance, may be transmitted to the child subtly and unintentionally, without either the parent or the child being fully aware of the process. In addition, without intending to, a spouse may influence the medical adherence of a mate by virtue of tangential statements, modeling, and attentiveness. This may be the product of the nested hierarchies of social context described by Glass and McAfee (2006), where norms and attitudes are greatly shaped by higher-order contexts such as race, religion, neighborhood, and economic status.

Smoking provides a good example of the complexity and nested hierarchies of social influences. Smoking is addictive, so many experimental smokers go on to become regular smokers. Smoking initiation and maintenance are also socially mediated, owing to both proximal social influences and broad societal influences, mainly the substantial position of cigarettes and smoking in society. The tobacco industry is large and powerful and has managed to establish and enjoy the advantages of relatively modest taxes, weak and decentralized regulation, and government protection for growers and producers, allowing substantial promotion of tobacco products (Pollack and Jacobson, 2003). Until recently, cigarettes could be sold and smoked almost anywhere, and tobacco remains highly available, even to teenagers (Johnston, O'Malley, Bachman, and Schulenberg, 2007; Simons-Morton et al., 1999). This is not to mention the estimated $9 billion annually spent on advertising for tobacco products (Wakefield, Flay, Nichter, and Giovino, 2003). Tobacco advertising and popular media portray smoking as glamorous, sexy, mature, and rebellious, seemingly targeting youth and certain other vulnerable population groups (Wakefield et al., 2003). Consequently, virtually all teenagers in the United States are greatly exposed to cigarette advertising and have ready access to cigarettes, and the majority of high school seniors report at least trying smoking (Johnston et al., 2007). However, not all adolescents who try smoking become regular smokers, and both peers and parents provide important influences on this behavior (Simons-Morton, Chen, et al., 2004). Therefore, interpersonal interactions provide proximal and dynamic influence within the cultural context.

> Interpersonal interactions provide proximal and dynamic influence within the cultural context.

LEVELS OF INFLUENCE

Kobus (2003) described social influence as omnidirectional, in that it occurs at multiple levels, with each level impacting the rest. While these levels are nested, they also overlap and the extent of influence at each level often cannot be discerned (Glass and McAfee, 2006). Although influences closest to the individual may well be the strongest, these influences are likely to have been filtered through broader contexts and overlapping levels of proximal and distal influence. The influence of family and friends is filtered by various cultural influences, from national media to racial and religious sources. Further, individuals' selective consumption of culture, particularly media, influences what they perceive as normative, acceptable, and important. Broadly, the three levels of social influence are interpersonal, community, and cultural.

The interpersonal level includes close relationships such as family members and friends (close others). The community level is composed of social networks such as those formed at school, in the neighborhood, and in the workplace. The cultural level includes broader factors such as racial and religious group affiliation and media exposure. Media sources include programming and advertising from books, magazines, radio, television, movies, and the Internet. Bronfenbrenner (1979) provided a cogent description of how various social levels provide interactive influences on child development. Shown in Figure 3.2 is a conceptualization of concentric circles of social influences. Proximal others, such as family and close others, are likely to have the greatest social influence owing to the closeness of the relationships and the frequency of contact. However, other more proximal relationships may provide additional influence either directly on the individual or indirectly through their influence on others within the individual's social circle. Thus, levels are overlapping and influences are

FIGURE 3.2   *Levels of Social Influence on Health Behavior*

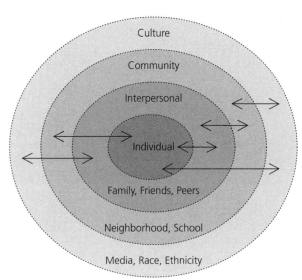

bidirectional, with individuals being exposed to various media source either with or without choosing to be.

As noted, family is the primary social unit for transmitting social values and norms (Grusec and Kuczynski, 1997; Oetting, 1999). In the United States, parents are expected to teach their children to respect authority and property and exercise self-control, among other values. Given the genetic similarities, opportunities for influence, and socially mediated roles of family members, it should not be surprising that there is a substantial association between family background and a wide range of health behaviors (Harding, 2003; McKinlay and Marceau, 2000).

The effect of parenting on children's behavior and outcomes has been well studied. Parents serve as models of health behaviors, such as nutritional choices (Cullen, Lara, and De Moor, 2002; Story, Neumark-Sztainer, and French, 2002) and substance use (Avenevoli and Merikangas, 2003; Simons-Morton and Haynie, 2003). Parenting itself is complex, involving both long-standing influences on behavior and values and proximal practices. Parenting practices that are appropriately demanding and responsive, known as authoritative parenting (Darling and Steinberg, 1993), have consistently been found to deter risky health behaviors such as substance use (Hyatt and Collins, 2000; Simons-Morton and Chen, 2005; Simons-Morton, 2007b), aggression (Simons-Morton, 2004; Simons-Morton, Chen, Hand, and Haynie, 2008), and problem behavior (Prelow, Bowman, and Weaver, 2007). Parents may exert indirect influence through their mediation of friend influences (Avenevoli and Merikangas, 2003; Simons-Morton, Haynie, Crump, Eitel, and Saylor, 2001). The mechanism for this may be either by managing friend selection (Kobus, 2003; Simons-Morton and Chen, 2005) or moderating friend influence (Deilman, Butchart, and Shope, 1993). Sibling behavior has been shown to be a powerful correlate of adolescent behavior independent of parent behavior (Rajan et al., 2003), particularly substance use (Brook, Brook, and Whiteman, 1999, Pomery et al., 2005; Windle, 2000), but it is difficult to sort out the extent to which these associations are due to genetics, parenting, or proximal social influences from various sources.

Friends are also important to consider, as they tend to share many dispositions and behaviors. Adolescents' behaviors, including problem behaviors such as substance use, are strongly associated with the behavior of close peers (Ennett and Bauman, 1994; Simons-Morton, Chen, et al., 2004). In part, adolescents make friends with those who have similar interests and outlooks and are introduced to certain behaviors and ways of thinking by their friends. The closeness of the peer is an important determinant of the degree of impact, and best friends are thought to exert the greatest influence (Kobus, 2003). Similarly, there is a strong association between adolescent reports of his or her own behavior and the number of friends he or she reports as engaging in the same behavior (Simons-Morton, 2007b). The processes by which close others influence behavior are based on group affiliation.

Like family and friends, other social groups tend to share common values, beliefs, and experiences. Some groups are based on a theme of uniformity, such as particular religious denominations or sports teams. Belonging to such a group fosters conformity, and a bond is created among members. Gang behavior is perhaps the extreme example of social conformity, but affiliation with less-organized groups or even vicarious identification with reputation-based (on politics, music preferences, attire, social activities, race, ethnicity, and the like) "crowds" can provide youth with a sense of social identity and means of comparing oneself with relevant others (Kobus, 2003). A relatively new behavior such as smoking among adolescents tends to diffuse based on exposure (associating with other youth who smoke) and on how the behavior is perceived and valued by one's friends and social group. There is evidence that the adoption of a behavior by those most centrally located in the crowd or group is more likely to increase the spread of the behavior throughout the group than adoption by less centrally located individuals, although this process is dynamic and complex (Collins, 1988).

Members of communities also share many characteristics, partly because families may select certain neighborhoods or lack the resources to select another neighborhood, but also because residents are affected by neighborhood characteristics. Neighborhood characteristics have been found to provide significant effects on alcohol and cigarette use when family and other factors were controlled (Rose et al., 2003). Violence is endemic in some poor urban neighborhoods (Lott, 2003), and residents of violent neighborhoods sometimes develop aggressive patterns of behavior that tend to perpetuate violence (Stewart, Schreck, and Simons, 2006). Religious affiliation and church attendance, considered here a proxy for membership in a community group, have been found to be protective against risk behaviors including substance use (Bjaranason, Thorlindsson, Sigfusdottire, and Welch, 2005; Perkins and Jones, 2004), sexual behaviors (Nonnemaker, McNeely, and Blum, 2003; Perkins and Jones, 2004), dating violence (Howard, Qiu, and Boekeloo, 2003) and aggression (Landau, Björkqvist, Lagerspetz, Österman, and Gideon, 2003; Nonnemaker et al., 2003), and the protective effects may be more pronounced in high-risk communities (Regnerus and Elder, 2003). Like reputation-based groups, communities can cross geographic boundaries, being composed of individuals from the same occupation, religion, political party, or with other common interests, with effects on attitudes and behavior similar to geographic neighborhoods.

The most distal and diffused level of social influence is culture. Culture refers to the shared belief system of a group defined by characteristics such as ethnicity, race, or nationality. As noted, culture is so entrenched that members are often not aware of the many cultural influences on their behavior (Glass and McAfee, 2006). Nevertheless, cultural influences are not totally uniform, as they are experienced and interpreted by members of the culture differently. Culture is transmitted through individual contact and impersonal mechanisms such as mass media. For example, ethnic identity is one way of identifying with one's cultural heritage and is often emphasized by parents (Hughes et al., 2006). Studies on ethnic identity with high-risk African American and Hispanic youth have found that having a strong sense of culture was protective against the debilitating effects of racial discrimination (Hughes et al., 2006; Townsend and Lanphier, 2007; Wong, Eccles, and Sameroff, 2003) and substance use (Scheier, Botvin, Diaz, and Ifill-Williams, 1997; Smith, Walker, Fields, Brookins, and Seay, 1999), and promoted better psychosocial adjustment (Smith et al., 1999; Wong et al., 2003). Culture is also transmitted through distal, impersonal mechanisms such as media. American youth are substantially exposed to print, television, the Internet, and other media, which influence their health attitudes and behavior (Dubow, Huesmann, and Greenwood, 2006; Collins, Elliot, Berry, Kanouse, and Hunter, 2003; Hofschire and Greenberg, 2002; Olson et al., 2007; Stockdale, 2001). There is also some promising evidence of the potential for intervening using mass media (Delgado and Austin, 2007; Reagan and Lee, 2007).

SOCIAL INFLUENCE PROCESSES

Basically, social influence is an information-processing activity. Social experiences provide information that is processed cognitively by individuals. However, people have varying social experiences and interpretations of their experiences. In part, both long-standing and immediate social contexts filter these experiences and their interpretations. Given the variability in social context, exposure, and interpretation, three general social influence processes operate: socialization, selection, and social norms (Table 3.2). These are not exclusive, in that they can occur simultaneously and may overlap and interact, though it is not always clear how these interactions operate; they may be uni- or bidirectional, direct or indirect, intended or unintended, proximal or distal, profound or subtle, lasting or fleeting. Here we describe these processes in relation to adolescent smoking.

The tendency of people who associate with one another to share common beliefs, attributes, and behavior, referred to as homophily, is well established (Ennett and Bauman, 1994; Eiser, Morgan, Gammage, Brooks, and Kirby, 1991; Kandel, 1978b). This similarity extends to a wide variety of demographic characteristics, including age, sex, ethnicity, religion, education, and social class (McPherson, Smith-Lovin, and Cook, 2001). For example, early adolescent smokers almost invariably have at least one smoking friend, while few nonsmokers report having a friend who smokes (Centers for Disease Control and Prevention, 2001). Both socialization and selection play a role in this. Although socialization tends to encourage an adjustment of beliefs to fit in with a social group, selection involves the development or retention of friendships based on beliefs that an adolescent already has. In the example of adolescent substance use, if beliefs or behaviors become contrasting among friends, typically an adolescent will either break off the friendship (deselection) or modify his or her drug behavior to maintain the friendship and reestablish homophily (socialization) (Kandel, 1978a). There is ample evidence for both socialization and selection with respect to the uptake among adolescents of substance use and other problem behaviors. Moreover, there is evidence that the processes of socialization and selection may be interactive (Urberg, Luo,

TABLE 3.2   Social Influence Processes.

	Socialization	Selection	Social Norms
Description	Inter-personal influence	Association with others who share common interests, attitudes, and behavior	Primary process by which socialization and selection influence behavior
Sources	Parents, friends, group affiliation, culture (distal, indirect)	Peers: overt group identity or actual affiliation or vicarious associations (with extraneous others known through media)	Parents, peers, group affiliations, social networks, context/culture, media
Direction	Others to individual; direct and intentional (friend offers a cigarette); indirect and unintentional (individual assumes smoking will make him or her "cool")	Mainly individual to others; can be direct and intentional (drug user seeks out friends who accept behavior and can give access to more substances); can be indirect and unintentional (adolescent experiments with drinking because he perceives that his close friends would approve).	Bidirectional and mutually reinforcing; direct and intentional (individual's peers smoke and offer cigarettes); indirect and unintentional (individual sees one peer smoking and might incorrectly assume that all peers smoke)
Actions	Persuasion, modeling, reinforcement, context management	Influence seeking, seeking approval of behaviors and views	Actual and perceived social norms
Mechanisms	Establish, reinforcement social norms, peer pressure	Social reinforcement, opportunity, modeling, social pressure	Interpretation of others views and behaviors; misperceptions
Protective factors	Parental behaviors monitoring and expectations	Parental monitoring and discouragement of friends who exhibit problem behaviors	Parental values; positive media messages

Pilgrim, and Degirmencioglu, 2003). Bauman and Ennett (1996), Arnett (2007), and others have described the complex nature of peer influences on smoking, where socialization by peers and selection interact with perceived social norms.

SOCIALIZATION

Description

Social experience teaches us how to think, feel, and behave—not exclusively, but powerfully and in a variety of aspects in our lives (Bandura, 1986). Parents socialize their children, group leaders socialize group members, and friends socialize one another. The primary mechanism for the process of socialization is social reinforcement. Some social influence is deliberate, for example, in the way a parent intentionally rewards, punishes, or ignores certain attitudes and behaviors of a child and the way peers encourage others to think and behave as they do. However, social influence can also be unintended and unwitting, as close others model behaviors and attitudes. Parent behavior serves as a model for child behavior, even if this is not the intent of the adult behavior. A child might learn problem-solving skills through parental instruction (direct socialization) and/or by watching parents deal with their own problems (indirect socialization through modeling). In the context of friendship groups, socialization is frequently viewed as peer pressure, where peers influence and compel others to take up certain attitudes and behaviors. However, peer influence can also be unintended and indirect. Merely the perception of social pressure may influence behavior, encouraging uniformity with the peer group.

Evidence of Effects

Similarity between the behavior of adolescents and friends is the most common way of assessing peer influence, and many studies have reported significant associations (Conrad, Flay, and Hill, 1992). Although there are limits to this approach (Urburg et al., 2003; Arnett, 2007), there is substantial evidence that association with substance-using friends leads to increases in adolescent substance use (Urberg, Degirmencioglu, and Pilgrim, 1997; Wills and Cleary, 1999). However, as noted, the discrete effects of socialization and selection are difficult to parcel out and are in all likelihood interactive. Certain groups of adolescents (particularly those with weak family and school bonds) may be more susceptible to peer influence than others (Urberg et al., 2003). Moreover, some qualitative studies have indicated that peer pressure is not always an overt factor in adolescent substance use uptake (Alexander, Allen, Crawford, and McCormick, 1999; Deniscombe, 2001).

There is growing evidence that protection against adolescent substance use can come in the form of authoritative parenting practices (primarily socialization effects), including monitoring (Dishion and Andrews, 1995) and other forms of parental involvement, expectations, and behaviors (Steinberg, Fletcher, and Darling, 1994; Simons-Morton and Chen, 2005). Both peer and parent influences appear to operate with respect to adolescent substance use (Simons-Morton, Chen, et al., 2004). Li and colleagues (2002) found that peer substance use had strong effects for adolescent use of the same type (such that smoking friends would influence smoking, and drinking friends, drinking); however, parental use was less directly correlated, but influenced a broader range of problem behaviors. For example, teens whose parents used marijuana were twice as likely to smoke, drink, and use marijuana.

SELECTION

Description

Selection is the process by which individuals tend to choose as friends those with whom they share common interests, views, and behaviors (Urberg, Degirmencioglu, and Tolson, 1998). This association could be based on something as relatively straightforward as proximity, which limits the potential friend pool, or gender. Adolescents, however, may choose friends with existing similarities in terms of attitudes related to sex, alcohol, smoking, success in school, and so on. Whether intentional or not, adolescents are influenced by those with whom they spend time, so the selection of friends has wide-reaching repercussions. Once selected, friends mutually reinforce one another's attitudes and behaviors.

Evidence of Effects

Although the selection of friends is complicated by adolescents' friendship-making potential, the proximity (neighborhood, school, and social activities) of possible friends, and other factors, there is substantial evidence that substance-using adolescents tend to increase their association with friends who also use these substances. Curran and colleagues (1997) found that associating with peers who drink leads to subsequent alcohol use (evidence of socialization), which, in turn, can lead to greater involvement with drinkers in the future (evidence for selection). Wills and Cleary (1999) found that early adolescents with friends who smoked were more likely to begin smoking a few years later (indicative of socialization), while Simons-Morton, Chen, et al. (2004) and Iannotti et al. (1996) found that early adolescents who smoked tended to have more friends who smoked a few years later on, an effect of selection.

Parents can provide protective effects against problem behavior by discouraging the selection of problem-behaving friends or mitigating the effects of these relationships. It has been shown for smoking (Simons-Morton, Chen, et al., 2004) and drinking (Simons-Morton and Chen, 2005) that sustained parent involvement, expectations, and monitoring mediated the association between adolescents and growth in the number of substance-using friends. Sustained authoritative parenting behaviors might be expected to alter peer influences partly by affecting adolescent attitudes about smoking or drinking, but also by affecting adolescents' perceptions about parental concern about this behavior. Hence, one way that parenting behavior protected against adolescent smoking and drinking was by controlling against an increase in friendships with adolescents who smoke. Parental discouragement of the development of friends who smoke or drink would alter perceptions about the acceptability of adolescent smoking and drinking, as well as reduce the availability of cigarettes and alcohol, as well as peer pressures on the adolescent to participate in the problem behaviors. In another vein, adolescents with parents who smoked were more likely to become affiliated with peers who also smoked (Engels, Vitaro, Blokland, de Kemp, and Scholte, 2004), perhaps illustrating the fact that teens will choose peers with similar social norms (and possibly reflecting a genetic propensity for addictive behaviors). Krosnick and Judd (1982) found that both peer and parent influences play a key role in impacting smoking behavior among preadolescents, while peers were somewhat more important than parents.

SOCIAL NORMS

Description

As noted, there are many influences on social norms. National and cultural norms probably have independent effects on behavior and are implicit in the development and outcomes of socialization and selection processes. Exposure to media is high among adolescents (Rideout, Roberts, and Goehr, 2005) and can provide both direct and indirect effects. Substance use marketing is directed at the behavior of potential young users (direct influence) and to their attitudes and subjective norms (indirect influence) so as to influence future behavior (Brown and Witherspoon, 2002). Proximal sources, mainly peers and parents, influence assumptions of what is "acceptable," directly through verbal communication and indirectly through modeling and nonverbal communication such as dress and music preferences. Mainly, associating with substance-using peers not only makes the substances more available, but also makes the behavior seem more normative (Dishion, Capaldi, Spracklen, and Li, 1995). Even the perception that substance use is acceptable and prevalent may increase adolescent use. In the abstract, smoking may not seem to an adolescent like a good thing, but when a friend does it, it may be easier to change perceptions about how bad smoking is than to change perceptions about a friend's judgment. Moreover, as smoking becomes more prevalent during adolescence, adolescents may reevaluate previous beliefs about smoking, and the effects of media and marketing influences related to smoking may increase (Wakefield et al., 2003). Therefore, adolescent development, macro-social influences, smoking prevalence (perceived and actual), and the proximal influences of socialization and selection probably interact.

Social norms may help to explain both selection and socialization effects. Both processes could operate independently of social norms, but conceptually, it makes sense that perceived social norms play a role in each process. With respect to socialization, an adolescent may perceive that it is socially normative and acceptable to smoke when it becomes evident that some peers are smoking. It may also be that just knowing a few other adolescents who smoke suggests to an adolescent that smoking is relatively common and acceptable. Moreover, as the prevalence of smoking increases with age, adolescents may perceive adolescent smoking in general and the offer of a cigarette specifically as more normative (Unger et al., 2001). Social norms also play out in selection processes. Adolescents select friends and identify with reputation-based groups based at least in part on the attitudes and behaviors they have in common. Normative perceptions of smoking may lead to a reevaluation of acceptability of adolescent smokers as friends. Of course, these processes work in the other direction as well, with perceived social norms, attitudes toward smoking, and association with peers who smoke or do not smoke, possibly altering the balance of motivation such that adolescents are less likely to smoke (Lucas and Lloyd, 1999; Maxwell, 2002). Social contexts have the potential to support nonsmoking, which is of great interest to prevention specialists.

Evidence of Effects

A number of studies have shown that the decision to try cigarettes was often more related to internally perceived peer pressure (for example, to avoid exclusion and to gain approval) than feeling overt pressure to accept the offer of a cigarette (Nichter, Nichter, Vuckovic, Quintero, and Ritenbaugh, 1997). Other evidence of the effect of social norms on behavior is provided by Berkowitz and Perkins (1986) in analyses of college student alcohol use. College students consistently overestimated the extent to which their peers were supportive of drinking behaviors, and student drinking was predicted by their estimation of the extent and acceptability of drinking.

While adolescents are reevaluating their normative perceptions with respect to both smoking and peers who smoke, parents remain influential with respect to smoking uptake. Of more interest is the effect of parenting behavior, which at least theoretically can influence adolescents' attitudes about smoking and its acceptability. Some research has shown that perceived parental expectations for adolescent behavior (subjective norms) are protective against substance use uptake (Simons-Morton and Chen, 2005). Moreover, media can influence adolescents on a wide variety of topics, including violence, sex, substance use, and nutrition (Brown and Witherspoon, 2002). Snyder et al. (2006) found that more exposure to alcohol advertisements lead to higher drinking levels among young people, revealing how the media might affect recognition of social norms.

Because peer influence is the single most important factor associated with smoking, at least when measured as the association between adolescent and peer smoking, a great deal of effort has gone into the development and evaluation of interventions to alter peer influence. Two main approaches include teaching adolescents peer pressure resistance skills and altering perceived social norms. Although there is evidence of the effectiveness of both approaches (Simons-Morton, Haynie, Saylor, Crump, and Chen, 2005; Botvin, Botvin, Baker, Dusenbury, and Goldberg, 1992; Botvin, Griffin, Diaz, and Ifill-Williams, 1999), a growing body of limited experimental evidence suggests that social norms approaches may be more important than peer pressure resistance (socialization) approaches. Notably, Hansen (1993) demonstrated that correcting normative beliefs was the critical element in an effective secondary school alcohol use prevention program. This finding has been replicated in a number of studies (Glider, Midvett, Mills-Novoa, Johannessen, and Collins, 2001; Foss, Deikman, Goodman, and Bartley, 2003). In the only comparison of peer pressure resistance and social norms approaches, the social norms approach had greater effects on smoking progression (McNeal, Hansen, Harrington, and Giles, 2004). Although more research is needed, it seems that social norms approaches may have at least as much potential to prevent smoking as peer pressure resistance approaches. Other interventions have targeted macro-level influences at the community level (Pentz et al., 1989), while others have attempted to improve adolescent media literacy by teaching adolescents how to evaluate and be dubious of advertising claims and media images (Johnston et al., 2007). A specific antismoking campaign, whose tactics included delivering straight facts about the consequences of smoking, as well as exposing tobacco companies' advertising techniques, was shown to increase antitobacco attitudes among youth over time, while a general, directive "just say no," campaign actually made youth more open to smoking (Farrelly et al., 2002).

TEENAGE PASSENGERS AND TEENAGE RISKY DRIVING

Having used adolescent substance use as the primary example throughout this chapter, it may be useful to return to the issue initially raised regarding the social influence of teenage passengers on teenage risky driving. Although there is considerably less literature on this topic than there is for substance use, it provides a rather unique and interesting example of possible social influences and how they might be studied.

To review, it is well established that crash rates of teenage drivers are highly elevated, particularly in the presence of passengers (Chen et al., 2000). It is also the case that risky driving behavior is higher in the presence of teen passengers (Simons-Morton, Lerner, et al., 2005). Crash rates of learners driving with parents, however, are very low, presumably because parents are controlling the situations in which learners practice driving and controlling the internal environment of the vehicle, and probably also provide a social influence on teenage driving attention and performance (Mayhew, Simpson, and Pak, 2003; Simons-Morton, 2007a). The fact that male and female teenage passengers have different effects, at least on male teenage drivers, with the presence of male passengers associated with greater risk taking among both males and female drivers, and the presence of female passengers associated with less risky driving among male drivers, suggests interesting social influence processes (Simons-Morton, Lerner, et al., 2005).

It is interesting to speculate on the possible influences of selection, socialization, and social norms on the increase in teenage risky driving behavior in the presence of teenage passengers. The selection effect would be that teenagers tend to have passengers who are like them and are supportive of their driving behavior, such that risk-taking drivers would tend to have risk-taking passengers. The socialization effect would be that male passengers exert overt peer pressure in the form of encouraging risky driving behavior, an influence that seems to be greatest on males, but also operates on females. Female passengers, on the other hand, may provide peer pressure by saying to the driver, "Slow down!" "Don't follow that car so closely!" or otherwise communicating their preference for safe versus risky driving. Of course, these same effects could occur through perceived social norms. Males may feel, rightly or wrongly, that their male passenger would expect and approve of risky driving while their female passengers' expectations and preferences would be for less risky driving behavior. These perceptions may be the result of information from previous experience driving with other male and female passengers, or they may result from general impressions of what males and females like rather than being based on good or correct information about passengers' actual normative expectations. We are currently conducting a study to learn more about these effects. Using a factorial design, young driver participants are asked to drive a course on a driving simulator several times, each time with a different passenger. The randomly assigned passenger is an instructor or a male or female teenager. The teenage passenger is subtly presented to the driver as being either risk-aversive or risk-accepting with a brief description of the passenger's general interests, and by the appearance of the passenger (conservative or "edgy"). This will allow us to learn more about the effect of perceived social norms on risky driving behavior.

In future experimental studies, we hope to learn more about selection effects and possible interactions between driver and passenger characteristics on risky driving behavior. It is quite possible and likely that certain driver and passenger combinations might provide more powerful social influences than others. That is, while it is the case that male passengers appear to increase and female passengers to reduce risky driving behavior, some adolescent males and some females may be more susceptible than others in this regard. This can be explored by recruiting high- and low-sensation seeking drivers and evaluating their driving behavior in a simulator while riding with passengers who are high- or low-risk taking.

There is also substantial evidence that parenting practices protect novice drivers from both risky driving and crashes (Simons-Morton, 2007a). Evidence from retrospective and cross-sectional studies show that teenagers whose parents set limits on initial driving privileges and establish strict expectations for safe driving performance engage in less risky driving behavior (Hartos, Eitel, and Simons-Morton, 2001) and have fewer tickets and crashes (Simons-Morton, Hartos, Leaf, and Preusser, 2006b). The explanation for the effects of parenting behavior on teenage risky driving behavior and driving performance is relatively straightforward. Because adolescents are relatively independent and spend much of their time unsupervised, it is difficult for parents to directly influence adolescent behavior. Therefore, the effects of parenting are likely indirect through adolescents' perceptions of parent expectations and how involved and attentive parents might be (Simons-Morton and Hartos, 2002). Indeed, one of the better predictors of adolescent behavior is parental knowledge about general adolescent behavior (Kerr and Stattin, 2000; Simons-Morton et al., in press). The level of parental knowledge about adolescent behavior probably reflects the amount of trust and communication, and frequent general communication leads to a good understanding by the teenager about the things that parents really care about (Kerr and Stattin, 2000). So we think teenagers whose parents are involved and concerned, and communicate this by setting limits on their newly licensed teenager, but by maintaining a high level of communication with their teenager on this and other behaviors, are likely to experience these parenting behaviors as sustained social influence to drive in a safe manner.

Our group has evaluated a series of interventions developed to increase parental management of teenage driving. The effectiveness of the Checkpoints Program has been demonstrated in several randomized trials (Simons-Morton, 2007a). The Checkpoints Program employs persuasive communications about the nature of teenage driving risk and the benefits and efficacy of parent limit-setting. The Checkpoints Parent-Teen Driving Agreement is an educational tool that facilitates parent-teenager communication about teenager driving privileges. It has several checkpoints coinciding with the first few months of driving, the next several months, and then the next several months for the first year of licensure. The idea is for parents to set very strict limits on newly licensed teenagers for the first month or so (for example, driving with no teenage passengers, during daylight only), and then gradually to allow greater driving privileges over time as teenagers gain greater driving experience and skill. The premises of the Checkpoints Program are that parents are concerned about the safety of novice teenage driving and tend to set some limits on their initial driving privileges, but these limits tend not to be very strict or to last long enough for teenagers to develop driving skills before they are exposed to more risky driving conditions, such as with teenage passengers and at night. By setting limits, parents not only reduce the amount of driving under higher risk driving conditions, but also establish the normative perception that driving is dangerous and that newly licensed teenagers are not as good at driving as they will become with experience. A key mediator of increased parent limit-setting is parents' perceptions that it is normative among parents to establish such limits (Simons-Morton, Hartos, Leaf, and Preusser, 2006a).

SUMMARY

In this chapter, we have discussed social influence processes, taking into account broad social contexts. Proximal social influences are likely to operate very differently depending on social context. The well-established effects of proximal social influences on adolescent smoking, for example, may need to be reexamined as the proximal social environment gradually becomes more favorable with respect to this behavior during the period of adolescence. We note that social influences affect a wide range of health behaviors and provide an essential perspective for understanding socially mediated behavior. Although there is substantial research on the topic and a great deal of relevant theory, there is no grand unifying theory of social influence. We offer only a broad conceptualization of the relationships between social influences and health behavior, suggesting that the influences of socialization, selection, and social norms overlap and interact. We propose a conceptualization that emphasizes cultural and interpersonal influences on exposure to and interpretation of information that influences socialization, selection, and social norms processes leading to behavior.

The various effects of proximal social influence processes on behavior have proven difficult to sort out and are complicated by the additional influences of social context. However, there is substantial evidence that social influences are powerfully associated with health behavior. Research is needed so that we can better understand the nature of these influences, although it seems clear that socialization, selection, and social norms are highly interactive and not entirely discrete processes. In particular, there is a great lack of experimental studies designed to evaluate the nature of social influences. Moreover, there are few studies comparing the relative effects of programs designed to alter susceptibility to peer and media pressures compared with those that are designed to alter normative expectations.

FUTURE DIRECTIONS

The effect of social influences on health behavior is a rich area of study and practice. A great deal remains to be learned from observational and experimental studies about the nature of social influences, particularly in the following two areas. First, there remains a need to learn more about how social influences work in varying social contexts. Many social psychology studies have been designed to tease out the variability in social influences on behaviors such as honesty and truthfulness in varying contexts, and if we are to develop better theory and better health promotion programs, more experimental research is needed. The second great research challenge will be to learn more about inter-individual and intra-individual variation in social influences in similar and variable social contexts. For example, we need to learn the extent to which teenage passengers affect the driving performance of risk-seeking versus risk-adverse teenage drivers and how that varies under varying social conditions such as late at night and with multiple passengers versus one teenage passenger. An abundance of good theory exists, but the emergence of a grand unifying theory emerging does not seem imminent. Nonetheless, with a broad understanding of social context in mind, most research on social influences is well-informed by SCT.

REFERENCES

Ajzen, I. (1988). *Attitudes, personality, and behavior*. Chicago: Dorsey Press.

Alexander, C. S., Allen, P., Crawford, M. A., and McCormick, L. K. (1999). Taking a first puff: Cigarette smoking experiences among ethnically diverse adolescents. *Ethnicity and Health, 4*, 245–257.

Andreasen, A.R. (1994). Social marketing: Definition and domain. *Journal of Marketing and Public Policy, 13*(1),108–114.

Arnett, J. J. (2000). Emerging adulthood: A theory of development from the late teens through the twenties. *American Psychologist, 55*(5), 469–480.

Arnett, J. J. (2007). The myth of peer influence in adolescent smoking initiation. *Health Education and Behavior, 34*, 594–607.

Avenevoli, S., and Merikangas, K. R. (2003). Familial influences on adolescent smoking. *Addiction, 98*, 1–20.

Bandura, A. (1986). *Social foundations of thought and action*. Englewood Cliffs, NJ: Prentice Hall.

Bauman, K. E., and Ennett, S. T. (1996). On the importance of peer influence for adolescent drug use: Commonly neglected considerations. *Addiction, 91*(2), 185–198.

Berkman, L. F. (2000). Social support, social networks, social cohesion and health. *Social Work Health Care*, *31*, 3–14.

Berkman, L. F., and Glass, T. (2000). Social integration, social networks, social support, and health. In L. Berkman and I. Kawachi (eds.), *Social epidemiology* (pp. 137–173). New York: Oxford University Press.

Berkman, L. F., and Kawachi, I. (2000). *Social epidemiology*. New York: Oxford University Press.

Berkowitz, A. D. (2004). An overview of the social norms approach. In L. Lederman, L. Stewart, F. Goodhart, and L. Laitman (eds.), *Changing the culture of college drinking: A socially situated prevention campaign*. Cresskill, NJ: Hampton Press.

Berkowitz, A. D., and Perkins, H. W. (1986). Problem drinking among college students: A review of recent research. *Journal of American College Health*, *35*, 21–28.

Bjarnason, T., Thorlindsson, T., Sigfusdottire, I. D., and Welch, M. R. (2005). Familial and religious influences on adolescent alcohol use: A multi-level study of students and school communities. *Social Forces*, *84*, 375–390.

Botvin, G. J., Griffin, K. W., Diaz, T., and Ifill-Williams, M. (2001). Preventing binge drinking during early adolescence: One- and two-year follow-up of a school-based preventive intervention. *Psychology of Addictive Behaviors*, *15*, 360–365.

Botvin, G. J., Griffin, K. W., Diaz, T., Miller, N., and Ifill-Williams, M. (1999). Smoking initiation and escalation in early adolescent girls: One-year follow-up of a school-based prevention intervention for minority youth. *Journal of the American Medical Women's Association*, *54*, 139–43, 152.

Bronfenbrenner, U. (1979). *The ecology of human development*. Cambridge, MA: Harvard University Press.

Brook, J. S., Brook, D. W., and Whiteman, M. (1999). Older sibling correlates of young sibling drug use in the context of parent-child relations. *Genetic, Social and General Psychology Monographs*, *125*, 451–468.

Brown, J. D., and Witherspoon, E. M. (2002). The mass media and American adolescents' health. *Journal of Adolescent Health*, *31*, 153–170.

Buchanan D. (2000). *An ethic for health promotion: Rethinking the sources of human well-being*. New York: Oxford University Press.

Centers for Disease Control and Prevention (2001). Youth tobacco surveillance—United States, 2000. *Morbidity and Mortality Weekly Report*, *50*, 1–84.

Chen, L., Baker, S. P., Braver, E. R., and Li, G. (2000). Carrying passengers as a risk factor for crashes fatal to 16- and 17-year-old drivers. *Journal of the American Medical Association*, *283*, 1578–1582.

Christakis, N. A., and Fowler, J. H. (2007). The spread of obesity in a large social network over 32 years. *New England Journal of Medicine, 357*, 370–379.

Cohen, S., and Syme, S. L. (1985). *Social support and health*. Orlando: Academic Press.

Collins, R. (1988). *Theoretical sociology*. New York: Harcourt Brace Jovanovich.

Collins, R. L., Elliott, M. N., Berry, S. H., Kanouse, D. E., and Hunter, S. B. (2003). Entertainment television as a healthy sex educator: The impact of condom-efficacy information in an episode of *Friends*. *Pediatrics*, *112*, 1115–1121.

Conrad, K. M., Flay, B. R., and Hill, D. (1992). Why children start smoking cigarettes: Predictors of onset. *British Journal of Addiction*, *87*, 1711–1724.

Cullen, K. W., Lara, K. M., and De Moor, C. (2002). Familial concordance of dietary fat practices and intake. *Family and Community Health*, *25*(2), 65–75.

Curran, P. J., Stice, E., and Chassin, L. (1997). The relation between adolescent alcohol use and peer alcohol use: A longitudinal random coefficients model. *Journal of Consulting and Clinical Psychology*, *65*, 130–140.

Darling, N., and Steinberg, L. (1993). Parenting style as context: An integrative model. *Psychological Bulletin*, *113*, 487–496.

Delgado, H. M., and Austin, S. B. (2007). Can media promote responsible sexual behaviors among adolescents and young adults? *Current Opinion in Pediatrics*, *19*, 405–410.

Deniscombe, M. (2001). Peer group pressure, young people, and smoking: New developments and policy implications. *Drugs: Education, Prevention, and Policy, 8*, 7–32.

Dielman, T. E., Butchart, A. T., and Shope, J. T. (1993). Structural equation model tests of patterns of family interaction, peer alcohol use, and intrapersonal predictors of adolescent alcohol use and misuse. *Journal of Drug Education*, *23*, 273–316.

Dishion, T. J., and Andrews, D. W. (1995). Preventing escalation in problem behaviors with high-risk young adolescents: Immediate and 1-year outcomes. *Journal of Consulting and Clinical Psychology*, *63*, 538–548.

Dishion, T. J., Capaldi, D., Spracklen, K. M., and Li, F. (1995). Peer ecology of male adolescent drug use. *Development and Psychopathology*, *7*, 803–824.

Dubow, E. F., Huesmann, L. R., and Greenwood, D. (2006). Media and youth socialization: Underlying processes and moderators of effects. In J. Grusec and P. Hastings (eds.). *The handbook of socialization* (pp. 404–432). New York: Guilford Press.

Durkheim, É. (1897). *Suicide: A study in sociology*. Glencoe, IL: Free Press.

Eiser, J. R., Morgan, M., Gammage, P., Brooks, N., and Kirby, R. (1991). Adolescent health behavior and similarity-attraction: Friends share smoking habits (really), but much else besides. *British Journal of Social Psychology*, *30*, 339–348.

Engels, R. C., Vitaro, F., Blokland, E. D., de Kemp, R., and Scholte, R. H. (2004). Influence and selection process in friendships and adolescent smoking behaviour: The role of parental smoking. *Journal of Adolescence*, *27*, 531–544.

Ennett, S. T., and Bauman, K. E. (1994). The contribution of influence and selection to adolescent peer group homogeneity: The case of adolescent cigarette smoking. *Journal of Personality and Social Psychology*, *67*, 653–663.

Farrelly, M. C., Healton, C. G., Davis, K. C., Messeri, P., Hersey, J. C., and Haviland, M. L. (2002). Getting to the truth: Evaluating national tobacco countermarketing campaigns. *American Journal of Public Health*, *92*, 901–907.

Fishbein, M., and Ajzen, I. (1975). *Belief, attitude, intention, and behavior: An introduction to theory and research*. Reading, MA: Addison-Wesley.

Forgas, J. P., and Williams, K. D. (2001). *Social influence: Direct and indirect processes*. Philadelphia: Psychology Press.

Foss, R., Deikman, S., Goodman, A., and Bartley, C. (2003). Enhancing a norms program to reduce high-risk drinking among first year students. University of North Carolina at Chapel Hill. Retrieved from http://www .hsrc.unc.edu/safety_info/alcohol/UNCSocialNormProject.pdf.

Gass, R. H. and Seiter, J. S. (2003). *Persuasion, social influence and compliance gaining* (2nd ed.). Boston: Pearson Education.

Glass, T. A., and McAfee, M. J. (2006). Behavioral science at the crossroads in public health: Extending horizons, envisioning the future. *Social Science and Medicine*, *62*, 1650–1671.

Glider, P., Midvett, S., Mills-Novoa, B., Johannessen, K., and Collins, C. (2001). Challenging the collegiate rite of passage: A campus-wide social marketing media campaign to reduce binge drinking. *Journal of Drug Education*, *31*(2), 207–220.

Grusec, J. E., and Kuczynski, L. (1997). *Parenting and the internalization of values: A handbook of contemporary theory*. New York: Wiley.

Hansen, W. B. (1993). School-based alcohol prevention programs. *Alcohol Research and Health*, *17*(1), 54–60.

Harding, D. J. (2003). Counterfactual models of neighborhood effects: The effect of neighborhood poverty on dropping out and teenage pregnancy. *American Journal of Sociology*, *109*, 676–719.

Hartos, J. L., Eitel, P., and Simons-Morton, B. (2001). Do parent-imposed delayed licensure and restricted driving reduce risky driving behaviors among newly licensed teens? *Prevention Science*, *2*, 113–122.

Hawkins, J. D., Catalano, R. F., and Miller, J. Y. (1992). Risk and protective factors for alcohol and other drug problems in adolescence and early adulthood: Implications for substance abuse prevention. *Psychological Bulletin*, *112*(1), 64–105.

Hawkins, J. D., and Weis, J. G. (1985). The social development model: An integrated approach to delinquency prevention. *Journal of Primary Prevention*, *6*, 73–97.

Hirschi, T. (1969). *Causes of delinquency*. Los Angeles: University of California Press.

Hofschire, L. J., and Greenberg, B. S. (2002). Media's impact on adolescents' body dissatisfaction. In J. Brown, J. Steele, and K. Walsh-Childers (eds.), *Sexual teens, sexual media* (pp. 125–149). Mahwah, NJ: Erlbaum.

House, J. S., Landis, K. R., and Umberson, D. (1988). Social relationships and health. *Science, 241*, 540–545.

Howard, D., Qiu, Y., and Boekeloo, B. (2003). Personal and social contextual correlates of adolescent dating violence. *Journal of Adolescent Health, 33*, 9–17.

Hughes, D., Rodriguez, J., Smith, E. P., Johnson, D. J., Stevenson, H. C., and Spicer, P. (2006). Parents' ethnic-racial socialization practices: A review of research and directions for future study. *Developmental Psychology, 42*, 747–770.

Hyatt, S. L., and Collins, L. M. (2000). Using latent transition analysis to examine the relationship between perceived parental permissiveness and the onset of substance use. In R. J. Rose, L. Chassin, C. C. Presson, and S. J. Sherman (eds.), *Multivariate applications in substance abuse research: New methods for new questions* (pp. 259–288). Mahwah, NJ: Erlbaum.

Iannotti, R. J., Bush, P. J., and Weinfurt, K. P. (1996). Perception of friends' use of alcohol, cigarettes, and marijuana among urban schoolchildren: A longitudinal analysis. *Addictive Behaviors, 21*, 615–632.

Institute of Medicine (2001). *Health and behavior: The interplay of biological, behavioral, and social influences*. Washington, D.C.: National Academy Press.

Institute of Medicine (2003). *The future of the public's health in the 21st century*. Washington, D.C.: National Academy Press.

Johnston, L. D., O'Malley, P. M., Bachman, J. G., and Schulenberg, J. E. (2007). *Monitoring the future: National survey results on adolescent drug use: Overview of key findings, 2006*. Bethesda, MD: National Institute on Drug Abuse.

Kandel, D. B. (1978a). Homophily, selection, and socialization in adolescent friendships. *The American Journal of Sociology, 84*, 427–436.

Kandel, D. B. (1978b). Similarity in real-life adolescent friendship pairs. *Journal of Personality and Social Psychology, 36*, 306–312.

Kazdin, A. E. (2001). *Behavior modification in applied settings* (6th ed.). Belmont, CA: Wadsworth.

Kerr, M., and Stattin, H. (2000). What parents know, how they know it, and several forms of adolescent adjustment: Further support for a reinterpretation of monitoring. *Developmental Psychology, 36*, 366–380.

Kobus, K. (2003). Peers and adolescent smoking. *Addiction, 98*, 37–55.

Krosnick, J. A., and Judd, C. M. (1982). Transitions in social influences at adolescence: Who induces cigarette smoking? *Developmental Psychology, 18*, 359–368.

Larson, N. I., Neumark-Sztainer, D., Hannan, P. J., and Story, M. (2007). Family meals during adolescence are associated with higher diet quality and healthful meal patterns during young adulthood. *Journal of the American Dietetic Association, 107*, 1502–1510.

Landau, S. F., Björkqvist, K., Lagerspetz, K.M.J., Österman, K., and Gieon, L. (2002). The effect of religiosity and ethnic origin on direct and indirect aggression among males and females: Some Israeli findings. *Aggressive Behavior, 28*, 281–298.

Lott, B. (2003). Violence in low-income neighborhoods in the United States: Do we care? *Journal of Aggression, Maltreatment and Trauma, 8*(4), 1–15.

Lucas, L., and Lloyd, B. (1999). Starting smoking: Girls' explanations of the influence of peers. *Journal of Adolescence, 22*, 647–655.

Maxwell, K. A. (2002). Friends: The role of peer influence across adolescent risk behaviors. *Journal of Youth and Adolescence, 31*, 267–277.

Mayhew, D. R., Simpson, H. M., and Pak, A. (2003). Changes in collision rates among novice drivers during the first months of driving. *Accident Analysis and Prevention, 35*, 683–691.

McKinlay, J. B., and Marceau, L. D. (2000). Upstream healthy public policy: Lessons from the battle of tobacco. *International Journal of Health Services, 30*, 49–69.

McNeal, R. B., Jr., Hansen, W. B., Harrington, N. G., and Giles, S. M. (2004). How all stars works: An examination of program effects on mediating variables. *Health Education and Behavior*, *31*, 165–178.

McNeill, L. H., Kreuter, M. W., and Subramanian, S. V. (2006). Social environment and physical activity: A review of concepts and evidence. *Social Science and Medicine*, *63*, 1011–1022.

McPherson, M., Smith-Lovin, L., and Cook, J.M. (2001). Birds of a feather: Homophily in social networks. *Annual Review of Sociology*, *27*, 415–444.

Nichter, M., Nichter, M., Vuckovic, N., Quintero, G., and Ritenbaugh, C. (1997). Smoking experimentation and initiation among adolescent girls: Qualitative and quantitative findings. *Tobacco Control*, *6*, 285–295.

Nonnemaker, J. M., McNeely, C. A., and Blum, R. W. (2003). Public and private domains of religiosity and adolescent health risk behaviors: Evidence from the National Longitudinal Study of Adolescent Health. *Social Science and Medicine*, *57*, 2049–2054.

Oetting, E. R. (1999). Primary socialization theory: Developmental stages, spirituality, government institutions, sensation seeking, and theoretical implications. V. *Substance Use and Misuse*, *34*, 947–982.

Oetting, E. R., and Donnermeyer, J. (1998). Primary socialization theory: The etiology of drug use and deviance. I. *Substance Use and Misuse*, *33*, 995–1026.

Olson, C. K., Kutner, L. A., Warner, D. E., Almerigi, J. B., Baer, L., Nicholi, A. M., et al. (2007). Factors correlated with violent video game use by adolescent boys and girls. *Journal of Adolescent Health*, *41*, 77–83.

Pentz, M. A., Dwyer, J. H., MacKinnon, D. P., Flay, B. R., Hansen, W. B., Wang, E. Y., et al. (1989). A multicommunity trial for primary prevention of adolescent drug abuse: Effects on drug use prevalence. *JAMA*, *261*, 3259–3266.

Perkins, D. F., and Jones, K. R. (2004). Risk behaviors and resiliency within physically abused adolescents. *Child Abuse and Neglect*, *28*, 547–563.

Pollack, H. A., and Jacobson, P. D. (2003). Political economy of youth smoking regulation. *Addiction*, *98*, 123–138.

Pomery, E. A., Gibbons, F. X., Gerrard, M., Cleveland, M. J., Brody, G. H., and Wills, T. A. (2005). Families and risk: Prospective analysis of familial and social influences on adolescent substance use. *Journal of Family Psychology*, *19*(4), 560–570.

Prelow, H. M., Bowman, M. A., and Weaver, S. R. (2007). Predictors of psychosocial well-being in urban African and European American youth: The role of ecological factors. *Journal of Youth and Adolescence*, *36*(4), 543–553.

Rajan, K. B., Leroux, B. G., Peterson, A. V., Bricker, J. B., Andersen, M. R., Kealey, K. A., et al. (2003). Nine-year prospective association between older siblings' smoking and children's daily smoking. *Journal of Adolescent Health*, *33*, 25–30.

Read, P. J, Wood, M. D., Davidoff, O. J. McLacken, J., and Campbell, J. F. (2002). Making the transition from high school to college: The role of alcohol-related social influence factors in students' drinking. *Substance Abuse 23*(1), 53–65.

Reagan, J., and Lee, M. J. (2007). Online technology, edutainment, and infotainment. In C. A. Lin and D. J. Atkin (eds.), *Communication, technology and social change: Theory and implications* (pp. 183–200). Mahwah, NJ: Erlbaum.

Regnerus, M. D., and Elder, G. H. (2003). Staying on track in school: Religious influences in high- and low-risk settings. *Journal of the Scientific Study of Religion*, *42*(4), 633–649.

Rideout, V., Roberts, D. F., and Goehr, U. G. (2005). *Generation M: Media in the lives of 8–18 year-olds*. Menlo Park, CA: The Henry J. Kaiser Family Foundation.

Rose, R. J., Viken, R. J., Dick, D. M., Bates, J. E., Pulkkinen, L., and Kaprio, J. (2003). It does take a village: Nonfamilial environments and children's behavior. *Psychological Science*, *14*, 273–277.

Scheier, L. M., Botvin, G. J., Diaz, T., and Ifill-Williams, M. (1997). Ethnic identity as a moderator of psychosocial risk and adolescent alcohol and marijuana use: Concurrent and longitudinal analyses. *Journal of Child and Adolescent Substance Abuse*, *6*(1), 21–47.

Simons-Morton B. G. (2004). The protective effect of parental expectations against early adolescent smoking initiation. *Health Education Research, 19*(5), 561–569.

Simons-Morton, B. G. (2007a). Parent involvement in novice teen driving: rationale, evidence of effects, and potential for enhancing graduated driver licensing effectiveness. *Journal of Safety Research, 38*, 193–202.

Simons-Morton, B. G. (2007b). Social influences on adolescent substance use. *American Journal of Health Behavior, 6*, 672–684.

Simons-Morton, B. G., and Chen, R. (2005). Latent growth curve analyses of parent influences on drinking progression among early adolescents. *Journal of Studies on Alcohol, 66*, 5–13.

Simons-Morton, B. G., Chen, R., Abroms, L., and Haynie, D. L. (2004). Latent growth curve analyses of peer and parent influences on smoking progression among early adolescents. *Health Psychology, 23*, 612–621.

Simons-Morton, B. G., Chen, R., Hand, L., and Haynie, D. (2008). Parenting behavior and adolescent conduct problems: Reciprocal and mediational effects. *Journal of School Violence, 7*(1):3–25.

Simons-Morton, B. G., Crump, A. D., Haynie, D. L., Saylor, K. E., Eitel, P., and Yu, K. (1999). Psychosocial, school, and parent factors associated with recent smoking among early-adolescent boys and girls. *Preventive Medicine, 28*(2), 138–148.

Simons-Morton, B. G., and Hartos, J. L. (2002). Application of authoritative parenting to adolescent health behavior. In R. DiClemente, R. Crosby, and M. Kegler (eds.), *Emerging theories and models in health promotion research and practice: Strategies for improving practice* (pp. 100–125). San Francisco: Jossey-Bass.

Simons-Morton, B. G., Hartos, J., Leaf, W., and Preusser, D. (2006a). Increasing parent limits on novice young drivers: Cognitive mediation of the effect of persuasive messages. *Journal of Adolescent Research, 21*, 83–105.

Simons-Morton, B. G., Hartos, J., Leaf, W., and Preusser, D. (2006b). Do recommended driving limits affect teen-reported tickets and crashes during the first year of teen independent driving? *Traffic Injury Prevention, 7*, 1–10.

Simons-Morton, B. G. and Haynie, D. L. (2003). Growing up drug free: A developmental challenge. In M.H. Bornstein, L. Davidson, C.L.M. Keyes, K. A. Moore, and Center for Child Well-being (eds.), *Well-being: Positive development across the life course* (pp. 109–122). Mahwah, NJ: Erlbaum.

Simons-Morton, B. G., Haynie, D. L., Crump, A. D., Eitel, P., and Saylor, K. E. (2001). Peer and parent influences on smoking and drinking among early adolescents. *Health Education and Behavior, 28*(1), 95–107.

Simons-Morton, B. G., Haynie, D. L., Saylor, K., Crump, A. D., and Chen, R. (2005). The effects of the Going Places program on early adolescent substance use and antisocial behavior. *Prevention Science, 6*, 187–197.

Simons-Morton, B. G., Lerner, N., and Singer, J. (2005). The observed effects of teenage passengers on the risky driving behavior of teenage drivers. *Accident Analysis and Prevention, 37*, 973–982.

Smith, E. P., Walker, K., Fields, L., Brookins, C. C., and Seay, R. C. (1999). Ethnic identity and its relationship to self esteem, perceived efficacy and prosocial attitudes in early adolescence. *Journal of Adolescence, 22*, 867–880.

Snyder, L. B., Milici, F. F., Slater, M., Sun, H., and Strizhakova, Y. (2006). Effects of alcohol advertising exposure on drinking among youth. *Archives of Pediatrics and Adolescent Medicine, 160*, 18–24.

Sorensen, G., Stoddard, A. M., Dubowitz, T, Barbeau, E. M., Bigby, J., Emmons, K. M., et al. (2007). The influence of social context on changes in fruit and vegetable consumption: Results of the healthy directions study. *American Journal of Public Health, 97*, 1216–1227.

Steinberg, L., Fletcher, A., and Darling, N. (1994). Parental monitoring and peer influences on adolescent substance use. *Pediatrics, 93*, 1060–1064.

Stewart, E. A., Schreck, C. J., and Simons, R. L. (2006). "I ain't gonna let no one disrespect me": Does the code of the street reduce or increase violent victimization among African American adolescents? *Journal of Research in Crime and Delinquency, 43*(4), 427–458.

Stockdale, J. E. (2001). The role of the media. In E. Houghton and A. M. Roche (eds.), *Learning about drinking* (pp. 209–242). Philadelphia: Brunner-Routledge.

Story, M., Neumark-Sztainer, D., and French, S. (2002). Individual and environmental influences on adolescent eating behaviors. *Journal of the American Dietetic Association, 102*(Suppl. 3), 40–51.

Townsend, T., and Lanphier, E. (2007). Family influences on racial identity among African American youth. *Journal of Black Psychology, 33*, 278–298.

Unger, J. B., Rohrbach, L. A., Cruz, T. B., Baezconde-Garbanati, L., Howard, K. A., Palmer, P. H. et al. (2001). Ethnic variation in peer influences on adolescent smoking. *Nicotine and Tobacco Research, 3*, 167–176.

Urberg, K. A., Degirmencioglu, S. M., and Pilgrim, C. (1997). Close friend and group influence on adolescent cigarette smoking and alcohol use. *Developmental Psychology, 33*, 834–844.

Urberg, K. A., Degirmencioglu, S. M. and Tolson, J. M. (1998). Adolescent friendship selection and termination: The role of similarity. *Journal of Social and Personal Relationships, 15*(5), 703–710.

Urberg, K. A., Luo, Q., Pilgrim, C., and Degirmencioglu, S. M. (2003). A two-stage model of peer influence in adolescent substance use: Individual and relationship-specific differences in susceptibility to influence.

Wakefield, M., Flay, B., Nichter, M., and Giovino, G. (2003). Role of the media in influencing trajectories of youth smoking. *Addiction, 98*(Suppl. 1), 79–103.

Wills, T. A., and Cleary, S. D. (1999). Peer and adolescent substance use among 6th-9th graders: latent growth analyses of influence versus selection mechanisms. *Health Psychology, 18*, 453–463.

Windle, M. (2000). Parental, sibling, and peer influences on adolescent substance use and alcohol problems. *Applied Developmental Science, 4*, 98–110.

Wong, C. A., Eccles, J. S., and Sameroff, A. (2003). The influence of ethnic discrimination and ethnic identification on African American adolescents' school and socioemotional adjustment. *Journal of Personality, 71*, 1197–1232

CHAPTER

4

SELF-ESTEEM ENHANCEMENT THEORY: PROMOTING HEALTH ACROSS THE LIFE SPAN

David L. DuBois
Brian R. Flay
Michael C. Fagen

SELF-ESTEEM, HEALTH, AND WELL-BEING

Self-esteem—commonly defined as overall feelings of self-worth (Harter, 1999)—is at once both a widely touted and often maligned construct. Historically, there is a long tradition of scholars and practitioners embracing the idea that a sense of positive self-regard is essential not only for emotional well-being and stability (Allport, 1955; Rogers, 1961), but also for the fulfillment of one's innate positive potential as a person (Branden, 1969; Maslow, 1954). During the 1980s, interest in self-esteem rose to a fever pitch and launched what has been referred to subsequently as a "self-esteem movement" in the United States (Twenge, 2006). A California task force established during this period captured much of the prevailing sentiment when it concluded that self-esteem "is the likeliest candidate for a social vaccine, something that inoculates against the lures of crime, violence, substance abuse, teen pregnancy . . . and educational failure" (California Task Force to Promote Self-Esteem and Social Responsibility, 1990, page 4). Optimism about the explanatory and healing power of self-esteem continues to be readily apparent today. Scores of studies are published each year investigating hypothesized links between feelings of self-worth and myriad aspects of health and well-being. Likewise, strategies to enhance self-esteem are featured with regularity in a wide range of interventions targeting different age groups. These efforts are based on the premise that feelings of personal worth can act as a psychological engine of sorts that propels us toward positive health and adaptation. Along the way, the groups and communities with whom high self-esteem individuals come into contact will benefit as well.

A growing chorus of criticism, however, has brought these long-standing assumptions about self-esteem into serious question. Noted psychologist Martin Seligman (1993), for example, has argued that a high or low level of self-esteem is simply an "epiphenomenon" or by-product of one's current health and adaptation and therefore entirely lacking in explanatory value. Others have gone further to propose a "dark side" (Baumeister, Smart, and Boden, 1994) for high self-esteem. These views have highlighted various ways in which an inflated (that is, unrealistically positive) sense of self may seriously compromise personal health and adjustment (Colvin and Block, 1994; Twenge, 2006) and, if challenged, trigger aggressive or violent behavior that imperils the welfare of others as well (Baumeister et al., 1994; Baumeister, Bushman, and Campbell, 2000). Such perspectives suggest that efforts directed toward enhancing self-esteem are likely not just to be ineffective, but actually exacerbate some of the very problems they are intended to help prevent. In her recent book, *Generation Me* (Twenge, 2006), psychologist Jean Twenge marshaled support for this perspective by presenting evidence that levels of both self-esteem and narcissism—a trait that involves tendencies toward excessive self-admiration and self-centeredness—have increased among young people in the United States during the same period of time that problems such as depression, anxiety, cynicism, and loneliness have been on the rise. To Twenge and others, the explanation for these seemingly paradoxical trends lies in our society's "culture of self-worth," in which holding oneself in high esteem has come to assume greater importance than personal accomplishment and productive engagement with others.

What is to be made of these polarizing views regarding self-esteem and its relationship to health and well-being? In this chapter, we present a new theory—self-esteem enhancement theory (SET)—that is intended to answer this question. Our goal in developing the theory was not to support one or the other side of the "self-esteem debate" (Edwards, 1995) that is outlined above. Rather, based on accumulating evidence that self-esteem can indeed be implicated in both favorable and unfavorable health and well-being, our aim is to provide a single, integrative framework that accounts for both possibilities. In doing so, our goal is to develop a set of testable and practical guidelines for enhancing self-esteem within health promotion interventions that will maximize benefits and minimize, if not eliminate, the potential for unwanted negative outcomes. SET thus most closely resembles what Glanz, Rimer, and Lewis (2002, page 26) refer to as a change theory or theory of action, in which the emphasis is on guiding the development of interventions (as contrasted with a theory of the problem, in which the focus is more on explanation and prediction of behavior).

In this chapter, we begin by presenting an overview of SET and the guidelines that it posits for the development of effective interventions. We then review empirical evidence for the effectiveness of esteem-enhancement interventions and the extent to which this evidence is consistent with the predictions of SET. Two health promotion interventions that are aligned with the guidelines of SET are described in detail. One of these interventions has been rigorously evaluated and thus provides a strong test of SET as a theory of change. We conclude by considering strengths and limitations of SET and promising directions for further refinement and application of the theory.

SELF-ESTEEM ENHANCEMENT THEORY

Self-esteem enhancement theory has its origins in recent research—much of it conducted in developmental, clinical, and social psychology—that has significantly advanced our understanding of the complex and dynamic structure of self-esteem, the processes that influence how it is formed and maintained, and its implications for health and well-being. SET includes five major sets of constructs: (a) contextual opportunities; (b) esteem formation and maintenance processes; (c) self-esteem; (d) health and well-being; and (e) modifying influences. The hypothesized associations among these sets of constructs within SET are depicted in Figure 4.1. As will be discussed, a key tenet of SET is that interventions should not focus simply on raising self-esteem, but rather should devote equal attention to implementing strategies that enable participants to cultivate a strong and healthy foundation for their feelings of self-worth.

FIGURE 4.1 Self-Esteem Enhancement Theory

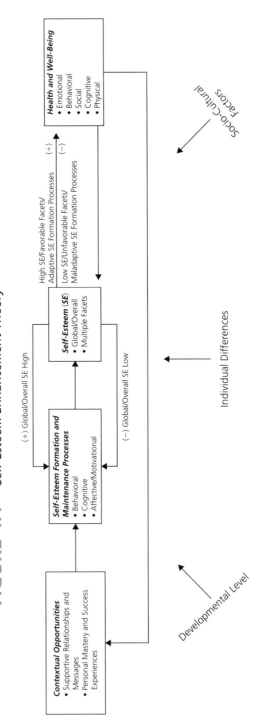

CONTEXTUAL OPPORTUNITIES

Overview

The Contextual Opportunities portion of the model is concerned with the individual's surrounding environment and whether it is conducive to developing and sustaining feelings of self-worth. Contextual opportunities can take two primary forms: (1) Supportive Relationships and Messages, and (2) Personal Mastery and Success Experiences. The focus on these two types of experiences is derived from research indicating that feelings of social acceptance and personal competence are fundamental determinants of self-esteem throughout life (Harter, 1999).

Supportive relationships are available when others in the individual's immediate social network (for example, friends, family, coworkers, classmates) interact with the person in a manner that can be expected to promote self-esteem. These interactions may include emotional support (empathy, love, caring), instrumental support (tangible aid and services), and informational support (advice, suggestions, and information). (For more in-depth discussion of these differing forms of support, see House, 1981.) Appraisal or esteem support, however, is assumed to be of particular importance (Heaney and Israel, 2002; House, 1981). This form of support involves the "provision of information that is useful for self-evaluation purposes, in other words, constructive feedback, affirmation, and social comparison" (Heaney and Israel, 2002, page 186). As is evident from this description, esteem support includes any social interactions that serve to validate a person's strengths and positive qualities. It also encompasses, however, situations in which feedback from others serves to highlight potentially more problematic aspects of one's personality or behavior that are not necessarily conducive to maintaining a high level of self-esteem. Expressing concern to a friend about her sedentary lifestyle thus may be supportive because it encourages her to become more active, a change that can be expected to help her feel better about herself (McDonald and Hodgdon, 1991). Supportive messages are assumed to be able to serve similar functions. This feedback, however, emanates from sources outside of the individual's immediate social network. Such sources include health educators and care providers, the media, and more informal channels of communication with members of one's community.

Opportunities for personal mastery and success are present when individuals have access to settings and activities in which they can both cultivate and demonstrate competence. Following an ecological model (Sallis and Owen, 2002), these opportunities may be present to varying degrees in each of the contexts in which individuals spend the bulk of their time every day (for example, home, school, work) as well as in the broader context of their surrounding communities. High self-esteem is most likely to result when individuals experience a sense of competence in pursuits to which they attach personal value or importance (Harter, 1999). This suggests that the competence-enhancing opportunities that exist within any individual's environment should be evaluated at least in part with respect to their degree of alignment with that person's interests and values. Thus, even though a school might provide a wide range of athletic programs, for a student with interest in other pursuits (for example, the arts) there may not be sufficient opportunities for skill building in areas most relevant to his or her self-esteem.

Implications for Intervention

Many esteem-enhancement programs have consisted of individual-level change strategies, such as exercises to help participants change their attitudes or feelings about themselves (Hattie, 1992). By contrast, SET assumes that it is important for interventions to adopt a more ecological orientation. A key goal should be to ensure that participants have sufficient opportunities in their environments to develop and maintain a high level of self-esteem. The assessment phase should consider the needs that participants may have for supportive relationships within their immediate social networks as well as for esteem-enhancing messages from other sources. Similarly, there should be attention given to whether the intended participants have access to settings and activities in which they can cultivate a sense of competence. Research suggests that experiences in multiple life domains and types of relationships each exert unique influences on self-esteem (Harter, 1999). A holistic and comprehensive approach thus may be necessary to fully address the esteem-enhancement needs of participants, especially within initiatives that have relatively broad goals such as promoting overall wellness.

> A key goal should be to ensure that participants have sufficient opportunities in their environments to develop and maintain a high level of self-esteem.

In designing these aspects of interventions, care should be taken to facilitate experiences that are likely to promote feelings of self-worth. Particular emphasis should be given to fostering relationships that will offer esteem-based forms of support, including both validation of strengths and constructive feedback on areas in need of change or improvement. Efforts also should be focused on building competence in areas that align with participant interests and values. In many instances, it may be feasible to generate esteem-enhancement opportunities through modifications to existing relationships or settings in participants' lives. Depending on the current environmental circumstances of the targeted population, however, it may be essential to introduce new social ties and additional avenues for building skills. The goals of the program should be kept in mind as well. In planning an exercise program, for example, it would be important to ensure both that participants interact with others who offer them support specifically for engaging in physical activity and that they have access to necessary facilities and instruction. Clearly, SET does not assume a one-size-fits-all approach to planning contextual opportunities for esteem enhancement. Rather, efforts should be guided by the principles outlined above, with specific content tailored to needs of the target population, program goals, and characteristics of the host setting and surrounding community.

SELF-ESTEEM FORMATION AND MAINTENANCE PROCESSES

Overview

Theorists (for example, James, 1890; Rosenberg, 1979) have long maintained that the desire to feel good about oneself is a universal and fundamental aspect of human functioning. An extensive body of research supports this idea (for a review, see Tesser, 2004). In SET, it is assumed that when individuals' efforts to achieve self-esteem are successful, these efforts will prove reinforcing and thus be repeated. By contrast, when feelings of worth are not experienced, the individual is expected to adjust his or her efforts in an attempt to better meet needs for self-esteem. These feedback loops are an important part of SET and are depicted in Figure 4.1.

Our need to experience a sense of self-worth may be satisfied primarily through efforts that are directed toward developing personal competencies and supportive, affirming relationships with others (Harter, 1999). This pattern may be established at an early age and then continued as a rewarding and effective means of maintaining positive feelings of self-regard. If the skills and relationships that are cultivated are such that they also promote overall health and well-being (an important assumption that will be discussed below), motivation for self-esteem then can assume a key role in fostering positive adaptation throughout the life span.

To some extent, however, all persons also rely on a variety of self-protective or self-enhancing strategies to preserve a favorable sense of self-regard (Blaine and Crocker, 1993; Kaplan, 1986; Rhodewalt, 2006; Rosenberg, 1979). As described by Kaplan (1986),

> Self-protective/self-enhancing responses are oriented toward the goal of (1) forestalling the experience of self-devaluing judgments and consequent distressful feelings (self-protective patterns) and (2) increasing the occasions for positive self-evaluations and self-accepting feelings (self-enhancing responses). (page 174)

Self-protective/self-enhancing strategies may involve self-referent cognitions, personal need-value systems, and personal behavior (Kaplan, 1986). Illustratively, when faced with a failure experience that threatens self-esteem, an individual may respond by not accepting responsibility for a role in the outcome (self-referent cognitions), by devaluing the importance of success in that area (personal need-value systems), and/or by seeking out alternative, less challenging activities (personal behavior). These are just a few of the myriad ways in which individuals have been found to attempt to both bolster and safeguard feelings of self-worth. (For a more extensive overview, see DuBois, Lopez, and Parra, 2004.)

Research points toward both favorable and unfavorable implications of self-protective/self-enhancing strategies for health and well-being. Findings concerning positive illusions about the self (which might be supported by a variety of self-protective/self-enhancing tendencies) are illustrative of this duality. Some research suggests that positive illusions can improve mood and increase both adaptive social behavior (for example, helping others) and effective problem solving (Taylor and Brown, 1988, 1994). Self-enhancing responses, furthermore, have been indicated to be helpful in coping with stressful life events, such as parental divorce (Mazur, Wolchik, Virdin, Sandler, and West, 1999) and sexual victimization (Taylor and Brown, 1988). Yet, there also are numerous studies in which individuals with inflated or unrealistically positive views of themselves have exhibited poorer outcomes (for reviews, see Colvin and Block, 1994; Harter, 2006; Tennen and Affleck, 1993). In this research inflated self-perceptions have been identified both directly via self-reported narcissistic tendencies (Baumeister et al., 2000) and more indirectly via comparisons with external criteria such as objective assessments of ability and the views of others who know the person well (Colvin, Block, and Funder, 1995; Hughes, Cavell, and Grossman, 1997; Shedler, Mayman, and Manis, 1994). In accordance with the findings of these investigations, theorists have noted a variety of liabilities that may be associated with positive illusions in self-perceptions. These include, for example, vulnerability to disconfirmation from others, the pressure of living up to an inflated self-image, limitations in self-understanding, and overconfidence leading to interpersonal difficulties (Blaine and Crocker, 1993; Colvin and Block, 1994; Harter, 2006; Tennen and Affleck, 1993). Positive illusions about the self appear to be especially likely to prove problematic when they are extreme (Baumeister, 1989) and when they are intertwined with self-protective strategies that are overtly maladaptive or that involve health-compromising behaviors such as aggression or drug use (Baumeister et al., 1996; DuBois et al., 2004; Kaplan, 1986).

Implications for Intervention

Interventions to enhance self-esteem typically have been concerned primarily with increasing feelings of self-worth among participants. From the preceding discussion, however, it is clear that the processes through which self-esteem are acquired and sustained may be an equally important concern. SET assumes that interventions oriented toward esteem enhancement should reflect this principle. It may be helpful in this regard to incorporate a psycho-educational component in which participants are made aware of the universal human need for self-esteem, how this can influence their thoughts, attitudes, and behaviors, and specific types of self-protective/self-enhancing strategies and their potential implications for health and well-being (DuBois, 2003). Armed with this type of information, participants may then be engaged in a self-assessment of the ways in which they strive to protect and increase their own self-esteem. Many of these processes are relatively subtle and may even be outside of conscious awareness. For this reason, a variety of strategies may be needed to facilitate optimal levels of insight. It may prove fruitful, for example, to have participants elicit feedback from significant others in their lives to provide an external perspective. Attitudes and behaviors that pose risks to health or well-being then can be targeted for personal improvement goals.

There also are likely to be instances in which particular esteem formation and maintenance processes can be prioritized for attention for entire groups or subgroups of participants. It appears, for example, that many adolescents who experience esteem-damaging forms of social rejection attempt to restore their feelings of self-worth via affiliation with more accepting, but deviant, peer groups. These same youth also may attempt to cope through aggression (as a form of retaliation against individuals or groups they hold responsible) or drug use (as a means of screening out negative thoughts and feelings about themselves) (Kaplan, 1986). Various commonalities in how self-esteem is safeguarded may be similarly present for groups that are reluctant to engage in particular health behaviors (for example, condom use, exercise). Such individuals often may seek to protect their self-esteem by overlooking information that would challenge the wisdom of their decisions or by discounting the importance of the behaviors involved.

The apparently fundamental nature of our motivation to feel good about ourselves underscores the importance, when necessary, of identifying adaptive strategies for fulfilling this need that can substitute for ones that pose threats to our health and well-being. To the extent that existing strategies are effective in safeguarding self-esteem (or simply are believed to be), it is unrealistic to expect them to be abandoned without a convincing demonstration that alternative strategies can serve the same end. Individuals who are prone to use rationalization (a self-protective/self-enhancing strategy) to justify engaging in risky behavior (for example, unprotected sexual activity) thus may need to be helped to see the potential for achieving a satisfying level of positive self-regard through more healthy lifestyle choices. Temporary lapses in self-esteem should be anticipated as an outgrowth of individuals relinquishing existing strategies for protecting feelings of self-worth as well as the trial and error process of becoming adept in more adaptive alternatives. SET assumes that interventions will need to provide participants with high levels of support and encouragement to ensure that they can overcome these potential barriers and avoid "relapse" to more reliable (but less adaptive) strategies for managing their self-esteem.

SELF-ESTEEM

Overview

Theoretically, overall feelings of self-worth provide a valuable foundation of emotional security and can facilitate effective coping and problem solving (Branden, 1969; Rosenberg, 1979). High levels of self-esteem thus may enhance health and well-being directly as well as by fostering resilience to stress and adversity (Mann, Hosman, Schaalma, and de Vries, 2004; Rutter, 1987). These benefits are suggested by research in which feelings of self-worth have been linked to outcomes such as happiness, life satisfaction, positive health practices, physical health, academic achievement, and job performance. Conversely, the relative absence of feelings of self-worth has been linked to emotional difficulties (most notably, depression, anxiety, and loneliness) as well as a wide range of other health concerns. The latter include eating disorders, obesity, high-risk sexual activity, substance use, violent behavior, victimization, and suicidal tendencies, and, among older adults, increased risk for all-cause mortality (for reviews, see DuBois and Flay, 2004; DuBois and Tevendale, 1999; Emler, 2001; Judge and Bono, 2001; A. Yarcheski, Mahon, T. J. Yarcheski, and Cannella, 2004). Several prospective studies have found initial levels of self-esteem to predict later outcomes, controlling for baseline levels of outcomes and/or other explanatory measures, thereby suggesting a potential causal contribution of feelings of self-esteem to later functioning. A recent study using data from the Dunedin Multidisciplinary Health and Development Study birth cohort (Trzesniewski et al., 2006), for example, found that adolescents with low self-esteem had significantly poorer mental and physical health, worse economic prospects, and higher levels of criminal behavior during adulthood, compared with adolescents with high self-esteem. These associations were not explained by adolescent depression, gender, or socioeconomic status.

At the same time, it is important to note that the associations between self-esteem and measures of functioning in other areas typically have been relatively modest in magnitude and (especially in prospective studies) have not consistently reached statistical significance. These aspects of findings have been emphasized by those who question the existence or practical importance of self-esteem's effects on health and well-being (see, for example, Baumeister, Campbell, Krueger, and Vohs, 2003; Goodson, Buhi, and Dunsmore, 2006). In several instances, higher levels of self-esteem have even been linked to problematic outcomes. For example, adolescents' feelings of self-worth have been associated positively with alcohol and drug use, earlier initiation of sexual intercourse, and delinquent behavior and gang involvement (DuBois and Tevendale, 1999). These findings are consistent with the potential discussed earlier for self-esteem to be supported by attitudes and behaviors that compromise functioning in other areas. SET attempts to account for all available research by assuming that a high level of overall self-esteem is generally facilitative of health and well-being, but that these benefits can be obscured when maladaptive strategies are relied on to acquire and sustain positive self-evaluations (DuBois and Flay, 2004).

Recent research has increasingly moved beyond overall feelings of self-worth to assess more specific facets of self-evaluation. These investigations have highlighted the importance of self-evaluations that are tied to particular domains or areas of experience (DuBois and Tevandale, 1999). Poor body image, for example, has been associated with greater risk for eating disorder symptomatology (for example, Jackson and Chen, 2008) as well as sexual risk behaviors (Wingood, DiClemente, Harrington, and Davies, 2002). Patterns of self-evaluation across multiple domains appear to be especially important (Harter, 1999). Among adolescents, for example, a profile in which peer-oriented sources of self-esteem predominate over family and school has been associated with greater involvement in problem behaviors such as substance use and fighting (DuBois and Silverthorn, 2004; DuBois, Burk-Braxton, Swenson, et al., 2002). Adolescents may come to rely on peers as a prevailing source of self-esteem in response to difficulties they experience deriving a sense of self-worth in their relationships with parents, teachers, and other adults (DuBois, Burk-Braxton, Swenson, et al., 2002). At the same time, when peer-oriented sources of self-esteem lag behind those pertaining to more adult-oriented domains, adolescents appear to be susceptible to emotional difficulties such as depression and anxiety (DuBois and Tevendale, 1999; Harter, 1999). There is also evidence that high levels of peer self-esteem can be important in promoting positive health behaviors among adolescents. More favorable self-evaluations of peer acceptance have been found to predict higher levels of metabolic control among adolescent girls with Type I diabetes (Maharaj, Daneman, Olmstead, and Rodin, 2004), for example, as well as disclosure of HIV status among HIV-positive adolescents (Wiener and Battles, 2006). Although complex, such patterns are consistent with the perspective that a balanced profile of positive self-evaluation across multiple domains is likely to be most conducive to overall health and well-being (Harter, 1999).

Research considering other specific facets of self-esteem has yielded further note-worthy findings. Several of these studies have focused on short-term patterns of change or instability in levels of self-esteem that are not likely to be reflected in traditional, trait-oriented assessments. In a study of 455 gay men (Martin and Knox, 1997), for example, self-esteem instability was found to be greater among those who had recently engaged in unprotected anal intercourse with non primary partners. The authors hypothesized that episodes of self-esteem injury might motivate some gay men to engage in risky sex. This interpretation is consistent with the view that insta-bility in feelings of self-worth may reflect a fragile or vulnerable sense of self and a reliance on counter-productive esteem-enhancement strategies (Kernis, Goldman, 2006). Other investigations have called attention to the health significance of more collective facets of self-evaluation that pertain to one's membership in different social groups, such as those defined by race, ethnicity, gender, or religion (Crocker, Luhtanen, Blain, and Broadnax, 1994). An investigation of African American adoles-cent girls (Salazar et al., 2004), for example, found that reports of a more positive ethnic identity (in conjunction with more favorable overall self-esteem and body image) were associated with attributes of partner communication about sex that, in turn, predicted greater frequency in refusal of unprotected sex. Such findings illustrate the potential for different facets of self-esteem to combine both with each other and with more general feelings of self-worth in shaping health behaviors and outcomes.

Implications for Intervention

It follows from the preceding discussion that within SET strategies focused directly on fortifying overall feelings of self-worth are a recommended component of esteem-enhancement interventions. A variety of affective and cognitive-behavioral techniques have been described that may be useful for this purpose (DuBois et al., 2004; Harter, 1999; Hattie, 1992). At the same time, in keeping with the generally limited explana-tory power of overall self-esteem, SET assumes that interventions should also target more specific facets of self-evaluation. Domain-specific self-evaluations appear to be influenced both by perceived attributes of the self in different areas (self-concept) and by the standards against which those attributes are judged (self-standards) (DuBois et al., 2000). It may be useful, therefore, to foster participants' appreciation of their strengths within relevant domains while simultaneously encouraging them to adopt standards or goals for themselves in those areas that are challenging, but realistic and attainable. Special attention should be given to strengthening those facets of participant self-esteem that are likely to be key determinants of the intended outcomes of the inter-vention (DuBois, 2003). In some instances, for example, it may be feasible to focus on self-evaluations that are directly tied to health behaviors of interest, such as self-care skills for chronic health conditions (see, for example, Wallston, Rothman, and Cherrington, 2007). Strategies that address multiple facets of participants' self-esteem in a more holistic manner also may be valuable (DuBois and Tevendale, 1999; Harter, 1999), especially within interventions that have comprehensive health promotion goals (Flay, 2002).

HEALTH AND WELL-BEING

Overview

The theory and research summarized in previous sections of this chapter indicate that self-esteem (along with its associated facets and supporting processes) has the potential to influence all major areas of health and well-being—emotional, behavioral, social, cognitive, and physical (Figure 4.1). Within each domain, effects may take the form of avoidance of (or increased susceptibility to) disorder, disease, and other health-compromising behaviors and states as well as promotion of (or decreases in) aspects of health and well-being that are associated with quality of life and fulfillment of personal potential. These assumptions align well with prevailing conceptualizations of health that emphasize physical, mental, and social aspects of well-being and that are not limited to the absence of disease or infirmity (World Health Organization, 1992).

As shown in Figure 4.1, different facets of health and well-being are also expected in SET to have reciprocal effects on self-esteem. This portion of the model is supported by research indicating that global and specific facets of self-esteem tend to be strengthened by positive outcomes or experiences such as life satisfaction (Huebner, Funk, and Gilman, 2000), exercise (McDonald and Hodgdon, 1991), academic achievement (Valentine and DuBois, 2005) and friendship quality (Keefe and Berndt, 1996) and diminished by those that are negative such as depression (Rosenberg et al., 1989), obesity (Strauss, 2000), and victimization (Egan and Perry, 1998). The resulting changes in self-esteem may then precipitate growth (or declines) in the same or related areas of health and well-being. This type of cyclical process in which outcomes feed back into self-esteem may allow its adaptive consequences to compound and accumulate over time to well beyond initial levels (DuBois and Tevendale, 1999).

Implications for Intervention

As noted, in SET self-esteem and associated processes are expected to have the potential to influence multiple domains of functioning. The model is therefore well-suited to comprehensive or broad-spectrum interventions in which the focus is on achieving improvements in a wide range of interrelated aspects of health and well-being. SET predicts that esteem-enhancement interventions will be most effective when they incorporate components geared directly toward strengthening different areas of health and well-being (DuBois, 2003). These types of programs will be better equipped to take advantage of bidirectional patterns of influence between self-esteem and desired outcomes, thereby increasing program effectiveness. Priority should be given in particular to health promotion strategies that have a demonstrated capacity to induce positive changes in self-esteem. Illustratively, if a reduction in the rate of obesity is a key goal, weight management strategies could be implemented that additionally show efficacy for improving self-esteem (Lowry, Sallinen, and Janicke, 2007). To help ensure beneficial effects on others, SET also proposes that interventions be designed to include health promotion activities that are explicitly prosocial in nature. This might entail engaging participants in volunteer activities such as community service or mentoring that are likely to be of value to all parties involved.

DEVELOPMENTAL, INDIVIDUAL, AND SOCIOCULTURAL DIFFERENCES

Overview

Differences in levels of self-esteem according to individual characteristics such as gender and ethnicity, age, and socioenvironmental and cultural factors all have received extensive examination. This literature reveals several trends, including lower self-esteem for females compared to males (Kling, Hyde, Showers, and Buswell, 1999) and for individuals of lower socioeconomic status (Twenge and Campbell, 2002). As noted at the outset of this chapter, broader sociocultural factors also have been suggested as responsible for rising levels of self-esteem among young people observed during the 1980s and 1990s. Trends observed in self-esteem often are qualified by interactions that suggest joint effects of individual, developmental, and social-cultural factors. Females, for example, appear to be especially susceptible to declines in self-esteem during adolescence (Zimmerman, Copeland, Shope, and Dielman, 1997), such that they lag farthest behind males in feelings of self-worth during this stage of development (Kling et al., 1999).

Similar variations are apparent across groups in more circumscribed self-esteem facets as well as in the processes relied on to form and maintain feelings of self-worth. Illustratively, females consistently report more negative body images than males (Harter, 1999). The magnitude of this difference, furthermore, has increased over time, thus suggesting an influence of sociocultural factors operating at a societal level (Feingold and Mazzella, 1998). With relevance to processes influencing self-esteem, Twenge, Zhang, and Im (2004) found evidence of an increase in external locus of control perceptions in the United States over the past several decades. This finding was interpreted as reflecting a likely increase in the use of a self-serving bias (which occurs when people attribute good events to themselves and bad events to outside forces). A trend toward increased use of self-enhancing strategies such as this would be consistent with the apparent rise in narcissism among young people during the same period of time (Twenge, 2006).

Other research has highlighted the potential for differential patterns of association among the constructs included in SET across groups. Several studies, for example, have examined the role of self-esteem among individuals exposed to high numbers of stressful events or other forms of environmental adversity. Under these circumstances, self-esteem appears to take on added importance as a resource facilitating positive outcomes (DuBois and Tevendale, 1999; Mann et al., 1995).

Implications for Intervention

SET assumes that interventions will be most effective when they take into account individual, developmental, and contextual sources of variation in the levels and inter-relationships of constructs in the model. In general, there are three ways in which this is expected to be beneficial. The first involves making a judgment as to the net effect that different characteristics of the target population are likely to have on the overall levels of self-esteem observed among program participants. This determination may have particularly important implications for planning components of interventions that are focused on processes for acquiring and maintaining self-esteem. For populations susceptible to low self-esteem, support for greater use of self-protective/self-enhancing strategies may be appropriate so as to ensure that adaptively high levels of self-esteem are attained. In contrast, where existing levels of self-esteem can be expected to be relatively high, it may be most beneficial to assist participants with critical evaluation of the attitudes and behaviors that support their positive self-evaluations and, where indicated, modifying these to be more conducive to their overall health and well-being.

Second, attention should be given to anticipated levels and interrelationships of other constructs within the model. This type of analysis may identify constructs likely to be at suboptimal levels for participants, such as opportunities for personal mastery needed to support self-esteem. Others may be highlighted because of their potential to be especially influential for a given group or population. In some instances, constructs may be important for both reasons and thus merit special consideration. A positive gender identity, for example, appears to be relatively less common among young adolescent females, while also being especially vital to this group's health and well-being (DuBois, Burk-Braxton, Tevendale, et al., 2002).

Finally, because a substantial amount of within-group variation can be expected for any population, tailoring to the needs of individual participants is assumed to be desirable in SET. As in applications of other health behavior theories (see, for example, Flay, Snyder, and Petraitis in this volume), this type of refinement may increase program effectiveness. In the case of esteem-enhancement interventions, tailoring to the participant's preexisting level of self-esteem may be especially important. For those who already enjoy high self-esteem, for example, an emphasis on increasing feelings of positive self-regard could inadvertently contribute to an inflated sense of worth that is not adaptive. Corresponding risks apply to situations in which intervention activities are not be well-matched to the needs of individuals with low self-esteem. A focus on curbing excesses in self-protective/self-enhancing strategies, for example, could lead those who are struggling with negative feelings of self-regard to become unduly inhibited in even the adaptive use of such strategies.

EMPIRICAL SUPPORT FOR SELF-ESTEEM ENHANCEMENT THEORY

In keeping with SET's status as a relatively new theory, no studies to date have been designed as a direct test of its utility as a framework for guiding intervention development. Several interventions, however, have targeted one or more of the core components of the model in ways that are largely consistent with the recommendations of SET. Table 4.1 provides an overview of the evidence in support of SET that can be gleaned from evaluations of these interventions. Along with information about study population and design, a key is provided indicating which components of SET were targets of each intervention. Findings are summarized with reference to effects on measures that pertain to different SET components.

TABLE 4.1 Empirical Evidence Supporting Self-Esteem Enhancement Theory (SET).

Citation	Population	Design	Intervention(s)	SET Intervention Target(s)	Findings[a]
O'Mara, Marsh, Craven and Debus (2006)	Children, adolescents	Meta-analysis of 145 experimental and quasi-experimental evaluations	Interventions to enhance self-concept/self-esteem	SE, DIF	SE: Overall positive impact ($d = .51$); effects stable from post-test to follow-ups ranging from 3 weeks to 14 months; largest effect sizes for interventions targeting a specific self-concept domain and effects assessed for that domain alone ($d = 1.16$); stronger effects for strategies utilizing praise and feedback ($d = 1.13$); similar effects for interventions attempting to change SE directly or indirectly (e.g., via skills training) DIF: Stronger effects for participants with pre-existing problems (e.g., low self-esteem, behavioral problems)
Haney and Durlak (1998)	Children, adolescents	Meta-analysis of 116 experimental and quasi-experimental evaluations	Interventions to enhance self-concept/self-esteem	SE, HWB, DIF	SE: Overall positive impact ($d = 27$); interventions specifically focused on changing self-concept/self-esteem more effective ($ds = .57$ vs. $.10$); interventions with empirical or theoretical rationale more effective HWB: Positive effects on behavioral, emotional, and academic outcomes; larger changes in SE associated with greater improvements in outcomes DIF: Stronger effects on SE for participants with pre-existing problems ($ds = 47$ vs. 09)

(opp = contextual opportunities; SFM = self-esteem formation and maintenance processes; SE = self-esteem; HWB = health and well-being; DIF: developmental, individual, and sociocultural differences)

(Continued)

TABLE 4.1 (Continued)

Hattie (1992)	Children, adolescents, adults	Meta-analysis of 89 evaluations	Interventions to enhance self-concept/self-esteem	SE, DIF	SE: Overall positive impact ($d = .37$); weaker effects on children ($d = .34$), preadolescents ($d = .23$), and adolescents ($d = .44$) compared to adults ($d = .56$); similar effects for interventions attempting to change SE directly or indirectly (for example, via enhancement of academic achievement) DIF: Stronger effects on SE for participants with preexisting problems and those from lower socioeconomic backgrounds
Blaine, Rodman and Newman (2007)	Adults	Meta-analysis of 77 evaluations	Weight-loss treatments	HWB, DIF	SE: Long-term effects on self-esteem for psychotherapy-based weight loss treatments; greater weight loss associated with greater effects HWB: Small average amounts of short- and long-term weight loss
Lowry et al. (2007)	Children, adolescents	Systematic review of 21 evaluations	Weight-management programs	HWB, DIF	SE: Evidence of increases in self-esteem or components of self-esteem in eighteen of twenty-one studies reviewed, with ten including control groups that did not experience equivalent improvements; authors concluded that weight change likely related to self-esteem improvements and that available research suggests domain-specific self-evaluations may be affected first (for example, body image) and then lead to global self-esteem improvements

(opp = contextual opportunities; SFM = self-esteem formation and maintenance processes; SE = self-esteem; HWB = health and well-being; DIF: developmental, individual, and sociocultural differences)

DiClemente et al. (2004); R. J. DiClemente (personal communication, December 15, 2007)	Adolescents (sexually active African-American females ages 14–18)	Randomized trial	SiHLE (HIV prevention program)	SE, HWB, DIF	SE: Improved ethnic identity for pregnant adolescents HWB: Condom use and incidence of new chlamydia infections and pregnancies
Flay, DuBois, and Ji (2007)	Children (elementary school students in grades 3–5)	Matched pairs randomized design involving fourteen urban schools	Positive Action (comprehensive school-based health promotion program)	OPP, SFM, SE, HWB	OPP: Parent and teacher rewards for prosocial behavior SFM: Use of adaptive and maladaptive esteem-formation processes SE: Peer and school domains of self-esteemHWB: Student character and prosocial behavior (for example, altruism, honesty, respect for rules), social competence, positive health behaviors, anxiety, initiation of substance use, violence-related behaviors, self-reported gradesNote: Results include noteworthy trends at p < 10, one-tailed level of significance.

(opp = contextual opportunities; SFM = self-esteem formation and maintenance processes; SE = self-esteem; HWB = health and well-being; DIF: developmental, individual, and sociocultural differences)

(Continued)

TABLE 4.1 (*Continued*)

Flay, Acock, Vuchinich, and Beets (2006)	Children (elementary school students in grades 1–6)	Matched pairs randomized design involving fourteen schools in Hawaii	Positive Action (comprehensive school-based health promotion program)	OPP, SFM, SE, HWB	OPP: Teacher, parent, and student ratings of school quality SFM: Attitudes toward positive behaviors and teacher-rated self-improvement behaviors SE: Teacher-rated self-concept HWB: Character and prosocial behavior (for example, honesty, responsibility, self-control), substance use, and teacher-rated disruptive behavior; at school level, academic achievement, absenteeism, and suspensions DIF: Violence-related behavior and sexual intercourse among boys, but not girls
Flay and Allred (2003)	Children, adolescents (elementary, middle, and high school students)	Quasi-experimental (matched control design at school level)	Positive Action (comprehensive school-based health promotion program)	SE, SFM, SE, HWB	HWB: Evidence of positive effects on academic achievement and disciplinary problems while receiving program in elementary school and long-term effects on levels of problem behavior (for example, substance use, violence), attendance, and achievement during middle and high school as well as post–high school (continuing education and employment)

(opp = contextual opportunities; SFM = self-esteem formation and maintenance processes; SE = self-esteem; HWB = health and well-being; DIF: developmental, individual, and sociocultural differences)

| Rhodes, Grossman, Resch (2000) | Young adolescents (ages 10–16) | Randomized trial | Big Brothers Big Sisters (mentoring program geared predominantly to youth from single-parent homes) | OPP, DIF | OPP: Quality of parent-child relationship
SMF: Improved valuing of school mediated by gains in parent-child relationship
SE: Improved perceived scholastic competence directly and mediated by gains in parent-child relationship; improved global self-worth mediated by gains in parent-child relationship
HWB: Improved grades and reduced skipping of school via pathways in which gains in valuing of school, perceived scholastic competence, and/or global self-worth mediated the effects of improved parent-child relationship on the outcomes |
| Rhodes, Reddy and Grossman (2005) | Young adolescents (ages 10–16) | Randomized trial | Big Brothers Big Sisters | OPP, DIF | OPP: Quality of parent-child relationship and decreased negative peer relations via gains in parent-child relationship
SE: Improved global self-worth via gains in parent-child relationship HWB
Reduced alcohol use via pathways in which gains in global self-worth mediated the effects of improved parent-child and peer relationships on this outcome
Note: All findings apply only to youth with mentoring relationships lasting twelve or more months |

(opp = contextual opportunities; SFM = self-esteem formation and maintenance processes; SE = self-esteem; HWB = health and well-being; DIF = developmental, individual, and sociocultural differences)

(Continued)

TABLE 4.1 *(Continued)*

DuBois et al. (2002)	Children, adolescents (ages 7–15)	Quasi-experimental	Big Brothers Big Sisters	OPP, DIF	OPP: Social support from significant nonparental adults SE: Effect (via significant adult social support) on composite measure reflecting global self-esteem and a positive and balanced profile of domain-specific self-evaluations HWB: Effects (via significant adult social support and SE) on reduced emotional and behavioral problems
Felner et al. (1993)	Young adolescents (grades 6–8)	Quasi-experimental	School Transitional Environment Project (STEP)	OPP	OPP: Positive effects on school experiences (for example, teacher support) and transition stress SE: Global self-esteem and peer, school, and family domain-specific self-evaluations HWB: School grades, depression, anxiety, and behavior problems
Faggiano et al. (2008)	Children, adolescents	Meta-analysis of twenty-nine experimental evaluations	School-based substance use prevention programs	OPP, HWB	SE: Small positive effect on self-esteem (Standardized Mean Difference = .22) for skill-based interventions compared to usual curricula HWB: Compared with usual curricula, skill-based interventions significantly reduced marijuana use (Relative Risk [RR] = .82) and hard drug use (RR = .45) Note: Studies showing effects on self-esteem included follow-up assessments ranging from two to five years.

(opp = contextual opportunities; SFM = self-esteem formation and maintenance processes; SE = self-esteem; HWB = health and well-being; DIF: developmental, individual, and sociocultural differences)

Stice and Shaw (2004)	Adolescents	Meta-analysis of fifty-one experimental and quasi-experimental evaluations	Eating disorder prevention programs	SFM, SE, HWB	SFM: Thin-ideal internalization SE: Body dissatisfaction HWB: Small to medium effects on body mass, dieting, negative affect, and eating pathology Note: Effects significant at both program termination and, with one exception (body mass), at follow-up
Hattie, Marsh, Neill, and Richards (1997)	Adolescents, adults	Meta-analysis of ninety-one evaluations	Adventure education programs	SE, HWB	SE: General self-concept (d 5 28) and domain-specific facets of self-concept such as independence (47), peer relations (28), and physical appearance (38); evidence of further gains in general and domain-specific self-concepts between end of program and follow-up assessments HWB: Diverse outcomes, including leadership (d 5 38), social competence (43), emotional stability (49), physical fitness (40), and academic achievement (50); evidence of sustained benefits at follow-up assessments Note: Follow-up assessments averaged 5.5 months from end of program.

(opp = contextual opportunities; SFM = self-esteem formation and maintenance processes; SE = self-esteem; HWB = health and well-being; DIF: developmental, individual, and sociocultural differences)

Note: Studies did not necessarily evaluate effects on all components of SET that were addressed by interventions; in some instances, evaluations also addressed components of SET that were not targeted by the intervention. For these reasons, SET intervention targets may include areas not represented in the summaries of study findings and vice-versa.

[a] Unless otherwise noted, all findings are in the direction of favorable effects of the intervention.

Several trends are noteworthy. First, as predicted by SET, interventions designed to increase contextual opportunities for developing and sustaining self-esteem (that is, supportive relationships/messages and personal mastery) have been found to foster improvements in this area. Notably, such improvements have occurred in tandem with greater reliance on adaptive strategies for seeking feelings of self-worth, gains in both overall and specific facets of self-esteem, and benefits within multiple domains of health and well-being. Interventions producing these types of effects include Positive Action, a comprehensive school-based health promotion program that also addresses other SET components (Flay et al., 2006, 2007; this program is described in greater detail in the following section of this chapter), and the Big Brothers Big Sisters mentoring program (DuBois, Neville, et al., 2002; Rhodes, Grossman, and Resch, 2000; Rhodes, Reddy, and Grossman, 2005), a program in which a supportive relationship with a nonparental adult is introduced into the life of a youth who is typically from a single-parent home.

Second, in further accordance with SET, benefits are evident for interventions with both youth and adults that directly target enhancements in self-esteem or self-concept (Haney and Durlak, 1998; Hattie, 1992; O'Mara et al., 2006). Findings include substantial improvements in specific domains of self-evaluation when intentionally targeted by programs (O'Mara et al., 2006), thus supporting the emphasis in SET on using intervention strategies that reflect a multidimensional conceptualization of self-esteem. It is also noteworthy that gains in self-esteem and self-concept for program participants have been found to be correlated with improvements in other areas of their functioning (Haney and Durlak, 1998). This pattern is directly supportive of the assumption in SET that interventions focused on esteem enhancement can contribute to substantial improvements in health and well-being.

Third, as can be seen in Table 4.1, several interventions that target one or more components of SET have demonstrated the types of comprehensive effects on health and well-being that are expected to be possible for programs designed in accordance with the model. These include favorable impacts on multiple domains of functioning (emotional, behavioral, cognitive, social, physical), effectiveness at problem prevention and health promotion, and improvements in areas that are likely to benefit others (for example, prosocial behavior). These trends are particularly salient for Positive Action (Flay et al., 2006, 2007), the intervention in Table 4.1 that to date most closely aligns with the principles and target areas of SET (for a summary of similar findings obtained in quasi-experimental evaluations of this program, see DuBois and Flay, 2004).

Fourth, available findings are consistent with the emphasis in SET on the potential value of directly targeting changes both in self-esteem and in different aspects of health and well-being within interventions. Of particular note are the sustained effects at follow-up assessments for interventions that have demonstrated immediate effects on both self-esteem and health/well-being (Faggiano et al., 2008; Flay and Allred, 2003; Hattie et al., 1997; Stice and Shaw, 2004). These results are consistent with the assumption in SET that changes in self-esteem and health/well-being can be mutually reinforcing over time and thus promote long-term impacts.

Finally, the research summarized in Table 4.1 provides some support for the prediction in SET that it is important to take into account the individual, developmental, and contextual circumstances of groups that are targeted for intervention. Interventions geared toward esteem enhancement, for example, have yielded notably stronger effects on the self-esteem of youth with preexisting problems (Haney and Durlak, 1998; Hattie, 1992; O'Mara et al., 2006). For these youth, who are likely to often exhibit deficits in self-esteem, traditional esteem-enhancement strategies may be a particularly good fit. Conversely, for those without identified adjustment difficulties, an alternative approach focused on ensuring that there is an adaptive basis for existing feelings of self-worth might be more beneficial. This would be consistent with the evidence that higher-functioning youth tend to receive limited benefits from participation in esteem-enhancement interventions in their current form. As predicted by SET, there is also a trend for favorable results to be obtained when intervention strategies are aligned with specific identified needs of participants. These include weight-management techniques for overweight youth and adults (Blaine et al., 2007; Lowry et al., 2007), school environment supports for youth undergoing the transition from elementary school to middle school (Felner et al., 1993), provision of adult role models for youth from predominantly single-parent homes (DuBois, Neville, et al., 2002; Rhodes et al., 2000, 2005), and promotion of positive gender and ethnic identity among African American female adolescents in an HIV prevention program (DiClemente et al., 2004).

CASE APPLICATIONS OF SET

As noted, as a relatively new theory the formal application of SET in the development of interventions has been limited. In this section, we describe the use of the theory to inform the design of GirlPOWER!, a mentoring program for ethnic minority young adolescent girls (DuBois et al., 2008). SET also may be a helpful tool for informing the evaluation of interventions that, although not necessarily developed specifically within this framework, are intended to influence many of the same processes. Our second case example illustrates this possibility using the Positive Action program referred to previously.

GirlPOWER!

GirlPOWER! is designed for ten- to thirteen-year-old girls and their female volunteer mentors. The program was developed in collaboration with an affiliate agency of Big Brothers Big Sisters of America (BBBSA) and is intended for implementation by BBBSA affiliates. The core component of GirlPOWER! is a year-long series of monthly, three-hour workshops in which up to fifteen Matches (mentor-youth pairs) participate as a group. Led by trained female facilitators, each workshop includes a mixture of one-on-one (mentor-youth), small-group, and larger group activities. Other program components include: (a) training modules for mentors and youth to prepare them for participation in the program; (b) semi structured activities for Matches to complete on their own between workshops that are thematically linked to curriculum content; (c) monthly supervision contacts with mentors; (d) parent involvement through participation in selected workshops, resource materials, and bimonthly agency contacts; and (e) a group reunion six months following the final workshop and at six-month intervals thereafter. Ongoing agency support for Match relationships is available until girls become too old for the agency's services. All program activities and content are organized around the concepts underlying the POWER acronym: Pride, Opportunities (for learning), Women-in-the-making, Energy and Effort, and Relationships.

As summarized in Table 4.2, the GirlPOWER! program is designed in accordance with the major principles of SET and addresses constructs within each domain of the model. (For a detailed description of the program, see DuBois et al., 2008.) The program's focus on helping girls to forge strong and enduring ties with their mentors and other group members is directly aligned with the emphasis in SET on providing contextual opportunities for supportive relationships and messages. The involvement of parents, furthermore, increases the potential for youth to experience increased esteem-enhancing interactions in their lives. A strong internal foundation for feelings of self-worth is fostered as well in GirlPOWER! through opportunities for cultivation of personal competencies. Program activities focus on building skills in areas such as problem solving, coping, and goal setting. Communication and teamwork skills are also honed throughout the program via collaborative projects and reflective discussions.

To support youth in pursuing routes to feelings of self-worth (that is, self-esteem maintenance and formation processes) that are adaptive, the concept of "healthy self-esteem" is introduced: "Feeling proud of yourself based on choices that are good for

TABLE 4.2   **Application of SET to GirlPOWER! and Positive Action.**

Construct	GirlPOWER!	Positive Action
Contextual Opportunities: Supportive Relationships and Messages	Mentoring relationship Supportive group experience Parent education	Reinforcement of positive behaviors by teachers, other school staff, and peers Family classes and at-home curriculum to support school components of program
Contextual Opportunities: Personal Mastery and Success Experiences	Skill building activities Collaborative projects and reflective discussions to strengthen communication and teamwork skills	Instruction in personal skills in areas such as self-control, social competence, stress management, and goal setting

Construct	GirlPOWER!	Positive Action
Self-Esteem Formation and Maintenance Processes	Introduction of concept of "healthy self-esteem" (feeling positive about yourself through attitudes and behaviors that are adaptive for self and others) Assistance with identifying and avoiding maladaptive self-protective/self-enhancing tendencies	Introduction of concept of motivation to feel good about oneself Assistance with identifying and avoiding maladaptive self-protective/self-enhancing tendencies through training in empathy toward others, self-honesty, and self-improvement
Self-Esteem	Thematic emphasis throughout program on pride in self and positive gender and ethnic identity Activities designed to strengthen domain-specific self-evaluations	Assistance with recognizing positive self attributes and behaviors Emphasis on importance of balanced positive self-perceptions across multiple domains
Health and Well-Being	Social connections Mood enhancement Positive health behavior Risk behavior prevention Academic success / career exploration	Peer relationships Positive health behavior Risk behavior prevention Academic achievement
Developmental, Individual, and Sociocultural Differences.	Content geared toward needs and strengths of target population (early adolescent ethnic minority females) Tailoring to individual youth facilitated through opportunities for choice in activities and mentor training/supervision	Separate curriculum for each grade level (K–12)

you, your future, and other people." Throughout the program, girls work with their mentors and other group members to apply this concept to different areas of their lives. Balanced attention is given to circumstances in which they may feel tempted to rely on maladaptive strategies for protecting or enhancing their self-esteem, such as engaging in risk behaviors (for example, substance use) or emotionally harmful interactions with peers (for example, relational aggression; Crick and Grotpeter, 1995) on the one hand, and those that offer opportunities to cultivate an adaptive foundation for feelings of worth, such as positive health behaviors (for example, exercise) and academic effort, on the other hand. POWER concepts, particularly Effort and Energy, serve to reinforce the theme that achieving and maintaining a high level of self-esteem in a healthy manner is possible, but also requires hard work.

As recommended by SET, direct strategies to promote self-esteem are a further important feature of GirlPOWER! The lead POWER concept of Pride serves to continually reinforce a message to participants of their unconditional worth and value as persons. In accordance with SET, several specific facets of self-esteem are also targeted in the program. These include self-evaluations tied to specific domains (school, peers, family, physical appearance) as well as both gender and ethnic identity. Body-image concerns, for example, are explored in the context of curriculum activities that focus on exercise and nutrition, with an emphasis on how media and other societal influences tend to perpetuate unhealthy and unrealistic ideals for women's physical appearance. In keeping with its status as an overarching goal of the program, promotion of gender identity is addressed at a more structural level by pairing each girl with a female mentor and establishing an all-female support group.

As discussed previously, design of programs to directly strengthen different aspects of health and well-being is recommended in SET. In GirlPOWER!, different portions of the curriculum focus on risk behavior prevention (substance use, violence, high-risk sexual behavior), promotion of positive health behaviors (exercise, healthy eating), and academic success/career exploration. The program also is geared toward enhancing the emotional well-being of participating girls by providing them with the opportunity to engage in enjoyable activities with others in a safe environment.

GirlPOWER!'s focus on early adolescent girls from ethnic minority backgrounds is consistent with the emphasis in SET on designing programs to be sensitive to developmental, individual, and sociocultural differences. As is evident from the examples provided, program content is geared toward those concerns that are likely to be especially relevant to girls as they undergo the transition to adolescence (for example, body image) as well as issues of particular importance for youth of color (for example, ethnic identity). The all-female composition of the group, furthermore, is intended to counter the tendency for girls' voices to be overshadowed or inhibited in mixed-gender settings (Gilligan, 1982). Tailoring to the needs of individual youth also is able to occur in a variety of ways in the program. When asked to complete activities on their own that support curricular objectives, for example, mentor-youth pairs have the opportunity to choose an activity they regard as most appropriate from a menu of several alternatives or simply design their own. Mentor training and supervision, furthermore, emphasize the need to be responsive to youth input and interests, as this has been found be an important factor in building strong mentoring relationships with young people (Rhodes and DuBois, 2006).

In a small-scale randomized control trial conducted for piloting and feasibility purposes by the first author, forty girls and their mentors were assigned to participate in GirlPOWER! or the traditional BBBSA community-based mentoring program. Preliminary results indicate significant differences favoring GirlPOWER! participants on multiple indicators of mentoring relationship quality as well as health and well-being benefits in the form of reduced affective/anxiety problems and increased exercise (Silverthorn et al., 2008). Improvements are also evident (standardized regression coefficient effect sizes of approximately .20 or greater, although not statistically significant in all cases owing to the small sample size) on measures of health knowledge and beliefs, overall feelings of self-worth, multiple domains of self-evaluation (peers, body image, sports/athletics), gender identity, coping self-efficacy, and aggressive/delinquent behavior. The benefits associated with participation in GirlPOWER! represent gains over and above those experienced by girls assigned to the standard BBBSA community-based mentoring model. The BBBSA program has well-documented benefits (Table 4.1) and is included in several registries of effective prevention programs (for example, Blueprints for Violence Prevention). Overall, initial findings for the GirlPOWER! program are promising and supportive of the value of designing interventions within the framework of SET.

Positive Action

Positive Action is a comprehensive school-based character and health promotion program (Allred, 1995). The basic underlying philosophy of the program, rooted in self-esteem motivation theory, is embodied in the Thoughts-Actions-Feelings Circle, according to which, "Our thoughts lead to actions, and those actions lead to feelings about ourselves, which lead to more thoughts" (*Components of the Positive Action Program*, Section 1, 2). Students are taught to understand this concept and are supported and reinforced in learning positive thoughts and behaviors that they can engage in as a basis for feeling good about themselves. Feelings of self-worth that result from a given set of actions are expected to prove intrinsically self-reinforcing and thus motivate continuation of those same behaviors. The program includes a K–12 classroom curriculum that is taught for fifteen to twenty minutes almost every day in every grade, together with schoolwide climate change, family involvement, and community components. A foundational introductory unit addresses the importance of forming and maintaining a positive self-concept. The remainder of the program focuses on actions for achieving positive feelings about the self in the areas of physical health, academic achievement, thinking and learning, self-management, social skills, self-honesty, and self-improvement.

Positive Action includes components that align remarkably well with SET (Table 4.2). The program, for example, is clearly designed to encourage youth to acquire and maintain positive feelings about themselves through adaptive behaviors.

Several units (for example, self-honesty) are also oriented toward helping youth avoid reliance on maladaptive self-protective and self-enhancing strategies for boosting their self-esteem. Although SET was not used to guide the development of Positive Action, the theory has proven valuable in guiding evaluation of the program. Based on analysis of the program within the framework of SET, a recent evaluation (Flay et al., 2007) incorporated measures of constructs relevant to each area of the model. These included teacher and parent reinforcement of youth for engaging in prosocial behavior (contextual opportunities for self-esteem), the youth's reliance on adaptive and maladaptive strategies for cultivating a sense of self-worth (self-esteem formation and maintenance processes), overall feelings of positive self-regard along with multiple domain-specific facets of self-evaluation (self-esteem), assets as well as liabilities in emotional, behavioral, social, and academic domains of adjustment (health and well-being), and preexisting variations across students in motivation for self-esteem that could affect responsiveness to the program (developmental, individual, and sociocultural differences). As noted previously, preliminary results are suggestive of effects on several of these measures (Table 4.1). Future analyses will examine such issues as whether improvements in self-esteem and esteem-formation processes mediate effects of the program on health and well-being outcomes, whether program effects on self-esteem and health/well-being are mutually reinforcing over time, and whether student levels of motivation for self-esteem moderate program effects, all of which would be consistent with assumptions of SET. As this example illustrates, SET offers a promising framework for strengthening the evaluation of esteem-enhancement interventions. Applications of this type are important because they have the potential to facilitate further development of programs and increase their effectiveness.

STRENGTHS AND LIMITATIONS OF SET

The chief strength of SET is that it provides a viable framework for resolving the ongoing debate over what role (if any) self-esteem should have in interventions to promote health and related outcomes. In concert with those on the "pro" side of this debate (and research supporting their views), SET assumes that feelings of self-worth do indeed matter for most if not all areas of well-being and adjustment. Efforts to ensure that individuals harbor a strong sense of their inherent value and dignity as persons therefore are regarded as prime candidates for inclusion in the design of any health education or promotion program. At the same time, in keeping with concerns expressed by those on the "con" side of the debate, SET assumes that the ways in which an individual achieves and sustains a high level of self-esteem are equally significant. If the beliefs, values, and behaviors involved are not adaptive, resulting feelings of self-worth may be associated with few net benefits and even adverse outcomes for both the individual and others.

Simply put, SET suggests that both the "ends" and the "means" of self-esteem are important and should be addressed in close coordination in

> Simply put, SET suggests that both the "ends" and the "means" of self-esteem are important and should be addressed in close coordination in interventions.

interventions. In so doing, SET offers a viable roadmap for how future health promotion initiatives can be organized either in their entirety or, in part, around goals of esteem-enhancement without being subject to the drawbacks of approaches that either overlook the motivational and health significance of self-esteem on the one hand or somewhat naively seek to cultivate feelings of self-worth among participants without due consideration to establishing a strong and adaptive supporting foundation for them on the other hand.

Several limitations of SET also deserve mention. First, as a relatively new theory, there have been few applications to date of SET to either the design or evaluation of health promotion interventions. The practical utility of the model for these purposes is in need of further clarification through its systematic use in a greater number of program development and evaluation efforts. Second, the supporting research for SET has focused to a large extent on children and adolescents and has involved primarily samples from the United States. The extent to which the model is viable for adults and those living in different countries and cultures is less well established, although available findings are generally supportive. Third, SET is presently limited by a lack of investigation of the mediational processes that are presumed to link the major constructs in the model to one another and to health outcomes. Notwithstanding the framing of SET as a theory of action, there is a need to better understand the empirical support that exists for these linkages. Finally, it must be acknowledged that the model is quite general in its present form. It does not, therefore, offer guidance at the level that typically would be required to fully inform intervention design and evaluation decisions.

FUTURE DIRECTIONS

Despite extensive investigation of self-esteem within psychology and other disciplines, it has remained mostly on the periphery of the health promotion literature. In the primary introductory text for the field, *Health Behavior and Health Education* (Glanz et al., 2002), neither self-esteem nor related terms such as self-evaluation or self-concept appear even once in the index. Several directions for future work with SET could be helpful in further establishing the relevance of the theory and, by implication, self-esteem to health promotion. One priority should be to explore the model's usefulness for informing the development of interventions that target major contemporary health threats such as obesity, addictions, diabetes, and HIV/AIDS.

Emphasis should be placed on identifying those facets of self-esteem and associated processes that are most closely linked with behavioral risk factors for different health outcomes and then targeting these in interventions. The influence of self-evaluative factors on aspects of psychological and emotional functioning has already received considerable attention and is relatively well documented. This suggests that application of SET to interventions with mental health aims, such as depression and suicide prevention, could prove especially fruitful and should be actively explored as well.

One priority should be to explore the model's usefulness for informing the development of interventions that target major contemporary health threats such as obesity, addictions, diabetes, and HIV/AIDS.

This chapter has discussed SET largely independent of other theories of health promotion. Yet, it could be useful to integrate concepts from SET into other models, especially those in which self-evaluative processes are assumed to have a role. The process of self-reevaluation in the Transtheoretical Model, for example, is posited to be important in allowing individuals to move from the stage of contemplation to one in which they are prepared to initiate a new behavior (Prochaska, Redding, and Evers, 2002). Incorporation of constructs and principles from SET into this portion of the model could serve to more fully elaborate the role of self-evaluative factors in decision making about behavior change. Building bridges between SET and other theoretical perspectives is likely to facilitate a broader range of applications of the model and serve the larger purpose of enhancing consideration of self-esteem and associated processes in health promotion.

SUMMARY

Self-esteem enhancement theory posits associations between the following key constructs: (a) contextual opportunities; (b) esteem formation and maintenance processes; (c) self-esteem; (d) health and well-being; and (e) modifying influences. The theory suggests that interventions should be designed to cultivate a strong and healthy foundation for people's feelings of self-worth. It also assumes that interventions will be most effective when they take into account individual, developmental, and contextual sources of variation in the levels and interrelationships of constructs in the model. Favorable results have been reported for several interventions that target one or more of the SET constructs in a manner that aligns with the recommendations of the theory. SET provides a framework for resolving debate regarding what role self-esteem should have in interventions to promote health. Future research should explore the model's usefulness for informing interventions addressing contemporary public health issues such as obesity, addictions, diabetes, and HIV/AIDS.

REFERENCES

Allport, G. W. (1955). *Becoming: Basic considerations for a psychology of personality.* New Haven, CT: Yale University Press.

Baumeister, R. F. (1989). The optimal margin of illusion. *Journal of Social and Clinical Psychology, 8,* 176–189.

Baumeister, R. F., Bushman, B. J. and Campbell, W. K. (2000). Self-esteem, narcissism, and aggression: Does violence result from low self-esteem or from threatened egotism. *Current Directions in Psychological Science, 9,* 26–29.

Baumeister, R. F., Campbell, J. D., Krueger, J. I., and Vohs, K. D. (2003). Does high self-esteem cause better performance, interpersonal success, happiness, or healthier lifestyles? *Psychological Science in the Public Interest, 4,* 1–44.

Baumeister, R. F., Smart, L., and Boden, J. M. (1996). Relation of threatened egotism to violence and aggression: The dark side of high self-esteem. *Psychological Review, 103,* 5–33.

Blaine, B., and Crocker, J. (1993). Self-esteem and self-serving biases in reactions to positive and negative events: An integrative review. In R. F. Baumeister (ed.), *Self-esteem: The puzzle of low self-regard* (pp. 55–85). New York: Plenum.

Blaine, B. E., Rodman, J., and Newman, J. M. (2007). Weight loss treatment and psychological well-being: A review and meta-analysis. *Journal of Health Psychology*, *12*, 66–82.

Blueprints for Violence Prevention. *Model Programs*. Retrieved April 5, 2008, from http://www.colorado .edu/cspv/blueprints/

Branden, N. (1969). *The psychology of self-esteem*. New York: Bantam Books.

California Task Force to Promote Self-Esteem and Personal and Social Responsibility. (1990). *Toward a state of esteem*. Sacramento: California State Department of Education.

Colvin, C. R., and Block, J. (1994). Do positive illusions foster mental health? An examination of the Taylor and Brown formulation. *Psychological Bulletin*, *116*, 3–20.

Colvin, C. R., Block, J., and Funder, D. C. (1995). Overly positive self-evaluations and personality: Negative implications for mental health. *Journal of Personality and Social Psychology*, *68*, 1152–1162.

Components of the Positive Action Program. (2003). Retrieved February 4, 2004, from http://www .positiveaction.net/programs/index.asp?ID1_1&ID2_1.

Crick, N. R., and Grotpeter, J. K. (1995). Relational aggression, gender, and social-psychological adjustment. *Child Development*, *66*, 710–722.

Crocker, J., Luhtanen, R., Blaine, B., and Broadnax, S. (1994). Collective self-esteem and psychological well-being among White, Black, and Asian college students. *Personality and Social Psychology Bulletin*, *20*, 503–513.

DiClemente, R. J., Wingood, G. M., Harrington, K. F., Lang, D. L., Davies, S. L., Hook, E. W., et al. (2004). Efficacy of an HIV prevention intervention for African American adolescent girls: A randomized controlled trial. *Journal of the American Medical Association*, *292*, 171–179.

DuBois, D. L. (2003). Self-esteem, adolescence. In T. P. Gullotta and M. Bloom (eds.) and T. P. Gullotta and G. Adams (section eds.), *Encyclopedia of primary prevention and health promotion* (pp. 953–961). New York: Kluwer Academic/Plenum.

DuBois, D. L., Burk-Braxton, C., Tevendale, H. D., Swenson, L. P., and Hardesty, J. L. (2002). Race and gender influences on adjustment in early adolescence: Investigation of an integrative model. *Child Development*, *73*, 1573–1592.

DuBois, D. L., Burk-Braxton, C., Swenson, L. P., Tevendale, H. D., Lockerd, E. M., and Moran, B. L. (2002). Getting by with a little help from self and others: Self-esteem and social support as resources during early adolescence. *Developmental Psychology*, *38*, 822–839.

DuBois, D. L., and Flay, B. R. (2004). The healthy pursuit of self-esteem: A comment on and alternative to the Crocker and Park formulation. *Psychological Bulletin*, *130*, 415–420.

DuBois, D. L., Lopez, C., and Parra, G. R. (2004). Cognitive therapy and the self. In M. A. Reinecke and D. A. Clark (eds.), *Cognitive therapy across the lifespan: Evidence and practice* (pp. 202–230). Cambridge, UK: Cambridge University Press.

DuBois, D. L., Neville, H. A., Parra, G. R., and Pugh-Lilly, A. O. (2002). Testing a new model of mentoring. In J. E. Rhodes (Ed.), *A critical view of youth mentoring* (New Directions for Youth Development: Theory, Research, and Practice, pp. 21–57). San Francisco: Jossey-Bass.

Dubois, D.L., & Silverthorn, N. (2004). Do deviant peer associations mediate the contributions of self-esteem to problem behavior during early adolescence? A 2-year longitudinal study. *Journal of Clinical Child and Adolescent Psychology*, 33, 382-388.

DuBois, D. L., Silverthorn, N., Pryce, J., Reeves, E., Sanchez, B., Silva, A., et al. (2008). Mentorship: The GirlPOWER! program. In C. W. Leroy and J. E. Mann (eds.), *Handbook of prevention and intervention programs for adolescent girls* (pp. 325–365). Hoboken, NJ: Wiley.

DuBois, D. L., and Tevendale, H. D. (1999). Self-esteem in childhood and adolescence: Vaccine or epiphenomenon? *Applied and Preventive Psychology*, *8*, 103–117.

DuBois, D. L., Tevendale, H. D., Burk-Braxton, C., Swenson, L. P., and Hardesty, J. L. (2000). Self-system influences during early adolescence: Investigation of an integrative model. *Journal of Early Adolescence*, *20*, 12–43.

Egan, S. K., and Perry, D. G. (1998). Does low self-regard invite victimization? *Developmental Psychology*, *34*, 299–309.

Edwards, R. (1995, May). Is self-esteem really all that important? *APA Monitor*, pp. 43–44.

Emler, N. (2001). *Self-esteem: The costs and consequences of low self-worth*. York, England: York Publishing Services.

Faggiano, F., Vigna-Taglianti, F. D., Versino, E., Zambon, A., Borraccino, A., and Lemma, P. (2008, May). School-based prevention for illicit drugs use: a systematic review. *Preventive Medicine*, *46*, 5, 385–396.

Feingold, A., and Mazzella, R. (1998). Gender differences in body image are increasing. *Psychological Science*, *9*, 190–195.

Felner, R. D., Brand, S., Adan, A. M., Mulhall, P. F., Flowers, N., Sartain, B., et al. (1993). Restructuring the ecology of the school as an approach to prevention during school transitions: Longitudinal follow-ups and extensions of the School Transitional Environment Project (STEP). *Prevention in Human Services*, *10*(2), 103–136.

Flay, B. R. (2002). Positive youth development requires comprehensive health promotion programs. *American Journal of Health Behavior*, *26*, 407–424.

Flay, B. R., and Allred, C. G. (2003). Long-term effects of the Positive Action program: A comprehensive, positive youth development program. *American Journal of Health Behavior*, *27* (Suppl. 1), S6–S21.

Flay, B. R., Acock, A., Vuchinich, S., and Beets, M. (2006). Progress report of the randomized trial of *Positive Action* in Hawaii: End of third year of intervention. Available from Positive Action, Inc. 264 4th Avenue South, Twin Falls, ID 83301.

Flay, B. R., DuBois, D. L., and Ji, P. (2007). Progress report of the randomized trial of *Positive Action* in Chicago: End of third year of intervention (Grade 5, Spring, 2007). Unpublished report, Department of Public Health, Oregon State University.

Gilligan, C. (1982). *In a different voice*. Cambridge, MA: Harvard University Press.

Glanz, K., Rimer, B., and Lewis, F. M. (eds.). (2002). *Health behavior and health education: Theory, research, and practice* (3rd ed.). San Francisco: Jossey-Bass.

Goodson, P., Buhi, E.R., and Dunsmore, S.C. (2006). Self-esteem and adolescent sexual behaviors, attitudes, and intentions: A systematic review. *Journal of Adolescent Health*, *38*, 310–319.

Haney, P., and Durlak, J. A. (1998). Changing self-esteem in children and adolescents: A meta-analytic review. *Journal of Clinical Child Psychology*, *27*, 423–433.

Harter, S. (2006). The self. In W. Damon and R. M. Lerner (Ed.-in-Chief) and N. Eisenberg (Vol. Ed.), *Handbook of child psychology: Vol. 3. Social, emotional, and personality development* (6th ed., pp. 505–570). Hoboken, NJ: Wiley.

Harter, S. (1999). *The construction of the self: A developmental perspective*. New York: Guilford Press.

Hattie, J. (1992). *Self-concept*. Hillsdale, NJ: Lawrence Erlbaum.

Hattie, J., Marsh, H. W., Neill, J. T., and Richards, G. E. (1997). Adventure education and outward bound: Out-of-class experiences that make a lasting difference. *Review of Educational Research*, *67*, 43–87.

Heaney, C. A., and Israel, B. (2002). Social networks and social support. In K. Glanz, B. Rimer, and F. M. Lewis (eds.), *Health behavior and health education: Theory, research, and practice* (3rd ed., pp. 185–209). San Francisco: Jossey-Bass.

House, J. S. (1981). *Work, stress, and social support*. Reading, MA: Addison-Wesley.

Huebner, E. S., Funk, B. A., and Gilman, R. (2000). Cross-sectional and longitudinal psychosocial correlates of adolescent life satisfaction reports. *Canadian Journal of School Psychology*, *16*, 53–64.

Hughes, J. N., Cavell, T. A., and Grossman, P. A. (1997). A positive view of self: Risk or protection for aggressive children? *Development and Psychopathology*, *9*, 75–94.

Jackson, T., and Chen, H. (2008). Predicting changes in eating disorder symptoms among Chinese adolescents: A 9-month prospective study. *Journal of Psychosomatic Research, 64*, 87–95.

James, W. (1890). The *principles* of *psychology*. New York: Holt.

Judge, T. A., and Bono, J. E. (2001). Relationship of core self-evaluations traits—self-esteem, generalized self-efficacy, locus of control, and emotional stability—with job satisfaction and job performance: A meta-analysis. *Journal of Applied Psychology. 86*, 80–92.

Kaplan, H. B. (1986). *Social psychology of self-referent behavior*. New York: Plenum.

Keefe, K., and Berndt, T. J. (1996). Relations of friendship quality to self-esteem in early adolescence. *Journal of Early Adolescence*, *16*, 110–129.

Kernis, M. H., and Goldman, B. M. (2006). Assessing stability of self-esteem and contingent self-esteem. In M. H. Kernis (Ed.), *Self-esteem issues and answers: A sourcebook of current perspectives* (pp. 77–85). New York: Psychology Press.

Kling, K. C., Hyde, J. S., Showers, C. J., and Buswell, B. N. (1999). Gender differences in self-esteem: A meta-analysis. *Psychological Bulletin*, *125*, 470–500.

Lowry, K. W., Sallinen, B. J., and Janicke, D. M. (2007). The effects of weight management programs on self-esteem in pediatric overweight populations. *Journal of Pediatric Psychology*, *32*, 1179–1195.

Maharaj, S., Daneman, D., Olmsted, M., and Rodin, G. (2004). Metabolic control in adolescent girls: Links to relationality and the female sense of self. *Diabetes Care*, 27, 709–715.

Mann, M., Hosman, C.M.H., Schaalma, H. P., and de Vries, N. (2004). Self-esteem in a broad-spectrum approach for mental health promotion. *Health Education Research*, *19*, 357–372

Martin, J., and Knox, J. (1997). Self-esteem instability and its implications for HIV prevention among gay men. *Health and Social Work*, *22*, 264–273

Maslow, A. H. (1954). *Motivation and personality*. New York: Harper.

Mazur, E., Wolchik, S. A., Virdin, L., Sandler, I., and West, S. (1999). Cognitive moderators of children's adjustment to stressful divorce events: The role of negative cognitive errors and positive illusions. *Child Development*, *70*, 231–245.

McDonald, D. G., and Hodgdon, J. A. (1991). *The psychological effects of aerobic fitness training: Research and theory*. New York: Springer-Verlag Publishing.

O'Mara, A. J., Marsh, H. W., Craven, R. G., and Debus, R. L. (2006). Do self-concept interventions make a difference? A synergistic blend of construct validation and meta-analysis. *Educational Psychologist*, *41*, 181–206.

Prochaska, J. O., Redding, C. A., and Evers, K. A. (2002). The Transtheoretical Model and Stages of Change. In K. Glanz, B. Rimer, and F. M. Lewis (eds.), *Health behavior and health education: Theory, research, and practice* (3rd ed., pp. 99–120). San Francisco: Jossey-Bass.

Rhodes, J. E., and DuBois, D. L. (2006). Understanding and facilitating the youth mentoring movement. *Social Policy Report*, *20*(3).

Rhodes, J. E., Grossman, J. B., and Resche, N. L. (2000). Agents of change: Pathways through which mentoring relationships influence adolescents' academic adjustment. *Child Development*, *71*, 1662–1671

Rhodes, J. E., Reddy, R., and Grossman, J. B. (2005). The protective influence of mentoring on adolescents' substance use: Direct and indirect pathways. *Applied Developmental Science*, *9*, 31–47.

Rhodewalt, F. (2007). Possessing and striving for high self-esteem. In M. H. Kernis (Ed.), *Self-esteem issues and answers: A sourcebook of current perspectives* (pp. 281–287). New York: Psychology Press.

Rogers, C. R. (1961). *On becoming a person: A therapist's view of psychotherapy*. Boston: Houghton Mifflin.

Rosenberg, M. (1979). *Conceiving the self*. New York: Basic Books.

Rosenberg, M., Schooler, C., and Schoenbach, C. (1989). Self-esteem and adolescent problems: Modeling reciprocal effects. *American Sociological Review*, *54*, 1004–1018.

Rutter, M. (1987). Psychosocial resilience and protective mechanisms. *American Journal of Orthopsychiatry*, *57*, 316–331.

Salazar, L. F., DiClemente, R. J., Wingood, G. M., Crosby, R. A., Harrington, K., Davies, S., Hook, E. W., and Oh, M. K. (2004). Self-concept and adolescents' refusal of unprotected sex: A test of mediating mechanisms among African American girls. *Prevention Science*. 5, 137–149

Sallis, J. F., and Owen, N. (2002). Ecological models of health behavior. In K. Glanz, B. Rimer, and F. M. Lewis (eds.), *Health behavior and health education: Theory, research, and practice* (3rd ed., pp. 462–484). San Francisco: Jossey-Bass.

Seligman, M.E.P. (1993). *What you can change and what you can't: The complete guide to successful self-improvement*. New York: Fawcett.

Shedler, J., Mayman, M., and Manis, M. (1994). The illusion of mental health. *American Psychologist, 48*, 1117–1131.

Silverthorn, N., DuBois, D. L., Pryce, J. M., Sanchez, B., Zmiewski, M., Hauber, S., et al. (2008, March). Can we improve on the "gold standard"? Evaluation of a program to enhance relationships in the Big Brothers Big Sisters program. In M. J. Karcher and S. Larose (Chair), *How do effective mentoring relationships work? A look inside the dyads*. Symposium presented at the Biennial Meeting of the Society for Research on Adolescence, Chicago, IL.

Stice, E., and Shaw, H. (2004). Eating disorder prevention programs: A meta-analytic review. *Psychological Bulletin, 130*, 206–227.

Strauss, R. (2000). Childhood obesity and self-esteem. *Pediatrics, 105,* e15.

Taylor, S. E., and Brown, J. D. (1988). Illusions and well-being: A social psychological perspective on mental health. *Psychological Bulletin, 103*, 193–210.

Taylor, S. E., and Brown, J. D. (1994). Positive illusions and well-being revisited: Separating fact from fiction. *Psychological Bulletin, 116*, 21–27.

Tennen, H., and Affleck, G. (1993). The puzzles of self-esteem: A clinical perspective. In R. Baumeister (Ed.), *Self-esteem: The puzzle of low self-regard* (pp. 241–262). New York: Plenum.

Tesser, A. (2004). Self-esteem. In M. B. Brewer and M. Hewstone (eds.), *Emotion and motivation* (pp. 184–203). Malden, MA: Blackwell Publishing.

Trzesniewski, K. H., Donnellan, M. B., Moffitt, T. E., Robins, R. W., Poulton, R., and Caspi, A. (2006). Low self-esteem during adolescence predicts poor health, criminal behavior, and limited economic prospects during adulthood. *Developmental Psychology, 42*, 381–390.

Twenge, J. M. (2006). *Generation Me: Why today's young Americans are more confident, assertive, entitled—and more miserable than ever before*. New York: Free Press.

Twenge, J. M., and Campbell, W. K. (2002). Self-esteem and socioeconomic status: A meta-analytic review. *Personality and Social Psychology Review, 6*, 59–71.

Twenge, J. M., Zhang, L., and Im, C. (2004). It's beyond my control: A cross-temporal meta-analysis of increasing externality in locus of control, 1960–2002. *Personality and Social Psychology Review, 8*, 308–319.

Valentine, J. C., and DuBois, D. L. (2005). Effects of self-beliefs on academic achievement and vice-versa: Separating the chicken from the egg. In H. Marsh and R. Craven (eds.), *International advances in self research* (Vol. 2, pp. 53–75). Greenwich, CT: Information Age.

Wallston, K., Rothman, R. L., and Cherrington, A. (2007). Psychometric properties of the Perceived Diabetes Self-Management Scale (PDSMS). *Journal of Behavioral Medicine, 30*, 395–401

Weiner, L.S., & Battles, H.B. (2006). Untangling the web: A close look at diagnosis disclosure among HIV-infected adolescents. *Journal of Adolescent Health, 38*, 307-309.

Wingood, G. M., DiClemente, R. J., Harrington, K., and Davies, S. L. (2002). Body image and African American females' sexual health. *Journal of Women's Health and Gender-Based Medicine, 11*, 433–439.

World Health Organization. (1992). *Basic documents* (39th ed.). Geneva: Author.

Yarcheski, A., Mahon, N. E., Yarcheski, T. J., and Cannella, B. L. (2004). A meta-analysis of predictors of positive health practices. *Journal of Nursing Scholarship, 36*, 102–108.

Zimmerman, M. A., Copeland, L. A., Shope, J. T., and Dielman, T. E. (1997). A longitudinal study of self esteem: Implications for adolescent development. *Journal of Youth and Adolescence, 26*, 117–141.

CONSERVATION OF RESOURCES THEORY: APPLICATION TO PUBLIC HEALTH PROMOTION

Stevan E. Hobfoll
Jeremiah A. Schumm

CONSERVATION OF RESOURCES THEORY: RESOURCES FOR PUBLIC HEALTH

In order to promote public health, communities and individuals must possess the resources necessary for engaging in healthy behavior. Conservation of resources (COR) theory (Hobfoll, 1988, 1989, 1998a) offers a framework for implementing public health promotion strategies by focusing on the resources of individuals and communities. **COR theory** provides a theoretical model for preventing **resource loss,** maintaining existing resources, and gaining resources necessary for engaging in healthy behaviors. In this chapter, we outline the theoretical principles of COR theory. We provide more detailed examples of the application of COR theory to HIV prevention on the group level and the treatment of **traumatic stress** on the community level. Finally, we discuss future directions for integrating COR theory into public health promotion with a view toward enhancing resiliency rather than focusing only on disease prevention.

ORIGINS OF COR THEORY

Bringing the Environment into Focus

COR theory was developed in response to the need to incorporate more fully both the objective and perceived environment into the process of coping with stress. Homeostatic and transactional models of stress and coping (for example, McGrath, 1970; Lazarus, 1966) defined stress as the perception of imbalance between coping capacity and the environment. These theories emphasized individuals' *perceptions* of imbalance to be important. Further, these cognitively based models suggest that individuals must perceive the consequences of the imbalance as important, asserting individual difference factors. By emphasizing perceptions and values when defining stress and coping capacity, secondary emphasis is placed on environmental contingencies.

In regard to developing public health promotion strategies, homeostatic and transactional models of stress and coping present problems in their conceptualization of coping demand and coping capacity. In homeostatic and transactional models, coping demand and capacity are not separately defined (Hobfoll, 1989). Coping capacity is defined as that which offsets coping demand. Demand is seen, in turn, as that which challenges coping capacity (Lazarus and Folkman, 1984). Clearly, this reasoning is circular and is solely a derivative of individual, idiographic perception. Because demand and capacity are not separately defined, they and the principles relating to them are not given to rejection. Therefore, if it is left to individual appraisal, it is difficult to assert which resources target groups will require and what common obstacles will impede their applying resources to goal-directed efforts. In addition, there are no anchor points for defining capacity and demand. Thus, it would be difficult for public health promotion efforts to define and target coping resources necessary for improving public health.

When addressing majority world health and health of the poor anywhere, a focus on appraisals denies the bitter reality of poverty and how it often undermines the resources that are required to promote health and well-being. Said another way, individuals' appraisals are particularly important when economic, social, and personal resources are adequate, but appraisal becomes less relevant when personal, social, and environmental obstacles are more substantive. Further, for all cultures, many appraisals are normative, and shared by large portions of the populations. So, for example, Marianismo, holding women as virginal or "fallen" dichotomously, is a powerful, shared social appraisal of women's expected role in many Latin Catholic cultures. But this shared appraisal should not be confused with individual idiographic appraisal, which is what cognitive-behavioral theories do.

Along with the problems in defining demand and capacity, de-emphasis of the objective environment in transactional and homeostatic models might be particularly problematic for public health promotion. Focusing on perceptions without closely considering the objective environment may lead to some demands remaining unnoticed, since individuals may be successfully coping in the course of the process. Individuals rich in resources may be unaware of stressful environmental circumstances, while those lacking resources may feel overwhelmed in dealing with the same situation. Since many threats to public health are a result of or are at least strongly influenced by environmental sources, it would serve public health promotion efforts to focus on objective environmental circumstances. Even when perceptions are to be taken into account, it is group and broad-based social perceptions that must be considered foremost, not individual differences.

COR theory bridges the cognitive and environmental viewpoints. Hobfoll (1988, 1989, 1998a; 2001) proposes that perceptions of most major stressful events of interest to public health promotion are universally held. For example, contraction of HIV and living through a natural disaster are events that are universally perceived as stressful. This is not to say that perceptions are unimportant in coping with such events. Perceptions can determine the strategies that one employs when attempting to offset the losses associated with these circumstances. However, COR theory argues that resources are the key components to determining individuals' appraisals of events as stressful, and resources define how individuals are able to cope with the situation. COR theory also would posit that resiliency processes must exist through actions that support health and well-being. These, in turn, will bring the kinds of successes that would support beliefs in efficacy and the reliance on a supportive social fabric. If realities do not underpin such perceptions they will be easily challenged and will be unlikely to translate to actual health gains.

DESCRIPTION OF COR THEORY

COR theory proposes that individuals seek to create circumstances that will protect and promote the integrity of the individual, nested in family, and nested in tribe (Hobfoll, 1998a). That is to say, the individual must always be viewed in a social context, and acts to protect and preserve the self and the attachments that establish self in social context relationship. The focus of COR theory is on reactions to the environmental events that affect resources. *Psychological distress* is thus defined as a reaction to the environment in which there is (a) threat of net loss of resources, (b) actual net loss of resources, or (c) lack of **resource gain** following the investment of resources. Loss or threat of loss of resources is particularly stressful because individuals are faced with diminished coping capabilities in handling future challenges. Lack of resource gain following investment is stressful because individuals have failed to increase their coping capabilities following expenditure of resources. Because individuals have invested resources without an increase in return, this lack of gain equates to resource loss. In each case, resources are the single unit necessary for understanding stress.

Resources are defined as objects, personal characteristics, conditions, or energies. Object resources are valued because of some physical aspect or because of their acquiring secondary status based on their rarity and expense. A small economy car has value because it provides transportation, whereas a BMW has increased value because it also indicates status. *Conditions* are resources that are valued and sought after. Marriage and tenure are examples of these. *Personal characteristics* are resources in that they generally aid stress resistance. *Personally held skills* are a second type of personal resource, especially as these skills relate to acquiring or protecting valued resources. As will be explored later in this chapter, mastery and optimism are personal resources that can affect people's resistance to stress. Energies are typically intrinsically valued in that they aid in the acquisition of other resources. Examples of these include time, money, and knowledge. In addition to resources being broadly defined, COR theory proposes that resources are interrelated and changes in one or more types of resources can affect the availability of other resources.

COR theory proposes the following principles in relation to change in resources:

1. Resource loss is more powerful than resource gain.
2. Resources must be invested in order to gain resources or prevent their loss.

Further, COR theory proposes that those already lacking in resources will be more vulnerable to the experience of loss spirals, while those with ample resources will have more opportunity for resource gain. In other words, COR theory suggests that initial loss leaves individuals, groups, and communities more vulnerable to the negative impact of ongoing resource challenges. Those endowed with greater resources will, of course, be more resilient, but ongoing resource loss will challenge even richly resource-endowed individuals or groups. Thus, loss spirals are a powerful force that is evident in individuals and communities already lacking resources. This principle is especially germane to people living in majority world economies. These economies have a broad base of poor individuals who live day to day. Adding gender-power politics, which in many cases are supported by violence and the threat of violence (Wingood and DiClemente, 1997), it can be seen that loss spirals will be especially significant for the poorest, those lacking power, and oftentimes for women.

COR theory also provides a framework for public health promotion by conceptualizing the resources critical in promoting public health. In addition, public health promotion efforts utilizing COR theory can target loss spirals and prevent future loss in individuals and communities. Finally, COR theory provides public health promotion with the framework to instill resources necessary to the individual and community for promoting public health. This in turn can be used to facilitate and foster individual and community resiliency. Where failure and lack of aid is widespread, the presence of advocacy, health-promoting intervention, and efforts that empower individuals can have a multiplicative effect that extends beyond the immediate intervention and target health outcome. On the community level, COR theory can be used equally well to examine and intervene in community-level resources and the processes that effect them (Zamani, Gorgievski-Dujivesteihn, and Zarafshani, 2006).

EMPIRICAL EVIDENCE FOR COR THEORY

Now that we have presented the basic theoretical origins and predictions of COR theory (Hobfoll, 1988, 1989, 1998a), we will outline research that supports its predictions. The studies that will be presented cut across several domains and settings and provide broad evidence for the theory's principles. In addition, the studies offer empirical support for COR theory in a variety of populations, suggesting that COR theory has been validated for application to assorted groups targeted by public health promotion. It is our contention that these studies show that interventions based on COR theory are capable not only of reducing the negative psychological reactions but that resource-based interventions are a key intervention strategy.

Finally, we wish to reassert the importance of considering individual and community-based resources when conceptualizing and implementing public health programs and policies. Much health promotion work has focused on "the mind" and behavior, because the pathways and obstacles to availability of resources have often been taken by health psychologists and those in public health as a given. Poverty, low social status, racism, unavailability of health care, and other fundamental conditions are often beyond the scope of many health promotion interventions. COR theory maintains that, at minimum, these fundamental resource conditions should remain foremost on our minds, both because they are necessary for the success of any program, and because failing to refer to them risks blaming the victim. No health promotion program can sidestep the resource reservoir that is ultimately available to people and the pathways that are often denied those who lack resources or the status that allows them to utilize what resources they might have.

Principle 1: Resource Loss Is More Powerful Than Resource Gain

COR theory proposes that resource loss is more salient than resource gain. Resource loss has been demonstrated to be a more powerful force than resource gain in a variety of cognitive, evolutionary, and psychosocial studies. Cognitive and evolutionary studies provide evidence for COR on a basic processing and evolutionary level. In turn, studies that focus on psychosocial outcomes provide evidence for the direct applicability of COR theory to outcomes of interest to public health promotion interventionists.

In the cognitive processing domain, several studies have supported the primacy of resource loss. In prospect theory, Tversky and Kahneman (1974) noted the steeper gradient for loss when compared to gain. Also, Tversky and Kahneman (1974) noted that an event involving loss engenders greater risk taking than a mathematical equivalent event involving gain. Individuals seem predisposed toward deciding against initiating events that have the potential for loss as compared to the potential for gain. It is important to note that this cognitive bias is not represented in people's awareness, that is, they do not know that they are making decisions based on the greater loss gradient.

In measuring brain activity, Cacioppo and colleagues (Cacioppo and Gardner, in press; Ito, Larsen, Smith, and Cacioppo, 1998) provide evidence for a *negativity bias* when perceiving aversive, appealing, or neutral stimuli. These authors view positive and negative emotional systems as being separate neuroanatomical pathways, and provide compelling evidence for greater processing energy elicited by negative stimuli. Their research suggests that negative or loss-related stimuli have a greater impact on processing efforts in the brain, and supports the lopsided impact of loss primacy at the neuroanatomical level.

Additional evidence for the disproportional impact of resource loss can be found in recent work in cognitive psychology on *immune neglect* (Gilbert, Pinel, Wilson, Blumberg, and Wheatley, 1998). Learning theory predicts that people should become conditioned to the fact that negative life events are typically overcome. In other words, people should learn to accurately perceive that adversity is usually conquered. They should not be as worried and as alarmed by threatening cues in the environment as they are. Contrary to this prediction, individuals continue to overestimate the degree of threat in potentially aversive events. In other words, they ignore the robustness of their *psychological immune system*. This is significant for predicting people's actions because their behavior is largely derived from their overreactive, oversensitive predictions concerning the emotional consequences of threatening events. Hence, this research on immune neglect suggests that the primacy of loss is not overcome through conditioning; we cannot learn not to overestimate loss and threat. What this suggests is that loss's impact must be occurring on a biological level, as it is resistant to environmentally based learning.

Although evolutionary explanations are generally unprovable, there is agreement among resource theorists that resource loss is primary because of its adaptive advantages for biological, attentional, psychological, and cultural systems (Carver and Scheier, 1998). The deep-seated biological nature of psychological reactions in trauma events provides evidence for the evolutionary importance of losses as they relate to survival (van der Kolk, 1996a, b). Specifically, traumatic events tend to imprint on the victim a memory for the event that alters the startle response to similar stimuli. In other words, whereas victims would normally exhibit an immediate, time-limited response that is accompanied by somatic and attentive arousal, this response is prolonged, accompanied with the smells, sounds, and sights of the event, and is rekindled as if during the original event by associated stimuli. Such a trauma constellation has been argued to have a biological basis, since on a psychological level, this reaction would appear to be counterproductive to functioning. This imprinted, hyper-vigilant reaction to trauma must serve the function of reminding the individual of the critical nature of the loss stimulus.

In addition to the cognitive-evolutionary evidence for the primacy of resource loss, evidence from psychosocial outcome literature also provides ample support for this principle. Studies have shown that resource loss in comparison to resource gain is a stronger predictor of negative psychological reactions such as anger, anxiety, and depression (for example, Hobfoll and Lilly, 1993; Lane and Hobfoll, 1992; Wells, Hobfoll, and Lavin, 1997, 1999). Lane and Hobfoll (1992) found in a longitudinal study of chronic obstructive-pulmonary disease patients that resource loss, but not resource gain, was predictive of outwardly expressed anger. Anger expression by these patients was concurrently related to anger expression of their significant others. Resource loss was found to be the major variable, compared to resource gain, in determining the anger of patients and subsequent anger of significant others. Thus, the amount of resources acquired by individuals has less influence in preventing distress than the effect of resource erosion has on causing distress.

In concluding the discussion of evidence for the primacy of resource loss, a particularly compelling series of studies by Holahan, Moos, Holahan, and Cronkite (1999, 2000) provided support for the long-term, powerful impact of resource loss. In these studies, interpersonal and personality resource losses were directly predictive of depressive symptoms over the course of extended periods of years. This relationship existed after controlling for initial symptoms of depression, in the first case in a community sample, and in the second instance in a clinically depressed sample. Critically, this study found that the impact of resource change entirely mediated the effect of life events on later depression. That is, only if resources were altered did life events influence changes in depression. This evidence again suggests resource loss's pervasive effect on the psychological well-being of individuals. Taken together with other evidence for the primacy of resource loss in predicting distress, it would appear that public health promotion efforts should target loss to prevent immediate and long-term negative psychological reactions as well as the behavioral manifestations that accompany them.

LOSS SPIRALS

As previously discussed, loss spirals tend to occur among individuals already lacking adequate resources or where initial resource loss renders people's resource reserves inadequate to meet subsequent, ongoing demand. King, King, Foy, Keane, and Fairbank (1999) provided compelling evidence for the negative impact of long-term loss spirals. In this study, a large sample of Vietnam veterans provided information regarding prewar risk factors such as family instability, war-zone stressors such as perceived threat during combat, and postwar resiliency-recovery variables such as social support. Using structural equation modeling, King et al. (1999) developed a model for predicting symptoms of post-traumatic stress disorder (PTSD) that was

FIGURE 5.1   *Model for Predicting Symptoms of PTSD*

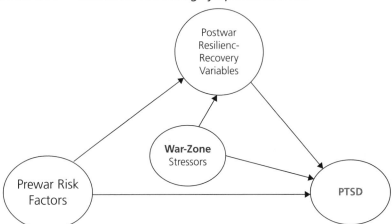

Source: Adapted from King et al., 1999.

consistent with the predictions made by COR theory (Figure 5.1). The authors found that individuals experiencing prewar loss tended to lack the postwar resiliency-recovery variables to help offset the stressors experienced during combat. In other words, lifelong loss spirals in combination with war-zone stressors exacerbated symptoms of PTSD. Notably, the model was highly effective in predicting PTSD, accounting for the majority of the variance in PTSD symptoms.

In a second study of middle-class pregnant women, Wells, Hobfoll, and Lavin (1999) found that women who had resource loss during later pregnancy were relatively unaffected by those events. In contrast, women who had resource loss both early and late in pregnancy were markedly negatively affected by the latter resource loss experiences. These findings indicate that these relatively well-resource-endowed women were resistant to resource loss if it was time-limited. Their likely underlying resource pools were adequate to respond in their defense. However, as **resource loss cycles** continued, there was deterioration in their ability to psychologically defend themselves and the negative sequelae in terms of increased anger and depressive mood were marked. This has important public health implications because these same factors have been linked to infant health (Rini, Dunkel-Schetter, Wadhwa, and Sandman, 1999).

These studies suggest that public health promotion efforts would be most effective when applied early to those at risk for experiencing future loss. Children lacking the economic, familial, and psychological resources to buffer future trauma are already being set up for potential downward psychosocial spiral. Moreover, the studies suggest that even those possessing substantive resource reservoirs are vulnerable if loss cycles are ongoing. Interventions targeting one or more of these categorized risk factors have the potential for preventing the vicious, snowballing loss cycle described in COR theory. For public health promotion efforts aimed at adult populations, an immediate focus in stopping resource loss would be extremely important in adults who have experienced a lifetime of such loss. Specific strategies for prevention, especially as they relate to preventing and minimizing trauma reactions, will be discussed in greater detail later in this chapter. Comprehensive studies such as that of King et al. (1999) highlight the importance of interrupting or preventing loss spirals for interventions targeting psychological distress.

Principle 2: Resources Must Be Invested to Gain Resources or Prevent Their Loss

Resources do not simply fall from the sky. Yet, most studies of resources as basic as self-efficacy and social support have uniformly ignored that the growth and maintenance of key resources requires a certain set of circumstances. Key resources depend on prior supportive environments, success histories, and the availabilities of pathways that allow success. It follows from COR theory that individuals must invest in order to acquire the reservoirs needed for buffering future loss, or they must receive resource investment from outside sources, be they parents, loved ones, work, or a favorable social system. According to predictions made by COR theory, resource gains are important in the context of loss. However, the key to understanding the empirical prediction made by this principle is *in the context of loss*. Gain cycles impact stress-related responses principally because such acquired resource reserves can serve to offset the losses.

A variety of personal resources have been shown to help offset the impact of resource loss. Self-efficacy is one such resource. Bandura (1997) defined self-efficacy as the view of self in the context of a specific challenge, such as the sense of mastering caretaking responsibilities with one's children. In prospective studies, self-efficacy has been found to be a personal resource that can help offset the losses associated with events ranging from minor hassles to major traumatic events (Bandura, 1997).

Another personal resource that has been shown to buffer resource loss is dispositional optimism. Scheier and Carver (1985, 1992; Carver and Scheier, 1998) have prospectively shown that surgery patients with higher dispositional optimism recover more quickly on both the physiological and the symptomatic levels. Thus, optimism might drive goal-oriented actions promoting health and have a more direct impact on people's well-being. Similar health-related outcomes have been found for self-esteem. People high in self-esteem are less likely to interpret difficulties as a function of their own inadequacies (Rosenberg, 1965). Women high in self-esteem, for example, have been found to be less negatively affected by complications of pregnancy (Hobfoll and Leiberman, 1987; Hobfoll, Nadler, and Leiberman, 1986). These studies suggest that public health promotion efforts would be wise to focus at the individual level on promoting gains in personal resources to provide a cushion for the powerful blows administered by resource loss.

Social resources have also been found to help buffer the effects of loss-related events. Social support has been an area of focus in this resource category. Social support is actually a complex construct that includes aspects such as the exchange of supportive interactions and the perception of the receipt of support (Sarason, Sarason, Shearin, and Pierce, 1987; Vaux, 1988). People higher in social support have been found to have better mental and physical health outcomes (Cohen and Wills, 1985; House, Landis, and Umberson, 1988; Vaux, 1988). Specifically related to physical health outcomes, recent experimental evidence convincingly shows that those with social support are less prone to infection (Cohen, Doyle, Skoner, Rabin, and Gwaltney, 1997). Thus, public health interventions should seek to increase not only the personal resources but also the social resources of the individual. Such efforts will become particularly important in the context of loss-related events such as physical illness or psychological trauma.

Although personal and social resources have been found to buffer loss, such resources have limited impact in the presence of major, ongoing loss cycles (Hobfoll and Lilly, 1993; Lane and Hobfoll, 1992). Although this notion was proposed in Principle 1 of COR theory, such reiteration serves to highlight the interaction in loss and gain cycles proposed by COR theory. In addition to COR theory predicting that gain will not have opposite and equal impact, it predicts that impacts of gain are not independent of loss. Again, gain is important mainly in that it is directly related to the potential for offsetting loss.

Studies by Wells, Hobfoll, and Lavin (1997, 1999) provide empirical evidence for the importance of resource gain in the context of loss. Pregnant women were followed prospectively to examine the impact of potential loss and gain cycles in a population experiencing potentially stressful life change. Consistent with Principle 1 of COR theory, resource loss but not resource gain was found to be directly related to changes in anger and depressive mood. However, related to Principle 2 of COR theory, resource gain became very important in women experiencing a great deal of resource loss. Specifically, women who experienced substantive gains were significantly less impacted by losses than those who had experienced no resource gain. This study provided support for the prediction that resource gains are important in offsetting loss, but gains do not have the same appreciable direct impact as resource losses.

In another study by Billings, Folkman, Acree, and Moskowitz (2000), AIDS caretakers who are experiencing severe resource loss cycles were found to be more psychologically resilient to the extent that they experienced resource gains with these same loved ones. One interpretation of this is that resource gains allow resource replenishment at this critical period. A further interpretation harks back to the early work of Viktor Frankl (1963), who noted that in the midst of tragedy, people seek to make positive meaning in order to sustain their plummeting psychological state. In making meaning, people attempt to create and focus on gains amidst tragedy and this may have a particularly sustaining effect. This would suggest that resource gain is in itself recuperative, and that individuals seek gains in order to sustain this recuperative impact.

Finally, a recent longitudinal study by Chang, Wong, and Tsang (2007) provides a caveat to the COR theory contention that gain cycles must be evaluated within the context of resource losses. Chang, Wong, and Tsang used COR theory to understand how the interaction of benefits (that is, resource gains) and costs (that is, resource losses) related to severe acute respiratory syndrome (SARS) might later impact the psychosocial resources of individuals and their family members in China who were exposed to SARS. Results showed that individuals who initially experienced both resource gains and losses following personal or family member SARS exposure had higher psychosocial resources at the eighteen-month follow-up. However, those who experienced initial benefits or resource gains without any initial costs or resource losses had *worse* psychosocial adjustment eighteen months later. These results highlight the COR theory proposition that resource gains are important within the context of offsetting loss. These findings are important in that they further advance this proposition by suggesting that following traumatic events, experiencing resource gains without the contextual backdrop of experiencing resource losses may create an illusory sense of positive growth. In this way, the experience of "no pain, all gain" may produce a false mind-set of having benefited from a traumatic event without translating this cognitive construction into meaningful action that improves coping resources. These findings support a secondary prevention approach to promoting resiliency in that individuals who are most likely to benefit from such public health interventions are those who have experienced resource loss as a result of physical or psychological trauma.

Both resource gain and loss are critical to understanding efforts to support resiliency and healthy behavior (as opposed to the mere lack of disease and distress, or not behaving in an unhealthy manner). Specifically, COR theory predicts that resiliency demands an ongoing, supported cycle of resource gain and a limited cycle of resource loss. Because resource loss is more powerful and faster moving than resource gain, gain cycles are by their nature fragile. To promote resiliency, gain cycles must be supported, fostered, and protected from the undermining nature of resource loss. This is especially a challenge for under resourced environments where the poor live, whether within developed countries or in economically underdeveloped countries.

CASE APPLICATION OF COR THEORY AS AN INTERVENTION

Although we have provided general suggestions regarding the application of COR theory to interventions, a case example will provide a concrete model for applying COR theory to public health promotion.

We will now present interventions aimed at reducing HIV/AIDS risk, as well as risk of violence among high-risk inner-city women. This program of research was reported in a series of publications by Hobfoll and colleagues (Britton, Levine, Jackson, Hobfoll, Shepherd, and Lavin, 1998; Hobfoll, 1998b; Hobfoll, Jackson, Lavin, Britton, and Shepherd, 1993; Hobfoll, Jackson, Lavin, Britton, and Shepherd, 1994a, b; Hobfoll, Jackson, Lavin, Johnson, and Schröder, 2002; Levine, Britton, James, Jackson, and Hobfoll, 1993; MacKenzie, Hobfoll, Ennis, Kay, Jackson, and Lavin, 1999) in which COR theory is described as part of intervention strategies aimed at reducing HIV risk activity. We note on the outset that it is not our intent to show that our intervention was more effective than other excellent models in the literature. Rather, we hope to highlight how a resource approach informs intervention.

Moreover, where our intervention is seen as similar to others that were derived from other theoretical perspectives, it may be argued that the resource perspective might be more fundamental to those perspectives than their authors have noted.

Specific Theoretical Assumptions of the Intervention

1. Change Is Resource-Driven, and Resources Are Interrelated The HIV reduction intervention strategies used by Hobfoll and colleagues were based on several theoretical underpinnings. A general guiding assumption based on COR theory was that changes were resource-driven (Hobfoll, 1998b). In order to produce changes in sexual behavior, it was assumed that individuals must be provided with the resources to produce those changes. In addition, personal, social, and socioeconomic resources were viewed as interconnected entities; that is, they tend to travel in caravans. This means that where one major resource is found, other key resources are likely to accompany it. Further, these caravans tend to cross from the self to the social domains. Therefore, interventions were developed that would provide these high-risk inner-city women with the personal, social, and economic resources necessary to practice safer sex behaviors.

Education about HIV and women's risk for contracting HIV was incorporated as an integral part of the interventions. It was assumed that if individuals were not convinced of the need for change, they were likely to take cognitive shortcuts such as minimizing their risk assessment (Hobfoll, 1998b). Efforts were made to relate the risk to a variety of outcomes for the women, such as the consequences that HIV might have for their health and their children. The interventions focused on convincing women of the potential negative impact of HIV on broad personal consequences.

If individuals did not have the resources necessary for change, they were also expected to engage in cognitive shortcuts (Hobfoll, 1998b). In other words, provision of education was viewed as a necessary, but not sufficient variable in changing the women's decision making about their risk for contracting HIV. If women were provided with the information on their HIV risk but not provided with the resources necessary to change this risk, it was expected that they would minimize their assessment of their personal risk for contracting HIV. Therefore, provision of the personal, social, and economic resources for changing sexual behavior was necessary for the women to change their personal risk assessment.

2. Empowerment Increases Resources Needed for Change Similar to the approach used by Wingood (see Chapter Fourteen in this volume), Hobfoll and colleagues viewed empowerment as a key to promoting safer sex behaviors in inner-city, pregnant women (Hobfoll, 1998b). The approach to empowerment used by Hobfoll and colleagues was based on the theory of **Gender and Power** (Connell, 1987) and defined empowerment as the interpersonal concept of relationships. In accordance with this theory, interventions emphasized ethnic and gender pride to increase women's sense of empowerment. It was assumed that such a strategy would increase the personal resources needed to instigate safer sex behaviors, such as the self-efficacy to negotiate with partners about using condoms. Thus, increasing pride was assumed to be a facet of the intervention that would have a direct impact on the personal and social resources of women.

3. Increasing Sense of Community and Attachment Helps Change Social Norms For poorer, inner-city women, raising the possibility of condom use with partners may raise the question of fidelity and endanger the women's romantic ties. Many of these women are not only connected romantically to their partners, but they rely on their partners to help provide economic support and a place to live. In order for women to successfully implement condom use, we encouraged women to engage support from both their partners and other women in the group. Interventions sought not only to raise women's sense of personal responsibility, but also responsibility toward their partners, other women in the group, their parents, and their children (or future children). Women were encouraged to think about their health and well-being as part of their key social attachments. They were also provided skills for encouraging this perspective with their partners. In this way, a sense of community responsibility was used to change social norms about safe sex.

4. Multiple Sessions Provide More Opportunity for Change A final theoretical assumption of Hobfoll and colleagues was that interventions should be spread over multiple sessions (Hobfoll, 1998b). Multiple sessions provided more opportunity for the women to increase their sense of community and empowerment. It was assumed that a single-session intervention would not allow the women to develop the social ties and pride necessary for producing adequate change in sexual practices. In addition, a multiple-session approach was assumed to provide more opportunity to increase the resources necessary for women to decide that safer sex behaviors were necessary and achievable. In general, a multiple-session approach was assumed to be a necessity for increasing the resources for change.

Of course, many interventions have used multiple sessions. The difference lies in that other interventions have tended to use multiple sessions to reach additional goals, with each session having a different objective. COR theory suggests that resource gain is slow and incremental. Hence, our interventions have tended to have fewer goals, but to work on each resource gain more intensively. Indeed, if we could convince women to come for more sessions, we would still not increase our number of resource targets, but instead work on each in more depth.

TWO RANDOMIZED, CONTROLLED CLINICAL TRIALS

First Generation Trial

Hobfoll and colleagues (Hobfoll, et al., 1994a) conducted a randomized clinical trial of the first generation of their intervention. Participants in this first trial were single, pregnant, inner-city women. The intervention was tailored toward impacting the specific resources necessary for these women to engage in safer sex.

The efficacy of the intervention was assessed through self-report and objective measures of behavior change. Participants completed a variety of self-report measures similar to those focused on other HIV prevention efforts (Fisher, Fisher, Misovich, Kimble, and Malloy, 1996). In addition, participants were provided condom credit cards through which they could obtain free condoms and spermicide from several local pharmacies, and pharmacies provided reports on the number of condoms and spermicide tubes obtained by participants. In summary, self-report and objective measures of safer-sex behavior were used to measure efficacy of this COR theory-based intervention.

Participants were randomly assigned to one of three groups: HIV prevention, health promotion, or no-intervention control. Intervention groups met for four sessions of one to two hours and included up to eight participants in addition to a female group leader. HIV prevention and health promotion interventions differed in that the HIV prevention group focused on sexual behavior, while the health promotion group focused on more general health-related behaviors such as turning down alcohol or smoking. Consistent with theoretical assumptions, interventions were multisession and provided the information and resources deemed necessary for change.

Various techniques were used to provide women with the social and personal resources necessary for initiating safer sex. Videotapes were created to support the curriculum and insure the integrity of the intervention across group leaders and over time. They were used to demonstrate and facilitate discussion of assertiveness, negotiation, and planning. Videotapes included actors representative of the target population, which was thought to enhance the effectiveness of the modeling techniques being demonstrated (Bandura, 1977). Consistent with the tenets of COR theory, videotapes were training based, that is, they encouraged participant skill practice, rather than passive viewing and discussion. In addition, discussion and practice of the modeled behaviors were thought to enhance the participants' sense of empowerment and community. In summary, a variety of techniques provided participants with the basic personal and social resources necessary for changing sexual behavior.

Related to the interactions based on modeled behavior, group discussion of previous sex-related mastery experiences were also viewed as essential to increasing the social and personal resources of women. These discussions helped group members develop a repertoire of strategies for engaging in safe sex or healthy behaviors and, therefore, to broaden women's personal resources. As with the videotape facet of the intervention, group discussions were thought to provide women with the resources necessary for enacting targeted behaviors, increasing participants' sense of empowerment and their sense of community.

Other facets of personal and social resources were also targeted through cognitive rehearsal and conditioning experiences. Participants cognitively rehearsed enacting target behaviors to help develop scripts for engaging in such behaviors in the future. Thus, cognitive rehearsal was another strategy used to increase women's personal resources necessary for engaging in safe sex. Interventions also incorporated aversive-conditioning experiences (Wolpe, 1958) paired with positive-conditioning experiences. For the aversive-conditioning experiences, participants were asked to imagine an unhealthy behavior (for example, unprotected sex) and aversive outcome (for example, becoming infected with HIV). Aversive conditioning was followed by a positive-conditioning experience in which participants paired a healthy behavior with a healthy outcome. The goals of the conditioning experiences were to increase mastery and change the group norms for healthy and unhealthy behaviors. Thus, techniques were adopted from the cognitive and behavioral literature in order to effectively target personal and social resources.

A final component of the intervention was the provision of condom credit cards to participants. These cards allowed women to obtain free latex condoms and spermicide from several pharmacies proximal to the clinic sites. Credit cards were valid from the time participants began the study until twelve months post-intervention (yoked to time for a no-intervention control group). Provision of the means for engaging in protected sex was viewed as necessary for instigating safer-sex behavior change. Not only were participants provided with the personal and social resources necessary for changes in sexual behavior, but the intervention also provided participants with the physical or economic resources necessary for instigating these changes.

Results provided strong support for the efficacy of the intervention. The HIV prevention group made greater overall gains within the outcome variables (HIV knowledge, safer sex intentions and behaviors, discussion of HIV and HIV prevention with partners, and condom and spermicide use) than the health promotion or no-intervention control group. Further, these effects were maintained at the six-month follow-up. These results provided support for the effectiveness of this particular intervention in increasing self-reported sex behaviors that are commonly examined in HIV prevention studies.

The HIV-focused intervention was found to be especially effective for promoting changes in objective behavior (that is, acquisition of condoms and spermicide). Women in the HIV intervention were found to be more likely to have used condom credit cards and to have obtained a greater number of condoms. Similar effects were found for the health-focused group; however, the effects were not as pervasive as the HIV-focused group. Thus, the HIV intervention produced the most pervasive changes in objective sex-related behavior. In conclusion, the HIV-focused intervention was broadly effective in promoting self-reported and objective changes in sex-related behaviors.

Second Generation Trial

In the second-generation randomized clinic trial, Hobfoll, Jackson, Lavin, Johnson, and Schröder (2002) incorporated negotiation skills training more centrally into the interventions. Negotiation training was hypothesized to increase women's resources for engaging in safer sex by increasing women's abilities to effectively engage their partners in safer sex. Interventions included non pregnant and pregnant women along with African American and European American women. Interventions also included facets tested in the previous generation of interventions (Hobfoll et al., 1994a) along with medical testing for sexually transmitted diseases (STDs). Thus, the second-generation trial attempted to expand the applicability of the interventions, and increase the resources of women, with major attention placed on the acquisition of negotiation skills.

Consistent with the first generation trial, women in the HIV prevention group were found to exhibit pervasive changes in self-reported and objective sexual behavior. In addition, women in the HIV prevention and health promotion groups were found to improve in the efficacy of their negotiation skills. Such an effect was anticipated, since both interventions targeted general negotiation skills. Finally, women in the HIV prevention group who had contracted an STD sometime earlier in their life showed reduction in point-prevalence of medically tested STDs, compared to women in the health promotion group, although no different than the no-intervention control. These results, provided further objective evidence for the effectiveness of this public health promotion strategy. In summary, the second-generation trial provided support for the efficacy of increasing women's resources for engaging in safer sexual behaviors.

Summary of Trials

The controlled clinical trials presented here highlight the importance of resource-driven change in public health promotion. Women were provided with the personal, social, and physical resources necessary for changing behavior. Interventions provided opportunities for increasing personal and social resources such as mastery, sense of community, and sense of empowerment. Further, opportunities for obtaining the physical resources (that is, condoms) necessary for behavior change were incorporated. In conclusion, a multifaceted intervention was shown to be effective in targeting the multiple resources necessary for engaging in healthy behaviors.

What is also important to note is where we failed to produce change. In this regard, women often reported limitations to change that were due to resource constraints. Their lack of economic viability, associated with their poor education and poor availability of good work often made them dependent on men who the women themselves felt were undesirable or unsafe. On a more day-to-day basis, women would miss sessions due to daycare limitations, or last-minute changes in their employers' requirements for their work. Having few work-related benefits (for example, insurance, guaranteed sick leave, or vacation time), they were often at employers' whim. Further, lack of transportation resources made attendance difficult for some women, especially in inclement weather. More major disruptions occurred where women lost their phone or housing. As many as 40 percent of these women had no "rights" to their housing, but were living at another's behest, and often lost their housing when interpersonal difficulties arose. At the same time as we attempt to alter women's resources, we must acknowledge greater social and economic factors that serve as obstacles to intervention.

FUTURE DIRECTIONS FOR EXPANDING COR THEORY

Application to Traumatic Stress

A second promising direction for extending the application of COR theory is in the realm of traumatic stress. Indeed, research has demonstrated the importance of resource loss in predicting psychological and physical health in victims of trauma. By evaluating efforts based on COR theory to date, we can also use this opportunity to explain how COR theory can be applied to community-level resources, and move beyond the individual focus.

As previously discussed in this chapter, King et al. (1999) found strong support for COR theory in their study of PTSD in Vietnam veterans. Long-term losses over the course of the veterans' lifetimes were found to account for the large majority of variability in PTSD diagnoses. In a study of victims of Hurricane Andrew, Ironson and colleagues (1997) found resource loss to be the best of a wide array of cognitive and psychological predictors of PTSD and general psychological distress. Resource loss was also found to have biological correlates in hurricane victims. Specifically, resource loss predicted lowered natural killer cell cytoxicity and increased white blood cell count, indicating an increase in immune system effort toward fighting infection.

Resource loss was further studied in response to the attacks on the World Trade Center in New York on September 11, 2001 (Hobfoll, Tracy, and Galea, 2006) and to the impact of ongoing terrorism in Israel (Hobfoll, Canetti-Nisim and Johnson, 2006; Hobfoll, Canetti-Nisim, Johnson, Varley, Palmieri, and Galea, 2008). In both instances psychosocial and material loss had major influence on post-traumatic stress and depression. This is important because theories pertaining to trauma and PTSD focus on peri-traumatic phenomena and cognitive-emotional reactivity, and not on the losses that people endure. These losses are in part cognitive, regarding hope, self-esteem, and belief in self-agency, but it is perhaps more surprising that people are largely affected by losses in material and job domains as well. Perhaps most to the point, the cognitive and material losses go hand in hand as predicted by COR theory. This has major relevancy for intervention as well, since correcting for resource losses and restoring losses are viable avenues for public health intervention (Hobfoll, Watson, et al., 2007).

Understanding of the process of resource loss as informed by COR theory can also aid the study of resiliency processes. A recent study by Bonanno, Galea, Bucciarelli, and Vlahov (2007) found that resource losses experienced by New York City residents following the September 11, 2001 terrorist attacks were important not only in predicting PTSD symptoms, but also were a central predictor in classifying which individuals demonstrated resilience in the context of these traumatic events. Predictions made by COR theory have implications not only for prediction but also promotion of the health and resilience of trauma victims.

Research has also demonstrated that resource loss is the key variable in predicting ability to cope with natural disasters. Freedy and colleagues (Freedy, Saladin, Kilpatrick, Resnick, and Saunders, 1994; Freedy, Shaw, Jarrell, and Masters, 1992) studied individuals in several types of natural disasters (hurricanes and earthquakes). Freedy et al. (1992, 1994) found resource loss was the most important variable in predicting motivation to cope with these natural disasters. This research suggests that public health promotion should focus on minimizing or eliminating resource loss, when possible, in order to increase individuals' motivation for coping and ability to cope with disasters.

Our line of research among economically disadvantaged, inner-city women suggests that resource loss is a key variable impacting women's lives in the context of traumatic events. In a study of women attending an inner-city substance-use treatment program, Schumm, Hobfoll, and Keogh (2004) found that recent interpersonal losses were associated with higher PTSD severity after accounting for the impact of childhood trauma and adult rape. Building on these results, Schumm, Stines, Hobfoll, and Jackson (2005) examined the interaction between child abuse and resource loss among a community sample of inner-city women. Results from this longitudinal study showed that women who experienced higher levels of childhood physical abuse were more psychologically damaged by resource loss spirals occurring during the course of the study (see also Johnson, Palmieri, Jackson, and Hobfoll, 2007). This effect, known as the "kindling hypothesis," suggests that childhood traumas can act like experiential kindling, such that resource loss spirals experienced later in life by abuse survivors are likely to quickly ignite and lead to a high amount of psychological distress. Finally, we examined the interaction of cumulative traumas experienced over the life span, and levels of social support resources in a large community sample of women (Schumm, Briggs-Phillips, and Hobfoll, 2006). Findings from this study showed that social support was most compromised among women who experienced traumas in both childhood and adulthood, versus those who experienced trauma during one or none of these developmental periods. Yet social support was shown to have the most impact in buffering PTSD among women who experienced traumas during both childhood and adulthood, versus those who experienced traumas in one or none of these periods. Findings from this study lend further support to the COR theory prediction that cumulative traumas are likely to cause resource loss spirals and, thereby, leave survivors deprived of important coping resources. Findings from these studies also suggest that public health interventions should be aimed at halting loss spirals that can quickly accumulate as a result of trauma histories.

Thus, it would do well to apply this work, for example, to an understanding of secondary losses experienced by people with HIV/AIDS and how loss cycles following trauma lead to exposure to HIV/AIDS. In a recent study, Simalyi, Kalichman, Strebel, Cloete, Henda, and Mqeketo (2007) found that persons in South Africa living with HIV/AIDS experienced further loss of sense of well-being, increased sense of stigma, with one in five losing their jobs, and subsequent increases of emotional distress. Likewise, it follows from COR theory that HIV/AIDS and poverty will be linked, with poverty-related stressors increasing risk for HIV exposure. In this light, Kalichman, Simbayi, Kagee, Toefy, Jooste, Cain, et al. (2006) found that HIV/AIDS risks were closely associated with indicators of poverty in South Africa. This research is excellent, but we believe would be further aided by noting COR theory, or other comprehensive theories that link resources, resource loss, emotional reactions, and health behavior. Otherwise, studies take a rather atheoretical epidemiological approach that limits the potential for intervention as to where to intervene and how theory can inform such intervention in these resource loss cycles.

In this regard, the nature of losses following traumatic events makes the mobilization and provision of resources especially important (Kaniasty and Norris, 2001; Norris and Kaniasty, 1996). Traumatic stress involves rapid loss of highly valued resources (Hobfoll, 1991). Those with few existing resources prior to the trauma have greater difficulty in coping with the effects of the traumatic loss and are at greater risk for clinical trauma reactions such as post-traumatic stress disorder (PTSD) or depression. In addition, the rapidness of losses during trauma, the unexpected nature of those losses, and the excessive demands of the traumatic event further burdens those with little existing resources (Hobfoll, 1991). Therefore, the mobilization and provision of resources to offset the losses resulting from trauma is critical for intervention strategies.

Application to Trauma Interventions

On the community level, COR theory can capture and guide collective efforts for coping with large-scale traumatic events (for example, earthquakes, nuclear disasters). It is helpful to categorize of community resources for the purpose of targeting multiple resources (Monnier and Hobfoll, 2000). Examples of personal characteristics of the community that might be targeted are community pride and cohesion (Monnier and Hobfoll, 2000). Increasing and mobilizing community pride and cohesion can help the community work together and increase collective coping efforts. Resources such as bridges, roads, and industries can be conceptualized as community object resources (Monnier and Hobfoll, 2000). The impact of object resources permeates short-term and long-term coping ability of the community. Along with community personal and object resources, communities' conditional resources such as availability of employment and emergency services might be important foci of trauma intervention efforts. Finally, resources such as money, heating, and transportation and fuel costs are energy resources that can be targeted by community-level interventions. In all, COR theory provides interventionists with useful ways of organizing facets of the intervention into conceptual categories and helps interventionists arrange mobilization efforts directed to these conceptual categories.

In addition to conceptualizing which resource categories to target, interventionists should proceed through several steps when helping communities and individuals cope with trauma (Monnier and Hobfoll, 2000). First, the focus should be on estimating the extent of the loss. For community-level trauma, this step might center on measuring the loss of people and property. Second, the availability of resources for dealing with the loss should be assessed (Monnier and Hobfoll, 2000). Emergency services might be needed to limit immediate trauma-related loss while mental health professionals might be mobilized to help individuals deal with the loss and limit clinical trauma reactions. Third, interventionists should consult with community leaders to become educated on the scope of the trauma and coping strategies that can be used by the community (Monnier and Hobfoll, 2000). Community leaders can help interventionists prioritize the most important community resources. Interventions can most successfully be developed using COR theory to guide the categorization of resources and following descriptive steps in administering the intervention.

To help communities and individuals cope with trauma, prevention efforts need to involve initiating **resource gain cycles** prior to the traumatic event (Monnier and Hobfoll, 2000). For example, helping communities gain the emergency services needed to cope with disasters will provide the community with immediate resources necessary for coping with disasters when they occur. Along with using the conceptual resource categories of COR theory for developing a strategy when trauma occurs, intervention-ists can use the conceptual categories to organize and target prevention efforts.

Theoretical Integration with COR Theory

Along with expanding COR theory into the domain of trauma, another promising direction is to investigate the efficacy of COR theory in combination with other theoretical approaches. COR theory provides a framework for ensuring that resources are in place for effectively integrating specific intervention approaches focused on specific interpersonal, cognitive, or behavioral strategies.

Integrating the Theory of Gender and Power with COR Theory As previously detailed in this chapter, Hobfoll and colleagues have integrated the theory of gender and power (Connell, 1987) along with the tenets of COR theory to develop an effec-tive approach to help inner-city women increase safer-sex behaviors. The theory of gender and power focuses on interpersonal resources, especially power within male-female relationships. Such an approach is especially important when considering the resource needs of historically disempowered groups such as minority inner-city women or women experiencing a lifetime of resource loss spirals.

Hobfoll, Bansal, and other authors (2002) found that childhood resource loss in the form of abuse has long-term impact on women's risk for contracting STDs. This suggests that women experiencing the tragic interpersonal loss cycles associated with abuse might have lacked the opportunities to develop the interpersonal resources nec-essary for enacting safe sex. In this study, women with a history of childhood physi-cal abuse also displayed higher levels of anger and depressive mood. This distress might have contributed to negative interactions between the women and their partners and further eroded the women's abilities to negotiate safer sex. In summary, child-hood abuse appears to initiate loss cycles that counteract women's efforts to develop and utilize interpersonal resources and power within their romantic relationships that are necessary for engaging in safe sex.

Therefore, a promising area of future research is to help women who have expe-rienced abuse gain the additional interpersonal resource strategies necessary for enacting safer-sex behaviors. Integrating the theory of gender and power (Connell, 1987) into COR theory, future interventions should help women gain interpersonal power within the romantic relationship. Interventions should incorporate strategies such as increasing the women's assertiveness skills along with increasing skills in negotiation and sense of mastery. This approach will provide women with a better stance within the relationship from which negotiation of safer sex can be effectively implemented.

Integrating the IMB Model with COR theory Another model that can be combined with COR theory to formulate public health interventions is the Information-Motivation-Behavioral Skills (IMB) model (see Chapter Two in this volume). The IMB model can be used to conceptualize the important target variables necessary for change (that is, possession of necessary information, motivation, and behavioral skills). COR theory can be used in conjunction with the IMB model to guide the provision of coping resources necessary for increasing the targets viewed to be necessary for behavior change.

For example, the IMB model predicts that in order for individuals to practice safer sex, they must possess the necessary information, motivation, and behavioral skills for engaging in safer-sex behavior. COR theory predicts that in order for individuals to become motivated for engaging in safer sex, they must possess the necessary resources for such behavior. Public health promotion efforts using these combined strategies would focus on increasing the knowledge, motivation, and specific behavioral resources relevant to safer sex while eliminating loss or threat of loss to these resources. Interventionists utilizing these two theoretical approaches will be provided with specific conceptual guidance for which variables to target and how to provide the resources necessary for changing these target variables.

Integrating Decision-Making Theories with COR Theory Decision-making theories can also be used in conjunction with COR theory to guide specific techniques used for information and motivation delivery. For interventions using COR theory in conjunction with decision-making theories, COR theory can be used as the encompassing model for providing individuals with the resource necessary for change. The decision-making models can be used within the framework of COR theory to deliver the necessary personal and conditional resources for change (for example, making a decision to enact behavior change and maintaining the motivation for change).

When people evaluate their options for health decisions, it would be helpful to clarify for them that they may potentially overweight negative outcomes, and minimize the possibility of gains they might make. This would be vital information for helping individuals to identify a list of options for changing their health, identify and weigh the consequences of those options, become informed on the probability of the consequences, and make a decision as to which option to pursue. COR theory can be used in conjunction to help individuals assess the resources necessary for changing their health and provide individuals the resources necessary for enacting logical options for changing health-related behavior.

In addition to incorporating behavior decision theory with COR theory, public health promotion efforts might integrate the Elaboration Likelihood model (see Chapter Seven in this volume) with COR theory. The Elaboration Likelihood model provides predictions on how to effectively frame information relevant to changing health-related behavior. Thus, the Elaboration Likelihood model can be used to guide efforts to encourage individuals to engage in healthy behaviors, while COR theory can be used to help provide individuals with the resources necessary for enacting and maintaining healthy behaviors.

A final example of a decision-making theory that can be combined with COR theory is the Precaution Adoption Process (PAP) model. The PAP model provides descriptions of the stage processes through which individuals will progress when deciding to engage in health-related behaviors. According to the PAP model, interventions will be most effective when tailored to the current stage of the individual. Therefore, the PAP model can be used to provide and frame the appropriate information for helping individuals move toward making healthy choices. COR theory can be combined with the PAP model to provide people with the resources necessary for progressing through the decision-making stages and to provide people with the resources necessary to act upon health-conscious decisions. Resource realities must again always be considered, as faced with difficult obstacles, individuals' motivation will decline. Therefore, paths of less resistance can be more effectively identified if people's resources and resource fit to their environment are acknowledged.

In summary, decision-making approaches can provide interventionists with the specific techniques for encouraging individuals to engage in healthy decisions. COR theory can help interventionists provide individuals with the resources necessary for enacting and maintaining healthy decisions. A combination of decision-making theory with COR theory can help interventionists develop the tools necessary for changing people's decisions, motivations, and resources for changing health-related behaviors.

THEORETICAL OVERLAP AND LIMITATIONS OF COR THEORY

Although COR theory has many unique aspects and is increasingly well documented in the stress literature, it also has many properties that overlap with other theories and models. This, in part, stems from the fact that resource ideas have been pervasive since Rabkin and Struening (1976) noted that stress itself accounted for relatively little variance in outcomes, and that people's resources moderated stress's impact. It is also the case that COR theory itself has been in the literature for twenty years and is quite well referenced as the leading pan-resource theory. As such, the implications of COR theory may have filtered down to many interventions that acknowledge the stressful nature of many public health crises.

Finally, we would acknowledge the limitations of COR theory. The most germane one to the current discussion is that COR theory outlines a general process, but does not specify which resources are most relevant in any given domain. For this, a study of that domain's ecology is critical (Kelly, 1966). In this regard, every health domain has a working ecology that defines how resources are naturally exchanged and interact prior to intervention. Further, an understanding of such ecologies not only highlights what resources need to be altered to effect health changes, but also what resources and ecological conditions are likely to be resistant to change or even implacable. COR theory emphasizes objective elements of the ecology and the resources available to individuals. Other theories and models are relevant for any intervention, as in our own efforts where we have incorporated cognitive-behavioral models and other theories in order to complement COR theory in practice. As is so often the case, marriage to any single model is typically too narrow for the real-world demands of health crises and responsive intervention efforts.

Strengths and Limitations of the Theory

COR theory has proven to be one of the two major theories explaining stress and behavior. It is especially well supported where stressors are objective or have major objective components. It is also a highly specific theory, making particular hypotheses which aid both research and practice. The COR model also integrates personal, social, and environmental factors which are critical in altering health behavior in stress and coping work and as applied to health behaviors such as threat of HIV/AIDS. The theory is not seen as a stand-alone theory, however. Rather, it must be integrated into the social and behavioral ecology of situations in order to be effectively applied. Where stress is more a matter of perception and appraisal, such as where stress is caused by more internal factors (for example, neuroticism), more clinically based theories may be more effectively applied.

SUMMARY

COR theory was developed as a response to the need to incorporate the environment as a more integral part of the stress and coping process. COR theory emphasizes change in resources as the key to stress and suggests that resource losses are more powerful than resource gains. In addition, COR theory states that resource gains serve to buffer against future loss and are the key to resiliency and health (as opposed to illness). Predictions made by COR theory have been empirically supported in a variety of populations, and COR theory has been shown to be an effective framework for HIV prevention. Application of COR theory also appears promising in the area of developing interventions for coping with traumatic events. Another promising area of research appears to be in combining COR theory with theories targeting specific variables important in public health promotion. COR theory provides the conceptual framework for providing people with the necessary resources for coping with stress and engaging in and maintaining healthy behaviors.

REFERENCES

Bandura, A. (1977). *Social learning theory.* Englewood Cliffs, NJ: Prentice-Hall.

Bandura, A. (1997). *Self efficacy: The exercise of control.* New York: W. H. Freeman and Company.

Billings, D. W., Folkman, S., Acree, M., and Moskowitz, J. T. (2000). Coping and physical health during caregiving: The roles of positive and negative affect. *Journal of Personality and Social Psychology, 79*(1), 131–142.

Bonanno, G. A., Galea, S., Bucciarelli, A., and Vlahov, D. (2007). What predicts psychological resilience after disaster? The role of demographics, resources, and life stress. *Journal of Consulting and Clinical Psychology, 75,* 671–682.

Britton, P. J., Levine, O. H., Jackson, A. P., Hobfoll, S. E., Shepherd, J. B., and Lavin, J. P. (1998). Ambiguity of monogamy as a safer-sex goal among, single, pregnant, inner-city women. *Journal of Health Psychology*, *3*(2), 227–232.

Cacioppo, J. T., and Gardner, W. L. (in press). Emotion. *Annual Review of Psychology*, *50*.

Carver, C. S., and Scheier, M. F. (1998). *On the self-regulation of behavior*. New York: Cambridge University Press.

Chang, C., Wong, W., and Tsang, K. W. (2007). Perceptions of benefits and costs during SARS outbreak: An 18-month prospective study. *Journal of Consulting and Clinical Psychology*, *74*, 870–879.

Cohen, S., Doyle, W. J., Skoner, D. P. Rabin, B. S., and Gwaltney, J. M. (1997). Social ties and susceptibility to the common cold. *Journal of the American Medical Association*, *277*, 1940–1944.

Cohen, S., and Wills, T. A. (1985). Stress, social support, and the buffering hypothesis. *Psychological Bulletin*, *98*, 310–357.

Connell, R. W. (1987). *Gender and power*. Stanford, CA: Stanford University Press.

Fisher, J. D., Fisher, W. A., Misovich, S. J., Kimble, D. L., and Malloy, T. E. (1996). Changing AIDS risk behavior: Effects of an intervention emphasizing AIDS risk reduction information, motivation, and behavioral skills in a college student population. *Health Psychology*, *15*(2), 114–123.

Frankl, V. E. (1963). *Man's search for meaning*. Boston: Beacon.

Freedy, J. R., Saladin, M. E., Kilpatrick, D. G., Resnick, H. S., and Saunders, B. E. (1994). Understanding acute psychological distress following natural disaster. *Journal of Traumatic Stress*, *7*, 257–273.

Freedy, J. R., Shaw, D., Jarrell, M., and Masters, C. (1992). Toward an understanding of the psychological impact of natural disasters: An application of the Conservation of Resources stress model. *Journal of Traumatic Stress*, *5*, 441–454.

Gilbert, D. T., Pinel, E. C., Wilson, T. D., Blumberg, S. J., and Wheatley, T. P. (1998). Immune neglect: A source of durability bias in affective forecasting. *Journal of Personality and Social Psychology*, *75*, 617–638.

Hobfoll, S. E. (1988). *The ecology of stress*. New York: Hemisphere.

Hobfoll, S. E. (1989). Conservation of resources: A new attempt at conceptualizing stress. *American Psychologist*, *44*, 513–524.

Hobfoll, S.E. (1991). Traumatic stress: A theory based on rapid loss of resources. *Anxiety Research*, *4*, 187–197.

Hobfoll, S. E. (1998a). *Stress, culture, and community: The psychology and philosophy of stress*. New York: Plenum.

Hobfoll, S. E. (1998b). Ecology, community, and AIDS prevention. *American Journal of Community Psychology*, *26*(1), 133–144.

Hobfoll, S. E. (2001). The Influence of culture, community, and the nested-self in the stress process: Advancing Conservation of Resources Theory. Lead article. *Applied Psychology*, *50*, 337–370.

Hobfoll, S. E., Bansal, A., Schurg, R., Young, S., Pierce, C. A., Hobfoll, I., and Johnson, R. (2002). The impact of perceived child physical and sexual abuse history on Native American women's psychological well-being and AIDS risk. *Journal of Consulting and Clinical Psychology*, *70*, 252–257.

Hobfoll, S. E., Canetti-Nisim, D., and Johnson, R. J. (2006). Exposure to terrorism, stress-related mental health symptoms, and defensive coping among Jews and Arabs in Israel. *Journal of Consulting and Clinical Psychology*, *74*, 207–218.

Hobfoll, S. E., Canetti-Nisim, D, Johnson, R. J., Varley, J., Palmieri, P. A., and Galea, S. (2008). The association of exposure, risk and resiliency factors with PTSD among Jews and Arabs exposed to repeated acts of terrorism in Israel. *Journal of Traumatic Stress*, *21*, 22–29.

Hobfoll, S. E., Jackson, A. P., Lavin, J., Britton, P. J., and Shepherd, J. B. (1993). Safer sex knowledge, behavior, and attitudes of inner-city women. *Health Psychology*, *12*(6), 481–488.

Hobfoll, S. E., Jackson, A. P., Lavin, J., Britton, P. J., and Shepherd, J. B. (1994a). Reducing inner-city women's AIDS risk activities: A study of single, pregnant women. *Health Psychology*, *13*(5), 397–403.

Hobfoll, S. E., Jackson, A. P., Lavin, J., Britton, P. J., and Shepherd, J. B. (1994b). Women's barriers to safer sex. *Psychology and Health*, *9*, 233–252.

Hobfoll, S. E., Jackson, A. P., Lavin, J., Johnson, R., and Schröder, K.E.E. (2002). Effects and generalizability of communally-oriented HIV/AIDS prevention versus general health promotion group for single, inner-city women in urban clinics. *Journal of Consulting and Clinical Psychology*, *70*, 950–960.

Hobfoll, S. E., and Leiberman, J. (1987). Personality and social resources in immediate and continued stress-resistance among women. *Journal of Personality and Social Psychology*, *52*, 18–26.

Hobfoll, S. E., and Lilly, R. S. (1993). Resource conservation as a strategy for community psychology. *Journal of Community Psychology*, *21*, 128–148.

Hobfoll, S. E., Nadler, A., and Leiberman, J. (1986). Satisfaction with social support during crisis: Intimacy and self esteem as critical determinants. *Journal of Personality and Social Psychology*, *51*, 296–304.

Hobfoll, S. E., Tracy, M., and Galea, S. (2006). The impact of resource loss and "traumatic growth" on probable PTSD and depression following terrorist attacks. *Journal of Traumatic Stress*, *19*, 867–878.

Hobfoll, S. E., Watson, P, Bell, C. C., Bryant, R. A., Brymer, M. J., Friedman, M. J., Friedman, M., Gersons, B.P.R., de Jong, J.T.V. M., Layne, C. M., Maguen, S., Neria, Y., Norwood, A. E., Pynoos, R. S., Reissman, D., Ruzek, J. I., Shalev, A. Y., Solomon, Z., Steinberg, A. M., and Ursano, R. J. (2007). Five essential elements of immediate and mid-term mass trauma intervention: Empirical evidence. *Psychiatry: Biological and Interpersonal Issues*, *70*, 283–315.

Holahan, C. J., Moos, R. H., Holahan, C. K., and Cronkite, R. C. (1999). Resource loss, resource gain, and depressive symptoms: A 10-year model. *Journal of Personality and Social Psychology*, *77*, 620–629.

Holahan, C. J., Moos, R. H., Holahan, C. K., and Cronkite, R. C. (2000). Long-term posttreatment functioning among patients with unipolar depression: An integrative model. *Journal of Consulting and Clinical Psychology*, *68*(2), 226–232.

House, J., Landis, K., and Umberson, D. (1988). Social relationships and health. *Science*, *241*, 540–545.

Ironson, G., Wynings, C., Schneiderman, N., Baum, A., Rodriguez, M., Greenwood, D., et al. (1997). Post-traumatic stress symptoms, intrusive thoughts, loss, and immune function after Hurricane Andrew. *Psychosomatic Medicine*, *59*, 128–141.

Ito, T. A., Larsen, J. T., Smith, N. K., and Cacioppo, J. T. (1998). Negative information weighs more heavily on the brain: The negativity bias in evaluative categorizations. *Journal of Personality and Social Relationships*, *75*, 887–900.

Johnson, D. M. Palmieri, P. A., Jackson, A. P., and Hobfoll, S. E. (2007). Emotional numbing weakens abused inner-city women's resiliency resources. *Journal of Traumatic Stress*, *20*, 197–206.

Kalichman, S. C., Simbayi, L. C., Kagee, A., Toefy, Y., Jooste, S., Cain, D., Cherry, C. (2006). Associations of poverty, substance use, and HIV transmission risk behaviors in three South African communities. *Social Science and Medicine*, *62*, 1641–1649.

Kaniasty, K. and Norris, F. H. (2001). Social support dynamics in adjustment to disasters. In B.R. Sarason and S. Duck (eds.), *Personal relationships: Implications for clinical and community psychology* (pp. 201–224). Chichester, UK: Wiley.

Kelly, J. G. (1966). Ecological constraints on mental health services. *American Psychologist*, *21*, 535–539.

King, D. W., King, L. A., Foy, D. W., Keane, T. M., and Fairbank, J. A. (1999). Posttraumatic stress disorder in a national sample of female and male Vietnam veterans: Risk factors, war-zone stressors, and resilience-recovery variables. *Journal of Abnormal Psychology*, *108*, 164–170.

Lane, C., and Hobfoll, S. E. (1992). How loss affects anger and alienates potential supporters. *Journal of Consulting and Clinical Psychology*, *60*, 935–942.

Lazarus, R. S. (1966). *Psychological stress and the coping process*. New York: Springer.

Lazarus, R. S., and Folkman, S. (1984). *Stress, appraisal, and coping*. New York: Springer.

Levine, O. H., Britton, P. J., James, T. C., Jackson, A. P., and Hobfoll, S. E. (1993). The empowerment of women: A key to HIV prevention. *Journal of Community Psychology*, *21*, 320–334.

MacKenzie, J. E., Hobfoll, S. E., Ennis, N., Kay, J., Jackson, A., and Lavin, J. (1999). Reducing AIDS risk among inner-city women: A review of the collectivist empowerment AIDS prevention (CE-AP) program. *Journal of the European Academy of Dermatology and Venereology*, *13*, 166–174.

McGrath, J. E. (1970). A conceptual formulation for research on stress. In J. E. McGrath (Ed.), *Social and psychological factors in stress* (pp. 10–21). New York: Holt, Rinehart, and Winston.

Monnier, J. and Hobfoll, S. E. (2000). Conservation of resources in individual and community reactions to traumatic stress. In S. Yehuda and K. McFarlane (eds.), *International Handbook of Human Response to Trauma* (pp. 325–336). New York: Plenum Publishers.

Norris, F. H. and Kaniasty, K. (1996). Received and perceived social support in times of stress: A test of the social support deterioration deterrence model. *Journal of Personality and Social Psychology, 71*(3), 498–511.

Rabkin, J. G., and Struening, E. L. (1976). Life events, stress and illness. *Science, 194*, 1013–1020.

Rini, C. K., Dunkel-Schetter, C., Wadhwa, P. D., and Sandman, C. A. (1999). Psychological adaptation and birth outcomes: The role of personal resources, stress, and sociocultural context in pregnancy. *Health Psychology, 18*(4), 333–345.

Rosenberg, M. (1965). *Society and adolescent self-image*. Princeton, NJ: Princeton University Press.

Sarason, I., Sarason, B., Shearin, E. and Pierce, G. (1987). A brief measure of social support: Practical and theoretical implications. *Journal of Social and Personal Relationships, 4*, 497–510.

Scheier, M. F., and Carver, C. S. (1985). Optimism, coping, and health: Assessment and implications of generalized outcome expectancies. *Health Psychology, 4*, 219–247.

Scheier, M. F., and Carver, C. S. (1992). Effects of optimism on psychology and physical well-being: Theoretical overview and empirical update. *Cognitive Therapy and Research, 16*, 201–228.

Schumm, J. A., Briggs-Phillips, M. L., and Hobfoll, S. E. (2006). Abuse and assault of women over the lifespan: The cumulative impact of multiple traumas on PTSD and depression. *Journal of Traumatic Stress, 19*, 825–836.

Schumm, J. A., Hobfoll, S. E., and Keogh, N. J. (2004). Revictimization and interpersonal resource loss predicts PTSD among women in substance use treatment. *Journal of Traumatic Stress, 17*, 173–181.

Schumm, J. A., Stines, L. R., Hobfoll, S. E., and Jackson, A. P. (2005). The double-barreled burden of child abuse and current stressful circumstances on adult women: The kindling effect of early traumatic experience. *Journal of Traumatic Stress, 18*, 467–476.

Simalyi, L. C., Kalichman, S., Strebel, A., Cloete, A., Henda, N, and Mqeketo, A. (2007). Internalized stigma, discrimination, and depression among men and women living with HIV/AIDS in Cape Town, South Africa. *Social Science and Medicine, 64*, 1823–1831.

Tversky, A., and Kahneman, D. (1974). Judgment under uncertainty: Heuristics and biases. *Science, 185*, 1124–1131.

van der Kolk, B. A. (1996a). The body keeps the score: Approaches to the psychobiology of posttraumatic stress disorder. In B. A. van der Kolk, A. C. McFarlane, and L. Weisaeth (eds.), *Traumatic stress: The effects of overwhelming experience on mind, body, and society* (pp. 214–241). New York: Guilford Press.

van der Kolk, B. A. (1996b). Trauma and memory. In B. A. van der Kolk, A. C. McFarlane, and L. Weisaeth (eds.), *Traumatic stress: The effects of overwhelming experience on mind, body, and society* (pp. 279–302). New York: Guilford Press.

Vaux, A. (1988). *Social support: Theory, research and intervention*. New York: Praeger Publishers.

Wells, J., Hobfoll, S. E., and Lavin, J. (1997). Resource loss, resource gain, and communal coping during pregnancy among women with multiple roles. *Psychology of Women Quarterly, 21*(4), 645–662.

Wells, J., Hobfoll, S. E., and Lavin, J. (1999). When it rains, it pours: The greater impact of resource loss compared to gain on psychological distress. *Personality and Social Psychology Bulletin, 25*, 1172–1182.

Wingood, G. M., and DiClemente, R. J. (1997). The effects of an abusive primary partner on the condom use and sexual negotiation practices of African-American women. *American Journal of Public Health, 87*, 1016–1018.

Wolpe, J. (1958). *Psychotherapy by reciprocal inhibition*. Stanford, CA: Stanford University Press.

Zamani, G. H., Gorgievski-Dujivesteihn, M. J., and Zarafshani, K. (2006): Towards a multilevel understanding based on conversation of resources theory. *Human Ecology, 34*, 677–692.

CHAPTER

6

SELF-DETERMINATION THEORY: PROCESS MODELS FOR HEALTH BEHAVIOR CHANGE

Michelle S. Fortier
Geoffrey C. Williams
Shane N. Sweet
Heather Patrick

BRIEF OVERVIEW OF SELF-DETERMINATION THEORY

Self-determination theory (SDT) (Deci and Ryan, 1985, 2002) is an individual-level theory of human motivation which postulates that humans are innately oriented toward growth and health (Deci and Ryan, 2002). It uses "empirical methods while employing an organismic meta-theory that highlights the importance of humans' evolved inner resources for personality development and behavioral self-regulation" (Ryan and Deci, 2000, page 68).

This chapter aims to review the literature on SDT and health behaviors in adults and to provide strategies for practitioners endeavoring to promote healthy lifestyles. Indeed, SDT is being increasingly used for understanding and promoting health behaviors (Fortier, Sweet, O'Sullivan, Blanchard, and Williams, 2007; Williams, McGregor, Sharp, Levesque, Kouides, Ryan, et al., 2006a). Two of these that have been of particular interest in our research programs over the past decade and that we will be highlighting in this chapter are: **physical activity** and **abstinence from tobacco**.

First the mini-theories of SDT will be presented. This will be followed by a literature review describing research findings in these areas. Case applications of the theory to tobacco dependence treatment and physical activity counseling will also be provided. Finally, strengths and limitations will be discussed, along with the provision of future directions.

ORIGINS OF SELF-DETERMINATION THEORY

An Organismic Meta-Theory

SDT is grounded in a humanistic perspective and is based on the premise that humans have an innate tendency toward growth, integration, and health. Growth occurs by seeking optimal challenges, discovering new perspectives, expressing one's interests and talents, and stretching one's capacities. Active growth and well-being are further complemented by a tendency to try to integrate, synthesize, and organize these experiences within one's identity, self-concept, and self-esteem. This process of integration results in a coherent, consistent, and complete sense of self from which people act.

Basic Psychological Needs

Self-determination theorists also posit that human beings have psychological needs that, if supported, result in optimal development and the energization of behavior. Need theories are distinguishable by their perspective on the target of needs (physiological or psychological) and by their definition of needs (that is, nutrients necessary for growth versus any motivating force). Hull's (1943) drive theory is one salient example of a *physiological* need theory. According to this perspective, people have a set of innate physiological needs including food, water, and sex. The perspective outlined by Murray (1938) has provided much of the basis for theories on *psychological* needs. In contrast to the Hullian tradition, which suggests that needs are innate, Murray's perspective on psychological needs suggests that needs are acquired. According to Murray, a need is conceptualized as anything that moves an individual to action. The SDT (Deci and Ryan, 1985, 2000) perspective has focused on psychological needs—consistent with the Murray perspective—and has characterized these needs as innate, consistent with Hull's theory. SDT further defines psychological needs as "nutriments that are essential for ongoing psychological growth, integrity, and well-being" (Deci and Ryan, 2000, page 229). Based on this definition, three basic psychological needs are assumed to be innately present within humans: **autonomy, competence,** and **relatedness**. These three needs are defined and discussed in detail later.

ADVANTAGES OF SDT OVER OTHER INDIVIDUAL-LEVEL THEORIES

Research on motivation and health has been largely guided by three theoretical perspectives: social cognitive theory, goals theory, and the transtheoretical model. Social cognitive theory (Bandura, 1986) focuses primarily on the concept of self-efficacy: belief in one's capacity to attain goals in a particular domain. Self-efficacy, a similar concept to SDT's perceived competence, develops from experiences such as past performance, physiological states, observing others perform the behavior, and verbal persuasion (Feltz, 1988). Self-efficacy then serves as the basis for initiation, engagement, and persistence in that behavior (Feltz, 1992). Like social cognitive theory, the goals approach (Duda, 1992; Nicholls, 1984; Nicholls, 1989) focuses on perceptions of competence. Goals theory suggests that people are motivated to develop competence and that to achieve competence, people can assume either a task-orientation or an ego-orientation. Task-orientation, also called mastery-orientation, focuses on the process involved in initiating, engaging in, and persisting at challenging activities (Duda, 1992; Ames, 1992) and has been associated with intrinsic motivation for the activity (Dweck, 1985). In contrast, ego- or performance-orientation focuses on achieving certain outcomes and performance evaluations. The transtheoretical model has two primary components: stages of change and processes of change (Prochaska and DiClemente, 1983). Stages of change represent individuals' readiness for behavior change. Processes of change represent the strategies people use to move through the stages of change. The strength of these theoretical perspectives is that they address important cognitive aspects related to behavior change such as perceptions of efficacy/competence and perceived readiness for change. However, they do not consider individuals' interest in or desire to perform the behavior or how characteristics of the social environment can affect individuals' interests or desires. SDT provides a more comprehensive theoretical framework through which to understand motivated behavior by addressing feelings of competence as well as needs for autonomy and relatedness. Simply feeling competent is not sufficient to promote optimal motivation (Markland, 1999; Markland and Hardy, 1997) or the persistence in behavior. Motivation and the persistence of behavior occur only when perceived competence is accompanied by the perception of autonomy. This is particularly important in health

FIGURE 6.1 *Visual Representation of Constructs from both SDT Mini-Theories*

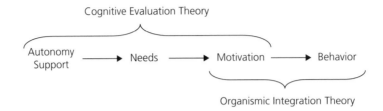

behavior change, where it is the persistence of behavior that is associated with health and quality of life. Also, it is important because autonomy is the unique element of SDT, setting it apart from other theories of motivation.

SDT MINI-THEORIES

In general, SDT proposes that humans have three basic psychological needs of autonomy, competence, and relatedness, and require them to be satisfied in order for the individual to be motivated for internal reasons and in turn achieve optimal growth and well-being. SDT presents itself through two main mini-theories (see Figure 6.1): **Organismic integration theory** (OIT) and **cognitive evaluation theory** (CET).

Organismic Integration Theory (OIT)

OIT focuses on the distinction between autonomous and controlled behaviors that reflects the degree to which behaviors are volitional and choiceful, resulting from interest in the behavior relative to behaviors that are the result of pressure and coercion, demand, or seduction. This distinction between autonomous and controlled behaviors represents a continuum rather than a dichotomy (Ryan and Connell, 1989; see Figure 6.2).

Behaviors that are the most controlled or the least autonomous are **externally regulated.** Externally regulated behaviors are engaged only to satisfy a demand (for example to follow rules) or to gain a reward (for example, abstaining from smoking to please a health provider). A second type of controlled motivation, **introjection,** involves engaging in behaviors out of a sense of guilt or obligation. A more autonomous form of regulation is **identification**, whereby the behavior is performed because people feel the behavior is important for them. The highest level of extrinsic autonomous regulation is **integrated**, whereby behaviors are performed because they are consistent with other personal goals and values (for example, exercising because of the value of being healthy, and because being healthy allows more positive family interactions). Finally, the most autonomous form of regulation is intrinsic. Behaviors that are **intrinsically regulated** are performed for their inherent enjoyment. In addition to the different types of motivational regulations, another component of OIT is the process of internalization. Internalization is the innate

FIGURE 6.2 *The Self-Determination Continuum Showing Types of Motivation with Their Regulatory Styles, Locus of Causality, and Corresponding Processes*

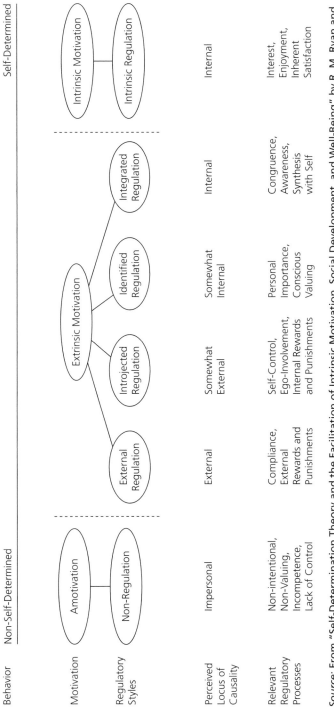

Source: From "Self-Determination Theory and the Facilitation of Intrinsic Motivation, Social Development, and Well-Being" by R. M. Ryan and E. L. Deci, 2000, *American Psychologist, 55*, p. 72. Copyright 2000 by American Psychological Association. Reprinted with permission.

process by which the self accepts greater autonomy and competence for a particular behavior over time. It is predicted that individuals have an inherent tendency to take on greater levels of autonomous self-regulations for behaviors new to them over time. For instance, an individual might start off engaging in a health behavior such as physical activity for controlled reasons such as weight loss. However if the internalization process is not hindered by external forces, the individual will naturally come to perform the behavior because they feel personally committed to their health, value physical activity, and in some cases even because they enjoy it. Finally, OIT also postulates that the more autonomous forms of motivation lead to positive consequences, whereas controlled motivation leads to less positive outcomes. This has been demonstrated in a great number of studies (Ryan and Deci; 2000), including those examining health behaviors as indicated below, and as reviewed previously (Williams, 2002; also see Fortier and Kowal, 2007 for a review on SDT and PA behavior change).

Cognitive Evaluation Theory (CET)

Three Psychological Needs CET has identified three essential needs for optimal psychological growth and well-being—competence, relatedness, and autonomy (Deci and Ryan, 2000). According to CET, a need for competence reflects the need to feel effective in one's efforts and capable of achieving desired outcomes. The need for relatedness involves a need to feel connected to and understood by others. Finally, autonomy reflects the need to feel volitional in one's actions, to fully and authentically endorse one's behaviors, and to act as the originator, or cause, of one's own behavior. A growing body of research based on both this conceptualization of psychological needs and on other perspectives provides evidence for the role of each of these needs in psychological health and well-being (Carver and Scheier, 2000; Deci and Ryan, 2000; Kernis, 2000).

Social Context: Autonomy Support CET suggests that the social context, in part, facilitates the innate human process of internalization and self-regulation. When the social context supports individuals' needs for competence, autonomy, and relatedness, individuals are more likely to come to regulate behaviors on their own, and thus lasting behavior change is more likely (Figure 6.3). The concept of autonomy support represents an interpersonal climate in which an authority figure (for example, physician, exercise professional) takes the perspective of the person under their charge into consideration, provides relevant information and effective opportunities for choice, and leads the individual to accept personal responsibility (for example, for health behaviors) by facilitating internalization. Autonomy support also includes interactions that involve asking the individual what he or she wants to achieve, encouraging questions, providing meaningful and satisfactory answers to questions, and refraining from judgment or evaluation when obtaining information about past behavior. Thus, autonomy support involves minimal pressure, criticism, and control (Reeve, 1998; Ryan, 1993; Williams, 2002).

FIGURE 6.3 *Proposed SDT Model for Internalization of Autonomous Self-Regulation and Perceived Competence*

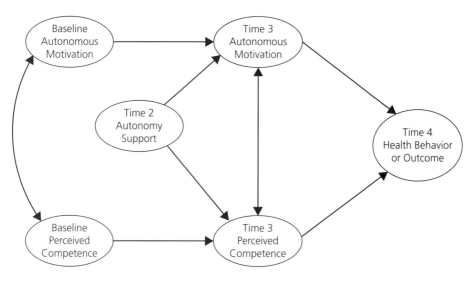

There are three elements crucial to autonomy-supportive contexts: providing a meaningful rationale for the prescribed behavior; acknowledging feelings and perspectives; and emphasizing choice and minimizing control. Results of an experiment in which these elements were manipulated demonstrated that each of these facilitating factors was associated with greater internalization or autonomous motivation for the prescribed behavior (Deci, Eghari, Patrick, and Leone, 1994). Thus, the contexts in which behaviors are prescribed have an important effect on whether behaviors are internalized. In the domain of health, physicians, exercise professionals, nurses, social workers, and other practitioners are in a unique position to facilitate autonomous motivation for health behavior change by providing contexts that support basic psychological needs, thus enhancing the likelihood of persistence, maintenance, and enjoyment (when possible) of prescribed health behaviors.

Autonomy Support and Motivational Interviewing

Motivational interviewing (MI) (Miller and Rollnick, 2002) is a clinical method based on client-centeredness (Rogers, 1951) that is intended to "enhance intrinsic motivation for change by resolving ambivalence" (Miller and Rollnick, 2002, page 25). While MI has been associated with stages of change (Prochaska, DiClemente, and Norcross, 1992) and social learning theory (Bandura, 1986), MI still lacks a comprehensive theoretical framework. Recently, SDT has been suggested as a possible explanatory theory that may account for changes that result from MI interventions (Foote, DeLuca, Magura, Warner, Grand, Rosenblum, and Stahl, 1999; Markland, Ryan,

Tobin, and Rollnick, 2005; Vansteenkiste and Sheldon, 2006). Both MI and SDT assume that humans have an innate tendency toward growth and psychological integration. MI provides an interpersonal climate that is autonomy-supportive and thus expected to facilitate change. The four active elements of MI include: expression of empathy, rolling with resistance, support of efficacy, and development of discrepancy. Each of these elements is considered autonomy-supportive. However, autonomy support in health care environments also emphasizes the support of patient initiative, and the provision of rationale and information giving, including when the practitioner provides a direct recommendation. Direct advice and information giving represent possible areas that autonomy-supportive, SDT-based practitioners may extend beyond MI-based practitioners. Specifically, SDT-based counseling in medicine extends beyond the issue of resolving ambivalence, by providing rationale, direct information (for example, about how the body works, the expected course of a disease) and advice. Without direct information giving, medical practitioners may well be perceived as controlling by withholding information that patients are open to internalizing directly, and they further run the risk of making the patient feel abandoned (Schneider, 1998). On the other hand, because ambivalence commonly occurs at some time during a treatment or a behavior change plan, medical practitioners should anticipate this and seek to identify it. Where ambivalence occurs, use of MI techniques is expected to facilitate autonomous self-regulation, as long as the other aspects of autonomy support are present. Empirical investigation is needed to inform the optimal practice of autonomy support in health care.

A recent empirical review of SDT and MI intervention trials attempting to facilitate health behavior change identified seven randomized controlled clinical trials that measured change in autonomous self-regulation and change in the targeted health behavior (Patrick, Williams, Fortier, Sweet, Halvari, Halvari, et al., 2008; Table 1). The review showed that both the four SDT and three MI interventions were efficacious in changing the health behavior over a six-month period of time. In addition, change in autonomous self-regulation also accounted for significant change in the health behavior independent of the effect of the interventions. However, only those interventions based on SDT accounted for significant change in autonomous self-regulation.

Thus, there may be unique elements of autonomy support that are necessary for promoting change in autonomy related to health behaviors that are not present in MI. One potential difference is that autonomous self-regulation of a behavior is increased when practitioners provide a menu of effective options for change, and direct information-giving with nonjudgmental structure to increase perceived competence. There are many possible reasons why the studies failed to detect an effect, including selection bias, or that the interventions did not accurately reflect the MI technique. At this point, there are too few clinical trials using these interventions and constructs to draw firm conclusions. SDT and MI have many common underlying principles, and the growing literature on them provides a ripe area for investigation.

TABLE 6.1 Intervention Trials of Self-Determination Theory in Health Care.

Outcome	Year Published	N	Findings
			SDT-Based Interventions
Tobacco Abstinence and Cholesterol Williams, McGregor, et al.	2006a and b		SDT intervention significantly increased autonomy support, autonomy competence, medication use, prolonged tobacco abstinence, and lowered LDL-cholesterol compared to community control. Thus, an SDT-based intervention has now been demonstrated to increase autonomy, perceived competence, and self-reported medication use.
Physical Activity Fortier, Sweet, et al.	2007	120	A randomized controlled trial assessed the impact of intensive autonomy-supportive physical activity counseling (six contacts over three months and brief physician counseling) compared to brief autonomy-supportive physician counseling alone. The intensive group perceived higher levels of autonomy support and autonomous self-regulation for physical activity at six weeks, and higher levels of physical activity at three months compared to the control group.
Dental Study Halvari and Halvari	2006	86	A randomized controlled trial demonstrated that dental patients who received sixty minutes of autonomy-supportive counseling in addition to usual care perceived greater autonomy support, autonomous motivation, and perceived competence. These motivation changes mediated the intervention's large effect on reduction in dental plaque and gingivitis over seven months.
Diet, Physical Activity, and Weight Loss Silva et al.	Under review	128	A randomized controlled trial assessed the impact of an SDT-based intervention to increase physical activity, improve diet, and reduce body mass index. The intensive group perceived higher levels of autonomous self-regulation, which mediated the intervention's effect on all three outcomes.

(Continued)

TABLE 6.1 (Continued)

MI-based Interventions

Physical Activity Resnicow et al.	2002	A randomized controlled trial assessed the impact of an MI-based intervention to increase physical activity among sedentary adults. The MI group evidenced greater increases in physical activity. MI intervention did *not* predict changes in autonomous self-regulation. However, changes in autonomous self-regulation independently predicted behavior change.
Fruit and vegetable intake Fuemmeler et al.	2006	A randomized controlled trial assessed the impact of an MI-based intervention to increase fruit and vegetable intake. The MI group perceived higher levels of autonomous self-regulation, which mediated the interventions' effect on two indicators of fruit and vegetable intake.
Fruit and vegetable intake Shaikh et al.	Under review	A randomized controlled trial assessed the impact of an MI-based intervention to increase fruit and vegetable intake. The MI group evidenced greater in-creases in fruit and vegetable intake. MI intervention did *not* predict changes in autonomous self-regulation. However, changes in autonomous self-regulation independently predicted behavior change.

Note: All results presented in this table were secondary analyses from their respective studies conducted for the empirical review.

It should be noted that SDT also has two other mini-theories: Causality orientation theory and **basic needs theory** (Deci and Ryan, 2002). Briefly, causality orientation theory posits the existence of individual differences in global (personality-level) motivational orientations, whereas basic needs theory gives a more detailed explanation of how the three basic psychological needs influence mental health and well-being.

SDT APPLICATIONS TO HEALTH BEHAVIORS

SDT has been applied to a variety of health behaviors, including attendance in an alcohol treatment program (Ryan, Plant, and O'Malley, 1995), participation in a weight-loss program (Williams, Grow, Freedman, Ryan, and Deci, 1996), adherence to medication prescriptions (Kennedy, Goggin, and Nollen, 2004; Williams, Rodin, Ryan, Grolnick, and Deci, 1998), diabetes self-management (Senécal, Nouwen, and White, 2000; Williams, Freedman, and Deci, 1998), cholesterol reduction (Williams, McGregor, Sharp, Kouides, Levesque, Ryan, and Deci, 2006b), abstinence from tobacco (Williams and Deci, 2001; Williams, Cox, Kouides, and Deci, 1999; Williams, Gagné, Ryan, and Deci, 2002), and physical activity (Fortier and Grenier, 1999; Fortier, Sweet, O'Sullivan, Blanchard, and Williams, 2007; Wilson, Rodgers, Blanchard, and Gessell, 2003). Most of these studies focused on motivation for behavior change as well as the treatment contexts in which health behavior change occurs. A study examined severely obese individuals in a twenty-six-week, medically supervised, very-low-calorie weight-loss program (Williams et al., 1996). Individuals who had more autonomous reasons for participating in the weight-loss program were more likely to attend weekly sessions and showed greater reduction of body mass index (BMI) throughout the program. It is important that autonomous motivation for participating in the program was associated with physical activity and weight loss maintenance at a two-year follow-up. During the program, individuals also provided their assessment of how autonomy-supportive they thought their program health providers were. Perceiving one's health provider as more autonomy-supportive predicted stronger autonomous reasons for participating, better attendance in the program, and greater long-term reduction in BMI. Additionally, path analyses indicated that autonomous regulation mediated the association between perceived autonomy support and better program attendance, as well as the association between autonomy support and greater long-term reduction in BMI.

Tobacco Abstinence

In studies of tobacco abstinence among adults, the benefits of autonomy-supportive contexts have been evident. Using the NCI Guidelines, Williams, Gagné, and colleagues (2002) tested whether having physicians use an autonomy-supportive or controlling manner in counseling their patients to quit smoking predicted tobacco abstinence. Smoking cessation was assessed at six, twelve, and thirty months using both self-reports and biochemical validation. The degree of physicians' support of autonomy was rated by independent coders using audiotaped recordings of patient consultations. Rated autonomy support predicted patients' autonomous self-regulation for smoking cessation. Both autonomous self-regulation for smoking cessation and perceived competence in turn independently predicted continuous abstinence over thirty months. Additional analyses demonstrated that when physicians were more autonomy-supportive, patients were more actively engaged with their physician (that is, they were more likely to ask questions, voice concerns, and so forth), and degree of engagement predicted smoking cessation rates (Williams and Deci, 2001).

Another study followed adults with chest pains over three years and investigated the impact of motivational variables on multiple health behaviors (Williams, Gagné, Mushlin, and Deci, 2005). Perception of health care providers' autonomy support was found to predict autonomous motivation. Subsequently, change in autonomous motivation predicted change in diet and physical activity and marginally predicted improvements in smoking over a three-year period.

Physical Activity

SDT has been increasingly used and recommended in the physical activity[1] area (Biddle and Nigg, 2000; Landry and Solomon, 2002). Overall, individuals who participate in physical activity for more internal reasons (that is, health, value, interest) generally have greater success at adhering to physical activity (Fortier and Kowal, 2007; Frederick-Recascino, 2002; Vallerand and Rousseau, 2001; Vallerand and Losier, 1999) than those that have more external controlled motivation. Specifically, Fortier and Grenier (1999), in a study with active adults who were members of a recreation/sport center, found that autonomous motivation was correlated to four-week physical activity adherence. In another study, Fortier, Sweet, Tulloch, Blanchard, Sigal, and Kenny (2009) investigated whether physical activity motivation of adults with Type 2 diabetes involved in a physical activity trial would become more autonomous as they progressed through the stages of change from contemplation to maintenance. Results indicated that overall, as individuals progressed through the stages, their autonomous motivation increased linearly. The relationship between autonomous motivation and physical activity has also been supported in other studies (Daley and Duda, 2006; Frederick-Recascino and Schuster-Smith, 2003; Wilson, Blanchard, Nehl, and Baker, 2006). The influence of specific types of motivational regulation, outlined by OIT, on physical activity has also been investigated. Specifically, Edmunds, Ntoumanis, and Duda (2006) recently revealed that introjected and identified regulations were both positively related to vigorous physical activity in a community-based adult sample, while other studies have demonstrated a relationship between both identified and intrinsic regulations on total physical activity (Wilson et al., 2003; Wilson, Rodgers, Fraser, and Murray, 2004).

---

[1]Physical activity will be used throughout the chapter. Physical activity includes leisure-time physical activity, sport, and structured exercise, which is in accordance with Caspersen, Powell, and Christenson's (1985) definition of physical activity: "any bodily movement produced by skeletal muscles that results in energy expenditure" (p. 126).

As described earlier, satisfaction of the three psychological needs and having an autonomy-supportive social context are expected to facilitate the internalization process of health behavior change. Research has only recently begun to focus on the influence of these needs in the physical activity domain. Kowal and Fortier (2000) investigated the relationship between psychological needs and motivation with master's level swimmers. Results indicated that situational perceptions of all three needs were related to situational autonomous motivation; however, only contextual perceptions of relatedness were found to predict contextual motivation. More recent studies have also supported the notion that psychological needs influence physical activity motivational regulations (Edmunds, Ntoumanis, and Duda, 2006; Edmunds, Ntoumanis and Duda, 2007; Wilson et al., 2003).

Autonomy support has also been investigated in the physical activity domain; however, most of these studies have been done with youth (Pelletier, Fortier, Vallerand, and Brière, 2001; Ntoumanis, 2005). In a recent study with active adults (Edmunds, Ntoumanis, and Duda, 2006), perceived autonomy support from an exercise professional was assessed to evaluate its influence on the psychological needs and on motivation. Perceived competence was found to mediate the relationship between autonomy support and intrinsic motivation, demonstrating the important role of autonomy support in fostering the psychological needs and autonomous motivation for physical activity.

These studies taken together provide strong support for both subtheories of SDT. However, the most stringent tests of theory are done with experimental/clinical trial studies.

RANDOMIZED CONTROLLED TRIALS OF SELF-DETERMINATION THEORY IN HEALTH CARE

As summarized in Table 6.1, five recently completed randomized controlled trials (RCTs) have demonstrated that SDT interventions were efficacious in significantly increasing autonomous self-regulation, the targeted health behaviors (tobacco abstinence, physical activity, medication adherence), and physiologic or physical health outcomes (LDL-cholesterol, tobacco abstinence, weight loss, gingivitis and dental plaque). Each of these interventions trained practitioners to act in an autonomy-supportive manner, thus linking theory to long-term health behavior and health outcomes. The components of autonomy support in these interventions were (1) eliciting and acknowledging patient perspective; (2) offering a clear rationale; (3) providing information in a nonjudgmental manner; (4) supporting patient initiative for change, or for not changing; (5) eliciting patient values and how changing the unhealthy behavior may affect those values; (6) minimizing control; and (7) providing effective options for change.

Four of these RCTs examining five different health outcomes (dental health, physical activity, weight, tobacco abstinence, LDL-cholesterol, and medication usage) revealed that SDT-based interventions consistently resulted in significant increases in autonomous self-regulation and perceived competence, thus confirming that the internalization of autonomous self-regulation and perceived competence can be facilitated with clinical interventions. In addition, the change in autonomous self-regulation and perceived competence accounted for significant change variance in those five health behaviors. Importantly, two of these studies (Williams, McGregor, et al., 2006b, Silva Teixeira, Markland, Minderico, Vieira, Castro, et al., 2007) involved multiple health behavior interventions which facilitated change in multiple outcomes.

The variance accounted for by the change in autonomous self-regulation was found to be independent of a separate effect of the intervention on these outcomes (Williams, Patrick, Sapp, Williams, Devine, Lafata, et al., 2007). Thus, practitioners who explicitly focus on the support of autonomy are not only meeting ethical standards of care (Beauchamp and Childress, 2001) and meeting the goals of the medical charter by respecting autonomy (ABIM Foundation, ACP-ASIM Foundation, European Federation of Internal Medicine, 2002), but at the same time are increasing the effect of the intervention on multiple health behavior outcomes known to improve the quality and length of life. In summary, health behavior intervention research based on SDT has shown that autonomy-supportive interventions increase autonomy and perceived competence, leading to improved diet, greater physical activity, abstinence from tobacco, weight loss, and medication use to reduce risk for cardiovascular disease and BMI.

Two examples of these RCTs are the "Smokers Health Study" (SHS; Williams, Miniccuci, Kouides, Levesque, Chirkov, Ryan, et al., 2002) conducted in the United States, and the Physical Activity Counseling trial (PAC; Fortier, Hogg, O'Sullivan, Blanchard, Reid, Sigal, et al., 2007) recently completed in Canada. In this section we will present the results of these trials and in the next section we will provide a detailed description of their interventions in order to facilitate knowledge transfer to health promotion contexts.

In the SHS, individuals who smoked more than five cigarettes a day were recruited to participate in the study and then randomized to either the community care group or the intensive SDT-based intervention group. The community care group was offered informational materials and was asked to consult their physician for more information on tobacco dependence. The intensive intervention group received the same information as the community care group, but also obtained four counseling sessions in a six-month period. The overall purpose of this trial was to determine whether the SDT-based intensive intervention had a greater influence on increasing the motivational constructs from SDT as well as reducing tobacco dependence when compared to the community care group. The intervention was perceived to be significantly more autonomy-supportive by smokers in the intensive group than smokers in the community care group. Smokers in the intensive group demonstrated greater levels of autonomous self-regulation for cessation and use of medications, and greater levels of perceived competence for stopping than the community care group. These increases in autonomous self-regulation and perceived competence over six months predicted prolonged abstinence at six, eighteen, and thirty months from baseline (Williams, McGregor, et al., 2006a, b; Williams, Niemiec, Patrick, Ryan, and Deci, 2007).

The purpose of the PAC trial was to determine the impact of integrating an SDT-trained physical activity counselor into the primary health care team. Specifically, we compared patients receiving brief (two- to four-minute sessions) autonomy-supportive physical activity counseling from their family physician or nurse practitioner, plus intensive three-month autonomy-supportive physical activity counseling from the physical activity counselor (intensive counseling group) with patients receiving only brief counseling (brief counseling group). Fortier, Sweet, O'Sullivan, Blanchard, and Williams (2007) investigated self-determination variables within the intervention phase of this RCT and found that individuals in the intensive counseling group showed greater levels of autonomous motivation at six weeks when compared to the brief counseling group, and that these translated into significantly higher levels of physical activity at the end of the intervention (thirteen weeks). Furthermore, path analyses showed that both autonomous self-regulation and perceived competence significantly predicted physical activity adoption, but only for the intensive counseling group.

Together, the findings from these studies suggest that when individuals are autonomously motivated toward a health behavior (for example, physical activity or tobacco abstinence), they are successful at improving it. Maintenance of these behaviors, in turn, is related to better health and lower health risks (Whitlock, Orleans, Pender, and Allan, 2002). Thus, autonomous self-regulation and perceived competence appear to be important predictors of health behavior change and subsequent health. These studies also demonstrated the importance of the social context. When health care practitioners and exercise professionals were perceived as autonomy-supportive, individuals became more autonomously self-regulated and felt more competent, which in turn predicted healthy behavior patterns. Thus, practitioners can improve individuals' health by interacting with them in ways that support their needs for autonomy and perceived competence. Importantly, this has been demonstrated in both experimental and non-experimental studies, thus suggesting that autonomy support plays an important causal role in increasing positive health behaviors.

CASE APPLICATIONS OF THE THEORY/MODEL

In this section, we provide a detailed description of the Smoker's Health Study (SHS) and Physical Activity Counseling (PAC) SDT-based interventions and also provide individual case examples. In an SDT-based intervention, the practitioner is trained to focus on enhancing patient autonomy as a clinical outcome in its own right (ABIM, 2002).

Tobacco Abstinence

Practitioners providing intensive treatment for tobacco dependence were taught these seven autonomy-supportive counseling behaviors in the SHS: (1) eliciting and acknowledging patient perspective; (2) offering a clear rationale for the recommended behavior; (3) providing information in a nonjudgmental manner; (4) supporting patient initiative for change, including for not changing; (5) eliciting patient aspirations and how changing the unhealthy behavior may affect those aspirations; (6) minimizing control; and (7) providing a menu of effective options for improving health. These style elements occur in the context of a traditional health assessment and treatment. For example, the tobacco abstinence treatment provided in the SHS was based on an integration of the Public Health Service's Clinical Practice Guideline recommendations for intensive treatment (Chapter 4, Fiore, Bailey, Cohen, Dorfman, Goldstein, Gritz et al., 2000) with an autonomy-supportive style. This was similar for PAC, where there was an integration with key physical activity promotion recommendations from the Task Force on Community Preventive Services (2001).

Once smokers consented to participate in the trial and were assigned to the intensive intervention, they met with a tobacco counselor individually for fifty minutes on the first visit and twenty to twenty-five minutes on follow-up visits. If smokers decided they wanted medical information or to use a medication to assist in a quit attempt, they were offered a choice of meeting with their own physician or with a physician provided by the study. This was done to increase smokers' experience of choice, with the intention of increasing perceived autonomy, competence, and relatedness. The initial fifty-minute visit included an introduction by the counselor, a brief overview of what they would be discussing, and the number of visits that were planned. The counselors then checked with the patients to see how they were feeling and if there were any immediate questions. Once questions were answered, a brief medical history was taken in what is often referred to as a patient-centered style (Rogers, 1951). After this information had been collected, clarified, and recorded, the counselor moved to elicit the smokers' story of tobacco use. Counselors were taught to interview in a manner that was positive and open to hearing the smokers' side of things. The counselors explicitly acknowledged that smoking may be enjoyable, relieve anxiety, and help the smoker concentrate if the smokers relayed those experiences, and that the smokers could continue to smoke without attempting to stop during the six-month intervention. In order to convey an openness to the common experience of ambivalence regarding continuing to smoke or not, counselors were taught to explore what the patient liked about smoking and what they didn't like about smoking. Answers were reflected back to the smokers in a summary reflection of the information elicited, with an acknowledgment that many smokers experienced both feelings of wanting to smoke and wanting to stop at the same time. Frequently, smokers indicated that they wanted to stop but did not feel able to. Counselors were taught to acknowledge smokers' feelings of incompetence, while remaining optimistic that the smokers could quit if it was desired. However, if the smokers indicated a desire to stop, the counselors would explore why they wanted to stop and how soon they wanted to try. If the smokers indicated they were afraid of particular diseases, counselors would acknowledge the affect displayed (for example, "You seem anxious when you mention cancer as a possibility"). In a similar manner, counselors explored what health benefits smokers felt they might receive if they stopped smoking. The counselors were taught to finish this segment of the interview on the health benefits that occur with abstinence from tobacco and to be optimistic that the smokers could stop if they wanted.

Motivations to Stop Counselors also asked the smokers to indicate how much they wanted to stop smoking, and how confident they were they could stop smoking completely on scales from 1 to 10. For example, if Mr. Smith indicated that he was a 5 on wanting to stop, counselors would ask "What keeps you from being an 3 [a number lower than what the smokers answered] on your wanting to stop?" This would be repeated regarding how confident they felt. The responses would be reflected back to the smokers. Once the interview elicited the smokers' motivations to stop, the counselors asked if the smokers wanted to stop and, if yes, what date they planned to stop on.

Problem Solving and Skills Building Once smokers indicated they wanted to stop in the next four weeks, the counselors utilized the skills building and problem solving techniques outlined in the *Public Health Service Clinical Practice Guideline* (Fiore et al., 2000, pages 37–39).

Planning Next Steps If smokers were planning to stop smoking, the end result of the counseling session was an individualized cessation plan that included behavioral techniques for dissociating smoking behaviors from the smokers' lives, and medications to temper withdrawal. A follow-up contact was planned during the first week of stopping to discuss how it was going and to make adjustments in the plan if needed. If the smoker did not plan to stop, the counselors would ask the smoker to schedule another contact to further discuss health and smoking.

Follow-Up The goals of the follow-up contacts were for the counselors to continue to support smoker autonomy about stopping or not, and to support competence by skill building and problem solving based on the specific difficulty the smokers were having. Counselors were taught to remain nonjudgmental of those who failed, as this is to be expected of the majority of smokers who try to stop. The counselors were taught to look for short successes and to acknowledge these efforts as important initiations and learning for the smoker. Additional attempts to stop were encouraged, but the counselors did not pressure the smokers to attempt again if they did not feel ready to do so for themselves. If the smokers had been successful in stopping completely, the counselors congratulated them on the success, and then asked the smokers to consider what additional planning was needed to handle the challenges to abstinence that lay ahead.

Physical Activity

For the PAC trial, we developed an SDT-based intensive physical activity counseling intervention model (Figure 6.4) to orient our intervention and to train our physical activity counselor. As shown, the intervention goal—to facilitate patient's autonomous motivation to foster greater and longer-term health behavior change—and the means—creation of an autonomy-supportive counseling climate—were very similar to those in the SHS.

What is innovative about this particular model is illustrating the intervention components encompassed in an autonomy-supportive style and showing which psychological need(s) they target. It also represents the concept of need sequencing. Indeed, in PAC, sequencing of the intensive counseling sessions was based on assumptions that in most cases, relatedness and autonomy/volition should be developed first, followed closely by competence/self-efficacy building. However, for some patients who had

FIGURE 6.4 *SDT-Based Intensive Physical Activity Counseling Intervention Model*

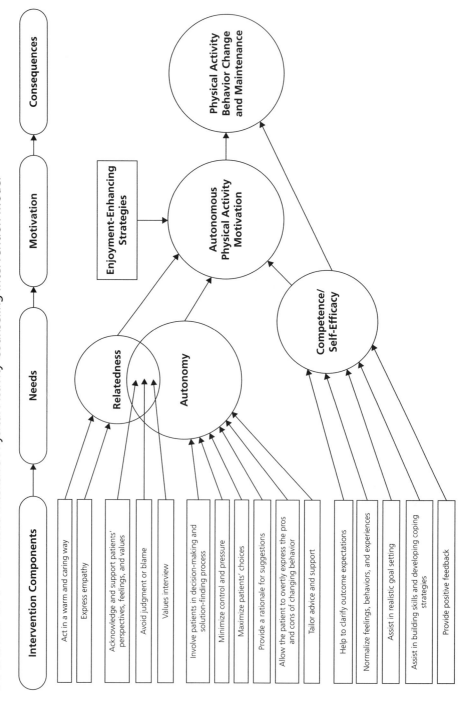

high initial levels of physical activity volition/motivation, competence building came earlier in the counseling process. This illustrates another key component of the PAC intervention: it was highly tailored to patients' needs. This is similar to the SHS, and aligns with recommendations in the physical activity promotion area (Task Force on Community Preventive Services, 2001).

One technique used in both the SHS and the PAC intervention was the values interview. Values interview (VI) is a technique where the practitioner asks the patient what his or her life strivings or aspirations are (for example, "Could you tell me two or three broad goals that you are seeking to achieve in your life?") and then takes each aspiration and asks the patient to reflect on and discuss how increasing physical activity or abstaining from smoking can help attain that aspiration and how it could prevent attaining that aspiration. Once answered, the counselor would thank the patient for providing a helpful illustration of how physical activity or smoking fit into the patient's life. As illustrated in Figure 6.4, VI is thought to build relatedness as the practitioner develops rapport with the patient by becoming more aware of his or her aspirations and by thanking the patient for sharing. This technique can also foster a sense of autonomy, as the practitioner acts in a neutral fashion and is not coercive or persuasive, but lets the patient overtly express their ambivalence by stating both the pros and cons of increasing their physical activity or abstaining from smoking. Finally, it can facilitate the internalization process (foster integration) as the patient realizes on his or her own that increasing their physical activity or abstaining from smoking can be an effective means of attaining their valued aspirations.

What was slightly different in the PAC intervention compared to the SHS was the distinction of fostering the needs within the counseling context and within the contextual (physical activity) setting and the addition of an enjoyment-enhancing component. Indeed, although counseling was individualized, in all sessions the physical activity counselor attempted to foster feelings of relatedness, autonomy, and competence in the patient and provided strategies to facilitate the needs in the physical activity context (for instance, suggesting finding physical activity buddies to build relatedness), as well as ensure that the physical activity experiences were as enjoyable as possible. Especially toward the end of the intervention, the physical activity counselor increasingly discussed enjoyment and assisted the patient in finding enjoyment-enhancing strategies to increase intrinsic motivation for physical activity and thus facilitate maintenance.

The PAC intervention followed the "Seven A's" interdisciplinary shared care model for PA counseling in primary care (Fortier, Tulloch, and Hogg, 2006). As such, the physical activity counselor was responsible for intensive counseling consisting of the Assess, Assist, and Arrange steps over the course of the three-month (six-session) intervention.

The Assess step (session one) involved in-depth questioning/exchange to get to know patients: their aspirations (via values interview), interests, medical history, past and current PA behaviors, PA motives (goal content) and further goal motives, competence/self-efficacy for behavior change, barriers, lifestyle, and social support networks. This step was designed to establish rapport and to individualize the intervention as well as to explore the pros and cons of PA behavior change.

The Assisting step continued over all sessions. In essence this step consisted of providing encouragement and support and helping patients become more active. Several common evidence-based strategies used to assist physical activity adoption and maintenance were incorporated (Kahn Ramsey, Brownson, Heath, Howze, Powell, et al., 2002). These included: (a) helping patients set appropriate weekly goals and determine potential barriers; (b) collaborative problem solving for potential strategies to overcome these barriers; (c) teaching and encouraging self-monitoring; (d) soliciting social support networks; (e) relapse prevention; and (f) linking patients with accessible physical activity services. Depending on the patient's needs/barriers, other strategies such as exploring ambivalence and challenging negative thoughts surrounding physical activity were also used. For instance, Mrs. Tremblay often mentioned to the counselor that she would have negative thoughts about her body and what people would think about her when going to the gym, so the counselor offered as an option that she write down her negative thoughts, practice thought stopping, and then replace these thoughts with more constructive ones. With time, this proved to be very helpful.

Following each in-person counseling session, all patients were provided with a form consisting of a standard combined goal sheet/action plan on one side and a self-monitoring tool for the next two weeks on the other. They were also provided with tailored tools and materials upon their departure from in-person sessions. For instance, Mr. Hébert, a very busy lawyer, was given a time-tracking tool to determine where physical activity would best fit into his busy schedule. Suggestions of specific physical activities, classes, or programs based on the patients' needs and preferences were made, and transitions were facilitated by the PAC. For example, Mrs. Patenaude had very much enjoyed dancing in her youth, so the counselor suggested she call up her neighborhood community center to see what dance classes they offered. She ended up taking a belly dance class twice a week with her best friend and loved it.

The final step was to Arrange for follow-up to determine progress and address any issues arising (for example, a new physical activity barrier). This was done at the beginning of each session for sessions two through six. This step was incorporated to modify PA goals and/or action plans and to ensure the patient was connected to the agreed-on external PA resource(s). Once winter arrived, the cold weather became an important barrier for Mr. Parent, who after brainstorming with the counselor decided to try mall walking twice a week with his wife. Reframing and normalizing difficulties with PA goals was an important component in building competence/self-efficacy.

While this section has focused on a tobacco dependence treatment intervention in the United States and a physical activity counseling intervention in Canada, SDT has been applied to many other health behaviors, as mentioned in the literature review, and in other countries, such as dental health in Norway (Halvari and Halvari, 2006) and weight loss in Portugal (Silva et al., 2007). Currently it is being used to develop another intervention aimed at physical inactivity in the United Kingdom. Owing to its many strengths (presented below) and growing popularity, we suspect it will be applied to other health threats, new populations, and in other countries in the near future.

SUMMARY

Strengths

SDT is a very versatile theory; it has been applied in numerous life contexts and for multiple outcomes: affects, cognitions, and behaviors (Deci and Ryan, 2002; Vallerand, 1997). In the health field, as illustrated in this chapter, it has been predictive of several health behaviors within varied populations. It is also a very well supported theory. Many investigations, including experimental and clinical studies, have provided empirical support for its postulates. SDT has been successfully used in health promotion contexts (Wilson, Evans, Williams, Mixon, Sirard, and Pate, 2005; Williams, Gagné et al., 2002) and recently has been combined with the recommended Seven A's model, which proposes key behavioral counseling steps (Fortier, Hogg, et al., 2007; Williams, McGregor, et al., 2006a). Moreover, as mentioned in the advantages section, SDT is the only individual-level theory that focuses on autonomy. Both the tobacco dependence guideline and the U.S. Preventive Services Task Force identify the importance of supporting patient autonomy in health behavior change counseling (Whitlock et al., 2002). Finally, SDT focuses on malleable individual factors that are amenable to change. As illustrated in this chapter, its core constructs—autonomous motivation and perceived competence—have been found to be modifiable from an intervention standpoint. Not only does SDT target changeable psychological variables, it also guides practitioners in the facilitation of these factors by postulating the mechanisms by which they change, predominantly via need satisfaction and autonomy

support. This is the main advantage of SDT over MI: SDT is a theory encompassing psychological and social processes, whereas MI is a technique. Finally, and importantly, research has shown that practitioners can be trained to use an autonomy-supportive counseling approach (Fortier, Sweet et al., 2007; Williams and Deci, 2001; Williams, Niemiec, Patrick, Ryan, and Deci, 2007; Williams, Gagné, et al., 2002; Williams, McGregor, et al., 2006a,b).

Limitations

SDT is an individual-level theory. It therefore does not make predictions or incorporate broader variables such as socioeconomic status and the physical environment that affect health and health behaviors (Marmot and Smith, 1997; Prus, 2007). SDT, however, has been recently incorporated within broader socioecological models to better elucidate health behaviors (McNeill, Wyrwich, Brownson, Clark, and Kreuter, 2006; O'Sullivan, Fortier, and Humphries, 2009). A second limitation is that some investigators have found ceiling effects in the SDT motivational variables when using the Treatment Self-Regulation Questionnaire for physical activity (Fortier, Sweet, et al., 2007; Fortier, Kowal, Lemyre, and Orpana, 2007). Investigating the different forms of motivational regulations separately (for instance, using the Behavioral Regulation Exercise Questionnaire-2; Markland and Tobin, 2004) might be one way of remedying this problem and would also allow a better understanding of the influence of the different types of regulations on health behaviors that have been recently recommended (Edmunds, Ntoumanis, and Duda, 2006; Wilson et al., 2003, 2004). Fortier and Sweet (2009) are currently analyzing data from the PAC trial to determine the influence of the different types of regulation on physical activity adoption (during the intervention) and maintenance (in the post-intervention phase) using hierarchical linear modeling (Raudenbush and Bryk, 2002).

FUTURE DIRECTIONS

One line of future direction is developing a checklist to determine whether a health promotion intervention is SDT-based or not and, if so, to what degree. This exists for motivational interviewing (Moyers, Martin, Catley, Harris, and Ahluwalia, 2003) and for evaluating to what extent a health promotion intervention is ecological or not (Richard, Potvin, Kishchuk, Prlic, and Green, 1996). Once this has been done, developing and implementing SDT training modules for practitioners (for example, physicians, exercise professionals, tobacco dependence counselors) would be the next logical step. Online training would be particularly useful to reach the largest number of practitioners possible, to standardize training and to allow international collaborations. This would also enable the application of SDT interventions to other important health-related areas, such as AIDS prevention, obesity treatment, and end-of-life care. In terms of research, we could investigate practitioners' uptake/adoption of autonomy support from these training sessions (dissemination trial similar to Eakin, Brown, Marshall, Mummery, and Larsen, 2004) and how this translates into individuals' improvements in autonomous self-regulation, health behavior change, and health.

Additional work should be done on the SDT intervention process model (Figure 6.4) to elaborate on the intervention components, better understand their effects and untangle the overlap between the needs. Investigating which strategy or strategies best facilitate improvements in autonomous motivation, perceived competence and subsequent health behavior change would be particularly useful from an intervention standpoint. Given that this might be highly individualized, qualitative research would be particularly useful in this regard. Another interesting direction would be to determine a threshold of autonomous motivation/self-determination for adoption and maintenance of health behavior change, similar to the work that is being done with self-efficacy at Stanford.

Future research should focus on further investigating the interplay between perceived competence and autonomous self-regulation over time, as some studies indicate that perceived competence is an antecedent of autonomous motivation (Edmunds, Ntoumanis, and Duda, 2006; Kowal and Fortier, 2000; Vallerand and Ratelle, 2002) while others have found perceived competence to be affected by autonomous motivation (Williams et al., 2006a; McNeill et al., 2006). Testing different mediational and/or moderational models is highly recommended.

More clinical trial research is needed on autonomy support in the health promotion context, especially by providers who deliver intensive interventions and thus have the opportunity to apply the approach over many sessions. Combining brief versus intensive behavior change counseling interventions with neutral versus autonomy-supportive approaches would provide a rigorous field test of SDT theory.

In order to explain more variance in health behavior change, integrating SDT with other individual-level theories and even other level health promotion theories would be useful. One such study is Sweet and Fortier's ongoing study (2007–2009) integrating self determination theory (Deci and Ryan, 1985, 2002) and social cognitive theory (Bandura, 1986) to understand physical activity maintenance in patients enrolled in a cardiac rehabilitation program. Incorporating self-regulation type variables between the SDT motivational variables and health behavior change outcomes along the lines of Koestner's work on implementation intentions (Koestner, Horberg, Gaudreau, Powers, Di Dio, Bryan, et al., 2006) would be especially helpful for investigating health behavior change maintenance.

REFERENCES

ABIM Foundation, ACP-ASIM Foundation, European Federation of Internal Medicine, (2002). Medical professionalism in the new millennium: A physician charter. *Annals of Internal Medicine*, *136*, 243–246.

Ames, C. (1992). Achievement goals, motivational climate, and motivational processes. In G. C. Roberts (ed.), *Motivation in sport and exercise*, pp. 40--57. Champaign, IL: Human Kinetics Books.

Bandura, A. (1986). *Social learning theory*. Englewood Cliffs, NJ: Prentice-Hall.

Beauchamp, T.L, and Childress, J.F., (2001). *Principles of biomedical ethics*. New York: Oxford University Press.

Biddle, S. J., and Nigg, C. R. (2000). Theories of exercise behavior. *International Journal of Sport Psychology*, *31*, 290–304.

Carver, C. S., and Scheier, M. F. (2000). Autonomy and self-regulation. *Psychological Inquiry*, *11*, 284–291.

Caspersen, C.J., Powell, K.E., and Christenson, G.M. (1985). Physical activity, exercise, and physical fitness: definitions and distinctions for health-related research. *Public Health Reports*, *100*, 126–131.

Daley, A. J., and Duda, J. L. (2006). Self-determination, stage of readiness of change for exercise, and frequency of physical activity in young people. *European Journal of Sport Science*, *6*(4), 231–243.

Deci, E. L., Eghari, H., Patrick, B. C., and Leone D. (1994). Facilitating internalization: The self-determination theory perspective. *Journal of Personality*, *62*, 119–142.

Deci, E. L., and Ryan, R. M. (1985). *Intrinsic motivation and self-determination in human behavior*. New York: Plenum.

Deci, E., and Ryan, R. (2002). *The handbook of self-determination research*. Rochester, NY: University of Rochester Press.

Duda, J. (1992) Motivation in sport settings: A goal perspective approach. In G. C. Roberts (ed.), *Motivation in sport and exercise*, pp. 57–92. Champaign, IL: Human Kinetics Books.

Dweck, C. S. (1985). Intrinsic motivation, perceived control, and self-evaluation maintenance: An achievement goal analysis. In C. Ames and RE Ames (eds.), *Research on motivation and education: the classroom milieu*. New York: Academic Press.

Eakin, E. G., Brown, W. J., Marshall, A. L., Mummery, K., and Larsen, E. (2004). Physical activity promotion in primary care. *American Journal of Preventive Medicine*, *27*, 297–303.

Edmunds, J., Ntoumanis, N., and Duda, J. L. (2006). A test of self-determination theory in the exercise domain. *Journal of applied social psychology*, *36*(9), 2240–2265.

Edmunds, J., Ntoumanis, N., and Duda, J. L. (2007). Adherence and well-being in overweight and obese patients referred to an exercise on prescription scheme: A self-determination theory perspective. *Psychology of Sport and Exercise. 8*, 722–740.

Feltz, D. (1988). Gender differences in the causal elements of self-efficacy on a high avoidance motor task. *Journal of Sport Psychology*, *10*, 151–166.

Feltz, D. (1992). Understanding motivation in sport: A self-efficacy perspective. In G. C. Roberts (ed.), *Motivation in sport and exercise*, pp. 93–106. Champaign, IL: Human Kinetics Books.

Fiore, M., Bailey, W., Cohen, S., Dorfman, S., Goldstein, M., Gritz, E., et al. (2000). *Treating tobacco use and dependence: Clinical practice guidelines*. Rockville, MD: U.S. Department of Health and Human Services, Public Health Service.

Foote, J., DeLuca, A., Magura, S., Warner, A., Grand, A., Rosenblum, A., and Stahl, S. (1999). A group motivational treatment for chemical dependency. *Journal of Substance Abuse and Treatment*, *17*, 181–192.

Fortier, M., and Grenier, M. (1999). Déterminants personnels et situationnels de l'adhérence à un programme d'exercice: Une étude prospective. *Revue STAPS*, *49*, 25–38.

Fortier, M. S., Hogg, W. E., O'Sullivan, T. L., Blanchard, C., Reid, R. D., Sigal, R. J., et al. (2007). The physical activity counselling (PAC) randomized controlled trial: Rationale, methods, and interventions. *Applied Physiology, Nutrition and Metabolism*, *32*, 1170–1185.

Fortier, M., and Kowal, J. (2007). The flow state and physical activity behavior change as motivational outcomes: A self-determination theory perspective. In M. S. Hagger and N.L.D. Chatzisarantis (eds.). *Intrinsic motivation and self-determination in exercise and sport* (pp. 113–126). Champaign, IL: Human Kinetics.

Fortier, M. S., and Sweet, S. (2009). [Influence of motivational regulations on physical activity adoption and maintenance in the physical activity counseling randomized controlled trial]. Unpublished raw data.

Fortier, M. S., Sweet, S., O'Sullivan, T. L., Blanchard, C., and Williams, G. C. (2007). A self-determination process model of physical activity adoption in the context of a randomized controlled trial. *Psychology of Sport and Exercise*, *8*, 741–757.

Fortier, M. S., Sweet, S., Tulloch, H., Blanchard, C., Sigal, R., and Kenny, G. (2009). Self-determination and exercise stage progression in individuals with type 2 diabetes: A longitudinal study. Manuscript submitted for publication.

Fortier, M., Tulloch, H. and Hogg, W. (2006). A good fit: Integrating physical activity counselors into family practice. *Canadian Family Physician*, *52*, 942–4, 947–9.

Frederick-Recascino, C. (2002). Self-determination theory and participation motivation research in the sport and exercise domain. In E. L. Deci and R. M. Ryan (eds), *The handbook of self-determination research* (pp. 277–298). Rochester, NY: The University of Rochester Press.

Frederick-Recascino, C. M., and Schuster-Smith, H. (2003). Competition and intrinsic motivation in physical activity: A comparison of two groups. *Journal of Sport Behavior*, *26*, 240–254.

Fuemmeler, B. F., Mâsse, L. C., Yaroch, A. L., Resnicow, K., Campbell, M. K., Carr, C., et al (2006). Psychosocial mediation of fruit and vegetable consumption in the body and soul effectiveness trial. *Health Psychology*, *25*, 474–83.

Halvari, A.E.M., and Halvari, H. (2006). Motivational predictors of change in oral health: An experimental test of self-determination theory. *Motivation and Emotion*, *30*, 295–306.

Hull, C. L. (1943). *Principles of behavior: An introduction to behavior theory*. New York: Appleton-Century-Crofts.

Kahn, E., Ramsey, L., Brownson, R., Heath, G., Howze, E., Powell, K., et al. (2002). The effectiveness of interventions to increase physical activity: A systemic review. *American Journal of Preventive Medicine*, *22*, 73–107.

Kennedy, S., Goggin, K., and Nollen, N. (2004) Adherence to HIV medications: Utility of the theory of self-determination. *Cognitive Therapy and Research*, *28*, 611–628.

Kernis, M. H. (2000). Substitute needs and the distinction between fragile and secure high self-esteem. *Psychological Inquiry*, *11*, 298–300.

Koestner, R., Horberg, E. J., Gaudreau, P., Powers, T., Di Dio, P., Bryan, C. et al. (2006). Bolstering implementation plans for the long haul: The benefits of simultaneously boosting self-concordance or self-efficacy. *Personality and Social Psychology Bulletin*, *32*, 1547–1558.

Kowal, J., and Fortier, M. S. (2000). Testing relationships from the hierarchical model of intrinsic and extrinsic motivation using flow as a motivational consequence. *Research Quarterly for Exercise and Sport*, *71*, 171–181.

Landry, J. B., and Solomon, M. A. (2002). Self-determination theory as an organizing framework to investigate women's physical activity behaviour. *Quest*, *54*, 332–354.

Markland, D. (1999). Self-determination moderates the effects of perceived competence on intrinsic motivation in an exercise setting. *Journal of Sport and Exercise Psychology*, *21*, 351–361.

Markland, D., and Hardy, L. (1997). On the factorial and construct validity of the Intrinsic Motivation Inventory: Conceptual and operational concerns. *Research Quarterly for Exercise and Sport*, *68*, 20–32.

Markland, D., Ryan, R. M., Jayne Tobin, V., and Rollnick, S. (2005). Motivational interviewing and self-determination theory. *Journal of Social and Clinical Psychology*, *24*(6), 811–831.

Markland, D. and Tobin, V. (2004). A modification to the behavioural regulation in exercise questionnaire to include an assessment of amotivation. *Journal of Sport and Exercise Psychology*, *26*, 191–196.

Marmot, M. G., and Smith, G. D. (1997). Socio-economic differentials in health. *Journal of Health Psychology*, *2*, 283–296.

McNeill, L. H., Wyrwich, K., Brownson, R., Clark, E., and Kreuter, M. (2006). Individual, social environmental, and physical environmental influences on physical activity among black and white adults: A structural equation analysis. *Annals of Behavioral Medicine*, *31*, 36–44.

Miller, W. R., and Rollnick, S. (2002). *Motivational interviewing: Preparing people for change* (2nd ed.). New York: The Guilford Press.

Moyers, T., Martin, T., Catley, D., Harris, K. J., and Ahluwalia, J. S. (2003). Assessing the integrity of motivational interviewing interventions: Reliability of the motivational skills code. *Behavioural and Cognitive Psychotherapy*, *31*, 177–184.

Murray, H. A. (1938). *Explorations in personality*. New York: Oxford University Press.

Nicholls, J. G. (1984). Achievement motivation: Conceptions of ability, subjective experience, task choice, and performance. *Psychological Review*, *91*, 328–346.

Nicholls, J. G. (1989). *The competitive ethos and democratic education*. Cambridge, MA: Harvard University Press.

Ntoumanis, N. (2005). A prospective study of participation in optional school physical education using a self-determination theory framework. *Journal of Educational Psychology*, *97*, 444–453.

O'Sullivan, T. L., Fortier, M., and Humphries, C. (2009). *Physical activity maintenance in middle aged women: A qualitative ecological study*. Manuscript submitted for publication.

Patrick, H., Williams, G. C., Fortier, M. S., Sweet, S. N., Halvari, A.E.M., Halvari, H., et al. (2008). Supporting autonomy in clinical interventions: Toward successful multiple-behavior change. Manuscript submitted for publication.

Pelletier, L. G., Fortier, M. S., Vallerand, R. J., and Brière, N. M. (2001). Associations among perceived autonomy support, forms of self-regulation, and persistence: A prospective study. *Motivation and Emotion*, *25*, 279–306.

Prochaska, J. O., and DiClemente, C. C. (1983). Stages and processes of self-change of smoking: Toward an integrative model of change. *Journal of Consulting and Clinical Psychology*, *51*, 390–395.

Prochaska, J. O., DiClemente, C. C., and Norcross, J. C. (1992). In search of how people change: Applications to the addictive behaviors. *American Psychologist*, *47*, 1102–1114.

Prus, S. G. (2007). Age, SES and health: A population level analysis of health inequalities over the lifecourse. *Sociology of Health and Illness*, *29*, 275–296.

Raudenbush, S. W., and Bryk, T. A. (2002). *Hierarchical linear models: Applications and data analysis methods* (2nd ed.). Thousand Oaks, CA: Sage.

Reeve, J. (1998). Autonomy support as an interpersonal motivating style: Is it teachable? *Contemporary Educational Psychology*, *23*, 312–330.

Resnicow, K., DiIorio, C., Blisset, D., Braithwaite, R. L., Perisamy, S., and Rahotep, S. (2002). Healthy body/healthy spirit: A church-based nutrition and physical activity intervention. *Health Education Research*, *17*, 562–573.

Richard, L., Potvin, L., Kishchuk, N., Prlic, H., and Green, L. W. (1996). Assessment of the integration of the ecological approach in health promotion programs. *American Journal of Health Promotion*, *10*, 318–328.

Rogers, C. R. (1951). *Client-centered therapy*. Boston: Houghton-Mifflin.

Ryan, R. M. (1993). Agency and organization: Intrinsic motivation, autonomy and the self in psychological development. In J. Jacobs (ed.), *Nebraska symposium on motivation: Developmental perspectives on motivation*, pp. 1–56. Lincoln, NE: University of Nebraska Press.

Ryan, R. M., and Connell, J. P. (1989). Perceived locus of causality and internalization: Examining reasons for acting in two domains. *Journal of Personality and Social Psychology*, *57*, 749–761.

Ryan, R. M., and Deci, E. L. (2000). Self-determination theory and the facilitation of intrinsic motivation, social development, and well-being. *American Psychologist*, *55*, 68–78.

Ryan, R., Plant, W., and O'Malley, S. (1995). Initial motivations for alcohol treatment: Relations with patient characteristics, treatment involvement and dropout. *Addictive Behaviors*, *20*, 279–297.

Schneider, C. E. (1998). *The practice of autonomy. Patients, doctors, and medical decisions.* New York; Oxford University Press.

Senécal, C., Nouwen, A., and White, D. (2000). Motivation and dietary self-care in adults with diabetes: Are self-efficacy and autonomous self-regulation complimentary or competing constructs? *Health Psychology*, *19*, 452–457.

Silva, M. N., Teixeira, P. J., Markland, D., Minderico, C. S., Vieira, P. N., Castro, M. M.,. (2007). Testing Self-Determination Theory for long-term exercise adherence and weight control: A randomized controlled trial. Unpublished manuscript University of Lisbon.

Sweet, S. N., and Fortier, M. S. (2007—2009). Self-determination theory and self-efficacy theory: Can they work together to predict physical activity adoption and maintenance in cardiac rehabilitation?. Ongoing study.

Task Force on Community Preventive Services. (2001). Increasing physical activity: A report on recommendations of the task force on community prevention services. *Morbidity and Mortality Weekly Report*, *50*(RR–18), 1–14.

Vallerand, R. J. (1997). Toward a hierarchical model of intrinsic and extrinsic motivation. In M. P. Zanna (ed.). *Advances in experimental social psychology* (pp. 271–360). New York: Academic Press.

Vallerand, R. J., and Losier, G. F. (1999). An integrative analysis of intrinsic and extrinsic motivation in sport. *Journal of Applied Sport Psychology*, *11*, 142–169.

Vallerand, R. J., and Ratelle, C. F. (2002). Intrinsic and extrinsic motivation: A hierarchical model. In E. L. Deci and R. M. Ryan (Eds), *The handbook of self-determination research* (pp. 37–64). Rochester, NY: The University of Rochester Press.

Vallerand, R. J., and Rousseau, F. L. (2001). Intrinsic and extrinsic motivation in sport and exercise: A review using the hierarchical model of intrinsic and extrinsic motivation. In R. N. Singer, H. A. Hausenblas and C. M. Janelle (eds.), *Handbook of sport psychology* (2nd ed., pp. 389–416). Toronto: Wiley.

Vansteenkiste, M., and Sheldon, K. S. (2006). There's nothing more practical than a good theory: Integrating motivational interviewing and self-determination theory. *British Journal of Clinical Psychology*, *45*, 63–82.

Whitlock, E. P., Orleans, T., Pender, N., and Allan, J. (2002). Evaluating primary care behavioral counseling interventions: An evidenced-based approach. *American Journal of Preventive Medicine*, *22*, 267–284. Available online at www.ajpm-online.net.

Williams, G. C. (2002). Improving patients' health through supporting the autonomy of patients and providers. In E. L. Deci and R. M. Ryan (Eds), *The handbook of self-determination research* (pp. 233–254). Rochester, NY: University of Rochester Press.

Williams, G. C., Cox, E. M., Kouides, R., and Deci, E. L. (1999). Presenting the facts about smoking to adolescents: The effects of an autonomy supportive style. *Archives of Pediatrics and Adolescent Medicine*, *153*, 959–964.

Williams, G., and Deci, E. (2001). Activating patients for smoking cessation through physician autonomy support. *Medical Care*, *39*, 813–823.

Williams, G. C., Freedman, Z. R., and Deci, E. L. (1998). Supporting autonomy to motivate glucose control in patients with diabetes. *Diabetes Care, 21*, 1644–1651.

Williams, G. C., Gagné, M., Mushlin, A. I., and Deci, E. L. (2005). Motivation for behavior change inpatients with chest pain. *Health Education*, *105*(4), 304–321.

Williams, G. C., Gagné, M., Ryan, R. M., and Deci, E. L. (2002). Facilitating autonomous motivation for smoking cessation. *Health Psychology*, *21*, 40–50.

Williams, G. C., Grow, V. M., Freedman, Z. R., Ryan, R. M., and Deci, E. L. (1996). Motivational predictors of weight loss and weight-loss maintenance. *Journal of Personality and Social Psychology, 20*, 115–126.

Williams, G. C., McGregor, H. A., Sharp, D. S., Kouides, R., Levesque, C. S., Ryan, R. M., et al. (2006b). Self-determination Multiple Risk Intervention Trial to improve smokers health. *Journal of General Internal Medicine, 21*, 1288–1294.

Williams, G. C., McGregor, H. A., Sharp, D. S., Levesque, C., Kouides, R. W., Ryan, R. M., et al. (2006a). Testing a self-determination theory intervention for motivating tobacco cessation: Supporting autonomy and competence in a clinical trial. *Health Psychology, 25*(1), 91–101.

Williams, G., Minicucci, D., Kouides, R., Levesque, C., Chirkov, V., Ryan, R., et al. (2002). Self-determination, smoking, diet, and health. *Health Education Research, 17*(5), 512–521.

Williams, G. C., Niemiec, C. P., Patrick, H., Ryan, R. M., and Deci, E. L. (2007). The importance of supporting autonomy in facilitating long-term tobacco abstinence. Unpublished manuscript. University of Rochester.

Williams, G. C., Patrick, H., Sapp, A., Williams, L. K., Devine, G., Lafata, J. E., et al. (2007). Adherence information and self-determination theory for reducing the health risks of diabetes. Unpublished manuscript. University of Rochester.

Williams, G. C., Rodin, G., Ryan, R., Grolnick, W., and Deci, E. (1998). Autonomous regulation and long-term medication adherence in adult outpatients. *Health Psychology, 17*, 269–276.

Wilson, D. K., Evans, A. E., Williams, J., Mixon, G., Sirard, J. R., and Pate, R. (2005). A preliminary test of a student-centered intervention on increasing physical activity in underserved adolescents. *Annals of Behavioral Medicine*, 30, 119–124.

Wilson, P. M., Blanchard, C., Nehl, E., and Baker, R. (2006). Predicting physical activity and outcome expectations in cancer survivors: An application of self-determination theory. *Psycho-Oncology, 15*, 567–578.

Wilson, P. M., Rodgers, W. M., Blanchard, C. M., and Gessell, J. (2003). The relationship between psychological needs, self-determined motivation, exercise attitudes, and physical fitness. *Journal of applied social psychology, 33*(11), 2373–2392.

Wilson, P. M., Rodgers, W. M., Fraser, S. N., and Murray, T.C. (2004). Relationship between exercise regulations and motivational consequences in university students. *Research Quarterly in Exercise and Sport, 75*, 81–91.

THE ELABORATION LIKELIHOOD MODEL OF PERSUASION: DEVELOPING HEALTH PROMOTIONS FOR SUSTAINED BEHAVIORAL CHANGE

Richard E. Petty
Jamie Barden
S. Christian Wheeler

INFLUENCING BEHAVIORAL CHANGE

Roughly half of all causes of mortality in the United States are tied to social and behavioral variables including smoking, alcohol use, diet and sedentary lifestyle (Institute of Medicine, 2000). Because of this, health promotion campaigns and research are typically designed to induce positive change in health-related behaviors. For example, a media campaign might attempt to convince people to use their seatbelts or to stop smoking. However, studies of the effectiveness of media and direct interventions have provided inconsistent results. In particular, efforts in critical areas such as drug and alcohol abuse and AIDS prevention have sometimes proven to be disappointing in terms of concrete successes. This challenge has led to a number of responses. Notably, there is a growing awareness of the importance of health promotion programs that establish sustained behavioral change, as distinct from merely having an impact on initiation of behavior change (Rothman, 2000). For example, between 2003 and 2007 the Office of Behavioral and Social Sciences Research awarded $53.8 million to support research investigating "Maintenance of Long-Term Behavioral Change" (Solomon, 2005). To understand why certain interventions with high face validity fail to provide sustained behavioral change, health promotion researchers and practitioners have sought insight from basic research on influence processes. In line with this view, funding agencies have identified the importance of uncovering the mechanisms underlying cause-effect relationships between specific intervention components and outcomes.

Experimental research has shown that attitudes represent one of the most important theoretical constructs that determine behavior (Eagly and Chaiken, 1993; Fishbein and Ajzen, 1975; Petty and Cacioppo, 1981). As most commonly conceived, an attitude is a relatively stable global evaluation of a person, object, or issue. Taking exercise behavior as an example, critical attitudes might include: Exercise is good; I feel favorable toward running on the weekends; I feel good enough about myself to believe I can start exercising. Thus, multiple attitudes held toward different objects at different levels of specificity (for example, the general concept of exercise, a specific behavior such as running, one's own self-efficacy) can impact the likelihood that any behavior is enacted (Petty, Baker, and Gleicher, 1991). Thus, one job of those interested in health promotion is to determine which attitudes are the most important for predicting a particular health behavior and which procedures are best used for changing those attitudes and obtaining sustained behavioral change.

Of course, a number of factors other than attitudes determine whether or not people engage in a certain behavior. These include social norms, (Goldstein and Cialdini, 2007; Fishbein and Ajzen, 1975), the strength of the attitude (Petty and Krosnick, 1995), feelings of self-efficacy and competence (Bandura, 1986), and prior behaviors and habits (Triandis, 1980; Wood and Neal, 2007). Although this might suggest that we should try to change these factors instead, many of these behavioral determinants result from attitudes as well. For example, when the attitudes of many people change, this changes social norms. Positive attitudes toward the self can increase feelings of self-efficacy making behavioral change more likely. Finally, the fact that past behaviors (habits) have a strong role in predicting current behaviors may be due in part to the impact of prior attitudes (Petty, Tormala, Briñol, and Jarvis, 2006). Thus, to change behavior, it is useful to understand how attitudes are changed.

Attitudes are most frequently measured using some type of direct self-report procedure such as asking a person how favorable or unfavorable and positive or negative they are toward some object or behavior such as wearing seat belts (see Eagly and Chaiken, 1993, for more detail about common attitude measurement procedures). More recently, attitudes have also been assessed with measures that tap the evaluation that automatically comes to mind when confronted with the issue (see Petty, Fazio, and Briñol, 2009). Because automatic attitudes can be influenced in the same ways as more deliberative attitudes (see Briñol, Petty, and McCaslin, 2009), we do not dwell on this distinction. Regardless of the measure employed, when planning a health promotion program, it is important to select the attitude or attitudes that the program intends to change and to measure each attitude separately to determine the success of the program. Depending on one's goals, it can be useful to measure attitudes toward a general idea (safe sex), a specific object (condom), or a behavior (using a condom). The success of a persuasive attempt is then measured by assessing change in the attitudes targeted. Change can be assessed in either a pre-post design or by comparing the attitudes of individuals who have and who have not received some persuasion treatment (Campbell and Stanley, 1964).

THE ELABORATION LIKELIHOOD MODEL OF PERSUASION

Contemporary scientific research on attitude change began in the 1940s as an extension of the U.S. military's effort during World War II to understand propaganda and persuasion (for example, see Hovland, Lumsdaine, and Sheffield, 1949). The most popular persuasion theory at the time was based on learning principles and viewed persuasion as a function of attention, comprehension, acceptance, and retention of the persuasive communication (Hovland, Janis, and Kelley, 1953). Early research guided by this framework identified many of the variables investigators continue to examine today as determinants of attitude change. That is, research focused on: features of the source of the message, Is the source attractive? Expert? A member of an in-group?; the message itself, Is the message complex? Composed of cogent arguments? Rational or emotional?; the recipient of the communication, Is the recipient in a good mood? Intelligent? Involved in the topic; and the context in which the message was presented, Is the environment quiet or distracting? Is the message on the radio, television, or the Internet?

As the number of persuasion studies began to grow, numerous inconsistencies in findings appeared. For example, increasing the same variable (for example, number of arguments, source expertise, use of fear) would increase persuasion in one experiment, decrease it in another, and have no effect in a third. Furthermore, numerous attitude change theories were developed to describe a number of processes through which persuasion could take place, but each theory only seemed to predict persuasion under certain conditions. Theories were also in disagreement about the effects of any one variable (for example, how does source expertise influence attitude change; see Petty, 1994).

The Elaboration Likelihood Model (ELM; Petty and Cacioppo, 1986) was developed to explain past inconsistencies in attitudes research. Whereas past models tended to emphasize one effect of a given variable and one process by which that effect occurred, the ELM organized multiple persuasion processes into two routes to attitude change. The central route involves change that occurs when people are relatively thoughtful in their consideration of the issue-relevant information presented. In contrast, the peripheral route to persuasion involves processes requiring relatively little thought about issue-relevant information. Instead, attitudes are changed by simple association processes (for example, classical conditioning) or the use of various mental shortcuts and heuristics. By noting that variables influence attitudes by different means at different points along an elaboration continuum, the ELM is able to explain seemingly inconsistent findings in the persuasion literature. After describing key ideas from the ELM, we discuss the utility of the model for understanding health communication.

Central Route Processing

As noted earlier, the ELM organizes attitude change processes into two routes to persuasion: the central route and the peripheral route. The central route to persuasion involves careful consideration of information pertaining to the attitude object and its relationship to pertinent knowledge stored in memory. Careful consideration of the issue-relevant information presented involves generating positive and/or negative thoughts toward the advocated position (for example, seat belt usage). Under the central route, the valence of those thoughts (whether positive or negative) is related to the direction of persuasion, and the extent to which the thoughts are new and more positive or negative than they were previously determines the extent of attitude change. The thoughts about the message make up the key component that links internal knowledge to the information presented in the message. Also, the more confidence people have in the thoughts that they generate under the central route, the more these thoughts determine a person's attitude (Petty, Briñol, and Tormala, 2002). Thus, if a person has many favorable thoughts but there is reason to doubt them, attitude change is unlikely. The focus of the thinking under the central route is often on the perceived desirability of the consequences in the communication and the perceived likelihood that these consequences will occur (Petty and Wegener, 1991; Fishbein and Ajzen, 2000).

Two conditions are necessary for effortful processing to occur—the recipient of the message must be both *motivated* and *able* to think carefully. A person's motivation to consider message arguments can be influenced by a number of variables, including the perceived personal relevance of the message (Petty and Cacioppo, 1979b) and whether the person enjoys thinking in general (their *need for cognition*; Cacioppo, Petty, and Morris, 1983). A person's ability to think can also be influenced by a number of variables, including the amount of distraction present in the persuasion context (Petty, Wells, and Brock, 1976), and the number of times the message is repeated (Cacioppo and Petty, 1979). If a person is both motivated and able to think about the issue-relevant information presented, the end result of this careful processing is an attitude that is well articulated, readily accessible, held with confidence, and integrated into the person's overall belief structure (Petty and Cacioppo, 1986).

Peripheral Route Processing

In our daily lives, we often lack either the motivation or the ability to thoughtfully consider every potential persuasive communication in the way characterized by the central route. Attitude change can occur nonetheless, because many persuasion processes require little to no consideration of substantive information. In the ELM, such processes are organized into the peripheral route, and they include reliance on simple cues available in the persuasion context as well as mental shortcuts called heuristics. The persuasion context can elicit an affective state (like happiness) that becomes associated with the advocated position through classical conditioning (Staats and Staats, 1958), or a mental shortcut might be used so that a message from an expert is judged based on the heuristic that, "experts are generally correct," rather than careful consideration of the substantive arguments (Chaiken, 1987). Another common method used when either motivation or ability is lacking is simply to count the number of arguments made rather than evaluating them based on their merit (Petty and Cacioppo, 1984). Although the peripheral route to persuasion does not involve thoughtful consideration of message content, it can be effective in leading to persuasion, at least in the short term.

For expository purposes, it has been convenient to break the processes of persuasion into two distinct routes. However, the ELM holds that persuasion occurs along an elaboration continuum. The continuum stretches from processes requiring no thinking, like subliminal classical conditioning that occurs outside of awareness, to processes requiring some effort, like counting arguments or making inferences based on one's experienced affect, to processes requiring careful consideration, such as listing the pros and cons to make an important life decision. Along much of the continuum, both peripheral and central processes take place and can influence attitudes simultaneously (Petty, 1994). But, as the elaboration likelihood increases, central route processes (that is, careful evaluation of issue-relevant information) tend to dominate in their impact on attitudes over more peripheral processes (for example, reliance on heuristics).

It is important to emphasize that the distinction between central and peripheral routes is made based on the extent of issue-relevant scrutiny and on how carefully the information is processed rather than on the type of information itself (Petty, Wheeler, and Bizer, 1999). As an example, information about the source of a message can have an impact on attitudes under either the central or the peripheral routes, depending upon whether the recipient has the motivation and ability to evaluate it carefully. If, for example, famous basketball player Magic Johnson is the source of a message about human immunodeficiency virus (HIV), and people use the heuristic, "famous is good," then persuasion will follow the peripheral route. However, if people are more persuaded because they realize that Magic

Johnson has contracted HIV and knows what he is talking about, then they are examining the central merits of Magic Johnson as a source as is likely to occur under the central route. Note that under the peripheral route, the use of Magic Johnson could be effective regardless of the message topic because if all one considers is his fame, and fame is good, this is constant across attitude objects. On the other hand, if one processes the source information carefully for relevance, Magic Johnson should be more effective in an HIV message (or for basketball shoes) than in a message for swimming pools.

Support for the Central and Peripheral Routes

There is extensive empirical support for the idea that persuasion can be governed by either central or peripheral route processing (see Petty and Cacioppo, 1986; Petty and Wegener, 1998a, for reviews). In one early and representative study, the presence or absence of a potential peripheral cue and the quality of the arguments, strong versus weak (as determined in pilot testing), were manipulated (Petty, Cacioppo, and Goldman, 1981). In this study, college students were given one of four persuasive messages that contained either: (a) strong and compelling arguments attributed to an expert source; (b) weak and specious arguments presented by an expert source; (c) strong and compelling arguments attributed to a nonexpert source; or (d) weak arguments attributed to a nonexpert source. No distractions were present during the procedure and the message was easily comprehended, so all participants had the ability to process the message. On the other hand, motivation to process the message was manipulated by informing some of the students that the proposal (supporting a change in campus policy) would take effect in a year (high relevance condition), whereas others were informed that the proposal would go into effect in ten years (low relevance condition). The high relevance condition should motivate effortful processing of the message (Petty and Cacioppo, 1979b). The low relevance condition offers little motivation to process the message, so low effort attitude change processes should have a greater impact on attitude change. This was in fact the observed pattern; those in the high motivation condition processed the message arguments, so their level of persuasion was greatly influenced by the manipulation of argument strength. Their attitudes toward the issue were based on whether the arguments offered good support for the advocated position or not. Those in the low personal relevance condition lacked the motivation to process the message thoroughly, and so their level of persuasion was a function of the expertise of the source rather than strength of the message. That is, they supported the policy change as long as the source was an expert, regardless of the quality of the arguments offered to support the policy.

Variables Influencing the Extent and Direction of Elaboration

Taken as a whole, the evidence supporting the ELM shows that a number of variables exist that can impact persuasion by influencing a message recipients' motivation or ability to think about the communication. In this way, these variables determine whether high or low effort processes are more likely to influence attitudes. For example, if a woman has a family history of breast cancer, then she might be motivated to think about a persuasive message about breast self-exams based on perceived self-relevance (Rothman and Schwarz, 1998). However, if the perceived self-relevance is so intense as to induce fear, defensive avoidance might occur (Janis and Feshbach, 1953). In addition to motivational variables, as noted earlier, ability variables also influence processing. For example, if the message is delivered in the hall of a busy hospital, the ability to think will be lowered. Variables that influence motivation and ability to think can be part of the *situation*, or they can be internal to the *person*.

The breast exam example mentioned variables that influence the *extent* of thinking (whether many or few thoughts are generated). Other variables influence the *direction* of thinking (whether thoughts are favorable or unfavorable to the message). For example, telling an audience that they are about to receive an attempt to persuade them on an important issue can bias responses to the message, because the audience becomes motivated to actively resist a change in their current opinion in order to maintain personal autonomy (Petty and Cacioppo, 1979a). Sometimes, however, when people want to change, they could be motivated to generate positive thoughts to the message. Similarly, if a person is put in a good mood when exposed to a message on an important topic, the good mood increases the likelihood of generating positive thoughts to the communication (Petty, Schumann, Richman, and Strathman, 1993). Thus, responses to a persuasive message are determined by both situational and personal factors that influence motivation or ability to think in ways that change the extent or direction of thinking.

Consequences of the Route to Persuasion

The route used to produce attitude change is critical, because central route attitude changes tend to have different consequences and properties than peripheral route attitude changes (Petty and Cacioppo, 1986). In general, attitudes that result from central route processes tend to be stronger than those from peripheral route processes. Strength refers not to the extremity of the attitude, but how consequential it is. As compared to weak attitudes, strong attitudes are more durable, because they persist over time and resist change when challenged by contrary information. In addition, strong attitudes guide thinking, and perhaps most important, strong attitudes guide behavior (Krosnick and Petty, 1995). As an example, consider an individual who engaged in thoughtful processing of a message on exercise resulting in a strong positive attitude toward engaging in exercise. Strong attitudes are more predictive of behavior, so thoughtful attitude change makes the initiation of exercise behavior more likely. In addition, because strong attitudes persist in memory, they are more likely to continue to influence behavior over time than weak attitudes. Furthermore, when a friend suggests forgoing exercise to "watch the game," the strong attitude will be resistant to change because it is based on more knowledge and held with greater confidence. It is also more likely to bias thinking in favor of the attitude, so the friend's statement may be reinterpreted as, "stay in and be a slob," increasing the likelihood of behavior maintenance. Thus, stronger attitudes produced through central route processes have a number of features that increase the chance of eliciting sustained behavioral change, as compared to attitudes changed the same amount by peripheral processes.

A number of studies provide evidence that attitudes resulting from more effortful thinking better predict behavioral intentions and guide actions than do attitudes resulting from little thinking. As one example, Brown (1974) assessed the attitudes of high school students toward various health-related behaviors such as using drugs, obeying traffic safety laws, and so forth. Students who reported giving the issues greater thought exhibited greater attitude-behavior consistency than those who reported giving the issues little thought.

Research on the "need for cognition" (a measure of the extent to which people engage in and enjoy thinking; Cacioppo and Petty, 1982), has also supported this proposition. For example, Cacioppo, Petty, Kao, and Rodriguez (1986) found that the attitudes toward presidential candidates of individuals who enjoy thinking were more predictive of their votes than the attitudes of individuals who did not enjoy thinking (see Cacioppo, Petty, Feinstein, and Jarvis, 1996, and Petty, Briñol, Loersch, and McCaslin, 2009, for reviews of work on need for cognition).

In these studies, existing attitudes based on high or low amounts of thought were examined. Other studies have created new attitudes by relatively thoughtful or non-thoughtful means and assessed how well the attitudes predict behavior. In one study, for example, (Sivacek and Crano, 1982; Experiment 2) undergraduate students were informed that their university was exploring the possibility of implementing senior comprehensive exams (an issue new to them), and they then read a message describing these exams. Then students reported their attitudes toward the proposal and were given the opportunity to sign petitions opposing the exams and to volunteer their services to a group that opposed the exams. The sample was divided into high and low relevance groups on the basis of the students' self-reports of whether the issue was high or low in perceived personal relevance (that is, would affect them or not). The high relevance group exhibited larger correlations between their attitudes toward senior comprehensive exams and their relevant behaviors (petition-signing/volunteering). That is, students for whom the message was more personally relevant demonstrated higher attitude-behavior consistency than students who considered the message less relevant. Based on the assumption that students in the high relevance group engaged in greater issue-relevant thought when forming their attitudes than students in the low relevance group (as would be expected based on numerous experiments (Petty and Cacioppo, 1990), this study supported the notion that more thoughtful attitudes are more predictive of behavior than less thoughtful attitudes. Other studies that have changed attitudes to a similar degree under conditions of high or low elaboration have also shown that more thoughtful attitude changes are more predictive of behavioral intentions and actions than are less thoughtful attitude changes (for example, Leippe and Elkin, 1987; Petty, Cacioppo, and Schumann, 1983). Thus, attitudes formed by the central route exhibit greater attitude-behavior consistency.

Research evidence also suggests that attitudes formed by the central route are more persistent over time and more resistant to counterpersuasive attempts than attitudes formed by the peripheral route. For example, in two studies (Haugtvedt and Petty, 1992) similar attitude changes were produced in individuals who differed in their need for cognition. In each study, college students were presented with a message containing strong arguments from a credible source, so there were two possible factors on which persuasion could be based. Both high and low need for cognition individuals became more favorable toward the position taken in the message, but what is critical is that they did so through different processes. Students who generally enjoy thinking changed based on a careful consideration of the high quality arguments. Low need for cognition students, who avoid thought, changed to the same extent, but because of the positive source cue. When attitudes toward the issue were examined just two days after the persuasive message, recipients low in need for cognition had returned to their initial positions, but high need for cognition students persisted in their new attitudes. In a second study, the students' new attitudes were challenged just a few minutes after they were created. Students with a high need for cognition resisted the message attacking their new attitudes to a greater extent than individuals with a low need for cognition.

Taken together, these results suggest that attitude change might have less enduring impact if it comes about through low rather than high amounts of issue-relevant thinking. Thus, although central route attitude changes are typically more difficult to produce than peripheral route changes, the benefits are considerable. A key contribution of the ELM is the proposition (and finding) that it is insufficient to know simply what a person's attitude is or how much change in attitude was produced. It is also important to know *how* the person's attitude was changed. Attitudes that are identical in valence can be quite different in terms of their underlying psychological antecedents (that is, how they were formed or changed) and consequences (for example, whether they predict behavior, see Petty, Haugtvedt, and Smith, 1995, for a review of persuasion and attitude strength research).

The difficulties of creating central route attitude change are familiar to health promotion researchers. For example, there are great challenges in engaging young adults in health-related topics like safe sex practices and substance abuse, simply because they often do not see them as personally relevant or important to their lives (Scott, 1996; Scott and Ambroson, 1994). Due to these challenges, it is tempting to suggest that use of peripheral cues and heuristics is the best way to create attitude change. However, as reviewed earlier, attitude change produced through peripheral route processes can represent an empty victory, since weak attitudes produce little in the way of tangible results. Instead, more needs to be done to understand what variables successfully engage the thoughtful processing of such messages in each population. One possible hybrid strategy is to use the peripheral route in combination with the central route. That is, one might make a health behavior (for example, using condoms) more acceptable to an unmotivated audience by the use of cues, and then when it is temporarily more desirable, more active processing techniques can be employed, such as getting people to justify their new attitudes in a role-playing exercise.

Before concluding our consideration of attitude strength, it is important to note that some recent research indicates that there may be a shortcut to strength by merely getting people to think that they have considered the issue thoughtfully in the absence of any real increases in thinking (Barden and Petty, 2008). In one study, for instance (Rucker, Petty, and Briñol, 2008), students were presented with one of two messages.

One message was a typical persuasive communication, which presented several arguments in favor of a proposal and one argument against it in a continuous stream. The second message was framed to make it more obvious that two sides of the issue were presented. That is, the pro arguments were organized in one column and the con argument was organized in another. Even though no new information appeared in the message that was simply framed as two-sided, and no additional thought was evident, participants perceived that they were more knowledgeable about the topic following this message. In addition, they were more confident in their opinions following this message. This recent research suggests that in addition to the likely structural benefits of increased thinking, such as greater attitude accessibility and attitude-belief consistency, there are also meta-cognitive benefits of thinking, such as perceptions of increased knowledge about an attitude issue and increased certainty in the validity of one's attitudes. Of most interest, these meta-cognitions can enhance the strength and impact of attitudes on their own (see Petty, Briñol, Tormala, and Wegener, 2007).

Multiple Roles of Variables in the ELM

We have seen that one critical aspect of the ELM is its identification of two routes to persuasion and the consequences of these routes. Another essential component of the ELM is that it allows for any one variable, such as the credibility of the message source, or the mood a person is in, to influence persuasion through different processes in different situations. The capacity of one variable to impact judgments through different processes explains how such simple variables as the credibility of the source or one's mood can produce complex outcomes. It also makes it essential to identify the conditions under which a variable influences attitudes by one process rather than another. We have hinted at the limited number of ways that variables can impact attitudes according to the ELM: by serving as a simple cue; by serving as an argument; and by affecting the amount or valence of one's thoughts. A final way in which variables can affect attitudes is by influencing the confidence people have in their thoughts. Thought confidence is important because it determines whether people will rely on the thoughts they have generated to form attitudes (Petty, Briñol, and Tormala, 2002).

Situations of low elaboration likelihood occur when people are unmotivated or unable to scrutinize the issue-relevant information presented. Under low elaboration conditions, then, persuasion-relevant variables such as a person's mood or the expertise of the source influence attitudes primarily through peripheral route processes. This is because people are either not motivated or not able to effortfully evaluate the merits of the information presented. Thus, if any evaluation is formed, it is likely to be the result of a relatively simple association or inference process that can occur without much cognitive effort (for example, "experts are correct"). For example, under low elaboration conditions, one's mood could serve as a simple cue either because the mood becomes associated with the advocated position through classical conditioning, or because people infer their attitude from their mood (for example, "I feel good, so I must like it," see Petty et al., 1993). Both of these peripheral processes assume that mood can influence attitudes without much issue-relevant thinking.

The ELM holds that under high elaboration conditions, however, people want to evaluate the merits of the arguments presented and they are able to do so. In these high elaboration situations, persuasion-relevant variables have relatively little impact by serving as simple cues. Instead the variable is scrutinized, like a message argument, and can result in attitude change if the variable provides information relevant to the merits of the attitude object (for example, an emotional factor such as how much you "love" someone is central to the merits of selecting a spouse and can serve as an argument in favor of marriage). Even variables not central to the merits of the object can influence attitudes under high processing conditions by biasing the direction of the thinking taking place. For example, people might be motivated to generate mostly favorable thoughts about the message if the source is credible (Chaiken and Maheswaran, 1994), or they might overestimate the likelihood that some good consequence mentioned in the message will happen if they are in a good mood (Wegener, Petty, and Klein, 1994). Finally, if thoughts are generated when people are in a good mood, or the source is expert, people might have more confidence in their thoughts than if the thoughts are generated when feeling bad (Briñol, Petty, and Barden, 2007) or are in response to an unknowledgeable source (Tormala, Briñol, and Petty, 2006). The more confidence one has in one's thoughts, the more these thoughts will impact attitudes.

In addition to the roles for variables when thinking is constrained to be high or low, variables can affect the amount of thinking itself when thinking is unconstrained by other variables. We previously noted that people are generally motivated to think more about messages of high rather than low personal relevance (Petty and Cacioppo, 1979b), and people are generally unable to carefully think about messages when distraction is high (Petty et al., 1976). But many other variables can influence the extent of thinking when the elaboration is not already constrained to be high or low. For example, the variables of source expertise and a person's mood can influence the extent of thinking in such situations. In these circumstances, people may be more motivated to pay attention to and to think about what an expert rather than a non-knowledgeable source advocates (Heesacker, Petty, and Cacioppo, 1983). Or, when in a happy mood, people will be more likely to think about a message that promises to be uplifting, but less likely to think about a message that promises to be depressing than individuals in a sad mood (Wegener, Petty, and Smith, 1995). This suggests that positive mood influences message processing, at least in part, due to mood management concerns (Isen and Simmonds, 1978; Wegener and Petty, 1996). That is, people in a positive mood tend to avoid message processing when they think it might attenuate their good feelings such as when the message is expected to be unpleasant (for example, on AIDS) or counter to one's own attitude, but they may engage in message processing when it will maintain or enhance their mood (see Wegener and Petty, 1996; Petty, Fabrigar, and Wegener, 2001, for a review of research on mood and persuasion).

Summary of the ELM

Figure 7.1 presents a schematic depiction of the ELM of persuasion and highlights the major features of the model. In the simplest sense, the ELM does three things.

FIGURE 7.1 *The Elaboration Likelihood Model of Persuasion*

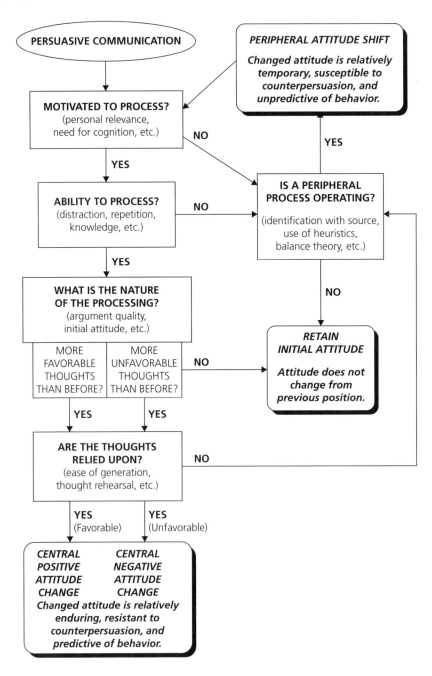

First, the ELM points to two routes to persuasion—a thoughtful and cognitively effortful route that occurs when the person is both motivated and able to think about the merits of the issue under consideration, and a less thoughtful route that occurs when motivation or ability are low. Second, the model points to consequences of these two routes. Thoughtful attitude changes are postulated to be more accessible to memory, confidently held, persistent over time, resistant to counterpersuasive attempts, and predictive of behavior. Third, the model specifies how variables have an impact on persuasion. That is, the model specifies certain roles that variables can play in the persuasion process. Variables can influence a person's motivation to think or one's ability to think. Variables can influence the valence of one's thoughts or the reliance on the thoughts generated. Finally, variables can serve as simple cues and change attitudes by one of several peripheral processes (for example, identification with the source, invocation of simple decision heuristics). With these features of the ELM in mind, we turn to the potential relevance of this model for health promotion.

USING THE ELM TO UNDERSTAND HEALTH COMMUNICATION EFFICACY

Over the past two decades, researchers in the area of health promotion have made use of the ELM to develop health promotion campaigns and interventions in areas including AIDS and condom use (Bakker, 1999; Carnaghi, Badinu, Castelli, Kiesner, and Bragantini, 2007; Dinoff and Kowalski, 1999; Helweg-Larsen and Collins, 1997; Igartua, Cheng, and Lopez, 2003; MacNair, Elliott, and Yoder, 1991; Mulvihill, 1996), exercise (Brock, Brannon, and Bridgwater, 1990; Jones, Sinclair, Rhodes, and Courneya, 2004; Rosen, 2000), dental flossing (Updegraff, Sherman, Luyster, and Mann, 2007), diet and nutrition counseling (Kerssens and van Yperen, 1996; Thompson, Baranowski, Cullen, and Baranowski, 2007; Wilson, 2007), substance abuse interventions (Scott, 1996; Scott and Ambroson, 1994), SARS education (Berry, Wharf-Higgins, and Naylor, 2007) smoking cessation (Quinlan and McCaul, 2000; Vidrine, Simmons, and Brandon, 2007), compliance in breast cancer screening (Drossaert, Boer, and Seydel, 1996; Holt, Lee, and Wright, 2008), maternal attitudes toward baby bottle tooth decay (Kanellis, Logan, and Jakobson, 1997), compliance with hospital infection control procedures (Bartzokas and Slade, 1991), prenatal care for low-income Mexican women (Alcalay, Ghee, and Scrimshaw, 1993), organ donor program participation (Skumanich and Kintsfather, 1996), and promoting road safety (Lewis, Watson, and White, 2008). Numerous dissertations pertaining to health promotion have also made use of the ELM in research related to phenomena such as promoting physical activity among middle school girls (Marks, 2004), preventing HIV/AIDS in a college-aged population (Spradlin, 2007), modifying patient requests for prescription drugs based on variations in the channel of communication (Lee, 2004), and changing smoking risk perceptions through tailored messages (Irvin, 2003).

As a general theory of information processing, the ELM has considerable utility for understanding the outcomes of different persuasive attempts on resulting attitudes and behaviors. Because attitudes are a primary determinant of behavior, especially when they are strong, producing attitude change can be a central focus of any health promotion program.

ELM Analysis of Message Tailoring

One area of health research in which the ELM has been fruitfully applied is in the domain of message tailoring. There is a large and growing literature on tailoring health communications. For example, one recent review found thirty empirical articles just on computer tailoring (Kroeze, Werkman, and Brug, 2006). Tailoring is generally defined as using any combination of information or attitude change strategy that is intended to reach one specific person based on characteristics that are unique to that person, related to the outcome of interest, and derived from an individual assessment (for example, see Kreuter, Farrell, Olevitch, and Brennan, 2000, p. 5). A related approach, often referred to as "targeting" involves aiming messages at particular groups of people based on identifiable characteristics (for example, race, gender). Although we focus our analysis on tailoring, the same principles are likely to apply to targeting.

Despite occasional contradictory results (for example, Quinlan and McCaul, 2000), the bulk of research has indicated that matching health messages to personal character-istics can increase the effectiveness of the messages in changing attitudes and behavior (see Kreuter et al., 2000; Kroeze et al., 2006 for reviews). Although tailoring strategies have generally been successful, little is known about *why* tailoring is an effective strat-egy. Moreover, little is known about what differentiates the situations in which tailoring will or will not be effective in generating short-term or long-term behavioral change.

In this final section, we use the ELM to examine some mechanisms by which message tailoring could work and provide illustrative examples.[1] In additional, we speculate about conditions that are likely to maximize the effectiveness of message tailoring as well as those in which tailoring might lead to null or even reversed effects.

Tailoring As just noted, tailoring typically refers to those instances in which the arguments contained in health communications are altered to match the particular concerns of the message recipient. For example, a pretest of Susie's concerns about condom use might indicate that she believes that they are awkward and inhibit plea-sure. Susie might be less concerned about the cost of condoms or about their efficacy in preventing pregnancy or disease. A message tailored to Susie, then, would address the social and physical issues associated with condom use while leaving out informa-tion about their efficacy or cost.

Tailoring procedures can be utilized to match not only the types of concerns an indi-vidual has about a particular health behavior, but also to the individual's stage of behav-ioral change. Stages of change models hold that there are a number of qualitatively distinct stages through which an individual must pass when adopting a health behavior (Prochaska, DiClemente, and Norcross, 1992; Weinstein, Rothman, and Sutton, 1998). For example, the transtheoretical model (Prochaska et al., 1992) suggests that individuals

---

[1]A complete review of message tailoring work is beyond the scope of this chapter.

pass through five distinct stages (precontemplation, contemplation, preparation, action, and maintenance) on the path to behavioral change, and that messages that match the individual's stage of change should be more effective in changing behavior. With some exceptions, the available literature generally indicates that this is the case.[2]

In theory, tailoring could include virtually any personal aspect of the individual. Although most tailoring approaches focus on the specific health concerns of the target of persuasion, tailoring could also include a variety of psychological variables (Salovey, 2005), such as self-efficacy (Brug, Steenhuis, Van Assema, and De Vries, 1996) attributional style (Strecher et al., 1994), or perceptions of time (Kreuter, Lukwago, Bucholtz, Clark, and Sanders-Thompson, 2003). When a message is tailored to a characteristic of a person that is shared with many others (for example, one's general personality traits, race, gender, or religion), tailoring is the same as targeting.

Matching Effects The finding that tailoring arguments to personal health concerns and other related characteristics can increase persuasion bears more than superficial similarity to findings in the persuasion literature showing that matching a persuasive message to various facets of the person can enhance the likelihood of attitude change. For example, matching a message to the functions of an individual's attitude can increase persuasion (for example, providing image-related arguments to a person concerned about social image; see Shavitt, 1989; Snyder and DeBono, 1985). Likewise, making an emotional appeal to a person whose attitude is based on emotion can be more effective than making a more rational or cognitive appeal (see Edwards, 1990; Priester, Wegener, Petty, and Fabrigar, 1999). Finally, matching a message to one's group identity can be effective (for example, framing the message as "for men" or "for women" for individuals highly identified with their gender; see Fleming and Petty, 2000; Mackie, Worth, and Asuncion, 1990).

As noted earlier, researchers in the health domain have drawn a distinction between *targeting* (matching the message to characteristics of a specified population), and *tailoring* (matching the message to a particular individual based upon an individual assessment; Kreuter, Bull, Clark, and Oswald, 1999). A third distinction that is sometimes made is *personalization*, in which a person's name is used in the message. Tailoring is the most specific of the "matching" approaches, in that many tailoring studies provide individuals with specific feedback about their personal risk and reasons for engaging in a particular behavior (Brug and de Vries, 1999). This information is not part of the simpler personalization and targeting approaches and likely contributes substantially to the success of tailoring procedures. Despite meaningful differences in the basis of the matching, we believe that the various matching approaches share important underlying conceptual similarities, namely, their common linkage to the self-characteristics of the respondent. Petty, Wheeler, and Bizer (2000) reviewed matching effects in a variety of social psychological research traditions,

---

[2] It should be noted that out aim here is not to assess the validity of stage models. As noted by Weinstein, Rothman, and Sutton (1998), the fact that personalization or tailoring can alter persuasion outcomes does not bear on the validity of stage models.

including attitude function matching, self-schema matching, group identity matching, and affect/cognition matching. Petty et al. (2000) noted that despite much diversity in the kinds of matching used, there was remarkable similarity in the outcomes observed, and this was attributed to the fact that each kind of matching established a link between the message or issue and some aspect of the self.

Matching Under Low Elaboration Conditions In line with the multiple roles postulate of the ELM, linking a message to some aspect of the self could influence persuasion in a number of different ways. Under low elaboration conditions, the match could act as a simple cue. That is, a person might think: "If it's for me (or relates to me or is similar to me), then I like it." This notion derives support from the numerous findings indicating that objects or ideas that are associated with the self are preferred to those that are not. Thus, individuals prefer products that they own to those that they do not, whether the products were chosen by the individual (for example, Brehm, 1956) or received as an unselected gift (for example, Kahneman, Knetsch, and Thaler, 1991). Individuals prefer arguments that they have generated to those that others have generated (for example, Greenwald and Albert, 1968) and even prefer the first letters in their own names to other letters of the alphabet (Nuttin, 1985). Given the typically high self-esteem that most individuals possess (see Taylor and Brown, 1988), it is not surprising that the self serves as a positive cue so frequently (an "own-ness" bias, Perloff and Brock, 1980). Some recent research even suggests that the transfer of positivity (or negativity) from the self to associated objects can occur automatically without one's awareness (Gawronski, Bodenhausen, and Becker, 2007).

Thus, under low elaboration conditions, matching a message to some aspect of the individual's self (for example, one's concerns, values, goals, groups, possessions, and so on) could act as a positive cue in the absence of much issue-relevant thinking. Although this cue strategy could be fruitful in the short run, as noted earlier, durable attitude change is more likely when a message is processed under high elaboration conditions. By engaging in active elaboration regarding the message topic, the individual forges more linkages between the new information and knowledge already stored in memory. Greater elaboration is therefore likely to render the resulting attitude more persistent, more resistant, and more likely to influence thought and behavior.

Matching Under Moderate Elaboration Conditions When baseline elaboration likelihood conditions are moderate (that is, motivation and ability factors are not constrained to be high or low), a persuasion variable can act to increase the amount of thinking that takes place. For example, we already noted that a variable that increases the perceived personal relevance of a message can increase the extent to which an individual thinks carefully about all of the issue-relevant information presented (Petty and Cacioppo, 1979b). Indeed, one of the most common findings in the social psychological literature on matching messages to the self is that such matching increases processing of the communication (for example, Petty and Wegener, 1998b; Updegraff et al., 2007; Wheeler, Petty, and Bizer, 2005). In line with this prediction, a number of studies in the health literature have provided evidence consistent with the idea that tailoring a message to the recipient can increase elaboration.

For example, Brug et al., (1996) found that tailored messages were perceived by recipients as more personally relevant and as written especially for them. Perhaps because of this increased perception of relevance, tailored messages are more likely to be read by the recipients, more likely to be attended to, and result in greater recall for the message content (Brug, et al., 1996; Brug, Glanz, Van Assema, Kok, and van Breukelm, 1998; Campbell et al., 1994; Heimendinger et al., 2005; Oenema, Tan, and Brug, 2005; Ruiter, Kessels, Jansma, and Brug, 2006; Skinner, Strecher, and Hospers, 1994; see Brug, Campbell, and Van Assema 1999; Skinner, Campbell, Rimer, Curry, and Prochaska, 1999, for reviews).

Tailoring Under High Elaboration Conditions Under high elaboration conditions, tailoring or matching a message to an individual could lead to biased message processing. For example, arguments that are tailored to address individual concerns (for example, about "cost") could be perceived to be stronger than those that are not so tailored (for example, about "social benefits"), even though there are no differences (or even a reverse difference) in actual argument quality. Consider, for example, that people may be more likely to fill in positive interpretations for matched than mismatched arguments. Alternately, tailored arguments could address health concerns about which the individual has a biased store of issue-relevant knowledge. This could lead to an ability bias even when the individual has an accuracy motivation. That is, the person's biased store of knowledge might enable the person to see the merits in some types of arguments more easily than other types. Finally, people might have more confidence in the thoughts that they generate to tailored rather than non-tailored messages, leading thoughts in response to those messages to have a greater impact on attitudes (see Cesario, Grant, and Higgins, 2004).

Illustrative Research on Tailoring

In a prototypical tailoring experiment, Oenema et al., (2005) collected an initial set of data on Dutch participants' fat, fruit, and vegetable intake, as well as a variety of demographic and general information (for example, height, weight, and so on). Participants were assigned to one of three conditions (tailored, generic, or control). Tailored message participants received a communication providing feedback about their food intake and its relationship to that of peers, as well as information about how to change or maintain eating habits depending on the person's current intake and motivation to change. Generic message participants received information stressing the importance of a diet low in fat and high in fruits and vegetables diet and information about how to change eating habits based upon common Dutch consumption patterns. Control participants did not receive any health information. Results indicated that the tailored message was perceived to be more personally relevant, more individualized, and newer than the generic nutrition information. Additionally, participants in the tailored information group spent more time with the information than did generic information participants. Most importantly, intention to change was greater among the tailored-message participants than those in either of the control groups. Mediation analyses indicated that these differential intentions were mediated by perceptions of personal relevance and by perceived individualization. The increased reading time suggests that the perceived relevance led recipients to engage in greater processing of the message and thus change in this instance probably occurred because of central route processing.

Although many studies within the health literature have tailored arguments to match the specific dimensions of concern the individual had expressed in that particular health domain, messages have also been matched on the basis of other, more general, characteristics. For example, Brock and colleagues (1990) conducted a study in which they tailored persuasive messages to match the self-schemas of the message recipients. To create the tailored messages, they first contacted a pool of over seven thousand former customers of a weight-loss company with a letter from the (fictitious) "Center for Personality Research." Using a card-sorting procedure and adjective-rating task, participants indicated their overall personality types. Brock et al. (1990) used these data to classify participants into one of four "schema sets" (for example, warm-communicative-compassionate). These same individuals were later sent a packet of materials from the weight-loss company. The materials included an insert that was tailored to either match or mismatch the schema set of the recipient and a business reply card that could be used to reactivate membership with the company. Control group participants received an insert designed to be neutral with regard to schema set. Results indicated that individuals who received an insert stringently matched to their schema set were over 12 percent more likely to return the business reply card than were individuals who received a mismatched insert. These results lend support to the hypothesis that tailoring messages to individuals' self-schemas can be an effective means of tailoring.

In addition, some work has shown that simply tailoring the message format to match some aspect of the recipient can increase persuasion. For example, Bakker (1999) reasoned that individuals who are high or low in their need for cognition (Cacioppo et al., 1982) would respond differently to messages presented in a way that made them appear easy or more difficult to process. As noted earlier, need for cognition is an individual difference variable that corresponds to a person's propensity to engage in and enjoy effortful cognitive activities (Cacioppo et al., 1982). In this experiment, high school students were exposed to one of two messages about AIDS and STDs. Although the messages contained essentially the same information, one message was presented in a concise, written format, whereas the other message was presented in a cartoon format. Bakker (1999) reasoned that low need for cognition individuals should be particularly motivated to think about the cartoon message because it would appear easier and more enjoyable to process. High need for cognition individuals, on the other hand, could be more motivated to process the written message because it would appear to be more interesting and important. He reasoned that the cartoon message could actually inhibit persuasion among high need for cognition participants by creating additional distraction or by leading to negative cognitive responses (for example, about the potentially "childish" or simplistic nature of the message format). Results indicated that participants in both the cartoon and written message conditions had significantly more knowledge about AIDS after reading the message than participants in a no-message control group. However, analyses on attitudes toward condom use indicated a main effect of message type as well as a significant need for cognition by message type interaction. The main effect indicated that individuals in both the cartoon and written message conditions showed more positive attitudes towards condom use than participants in the no-message control group. The interaction, however, indicated that low need for cognition individuals expressed more positive attitudes toward condom use after reading the cartoon message than the written message, and high need for cognition individuals indicated more positive attitudes toward condom use after reading the written message than the cartoon message. Thus, message format appears to be an additional type of tailoring or matching variable that can have a significant impact on health attitudes and behaviors.

Interpreting Tailoring Research

The examples of tailoring research just described demonstrate self-matching effects with three different types of manipulations. Oenema, et al. (2005) tailored their arguments to match the specific concerns of the message recipients (the most typical tailoring procedure); Brock et al. (1990) matched the arguments to aspects of the individuals' personality schemas; and Bakker (1999) matched the format of the message to the individuals' cognitive processing style. Though it is certainly possible to obtain similar findings for very different reasons, it is possible that each of these results shares an important underlying similarity. That is, each of the studies reviewed above matched an aspect of the persuasive message to a corresponding aspect of the message participant and may have therefore influenced persuasion as a result of the self-match.

Although each of the studies found increased persuasion under matched, rather than mismatched, conditions the precise mechanism responsible for each finding is not entirely clear. Recall that according to the ELM, a given variable like a message match can produce attitude change by different mechanisms, depending on the overall level of elaboration present in the persuasion context. Consequently, additional manipulations and measures are necessary to draw strong inferences about the processes operating in each experiment. The authors of the experiments just reviewed all favored the explanation that matching increased thinking about the message, and this idea has strong support in both the basic persuasion literature on matching (Fujita et al., 2008; Petty and Wegener, 1998b; Wheeler et al., 2005) as well as the health communication literature on tailoring (Brug, et al., 1999; Skinner et al., 1999; Updegraff et al., 2007). If one assumes that in the studies just reviewed the arguments presented were strong and that elaboration was not constrained at high or low levels by other variables, this explanation would be quite plausible and consistent with the ELM. However, other researchers have provided support for the idea that self-matching can have other effects besides increasing elaboration, such as biasing elaboration in a favorable direction (Cacioppo, et al., 1982; Lavine and Snyder, 1996), serving as a peripheral cue (DeBono 1987), or affecting thought confidence (Cesario et al., 2004). Thus, in the absence of empirical process indicators, multiple explanations for the findings previously presented are possible. For example, in the Bakker (1999) study, was a cartoon more effective than a written message for individuals low in need for cognition because the cartoon served as a simple positive cue, or because it motivated increased processing of the strong message arguments because of its apparent simplicity? Recent research suggests that simply describing a message as simple to understand is sufficient to increase the information processing activity of individuals low in need for cognition (See, Petty, and Evans, in press). Given that individuals low in need for cognition generally avoid thinking, it seems unlikely that the cartoon served in one of the roles reserved for high elaboration conditions, such as biasing the ongoing processing or affecting thought confidence. In any case, the multiple roles reviewed previously in this chapter provide examples of how the same effects could be obtained via different processes under different elaboration conditions. As noted earlier, the ELM holds that it is important to understanding the underlying processes of change because of the strength consequences that follow from the different processes.

Despite the strong support for greater perceived relevance of and attention to tailored messages, the underlying mechanism behind many tailoring studies remains ambiguous. For example, the greater perceived relevance and individualization in the Oenema et al. (2005) experiments could have led to more positive behavioral intentions for all of the reasons outlined above. Personal relevance and individualization could have served as a cue (for example, "This is for me, so I like it!"), as a motivator of greater elaboration, as a high-elaboration biasing agent, or as a magnifier of confidence in any favorable thoughts generated. Hence, measures of perceived relevance may not be sufficient to conclusively determine the underlying mechanism.

Other studies have provided more conclusive evidence for the proposed mechanism of greater elaboration. For example, Kreuter et al. (1999) found that participants generated more positive thoughts in response to tailored messages. Though not significant, results further suggested that the total number of thoughts generated in response to the message was highest among individuals who read the tailored messages. Thus, it seems plausible that, in the Kreuter et al. (1999) experiment, at least, tailoring increased message elaboration.

Similarly, Ruiter et al. (2006) used a subtle means to assess information processing. Specifically, they exposed participants to a tailored or nontailored message while they were simultaneously engaged in a secondary, tone-detection task. The task required them to listen to a series of high and low tones and push a button whenever they heard the (infrequent) high tone. A dependent variable in the study was a measurement of participants' P300 EEG responses, which are a pattern of brain activation associated with attending to infrequent or novel events. The authors reasoned that if greater allocation was devoted to the message (relative to the tone task), it should be reflected in smaller P300 responses. That is, if participants were paying more attention to the tailored message (and hence, less attention to the tone task), one should find smaller P300 responses to the infrequent high tones in the tailored versus the nontailored message conditions. This is what they observed. This type of measure has the added benefit of being an unobtrusive implicit measurement, rather than a self-reported one.

From the standpoint of understanding the processes responsible for self-matching effects, it would be very useful to include a manipulation of argument quality in future research designs.[3] Argument-quality manipulations can provide an additional source of information about the role of the variable by indicating the extent of elaboration (Petty and Cacioppo, 1986). That is, if a variable (like tailoring) increases persuasion equally when both strong and weak arguments are presented, and argument quality makes little difference, then tailoring is likely to be operating as a peripheral cue. If, on the other hand, tailoring increases sensitivity to differences in argument quality, then it may be increasing objective message elaboration. If such were the case, tailoring would increase persuasion when the message arguments were strong, but would decrease persuasion when the message arguments were weak. When an argument-quality main effect is found in conjunction with a main effect of the experimental variable, the variable may be biasing the already high levels of elaboration. Of course, to fully examine the multiple roles for message tailoring, it would be necessary to include a manipulation of tailoring and argument quality along with a manipulation of the extent of thinking.

It is also useful to assess ancillary measures such as the number and valence of thoughts generated and the confidence people have in their thoughts to help determine the underlying processes of persuasion. Additional measures of cognitive processing such as message recall, reading times, or self-reported effort can provide further information about the extent of elaboration, though they are imperfect when utilized in isolation.

Of course, using multiple manipulations and measurements can be difficult to achieve in practice. Field settings can often provide pragmatic limitations on the types of manipulations and measures that one is able to implement. More important, sometimes there would be ethical concerns associated with providing weak arguments for engaging in positive health behaviors. No doubt, this is likely one of the reasons for the limited use of argument quality manipulations in health communication research to date. However, argument-quality manipulations have been used in some experiments (for example, see Rosen, 2000; Updegraff et al., 2007), and when combined with a thorough debriefing including distribution of appropriate materials, argument quality effects can provide important insight into the functioning of variables like tailoring. More likely, treatments can be pilot tested in a controlled laboratory context in which strong and weak arguments are used in order to understand the mechanisms behind an effect (for example, is the variable operating as a cue or increasing thinking). Then, once the desired outcome is obtained, the treatment can be taken to the field where only strong arguments would be used.

---

[3]It might be argued that tailoring itself constitutes a manipulation of argument quality. However, the goal of most tailoring research is to uncover the dimensions of an object or issue that are important for a person (for example, price, social consequences, and so on). The information that is presented on these dimensions, however, can constitute strong (for example, "this treatment is less expensive than all others") or weak (for example, "this treatment costs just slightly more than all others") evidence in favor of the position advocated (see Petty and Wegener, 1998b).

IMPLICATIONS FOR PRACTITIONERS

This chapter has reviewed the theoretical underpinnings of the ELM of persuasion, along with some relevant empirical support. In addition, we provided examples of social psychological and health-related research examining the effects of message tailoring or self-matching, and discussed the possible mechanisms by which these effects occur. In concluding this chapter, we briefly provide suggestions for using the ELM to derive more effective health communications and persuasion interventions.

First, to effect durable and meaningful attitude change, practitioners should attempt to increase the elaboration of the message recipients—the extent to which people relate the ideas in the message to their prior knowledge and beliefs (Petty and Cacioppo, 1986). A common problem noted by researchers in the area of health communication is that recipients of health messages are often unmotivated to carefully process the materials they receive (Scott, 1996; Scott and Ambroson, 1994). This might lead some scholars to forward the suggestion that developers of health messages should put their energies toward injecting peripheral cues into their communications. Although, this could have a positive short-term impact, long-lasting attitude changes are unlikely to result from this strategy. Instead, procedures that increase the formation of highly elaborated, accessible, well-integrated, and confidently held attitudes will be more likely to result in actual and sustained behavioral change.

One means of inducing elaboration is by increasing the perceived personal relevance of the communication (Johnson and Eagly, 1989; Petty and Cacioppo, 1979b). As reviewed above, different kinds of message matching or tailoring could be effective in this regard (Kreuter et al., 1999; Petty, Wheeler, and Bizer, 2000), even for those who are prone to engaging in low-effort cognitive strategies (Bakker, 1999; Wheeler et al., 2005). Making individuals feel personally responsible or accountable for their own health outcomes could likewise increase attention to health-related communications (see Petty, Harkins, and Williams, 1980; Tetlock, 1983). Additionally, if individuals feel that their current health beliefs or practices place them in the minority, they may elaborate more on the message to resolve the surprise that can result from being discrepant from others (Baker and Petty, 1994). Other variables that have had an impact on message elaboration have been reviewed extensively elsewhere (see Petty and Wegener, 1998a; Petty, Wheeler, and Tormala, 2003), and could prove useful in health communication campaigns.

In addition to these motivational variables, ability variables can also affect message elaboration. Thinking about health communications should be higher when the communications are presented in a medium that permits self-pacing (for instance, by using written, rather than audio or video media; Chaiken and Eagly, 1976), in an environment without distractions (Petty, Wells, and Brock, 1976), and in language that is easily understood by the recipients (Hafer, Reynolds, and Obertynski, 1996). Because the language used to describe health conditions and treatments is often quite technical, this latter prescription may require pretesting on the recipient population to ensure that the language is not perceived to be too technical. Perceptions that the message is too technical can decrease elaboration by affecting perceived ability to process it, even though actual ability may be adequate for elaborative processing (see, for instance, Yalch and Elmore-Yalch, 1984). The educational background of the targets of many health communications could inhibit their ability to process verbal information, and such limitations should be taken into account.

High levels of elaboration will increase the impact of argument quality. Thus, the use of strong arguments is another important aspect of any health intervention. Argument strength can be determined by pretesting arguments on subsets of the target population. Particularly effective messages can be developed when the concerns of the target population are measured and arguments are developed to address each concern. More fine-grained procedures can be used to isolate subpopulations of the larger population that share similar concerns. For example, single individuals with multiple partners may be more interested in condom efficacy for preventing sexually transmitted diseases, whereas married individuals with a single partner may be more interested in condom efficacy for preventing pregnancy. Once developed, the tailored arguments can be pretested, not only to ensure that they are perceived as cogent by the target segments, but that they also elicit favorable thoughts rather than counterarguments. Adjustments can be made on the basis of such pretests before a more wide-scale distribution of the materials is undertaken. Argument tailoring can thus serve as one means of ensuring that each population receives arguments that are perceived to be relevant and are compelling (Kreuter et al., 2000). Recent technological advances have made tailoring procedures increasingly efficient and affordable. Of course, as we noted above, tailoring the message arguments is only one type of self-matching strategy that might be used effectively to increase message elaboration and effectiveness.

Last, assessment of the intervention's efficacy should be conducted, and adjustments should be made on the basis of the findings. An important element in such an assessment is a measure of the recipients' attitudes. As noted earlier, message learning can occur in the absence of attitude change (Helweg-Larsen and Collins, 1997; MacNair et al., 1991), and differing levels of attitude change can occur with equal increases in knowledge (Bakker, 1999). Also, since not all attitude change is the same, indicators of the strength of the changed attitude, such as the accessibility of the attitude or the confidence in the attitude, should also be assessed (Petty and Krosnick, 1995).

SUMMARY

This chapter has presented the ELM as a useful framework for interpreting and predicting the impact that health communications have on subsequent attitudes and behavior. The model proposes that attitudes can be formed as the result of different types of processes. Peripheral route processes are those that involve minimal cognitive effort and instead rely on superficial cues or heuristics as the primary bases for attitude change. Central route processes are those that involve effortful cognitive elaboration and rely on careful scrutiny of issue-relevant information and one's own cognitive responses as the primary bases for attitude change. Although each category of process can sometimes result in attitudes with similar valence, the two routes to change typically lead to attitudes with different consequences. High effort central route processes are more likely to lead to attitudes that are persistent over time, resistant to counterattack, and influential in guiding thought and behavior than are peripheral route processes. Because enduring attitude and behavioral change is likely to be a key goal of any health communication campaign, promoting attitude formation via central route processes is important. Consequently, using techniques that increase the perceived relevance of the communication and the quality of the arguments will promote achievement of a health promotion program's goals. A thorough understanding of these principles should result in more effective health communication campaigns thereby favorably influencing public health.

REFERENCES

Ajzen, I., and Fishbein, M. (2000). Attitudes and the attitude-behavior relation: Reasoned and automatic processes. In W. Stroebe and M. Hewstone (eds.), *European Review of Social Psychology* (Vol. 11, pp. 1–33). New York: Wiley.

Alcalay, R., Ghee, A., and Scrimshaw, S. (1993). Designing prenatal care messages for low-income Mexican women. *Public Health Reports*, 108 (May-June), 354–362.

Baker, S. M., and Petty, R. E. (1994). Majority and minority influence: Source position imbalance as a determinant of message scrutiny. *Journal of Personality and Social Psychology*, *67*(1), 5–19.

Bakker, A. B. (1999). Persuasive communication about AIDS prevention: Need for cognition determines the impact of message format. *AIDS Education and Prevention*, *11*(2), 150–162.

Bandura, A. (1986). *Social Foundations of Thought and Action*. Englewood Cliffs, NJ: Prentice-Hall.

Barden, J., and Petty, R. E. (2008). The mere perception of elaboration creates attitude certainty: Exploring the thoughtfulness heuristic. *Journal of Personality and Social Psychology*, *95*, 489–509.

Bartzokas, C., and Slade, P. (1991). Motivation to comply with infection control procedures. *Journal of Hospital Infection*, *18* Suppl A (June), 508–14.

Berry, T. R., Wharf-Higgins, J., and Naylor, P. J. (2007). SARS wars: An examination of the quantity and construction of health information in the news media. *Health Communication*, *21*, 35–44.

Brehm, J. W. (1956). Post-decision changes in the desirability of alternatives. *Journal of Abnormal and Social Psychology*, *52*, 384–389.

Briñol, P., Petty, R. E., and Barden, J. (2007). Happiness versus sadness as a determinant of thought confidence in persuasion: A self-validation analysis. *Journal of Personality and Social Psychology*, *93*, 711–727.

Briñol, P., Petty, R. E., and McCaslin, M. (2009). Changing attitudes on implicit versus explicit measures: What is the difference?. In R. E. Petty, R. H. Fazio, and P. Briñol (Eds.). *Attitudes: Insights from the new implicit measures* (pp. 285–326). New York: Psychology Press.

Brock, T. C., Brannon, L. A., and Bridgwater, C. (1990). Message effectiveness can be increased by matching appeals to recipients' self-schemas: Laboratory demonstrations and a national field experiment. In S. J. Agres and J. A. Edell (eds.), *Emotion in advertising: Theoretical and practical explorations*. (pp. 285–315). New York: Quorum Books.

Brown, D. W. (1974). Adolescent attitudes and lawful behavior. *Public Opinion Quarterly*, *38*(1), 98–106.

Brug, J., Campbell, M., and Van Assema, P. (1999). The application and impact of computer-generated personalized nutrition education: A review of the literature. *Patient Education and Counseling*, *36*(2), 145–156.

Brug, J., Glanz, K., Van Assema, P., Kok, G., and van Breukelen, G.J.P. (1998). The impact of computer-tailored feedback and iterative feedback on fat, fruit, and vegetable intake. *Health Education and Behavior*, *25*(4), 517–531.

Brug, J., Steenhaus, I., Van Assema, P., and de Vries, H. (1996). The impact of computer-tailored nutrition intervention. *Preventive Medicine*, *25*, 236–242.

Cacioppo, J. T., and Petty, R. E. (1979). Effects of message repetition and position on cognitive response, recall, and persuasion. *Journal of Personality and Social Psychology*, *37*, 97–109.

Cacioppo, J. T., and Petty, R. E. (1982). The need for cognition. *Journal of Personality and Social Psychology*, *42*, 116–131.

Cacioppo, J. T., Petty, R. E., Feinstein, J. A., and Jarvis, W.B.G. (1996). Dispositional differences in cognitive motivation: The life and times of individuals varying in need for cognition. *Psychological Bulletin*, *119*(2), 197–253.

Cacioppo, J. T., Petty, R. E., Kao, C. F., and Rodriguez, R. (1986). Central and peripheral routes to persuasion: An individual difference perspective. *Journal of Personality and Social Psychology*, *51*(5), 1032–1043.

Cacioppo, J. T., Petty, R. E., and Morris, K. J. (1983). Effects of need for cognition on message evaluation, recall, and persuasion. *Journal of Personality and Social Psychology*, *45*(4), 805–818.

Campbell, D. T., and Stanley, J. C. (1966). *Experimental and quasi-experimental designs for research*. Chicago: Rand McNally.

Campbell, M. K, DeVellis, B. M., Strecher, V. J., Ammerman, A. S., DeVillis, R. F., Sandler, R. S. (1994). Improving dietary behavior: The effectiveness of tailored messages in primary care. *American Journal of Public Health*, *84*(5), 783–787.

Carnaghi, A., Cadinu, M., Castelli, L., Kiesner, J., and Bragantini, C. (2007). The best way to tell you to use a condom: The interplay between message format and individuals' level of need for cognition. *AIDS Care*, *19*(3), 432–440.

Cesario, J., Grant, H., and Higgins, E. T. (2004). Regulatory fit and persuasion: Transfer from "feeling right." *Journal of Personality and Social Psychology*, *86*, 388–404.

Chaiken, S. (1987). The heuristic model of persuasion. In M. P. Zanna and J. M. Olson (eds.), *Social influence: The Ontario symposium, Vol. 5*. (pp. 3–39). Hillsdale, NJ: Erlbaum.

Chaiken, S., and Eagly, A. H. (1976). Communication modality as a determinant of message persuasiveness and message comprehensibility. *Journal of Personality and Social Psychology*, *34*(4), 605–614.

Chaiken, S., and Maheswaran, D. (1994). Heuristic processing can bias systematic processing: Effects of source credibility, argument ambiguity, and task importance on attitude judgment. *Journal of Personality and Social Psychology*, *66*(3), 460–473.

Dinoff, B. L., and Kowalski, R. M. (1999). Reducing AIDS risk behavior: The combined efficacy of protection motivation theory and the Elaboration Likelihood Model. *Journal of Social and Clinical Psychology*, *18*(2), 223–239.

DeBono, K.G. (1987). Investigating the social-adjustive and value-expressive functions of attitudes: Implications for persuasion processes. *Journal of Personality and Social Psychology*, *52*, 279–287.

de Vries, H., Brug, J. (1999). Computer-tailored interventions motivating people to adopt health promoting behaviors: Introduction to a new approach. *Patient Education and Counseling*, *36*, 2, 99–105.

Drossaert, C.H.C., Boer, H., and Seydel, E. R. (1996). Health education to improve repeat participation in the Dutch breast cancer screening program: Evaluation of a leaflet tailored to previous participants. *Patient Education and Counseling*, *28*(2), 121–131.

Eagly, A. H., and Chaiken, S. (1993). *The psychology of attitudes*. Fort Worth, TX: Harcourt Brace.

Edwards, K. (1990). The interplay of affect and cognition in attitude formation and change. *Journal of Personality and Social Psychology*, *59*(2), 202–216.

Fishbein, M., and Ajzen, I. (1975). *Belief, attitude, intention, and behavior: An introduction to theory and research*. Reading, MA: Addison-Wesley.

Fleming, M. A., and Petty, R. E. (2000). Identity and persuasion: An elaboration likelihood approach. In M. A. Hogg and D. J. Terry (eds.), *Attitudes, behavior, and social context: The role of norms and group membership* (pp. 171–199). Mahwah, NJ: Erlbaum.

Fujita, K., Tal, E., Chaiken, S., Trope, Y., and Liberman, N. (2008). Influencing attitudes toward near and distant objects. *Journal of Experimental Social Psychology*, 44, 562–572.

Gawronski, B., Bodenhausen, G. V., and Becker, A. P. (2007). I like it, because I like myself: Associative self-anchoring and post-decisional change of implicit evaluations. *Journal of Experimental Social Psychology, 43,* 221–232.

Goldstein, N. J., and Cialdini, R. B. (2007). Using social norms as a lever of social influence. In A. R. Pratkanis (ed.), *The science of social influence: Advances and future progress* (pp. 167–191). New York: Psychology Press.

Greenwald, A. G., and Albert, R. D. (1968). Acceptance and recall of improvised arguments. *Journal of Personality and Social Psychology, 8,* 31–34.

Hafer, C. L., Reynolds, K. L., and Obertynski, M. A. (1996). Message comprehensibility and persuasion: Effects of complex language in counterattitudinal appeals to laypeople. *Social Cognition, 14*(4), 317–337.

Haugtvedt, C. P., and Petty, R. E. (1992). Personality and persuasion: Need for cognition moderates the persistence and resistance of attitude changes. *Journal of Personality and Social Psychology, 63*(2), 308–319.

Heesacker, M., Petty, R. E., and Cacioppo, J. T. (1983). Field dependence and attitude change: Source credibility can alter persuasion by affecting message-relevant thinking. *Journal of Personality, 51*(4), 653–666.

Heimendinger, J., O'Neill, C., Marcus, A., Wolfe, P., Julesburg, K., Morra, M., Allen, A., Davis, S., Mowad, L., Perocchia, R., Ward, J., Strecher, V., Warnecke, R., Nowak, M., Graf, I., Fairclough, D., Bryant, L., and Lipkus, I. (2005). Multiple tailored messages are effective in increasing fruit and vegetable consumption among callers to the cancer information service. *Journal of Health Communication, 10*(18), Supplement 1, 65–82.

Helweg-Larsen, M., and Collins, B. E. (1997). A social psychological perspective on the role of knowledge about AIDS in AIDS prevention. *Current Directions in Psychological Science, 6*(2), 23–26.

Holt, C. L., Lee, C., and Wright, K. (2008). A spiritually based approach to breast cancer awareness: Cognitive response analysis of communication effectiveness. *Health Communication, 23,* 13–22.

Hovland, C. I., Janis, I. L., and Kelley, H. H. (1953). *Communication and persuasion.* New Haven, CT: Yale University Press.

Hovland, C. I., Lumsdaine, A. A., and Sheffield, F. D. (1949). *Experiments on mass communication.* Princeton, NJ: Princeton University Press.

Igartua, J. J., Cheng, L., and Lopes, O. (2003). To think or not to think: Two pathways towards persuasion by short films on AIDS prevention. *Journal of Health Communication, 8*(6), 513–528.

Institute of Medicine (Division of Health Promotion and Disease Prevention). (2000). Promoting health: Intervention strategies from social and behavioral research. In B. D. Smedley and S. L. Syme (eds), *Committee on capitalizing on social science and behavioral research to improve the public's health.* Washington, DC: National Academy Press.

Irvin, J. E. (2003) Construction of smoking-relevant health risk perceptions among college students: The influence of need for cognition and message content. *ProQuest Digital Dissertations database.* (Publication No. AAT 3151228).

Isen, A. M., and Simmonds, S. F. (1978). The effect of feeling good on a helping task that is incompatible with good mood. *Social Psychology, 41*(4), 346–349.

Janis, I. L., and Feshback, S. (1953). Effects of fear arousing communications. *Journal of Abnormal and Social Psychology, 48,* 78–92.

Johnson, B. T., and Eagly, A. H. (1989). Effects of involvement on persuasion: A meta-analysis. *Psychological Bulletin, 106*(2), 290–314.

Jones, L. W., Sinclair, R. C., Rhodes, R. E., and Courneya, K. S. (2004). Promoting exercise behaviour: An integration of persuasion theories and the theory of planned behavior. *British Journal of Health Psychology, 9*(4), 505–521.

Kahneman, D., Knetsch, J., and Thaler, R. (1991). The endowment effect, loss aversion, and status quo bias. *Journal of Economic Perspectives, 5,* 328–338.

Kanellis, M. J., Logan, L. L., and Jakobson, J. (1997). Changes in maternal attitudes toward baby bottle tooth decay. *Pediatric Dentistry, 19*(1), 57–60.

Kerssens, J. J., and van Yperen, E. M. (1996). Patient's evaluation of dietetic care: Testing a cognitive-attitude approach. *Patient Education and Counseling, 27*(3), 217–226.

Kreuter, M. W., Bull, F. C., Clark, E. M., and Oswald, D. L. (1999). Understanding how people process health information: A comparison of tailored and nontailored weight-loss materials. *Health Psychology*, *18*(5), 487–494.

Kreuter, M. W., Farrell, D., Olevitch, L., and Brennan, L. (2000). *Tailoring health messages: Customizing communication with computer technology*. Mahwah, NJ: Erlbaum.

Kreuter, M. W., Lukwago, S. N., Bucholtz, D. C., Clark, E. M., and Sanders-Thompson, V. (2003). Achieving cultural appropriateness in health promotion programs: Targeted and tailored approaches. *Health Education and Behavior*, *30*, 2, 133–146.

Kroeze, W., Werkman, A., and Brug, J. (2006). A systematic review of randomized trials on the effectiveness of computer-tailored education on physical activity and dietary behaviors. *Annals of Behavioral Medicine*, *31*(3), 205–223.

Krosnick, J. A., and Petty, R. E. (1995). Attitude strength: An overview. In R. E. Petty and J. A. Krosnick, et al. (eds.), *Attitude strength: Antecedents and consequences*. (pp. 1–24). Mahwah, NJ: Erlbaum.

Lavine, H., and Snyder, M. (1996). Cognitive processing and the functional matching effect in persuasion: The mediating role of subjective perceptions of message quality. *Journal of Experimental Social Psychology*, *32*, 580–604.

Lee, A. L. (2004) Effects of mass, interpersonal and hybrid communication on patients' requests for prescription drugs. *ProQuest Digital Dissertations database*. (Publication No. AAT 3140355).

Leippe, M. R., and Elkin, R. A. (1987). When motives clash: Issue involvement and response involvement as determinants of persuasion. *Journal of Personality and Social Psychology*, *52*(2), 269–278.

Lewis, I., Watson, B., and White, K. M. (2008). An examination of message-relevant affect in road safety messages. *Transportation Research Part F: Traffic Psychology and Behaviour*, *11*, 403–417.

Mackie, D. M., Worth, L. T., and Asuncion, A. G. (1990). Processing of persuasive in-group messages. *Journal of Personality and Social Psychology*, *58*, 812–822.

MacNair, R. R., Elliott, T. R., and Yoder, B. (1991). AIDS prevention groups as persuasive appeals: Effects on attitudes about precautionary behaviors among persons in substance abuse treatment. *Small Group Research*, *22*(3), 301–319.

Marks, J. T. (2004) A comparison of Web and print media for physical activity promotion among middle school girls. *ProQuest Digital Dissertations database*. (Publication No. AAT 3140366).

Mulvihill, C. (1996). AIDS education for college students: review and proposal for a research-based curriculum. *AIDS Education and Prevention*, *8* (Feb), 11–25.

Nuttin, J. M. (1985). Narcissism beyond Gestalt and awareness: The name letter effect. *European Journal of Social Psychology*, *15*(3), 353–361.

Oenema, A., Tan, F., and Brug, J. (2005). Short-term efficacy of a Web-based computer-tailored nutrition intervention: Main effects and mediators. *Annals of Behavioral Medicine*, *29*(1), 54–63.

Perloff, R. M., and Brock, T. C. (1980). And thinking makes it so: Cognitive responses to persuasion. In M. Roloff and G. Miller (eds.), *Persuasion: New directions in theory and research* (pp. 67–100). Beverly Hills, CA: Sage.

Petty, R. E. (1994). Two routes to persuasion: State of the art. In G. d'Ydewalle and P. Eelen (eds.), *International perspectives on psychological science, Vol. 2: The state of the art*. (pp. 229–247). Hillsdale, NJ: Erlbaum.

Petty, R.E., Baker, S., and Gleicher, F. (1991). Attitudes and drug abuse prevention: Implications of the Elaboration Likelihood Model of persuasion. In L. Donohew, H.E. Sypher and W.J. Bukoski (eds.), *Persuasive communication and drug abuse prevention* (pp. 71–90). Hillsdale, NJ: Erlbaum.

Petty, R. E., Briñol, P., Loersch, C., and McCaslin, M. J. (2009). The need for cognition. In M. R. Leary and R. H. Hoyle (Eds.), *Handbook of individual differences in social behavior* (pp. 318–329). New York: Guilford Press.

Petty, R. E., Briñol, P., and Tormala, Z. L. (2002). Thought confidence as a determinant of persuasion: The self-validation hypothesis. *Journal of Personality and Social Psychology*, *82*(5), 722–741.

Petty, R. E., Briñol, P., Tormala, Z. L., and Wegener, D. T. (2007). The role of meta-cognition in social judgment. In E. T. Higgins and A. W. Kruglanski (eds.), *Social psychology: Handbook of basic principles* (2nd ed.). New York: Gilford Press.

Petty, R. E., and Cacioppo, J. T. (1979a). Effects of forewarning of persuasive intent and involvement on cognitive responses and persuasion. *Personality and Social Psychology Bulletin, 5*(2), 173–176.

Petty, R. E., and Cacioppo, J. T. (1979b). Issue involvement can increase or decrease persuasion by enhancing message-relevant cognitive responses. *Journal of Personality and Social Psychology, 37*(10), 1915–1926.

Petty, R. E., and Cacioppo, J. T. (1981). *Attitudes and persuasion: Classic and contemporary approaches.* Dubuque, IA: W. C. Brown.

Petty, R. E., and Cacioppo, J. T. (1984). The effects of involvement on responses to argument quantity and quality: Central and peripheral routes to persuasion. *Journal of Personality and Social Psychology, 46*(1), 69–81.

Petty, R. E., and Cacioppo, J. T. (1986). The Elaboration Likelihood Model of persuasion. In L. Berkowitz (ed.), *Advances in experimental social psychology* (Vol. 19, pp. 123–205). New York: Academic Press.

Petty, R. E., and Cacioppo, J. T. (1990). Involvement and persuasion: Tradition versus integration. *Psychological Bulletin, 107*(3), 367–374.

Petty, R. E., Cacioppo, J. T., and Goldman, R. (1981). Personal involvement as a determinant of argument-based persuasion. *Journal of Personality and Social Psychology, 41*(5), 847–855.

Petty, R. E., Cacioppo, J. T., and Schumann, D. (1983). Central and peripheral routes to advertising effectiveness: The moderating role of involvement. *Journal of Consumer Research, 10*(2), 135–146.

Petty, R. E., Fabrigar, L. R., and Wegener, D. T., (2001). Emotional impact on attitudes and attitude change. In R. J. Davidson, H. H. Goldsmith, and K. R. Scherer (eds.), *Handbook of affective sciences.* Cambridge, UK: Cambridge University Press.

Petty, R. E., Fazio, R. H., and Briñol, P. (eds.). (2009). *Attitudes: Insights from the new implicit measures.* New York: Psychology Press.

Petty, R. E., Harkins, S. G., and Williams, K. D. (1980). The effects of group diffusion of cognitive effort on attitudes: An information-processing view. *Journal of Personality and Social Psychology, 38*(1), 81–92.

Petty, R. E., Haugtvedt, C. P., and Smith, S. M. (1995). Elaboration as a determinant of attitude strength: Creating attitudes that are persistent, resistant, and predictive of behavior. In R. E. Petty and J. A. Krosnick (eds.), *Attitude strength: Antecedents and consequences.* (pp. 93–130). Mahwah, NJ: Erlbaum.

Petty, R. E., and Krosnick, J. A. (eds.). (1995). *Attitude strength: Antecedents and consequences.* Mahwah, NJ.: Erlbaum.

Petty, R. E., Schumann, D. W., Richman, S. A., and Strathman, A. J. (1993). Positive mood and persuasion: Different roles for affect under high- and low-elaboration conditions. *Journal of Personality and Social Psychology, 64*(1), 5–20.

Petty, R. E., Tormala, Z. L., Briñol, P., and Jarvis, W.B.G. (2006). Implicit ambivalence from attitude change: An exploration of the PAST model. *Journal of Personality and Social Psychology, 90*, 21–41.

Petty, R. E., and Wegener, D. T. (1991). Thought systems, argument quality, and persuasion. In R.S.J. Wyer and T. K. Srull (eds.), *The content, structure, and operation of thought systems.* (pp. 147–161), Hillsdale, NJ: Erlbaum.

Petty, R. E., and Wegener, D. T. (1998a). Attitude change: Multiple roles for persuasion variables. In D. T. Gilbert, S. T. Fiske, and G. Lindzey (eds.), *The handbook of social psychology* (4th ed, Vol. 1, pp. 323–390). New York: McGraw-Hill.

Petty, R. E., and Wegener, D. T. (1998b). Matching versus mismatching attitude functions: Implications for scrutiny of persuasive messages. *Personality and Social Psychology Bulletin, 24*, 227–240.

Petty, R. E., Wells, G. L., and Brock, T. C. (1976). Distraction can enhance or reduce yielding to propaganda: Thought disruption versus effort justification. *Journal of Personality and Social Psychology, 34*(5), 874–884.

Petty, R. E., Wheeler, S. C., and Bizer, G. Y. (1999). Is there one persuasion process or more? Lumping versus splitting in attitude change theories. *Psychological Inquiry, 10*, 156–163.

Petty, R. E., Wheeler, S. C., and Bizer, G. Y. (2000). Attitude functions and persuasion: An elaboration likelihood approach to matched versus mismatched messages. In G. R. Maio and J. M. Olson (eds.), *Why we evaluate: Functions of attitudes.* (pp. 133–162). Mahwah, NJ: Erlbaum.

Petty, R. E., Wheeler, S. C., and Tormala, Z. L. (2003). Persuasion and attitude change. In T. Millon and M. J. Lerner (eds.), *Handbook of psychology: Volume 5: Personality and social psychology* (pp. 353–382). Hoboken, NJ: Wiley.

Priester, J., Wegener, D., Petty, R., and Fabrigar, L. (1999). Examining the psychological process underlying the sleeper effect: The elaboration likelihood model explanation. *Media Psychology*, *1*(1), 27–48.

Prochaska, J. O., DiClemente, C. C., and Norcross, J. C. (1992). In search of how people change: Applications to addictive behaviors. *American Psychologist*, *47*(9), 1102–1114.

Quinlan, K. B., and McCaul, K. D. (2000). Matched and mismatched interventions with young adult smokers: Testing a stage theory. *Health Psychology*, *19*(2), 165–171.

Rosen, C. S. (2000). Integrating stage and continuum models to explain processing of exercise messages and exercise initiation among sedentary college students. *Health Psychology*, *19*(2), 172–180.

Rothman, A. J. (2000). Toward a theory-based analysis of behavioral maintenance. *Health Psychology*, *19*(Suppl 1), 64–69.

Rothman, A. J., and Schwarz, N. (1998). Constructing perceptions of vulnerability: Personal relevance and the use of experiential information in health judgments. *Personality and Social Psychology Bulletin*, *24*, 1053–1064.

Rucker, D. D., Petty, R. E., and Briñol, P. (2008). What's in a frame anyway? A meta-cognitive analysis of the impact of one versus two sided message framing on attitude certainty. *Journal of Consumer Psychology*, *18*, 137–149.

Ruiter, R.A.C., Kessels, L.T.E., Jansma, B. M., and Brug, J. (2006). Increased attention for computer-tailored health communications: An event-related potential study. *Health Psychology*, *25*(3), 300–306.

Salovey, P., Bibace, R., Laird, J. D., Noller, K. L., and Valsiner, J. (2005). *Promoting prevention and detection: Psychologically tailoring and framing messages about health*. Westport, CT: Praeger.

Scott, C. G. (1996). Understanding attitude change in developing effective substance abuse prevention programs for adolescents. *School Counselor*, *43*(3), 187–195.

Scott, C. G., and Ambroson, D. L. (1994). The rocky road to change: Implications for substance abuse programs on college campuses. *Journal of American College Health*, *42*(6), 291–296.

See, Y.H.M., Petty, R. E., and Evans, L. M. (in press). The impact of perceived message complexity and need for cognition on information processing and attitudes. *Journal of Research in Personality*.

Shavitt, S. (1989). Operationalizing functional theories of attitude. In A. R. Pratkanis, S. J. Breckler, and A. G. Greenwald (eds.), *Attitude structure and function*, (pp. 311–338). Hillsdale, NJ: Erlbaum.

Sivacek, J., and Crano, W. D. (1982). Vested interest as a moderator of attitude-behavior consistency. *Journal of Personality and Social Psychology*, *43*(2), 210–221.

Skinner, C. S., Campbell, M. K., Rimer, B. K., Curry, S., and Prochaska, J. O. (1999). How effective is tailored print communication? *Annals of Behavioral Medicine*, *21*(4), 290–298.

Skinner, C. S., Strecher, V. J., and Hospers, H. J. (1994). Physician recommendations for mammography: Do tailored messages make a difference? *American Journal of Public Health*, *84*, 43–49.

Skumanich, S., and Kintsfather, D. (1996). Promoting the organ donor card: a causal model of persuasion effects. *Social Science and Medicine*, *43*(Aug), 401–408.

Snyder, M. and Debono, K. G. (1985). Appeals to image and claims about quality: Understanding the psychology of advertising. *Journal of Personality and Social Psychology*, *49*, 586–597.

Solomon, S. D. (2005). A new wave of behavior change intervention research. *Annals of Behavioral Medicine*, *29*, Special Supplement, 1–3.

Spradlin, K. (2007) Integration of the transtheoretical model of change and the elaboration likelihood model in approaching HIV/AIDS prevention. *Dissertation abstracts international: Section B: The sciences and engineering*, *68*(1-B), 672.

Staats, A. W., and Staats, C. (1958). Attitudes established by classical conditioning. *Journal of Abnormal and Social Psychology*, *67*, 159–167.

Strecher, V. J., Kreuter, M., Den Boer, D. J., and Kobrin, S. (1994). The effects of computer-tailored smoking cessation messages in family practice settings. *The Journal of Family Practice, 39*(3), 262–270.

Taylor, S. E., and Brown, J. D. (1988). Illusion and well-being: A social psychological perspective on mental health. *Psychological Bulletin, 103*, 193–210.

Tetlock, P. E. (1983). Accountability and the complexity of thought. *Journal of Personality and Social Psychology, 45*, 74–83.

Thompson, D., Baranowski, J, Cullen, K., and Baranowski, T. (2007). Development of a theory based internet program promoting maintenance of diet and physical activity change to 8 year old African American girls. *Computers and Education, 48*, 446–459.

Tormala, Z. L., Briñol, P., and Petty, R. E. (2006). When credibility attacks: The reverse impact of source credibility on persuasion. *Journal of Experimental Social Psychology, 42*, 684–691.

Triandis, H. C. (1980). Values, attitudes, and interpersonal behavior. In H. Howe and M. Pabe (eds.), *Nebraska symposium on motivation* (Vol. 27). Lincoln: University of Nebraska Press.

Updegraff, J. A., Sherman, J. K., Luyster, F. S., and Mann, T. L. (2007). The effects of message quality and congruency on perceptions of tailored health communications. *Journal of Experimental Social Psychology, 43*, 249–257.

Vidrine, J. I., Simmons, V. N., and Brandon, T. H. (2007). Construction of smoking-relevant risk perceptions among college students: The influence of need for cognition and message content. *Journal of Applied Social Psychology, 37*(1), 91–114.

Wegener, D. T., and Petty, R. E. (1996). Effects of mood on persuasion processes: Enhancing, reducing, and biasing scrutiny of attitude-relevant information. In L. L. Martin and A. Tesser (eds.), *Striving and feeling: Interactions among goals, affect, and self-regulation.* (pp. 329–362). Hillsdale, NJ: Erlbaum.

Wegener, D. T., Petty, R. E., and Klein, D. J. (1994). Effects of mood on high elaboration attitude change: The mediating role of likelihood judgments. *European Journal of Social Psychology, 24*(1), 25–43.

Wegener, D. T., Petty, R. E., and Smith, S. M. (1995). Positive mood can increase or decrease message scrutiny: The hedonic contingency view of mood and message processing. *Journal of Personality and Social Psychology, 69*(1), 5–15.

Weinstein, N. D., Rothman, A. J., and Sutton, S. R. (1998). Stage theories of health behavior: Conceptual and methodological issues. *Health Psychology, 17*, 290–299.

Wheeler, S. C., Petty, R. E., and Bizer, G. Y. (2005). Self-schema matching and attitude change: Situational and dispositional determinants of message elaboration. *Journal of Consumer Research, 31*, 787–797.

Wilson, B. J. (2007). Designing media messages about health and nutrition: What strategies are most effective? *Journal of Nutrition Education and Behavior, 39*, S13-S19.

Wood, W., and Neal, D. T. (2007). A new look at habits and the habit-goal interface. *Psychological Review, 114*(4), 843–863.

Yalch, R. F., and Elmore-Yalch, R. (1984). The effect of numbers on the route to persuasion. *Journal of Consumer Research, 11*(1), 522–527

8

AN INTEGRATIVE MODEL FOR BEHAVIORAL PREDICTION AND ITS APPLICATION TO HEALTH PROMOTION

Martin Fishbein

CHANGING BEHAVIORS EFFECTIVELY

How can we develop effective interventions to improve the public's health? As we all know, not all interventions are equally effective, and even worse, some may actually be counterproductive (see for example, Bushman and Stack, 1996; Hornik et al., in press). What behavioral science theory and research can do is provide guidelines for developing effective behavior change programs. Clearly, the more one knows about the factors that underlie the performance (or nonperformance) of any given behavior, the more likely it is that one can design a successful intervention to change or reinforce that behavior. By identifying a limited set of variables that account for a substantial proportion of the variance in any given behavior, the integrative model of behavioral prediction provides a framework for predicting, understanding, and changing any behavior (Fishbein, 2000; Institutes of Medicine, 2002; National Academy of Science, 2002).

The integrative model (IM) is the most recent formulation of the reasoned action approach to predicting and understanding human behavior. This approach, first introduced in 1967 (see Fishbein, 1967), underlies both the theory of reasoned action (Fishbein and Ajzen, 1975; Fishbein, 1980; Ajzen and Fishbein, 1980) and the theory of planned behavior (Ajzen, 1991). The IM was developed largely as a result of a 1991 National Institute of Mental Health workshop designed to identify similarities and differences among some of the major theories of behavioral prediction and change (see Fishbein et al., 2001). The IM clarifies how key variables from several theories can be viewed within a reasoned action framework. For example, the IM extends the theory of planned behavior by including descriptive as well as injunctive normative influences and by explicitly considering factors that may moderate the relationship between **intention** and behavior.

At the most basic level, a reasoned action approach to the explanation and prediction of social behavior assumes that people's behavior follows reasonably from their beliefs about performing that behavior. There are, however, some investigators who have questioned the basic assumption that human behavior can be described as reasoned. According to this critique, theories like reasoned action and planned behavior are too rational, failing to take into account emotions, compulsions, and other noncognitive or irrational determinants of human behavior (see for example, Armitage, Conner, and Norman, 1999; Gibbons, Gerrard, Blanton and Russell, 1998; Ingham, 1994; Morojele and Stephenson, 1994; Reyna and Farley, 2006; van der Pligt and de Vries, 1998). It must be recognized, however, that a reasoned action approach says nothing about rationality, nor does it deny the role of emotions. It merely assumes that once a set of beliefs is formed, these beliefs serve as the cognitive foundation from which attitudes, perceived social norms, perceptions of control, and ultimately intentions and behavior are assumed to follow (often automatically) in a reasonable and consistent fashion. These beliefs need not be veridical; they may be inaccurate, biased, or even irrational. Indeed, from our perspective, it is just as reasonable for a person to perform a given behavior because he or she believes that "my performing behavior X will stop the voices in my head" as it is for that person to behave because he or she believes that "my performing behavior X will reduce my chance of getting HIV" or that "my performing behavior X will please my parents" or that "my performing behavior X will make me feel proud of myself." Within a reasoned action approach, all of these beliefs are viewed as behavioral beliefs (or **outcome expectancies**) about personally performing the behavior in question, and, as we will see below, a person's **salient behavioral beliefs** about personally performing behavior X are assumed to contribute (often automatically) to the individual's attitude toward "My performing behavior X."

Although there are almost an infinite number of variables that may directly or indirectly influence the performance (or nonperformance) of any given behavior, the IM suggests that there are only a limited number of variables that need to be considered in order to predict, understand, change, or reinforce a given behavior. This limited set of variables is defined by, or represented in, four major theories of behavior and behavior change:

1. The Health Belief Model (Rosenstock, 1974; Becker 1974);
2. Social Cognitive Theory (Bandura, 1986, 1997);
3. The Theory of Reasoned Action (Fishbein and Ajzen, 1975; Ajzen and Fishbein, 1980); and
4. The Theory of Planned Behavior (Ajzen, 1991).

According to the original health belief model (see Rosenstock, 1974), one is unlikely to change behavior unless there is a good reason to do so. Thus, for a recommended behavior to be adopted one must feel personally susceptible to a severe and serious illness and one must believe that the benefits of following the recommended action outweigh the costs or other barriers to performance. For all practical purposes then, the original model identified two primary determinants of behavior: perceived risk (which is viewed as some function of perceived susceptibility and perceived severity) and behavioral beliefs, that is, beliefs about the consequences, the costs, and the benefits of performing the behavior in question.

Social cognitive theory (Bandura, 1986, 1997) also suggests two key determinants of behavior: behavioral beliefs and **self-efficacy**. According to this approach, one must be motivated to perform the behavior in question. That is, one must believe that performing the behavior will lead to more positive than negative outcomes. According to Bandura, these "**outcome expectancies**" may be physical (will protect me from AIDS), social (will please my spouse) or refer to self-standards (will make me feel guilty). In addition to being motivated, one must also believe that he or she has the necessary skills and abilities to perform the behavior and that performing the behavior is possible. That is, one must have a sense of personal agency or self-efficacy with respect to performing the behavior.

Although the health belief model and social cognitive theory linked their central constructs (that is, outcome expectancies, perceived risk, and self-efficacy) directly to behavior, the theory of reasoned action (Fishbein and Ajzen, 1975; Ajzen and Fishbein, 1980) assumed that behavior was primarily a function of a person's intention to perform the behavior and further, that the intention itself was a function of the person's attitude toward performing the behavior (that is, the extent to which the person felt positively or negatively about personally performing the behavior in question) and/or the person's subjective norm with respect to performing the behavior (that is, the extent to which the person perceived that their "important others" thought they should or should not perform the behavior). Moreover, the attitude toward performing a behavior is itself viewed as a function of the person's beliefs that performing the behavior will lead to various outcomes and the person's evaluation of those outcomes. To put this somewhat differently, in the theory of reasoned action, the behavioral beliefs (or outcome expectancies) of the HBM and SCT were viewed as determinants of attitudes that in turn served as potential determinants of intention and behavior. In a similar fashion, the subjective norm with respect to performing a behavior is viewed as a function of the person's beliefs that specific referent others think one should (or should not) perform the behavior and the person's general motivation to comply with those referents.

The theory of planned behavior (TPB, Ajzen, 1991) extended the TRA by adding the concept of perceived behavioral control as a predictor of both intention and behavior. It is important to note that, for all practical purposes, perceived behavioral control is essentially the same construct as Bandura's construct of self-efficacy. Ajzen (2005, p 118) has clearly stated that "perceived behavioral control" refers to "a sense of self-efficacy or ability to perform the behavior of interest." Indeed, there does not appear to be any real theoretical differences between perceived behavioral control and self-efficacy; both constructs refer to the belief (or perception) that one has the necessary skills and abilities to perform the behavior; that one can perform the behavior if one really wants to, even given various obstacles.

There does not appear to be any real theoretical differences between perceived behavioral control and self-efficacy.

In the TPB, behavior is viewed as a function of both intention and perceived behavioral control and intention is viewed as a function of attitude, subjective norm, and perceived behavioral control. Moreover, just as attitudes and subjective norms are based on underlying behavioral and **normative beliefs**, perceived behavioral control is viewed as a function of **control beliefs** (that is, beliefs that certain events or circumstances will be present when one performs the behavior) and perceived power (that is, the perception that those circumstances or events will make behavioral performance "easy" or "difficult.")

From the perspective of a reasoned action approach, these four theories suggest seven critical determinants of behavior:

1. intention
2. attitude
3. norms
4. self-efficacy/ perceived behavioral control
5. behavioral beliefs/cost-benefits/outcome expectancies
6. normative beliefs
7. control beliefs

Although it could be argued that there are at least three other important determinants of behavior that should be included on this list (perceived risk, mood and emotion, and knowledge), we will see below that according to the IM, these three variables, like many other important demographic and individual difference variables, are best seen as "background variables" that may or may not indirectly influence intentions and behavior.

DESCRIPTION OF THE INTEGRATIVE MODEL

According to the IM, intentions are the best predictors of whether one will or will not perform a given behavior. Empirical research over the past three decades has led to the recognition that specific behaviors can be predicted with considerable accuracy by appropriately assessing intentions to engage in the behaviors under consideration. Intentions can be conceptualized as a readiness to engage in a particular behavior. This readiness to act can find expression in such statements as: "I will engage in the behavior," "I intend to engage in the behavior," "I expect to engage in the behavior," "I am willing to engage in the behavior," "I will try to engage in the behavior," and so forth. In other words, as is the case for other psychological constructs, different indicators can be used to assess intention or readiness to perform a given behavior. Perhaps not surprisingly, some investigators have proposed that some of these expressions are better treated as distinct constructs rather than as indicators of a single construct, (see for example, Warshaw and Davis, 1985; Gibbons et al., 1998). This, however, is an empirical question and the evidence to date does not appear to support these distinctions. For example, most research on this issue has been devoted to a proposed distinction between behavioral intention and behavioral expectation or self-prediction. In this research, items such as "I intend to . . . ," "I will try to . . . ," and "I plan to . . ." are assumed to assess "intentions," while items such as "I expect to . . ." and "I will . . ." are assumed to assess "behavioral expectations" (Warshaw and Davis, 1985). It was hypothesized that behavioral expectations would be better predictors of behavior than behavioral intentions because the former are supposed to be more likely to take possible impediments to the performance of the behavior into account (Sheppard, Hartwick, and Warshaw, 1988; Warshaw and Davis, 1985).

Although the empirical data often indicate mean differences between items assessing "intentions" and items assessing "behavioral expectations," all of these items are highly correlated, and meta-analyses have failed to provide support for the superiority of behavioral expectation measures over measures of behavioral intention as predictors of behavior. For example, in a meta-analysis of studies concerned with the prediction of condom use, Sheeran and Orbell (1998) found no difference in the mean amount of variance accounted for by behavioral expectation (18 percent) and by behavioral intention (19 percent), and a meta-analysis of a much broader set of behaviors (Armitage and Conner, 2001) also found no difference in the predictive validity of "expectations" and "intentions."

Although there has been only a limited amount of research conducted on **willingness** to perform a behavior, the results again suggest that willingness, intention, and self-prediction are all indicants of the same underlying disposition. However, in their analysis of willingness, Gibbons, Gerrard, Blanton, and Russell (1998) proposed that unlike measures of intentions (or behavioral expectations), a measure of willingness is somehow capable of capturing nonintentional, reactive, and irrational influences on behavior. This is a somewhat strange claim given how "willingness" is measured. For example, in one of the first studies of "willingness," willingness to engage in unprotected sex was assessed by asking participants to "imagine being with their boyfriend or girlfriend who wanted to have sex but with no birth control available" and to *indicate how likely it was* that they would do each of the following: have sex but use withdrawal, not have sex, and have sex without any birth control. It is not at all clear why this measure of "willingness" (or more appropriately, the mean of three conditional intentions) would reflect the influence of nonintentional, nonrational factors. Indeed, it appears that people are perfectly capable of reporting how they are likely to react (that is, what they intend to do) in different hypothetical situations, and just as there is little empirical support for the distinction between intention and behavioral expectation, there is little evidence for a distinction between willingness and either of these intention measures. It is interesting to note that in some of their later studies, Gibbons, Gerrard, and their colleagues have either dropped the measure of "intention" (relying solely on "willingness" (see for example, Gerrard, Gibbons, Stock, Van de Lune, and Cleveland, 2005) or they have used a derived measure that combines willingness and behavioral expectation (see for example, Gibbons, Gerrard, Cleveland, Wills, and Brody, 2004). In sum, "intentions" refer to one's readiness to engage in a behavior and, like other psychological constructs, they can be assessed with multiple indicants.

In sum, "intentions" refer to one's readiness to engage in a behavior, and like other psychological constructs, they can be assessed with multiple indicants.

Many studies have substantiated the predictive validity of behavioral intentions. When appropriately measured, behavioral intentions account for an appreciable proportion of variance in actual behavior. Meta-analyses covering diverse behavioral domains have reported mean intention-behavior correlations ranging from a low of .45 to a high of .62 (Armitage and Conner, 2001; Notani, 1998; Shepherd, Hartwick, and Warshaw, 1988; Randall and Wolff, 1994; van den Putte, 1993). Studies in specific behavioral domains, such as condom use and exercise, have produced similar results, with intention-behavior correlations ranging from .44 to .56 (Albarracin, Johnson, Fishbein, and Muellerleile, 2001; Godin and Kok, 1996; Hausenblas, Carron, and Mack, 1997; Sheeran and Orbell, 1998). In a meta-analysis of these and other meta-analyses, Sheeran (2002) reported an overall correlation of .53 between intention and behavior.

The IM, however, recognizes that intentions do not always predict behaviors. That is, according to the IM, people may not perform a particular behavior, either because they have no intention of doing so, or because they intend to do so but are unable or unwilling to act on that intention. As can be seen in Figure 8.1 (which presents the integrative model of behavioral prediction), a lack of necessary skills or abilities or unanticipated barriers or environmental constraints may prevent people from carrying out their intention.

FIGURE 8.1   *The Integrative Model of Behavioral Prediction*

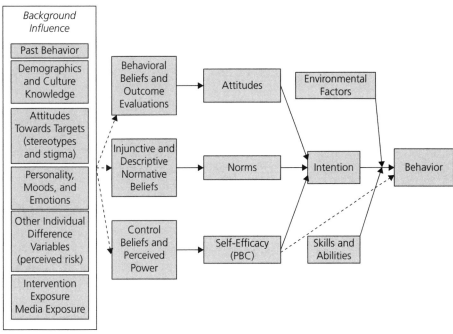

However, if people are not performing a behavior because they have little or no intention of doing so, the integrative model assumes that there are three primary determinants of intention: (1) the attitude toward performing the behavior in question; (2) normative influence or the amount of social pressure one feels vis-à-vis performing the behavior; and (3) one's sense of personal agency or self-efficacy with respect to performance of the behavior. Generally speaking, one's attitude toward performing the behavior in question reflects his or her overall feeling of favorableness or unfavorableness toward personally performing the behavior. The critical defining dimension of attitude is its bipolar evaluative nature; for example, "Do I like or dislike performing the behavior?" "Is my performing the behavior pleasant or unpleasant?" "Is my performing the behavior wise or foolish?"

The second major determinant of behavior is the perceived norm (or perceived normative pressure). A major addition to a reasoned action approach is the recognition that one's perception of the social norms or social pressure with respect to one's personally performing the behavior in question is based on descriptive as well as upon injunctive norms. That is, to fully understand perceived normative pressure, one must consider both the perception that "most people who are important to me" think I should or should not perform the behavior, and the perception that "most people like me" are or are not performing the behavior in question. We've probably all heard the expression, "do what I say, not what I do," yet both what is said (injunctive) and what is done (descriptive) are likely to shape one's perceptions of what is appropriate or acceptable behavior.

Finally, the third critical determinant of intention is one's sense of personal agency or self-efficacy with respect to performing the behavior in question. As described above, this sense of agency or self-efficacy refers to one's belief that one has the necessary skills and abilities to perform the behavior, even under a number of difficult circumstances. Self-efficacy is perhaps best represented by the belief that, "if I really wanted to, I could perform the behavior."

According to the IM, attitudes, perceived norms, and self-efficacy should account for a very substantial proportion of the variance in any intention. However, the relative importance of these three psychosocial variables as determinants of intention is expected to vary as a function of both the behavior and the population being considered. That is, there are some behaviors that are almost entirely driven by attitudinal considerations, whereas others may be primarily influenced by normative or efficacy considerations. Further, a behavior that is attitudinally driven in one culture or population may be normatively driven in another. In some instances, one or another of the three factors (attitude, norm, or self-efficacy) may not carry any significant weight in the prediction of intention. When this happens, it merely indicates that for the particular behavior and population under investigation, the factor in question is not an important consideration in the formation of intentions.

An important question to consider is, where do these attitudes, norms and feelings of self-efficacy come from? According to the IM (Figure 8.1), all three of these variables are themselves viewed as functions of underlying beliefs—about the outcomes of performing the behavior in question, about the normative proscriptions and/or behaviors of specific referents, and about specific barriers to, or facilitators of, behavioral performance. Thus, for example, the more one believes that performing the behavior in question will lead to "good" outcomes and prevent "bad" outcomes, the more favorable one's attitude will be toward performing the behavior. Algebraically this can be expressed as follows:

$$A_b = \Sigma b_i e_i$$

Where A_b = the attitude toward performing the behavior, b_i = the belief that performing the behavior will lead to outcome i, and e_i = the evaluation of outcome i.

Just as attitudes are based on behavioral beliefs, so too are perceptions of social pressure and self-efficacy based upon normative and control beliefs. That is, the more one believes that specific others are (or are not) performing the behavior in question and the more one believes that specific others think one should (or should not) perform the behavior, the more social pressure one will feel (or the stronger the perceived norm) with respect to performing (or not performing) the behavior. Similarly, the more one perceives that one can (that is, has the necessary skills and abilities) perform the behavior, even in the face of specific barriers or obstacles, the stronger will be one's sense of personal agency or perceived self-efficacy with respect to performing the behavior.

Each model is taken not as an accurate description of the way in which decisions are made, but rather as an ideal or normative model against which actual judgments and decisions can be compared.

Although one can algebraically express the relations between behavioral beliefs and attitude (for example, $A_b = \Sigma b_i e_i$) normative beliefs and perceived norms ($PNP = \Sigma nb_i$) and efficacy beliefs and self-efficacy (for example, $SE = \Sigma cb_i$), individuals are not expected to actually perform the mental calculations described by these models. Each model is taken not as an accurate description of the way in which decisions are made, but rather as an ideal or normative model against which actual judgments and decisions can be compared.

It is assumed that human decisions can be modeled as if a person were performing the specified calculations. Moreover, once an attitude, perceived norm, or perception of control has been formed, it is assumed to be accessible in memory and, as indicated above, depending upon the behavior in question, it may or may not have a directive influence on that behavior.

Figure 8.1 also shows the role played by more traditional demographic, personality, attitudinal, and other individual difference variables (such as perceived risk, moods, and emotions). According to the IM, these types of variables play primarily an indirect role in influencing behavior. For example, while men and women may hold different beliefs about performing some behaviors, they may hold very similar beliefs with respect to others. Similarly rich and poor, old and young, those from developing and developed countries, those who do and do not perceive they are at risk for a given illness, those with favorable and unfavorable attitudes toward family planning, or toward some religious or ethnic group, and so on, may hold different attitudinal, normative or control beliefs with respect to one behavior, but may hold similar beliefs with respect to another. Similarly, exposure to an intervention or a media campaign may or may not produce changes in an individual's beliefs. Thus, there is no necessary relation between these "external" or "background" variables and any given behavior.

Nevertheless, external variables such as cultural differences, moods, emotions, and differences in a wide range of values should be reflected in the belief structure underlying any given behavior. For example, it is well known that, in comparison to being in a bad mood, when one is in a good mood, one is more likely to believe that a given course of action will succeed and that "good things" will happen. Similarly if one is mad or angry, one is less likely to believe that "good things" will happen and, in addition, one is likely to have less positive or more negative evaluations of possible outcomes than someone who is happy or relaxed.

One advantage of a reasoned action approach is that it helps to explain why different background factors are related (or are not related) to a given behavior. For example, if men are found to be more likely to get colonoscopies than women, a reasoned action approach should be able to tell you why this is the case. That is, we should be able to identify the factors that are responsible for the different behaviors of men and women. For example, suppose both men and women had unfavorable attitudes toward getting a colonoscopy but felt considerable social pressure to do so. One possible explanation of the differential prevalence of this behavior in men and women could be that this behavior was driven primarily by normative considerations in men, but by attitudinal consideration in women. On the other hand, suppose that we found that while this behavior was primarily driven by attitudinal considerations in both men and women, men had more favorable attitudes toward "getting a colonoscopy" than did women. This would suggest that men and women had different behavioral beliefs about getting a colonoscopy. Further examination might reveal that while men believed that getting a colonoscopy could actually prevent colon cancer, women did not hold this belief. This would suggest that an appropriate intervention for women would be to address this belief.

To summarize, there are a number of background and cultural factors that may influence one's behavioral, normative and/or control beliefs about performing any given behavior. These beliefs (often automatically) lead to attitudes, perceived norms and feelings of self-efficacy, which, in turn, lead (again often automatically) to intentions and behavior.

Applying the Integrative Model

Next, it is important to consider how a reasoned action approach and the IM can help us to develop effective behavior change interventions. The first step in using a reasoned action approach is to clearly define (and describe) the behavior or behaviors in which you are interested. Unfortunately, this is not quite as easy as it may appear. First, it is important to recognize that there is a difference between specific behaviors (for example, walk for twenty minutes three times per week), behavioral categories (for example, exercise, diet), and behavioral goals or outcomes (for example, lose weight). Although the IM can predict and explain any intention (that is, to perform specific behaviors, to engage in a category of behavior, or to reach a specific goal), the prediction of a specific behavior from a behavioral intention is likely to be much more successful than is the prediction of engaging in a behavioral category or attaining a given outcome or goal. That is, it is much more likely that an intention will be highly correlated with whether one does or does not engage in a particular behavior than with whether one engages in a class of behaviors or attains a given goal. Thus whenever possible interventions should be directed at changing specific behaviors.

Second, one must recognize that the definition of a behavior involves four elements. More specifically, a behavior can be viewed as involving an *action* directed at a *target*, performed in a given *context*, at a certain point in *time*. Although the definition of action, target context and time is somewhat arbitrary, it is useful to clearly specify each element. For example, suppose that we ask a respondent whether she had a mammogram at the women's clinic in the past twelve months. Clearly, there are different ways of specifying this self-reported behavior:

Action	mammogram	Time
get	Context	in the past twelve months
Target	the women's clinic	

Alternatively, the behavior could have been defined as:

Action	get a mammogram

Target	(not specified)
Context	womens' clinic
Time	In the past twelve months

Note that one or more elements can be left unspecified. In addition, it is important to recognize that behaviors can be defined very specifically, for example, "Did you buy (action) Advil (target) at your local SavOn Drug store (context) between 5 and 7 PM on March 3 (time)?" Alternatively, behaviors can be defined in general terms, for example, "In the past six months (time), did you buy (action) a nonprescription pain reliever (target)?" The level of specificity of any given behavior should be determined by the nature of the problem one is investigating. Thus, sometimes one might be interested in understanding why women did or did not go to a specific venue for a mammogram during a particular time period, while on other occasions one may simply be trying to understand why some women did, while others did not, get a mammogram in the past year.

Irrespective of how one chooses to define a behavior, once that behavior has been defined, a reasoned action approach suggests that a change in any one of these elements changes the behavior under consideration. Thus, for example, from our perspective, getting a mammogram at the women's clinic is a different behavior than is getting a mammogram at University Hospital. That is, according to a reasoned action approach, one does not perform the same behavior in different contexts, but instead performs different behaviors. Similarly, using a condom with one's spouse is a very different behavior than is using a condom with a new or occasional partner, and using a condom for anal sex is a very different behavior than using a condom for vaginal sex. Equally important, smoking marijuana in the privacy of one's home is a different behavior than is smoking marijuana in public, and as we saw above, once a behavior is defined, a reasoned action approach suggests that the single best predictor of whether one will (or will not) perform the behavior in question is the person's intention to perform that behavior. However, for a measure of intention to accurately predict behavior, the intention measure must involve exactly the same four elements as the behavior itself. The requirement that measures of intention and behavior involve exactly the same action, target, context, and time elements is known as the principle of correspondence or compatibility (Ajzen, 1988; Ajzen and Fishbein, 1977). This does not mean that intentions and behaviors should be defined and measured at very specific levels; the principle simply suggests that the two variables, intention and behavior, should be measured at equivalent levels of generality or specificity. There is considerable evidence demonstrating that the greater the correspondence between measures of intention and behavior, the higher is the correlation between these two measures.

The requirement that measures of intention and behavior involve exactly the same action, target, context, and time elements is known as the principle of correspondence or compatibility.

Despite the fact that intentions are our best single predictors of whether one will or will not perform a given behavior, intentions do not always predict corresponding behaviors. Needless to say, very different interventions are necessary if one has formed an intention but is unable to act on it than if one has little or no intention of performing the behavior. In the former case, the intervention should be directed at skills training, at changing environmental factors. The latter may involve social engineering or teaching people how to avoid or get around such environmental barriers. However, if the problem is a lack of intention, then the intervention should be directed at developing or increasing intentions.

Unfortunately, when people are not performing behaviors we think they should perform, a typical reaction is to assume that people are not performing the "correct" behavior because they do not have enough knowledge to let them make the "correct" decision, or because they have the wrong attitude. Given this assumption, many interventions are designed to influence attitudes or to provide "appropriate" knowledge. Not surprisingly, more often than not, these interventions do not work. Clearly, if people already intend to perform the behavior in question but are not acting on those intentions, they are likely to already have enough knowledge and the "right" attitude, and thus it is unlikely that a knowledge-based intervention designed to change attitudes will be effective. The reason these people are not performing the behavior is either because they do not have the necessary skills and abilities or because there are internal or external barriers that are preventing them from acting on their intentions. In these cases, the appropriate intervention is not one designed to impart knowledge or to change attitudes, but one directed at skills-building or at helping people overcome or avoid barriers.

On the other hand, if people are not performing a behavior because they have little or no intention to do so, the problem is very different. As indicated earlier, according to a reasoned action approach, there are three primary determinants of intention: the attitude toward performing the behavior in question, normative influence or the amount of social pressure one feels vis-à-vis performing the behavior, and one's self-efficacy with respect to performing the behavior. The relative importance of these three psychosocial variables as determinants of intention will vary as a function of both the behavior and the population being considered.

Thus, before developing interventions to change intentions, it is important to first determine the degree to which that intention is under attitudinal, normative, or self-efficacy control in the population in question. It should be clear that very different interventions are needed for attitudinally controlled behaviors than for behaviors that are under normative influence or are strongly related to feelings of self-efficacy. Clearly, one size does not fit all, and interventions that are successful in one culture or population may be a complete failure in another.

Alternatively, if a behavior is primarily influenced by attitudinal, normative, or control considerations, how does one change these variables? As previously described and as can be seen in Figure 8.1, attitudes, perceived norms, and self-efficacy are all, themselves, functions of underlying beliefs—about the outcomes of performing the behavior in question, about the normative proscriptions and/or behaviors of specific referents, and about specific barriers to behavioral performance.

It is at the level of these underlying beliefs that the substantive uniqueness of each behavior becomes most evident. To put this somewhat differently, a change in any of the four elements defining the behavior is likely to have a large impact on the beliefs that need to be considered. For example, the barriers to using and/or the outcomes (or consequences) of using a condom for vaginal sex with one's spouse or main partner may be very different from those associated with using a condom for vaginal sex with a commercial sex worker or an occasional partner. Similarly, the beliefs about going to a women's clinic for a mammogram may be very different from beliefs about going to a university hospital or a private hospital, and the beliefs about taking an anti-depressant may be very different from beliefs about taking a diuretic.

Yet it is these behavioral, normative, and self-efficacy beliefs that must be addressed in an intervention if one wishes to change intentions and behavior. Although an investigator can sit in her or his office and develop measures of attitudes, perceived norms, and self-efficacy, she or he cannot tell you what a given population (or a given person) believes about performing a given behavior. Thus, one must go to members of that population to identify salient outcomes, referents, and barriers and facilitators. To put this somewhat differently, one must understand the behavior from the perspective of the population one is considering.

Using the Integrative Model to Design Interventions

In order to illustrate how the theory can be used to design interventions, consider a study that was designed to examine the role of attitudes, social pressure, and perceived self-efficacy as determinants of six different cancer-related behaviors (for a more complete description of this study, see Smith-McLallen and Fishbein, 2008). The items assessing the IM constructs were embedded within a larger survey regarding seeking and scanning for cancer-related information that took place between October 2005 and June 2006 (see Niederdeppe et al., 2007). Participants were 1,753 individuals (874 male, 879 female) ranging in age from forty to seventy years old, with an average age of 52.77 (SD = 8.42) from a nationally representative U.S. sample. With respect to race/ethnicity, 76.3 percent were white, non-Hispanic, 11.1 percent were black, non-Hispanic, 7.1 percent were Hispanic, 3.0 percent identified as more than two races, and 2.6 percent indicated "other."

Participants responded to a survey that contained questions assessing intentions, attitudes, perceived normative pressure, and self-efficacy regarding cancer screening and healthy lifestyle behaviors. Specifically, they responded to questions regarding getting a colonoscopy in the next year (or when it is next recommended), eating five or more servings of fruits and vegetables most days in the next year, dieting to control weight, and exercising at least three times in most weeks over the next year. Male participants also responded to questions regarding getting a PSA test for prostate cancer in the next year (or when it is next recommended), and female participants responded to additional questions about getting a mammogram in the next year (or when it is next recommended). Table 8.1 shows the variance accounted for and the standardized regression weights of attitudes, self-efficacy, and normative pressure as independent predictors of intentions to engage in each of the six behaviors.

Perhaps the first thing to notice is that the consideration of attitudes, normative pressure and perceived control significantly predicted intentions to engage in all six

TABLE 8.1 **Standardized Regression Weights and Variance Accounted for in Each of Six Cancer-Related Behaviors by Attitudes (ATT), Perceived Control (PBC), and Normative Pressure (NP).**

	Beta Weights and Variance Explained			
Behavior	ATT	PBC	NP	R2
Mammography	.244	.375	.289	.468
Colonoscopy	.242	.194	.458	.496
PSA test	.240	.224	.422	.496
Exercise	.343	.445	.079	.534
Eating f and v	.273	.260	.303	.441
Dieting	.338	.342	.245	.537

Note: All regression weights and R2 are significant.

behaviors, accounting for between 44 percent to 54 percent of the variance. But perhaps more important, and consistent with expectations, the relative importance of the three variables differed as a function of the behavior being considered. While all three variables contributed significantly to the prediction of most behaviors, it can be seen that normative pressure had very little influence on the intention to exercise. In marked contrast, normative pressure was, by far, the most important determinant of intentions to get a colonoscopy or to take a PSA test. What this suggests is that while an intervention designed to increase normative pressure to get a colonoscopy could be effective (for example, if it actually did increase normative pressure), an intervention designed to increase normative pressure to exercise (even if it successfully did increase perceived pressure to exercise) is unlikely to influence exercise behaviors.

As another example, suppose we were interested in reducing adolescents' intentions to engage in vaginal intercourse in the next twelve months. The data to be presented come from the first year of a three-year longitudinal study that is designed to investigate the impact of the media on adolescent sexual behavior. The sample is composed of 522 adolescents, 43 percent white and 41 percent black, 60 percent female, with equal numbers of fourteen-, fifteen-, and sixteen-year-olds. As part of the survey, respondents were asked to indicate their behavioral, normative, and self-efficacy beliefs about engaging in sexual intercourse in the next twelve months. These beliefs were identified through formative elicitation research conducted with a representative sample of the population prior to the development of the survey instrument. In addition, the survey instrument also assessed their intentions, attitudes, perceptions of normative pressure and self-efficacy with respect to this behavior. Consistent with the IM, attitude, norms, and perceived control explained 55 percent of the variance in the adolescents' intentions to have sex in the next twelve months. Perhaps more important from an intervention perspective, adolescents' intentions to engage in vaginal sex were primarily determined by attitudinal considerations. More specifically, the standardized regression weights for attitudes, norms and self-efficacy were .53, .22, and .07 respectively. This implies that the most effective intervention to reduce the likelihood that adolescents will engage in premarital sex in the next year would be one directed at decreasing adolescents' attitudes toward this behavior.

However, as indicated above, in order to do this it will be necessary to change adolescents' beliefs about the consequences of engaging in this behavior. But which beliefs should be changed? As described above, as part of a pilot study, the adolescents' salient beliefs about engaging in vaginal sex in the next twelve months were identified and were assessed in the survey. Consistent with an expectancy-value formulation, the sum of the b x e products ($\Sigma b_i e_i$) was correlated (.71) with the direct measure of attitude. This provides strong support for the notion that we were able to identify the beliefs underlying adolescents' attitudes toward engaging in sex. In order to develop an intervention, however, we need to know which of these beliefs distinguish between those who do and do not intend to engage in sex in the next twelve months. Table 8.2 shows the differences in behavioral beliefs between intenders and non-intenders, as well as the correlation between each belief and the intention to have sex.

It can be seen that each of the fourteen modal salient beliefs were significantly correlated with the intention to have sex with intenders significantly more likely than non-intenders to believe that "good" outcomes would occur, and that bad outcomes would not. Thus, if we want to reduce adolescents' intentions to have vaginal sex in the next twelve months, we can either increase beliefs that engaging in sex will lead to negative outcomes or decrease beliefs that engaging in sex will lead to positive outcomes. Note however, that this is not quite as simple as it sounds. If someone has had sex in the past, and believes that having sex will give them pleasure, please their partner, and increase their intimacy with their partner, it seems very unlikely that one will be able to develop an intervention to change these beliefs. Generally speaking, it will usually be difficult, if not impossible, to change beliefs that are based on direct experience. It may be possible, however, to craft an intervention that could successfully increase their beliefs that engaging in sex in the next year will lead to an increased risk of a sexually transmitted disease (STD) or pregnancy.

Generally speaking, interventions should address beliefs that are strongly and significantly related to the behavior in question, that is, beliefs that discriminate between those who do and do not intend to perform the behavior. In addition, as Hornik and Woolf (1999) have argued, you only want to address beliefs if a

TABLE 8.2 Differences in Behavioral Beliefs Between Intenders (n=155) and Non-Intenders (n=371).

	Do Not Intend	Intend	CCOR Relation with Intention
Give me pleasure	0.36	2.30**	.482**
Improve relationship	−0.70	0.99**	.441**
Please partner	1.05	2.17**	.335**
Increase intimacy with partner	0.47	1.64**	.302**
Gain friends respect	1.31	−1.02	.137*
Feel good about myself	0.98	0.39**	.381**
Give me an STD	0.79	−2.00**	−.321**
Give me HIV	0.98	−2.20**	−.318**
Hurt relationship with partner	0.81	−1.98**	−.318**
Make parents mad	1.55	0.59**	−.220**
Friends think badly	1.11	−2.25**	−.319**
Get pregnant	−0.92	−1.58**	−.143**
Lose virginity	1.80	−0.55**	−.434**
Be taken advantage of	1.00	−2.49**	−.404**

*p < .05 **p < .001
Scale ranges from −3 (extremely unlikely) to +3 (extremely likely).

substantial segment of the target population does not hold the "appropriate" belief. That is, you want to make sure that your intervention will change the beliefs of enough people to make a difference. Finally, and in some ways most important, you want to address beliefs that are "changeable." As Hornik and Woolf have suggested, you should be able to craft a convincing message—one supported by reasonable arguments and, if possible, hard data.

Although the IM can help to identify the critical behavioral, normative, or control beliefs that have to be addressed if one wishes to reinforce or change any given behavior, it is important to recognize that it does not tell us how to change those beliefs. Indeed, despite a large body of research on communication and persuasion, we know very little about the factors that influence why someone will accept or reject a given argument or piece of information. Thus it is critical that we very carefully test our interventions before we try to implement them in any population. If someone gave you a chemistry set, you wouldn't go down to your basement, mix a few chemicals together, declare you had a cure for AIDS, and then go out and start vaccinating people. Unfortunately, and all too often, people do sit around a table and come up with a behavioral intervention that they are ready and willing to implement. But just as one cannot "throw together" a vaccine, one cannot "throw together" an intervention. To begin with, an intervention should be based on sound empirical research pertaining to several questions: Who are the people failing to perform the behavior? Is the failure to perform the behavior due to a lack of intention, or to an inability to act on one's intention? If the latter, is the problem one of a lack of skills and abilities, or is it one of real or perceived environmental constraints? If the former, is the intention primarily a function of attitudes, perceived norms, self-efficacy, or some combination of these factors? What are the critical beliefs underlying the primary determinant? Finally, which of these beliefs should I address with my intervention? If you can answer these questions, you should be able to design an intervention that at least has a chance of being successful. However, even when carefully developed, one should never send a communication or intervene in some population without first carefully pretesting the message or the intervention. In essence, first determine whether the intervention will do what it's supposed to do or whether it will have some unanticipated effects.

In conclusion, let me suggest that we do know what we have to do in order to change a behavior. That is, we can identify the beliefs that would have to be changed or strengthened in order to change or reinforce a given behavior. In that sense, we really have come a long way in our understanding of why people behave the way they do. What we still need, however, are better theories of communication effects. In particular we need to understand the factors influencing whether a given piece of information will be accepted or rejected. I think this is the next major challenge for those of us who are interested in bringing about changes in behavior in order to improve the public's health.

SUMMARY

The integrative model (IM) is the most recent formulation of the reasoned action approach to predicting and understanding human behavior. A reasoned action approach assumes that people's behavior follows reasonably from their beliefs. Seven critical determinants of behaviors are: intention, attitude, norms, self-efficacy/perceived behavioral control, behavioral beliefs/cost-benefits/outcome expectancies, normative beliefs, and control beliefs. Attitude toward performing the behavior, normative influences, and one's sense of personal agency or self-efficacy with respect to performance of the behavior are the key aspects of the integrative model, and they each derive from underlying beliefs. In using the model to plan behavioral interventions, attention to target, action, context, and time is critically important. Further, different interventions are needed for attitudinally controlled behaviors compared to behaviors that are under normative influence or are strongly related to self-efficacy. Interventions should address beliefs that are strongly and significantly related to the behavior in question.

ACKNOWLEDGMENTS

This publication was made possible by NCI Grant 5P50CA095856–04 and NICHD Grant 5R01HD044136–05. Its contents are solely the responsibility of the author and do not necessarily represent the official views of NCI or NICHD. Much of the content of this chapter reproduces or is based upon previously published material (see for example, M. Fishbein, "A Reasoned Action Approach to Health Promotion," *Medical Decision Making* (in press).

REFERENCES

Ajzen, I. (1988). *Attitudes, personality, and behavior.* Chicago: Dorsey Press.

Ajzen, I., (1991). The theory of planned behavior; *Organizational Behavior and Human Decision Processes*, *50*, 179–211.

Ajzen, I., and Fishbein, M. (1977) Attitude behavior relations: A theoretical analysis and review of empirical research. *Psychological Bulletin*, *84*, 888–918.

Ajzen, I., and Fishbein, M. (1980). *Understanding attitudes and predicting social behavior.* Englewood Cliffs, NJ: Prentice Hall, pp. 278.

Albarracin, D., Johnson, B. T., Fishbein, M. and Muellerleile, P. A. (2001). Theories of reasoned action and planned behavior as models of condom use: A meta-analysis; *Psychological Bulletin*, *127*(1), 142–161.

A meta-analytic review. *British Journal of Social Psychology; 40*(4), 471–499.

Armitage, C. J., and Conner, M. (2001). Efficacy of the theory of planned behaviour: A meta-analytic review. *British Journal of Social Psychology*, *40*(4), 471–499.

Armitage, C. J., Connor, M., and Norman, P. (1999). Differential effects of mood on information processing: Evidence from the theories of reasoned action and planned behavior. *European Journal of Social Psychology*, *29*, 419–433.

Bandura, A. (1986). *Social foundations of thought and action: A social cognitive theory.* Englewood Cliffs, NJ: Prentice Hall.

Bandura, A. (1997). *Self-efficacy: The exercise of control.* New York: W H Freeman/Times Books/Henry Holt & Co.

Becker, M. H. (1974). The health belief model and personal health behavior. *Health Education Monographs*, *2*, 324–473.

Bushman, B. J., and Stack, A. D. (1996). Forbidden fruit vesus tainted fruit: Effects of warning labels on attraction to television violence. *Journal of Experimental Psychology: Applied*, *2*(3), 207–226.

Fishbein, M. (1967). Attitude and the prediction of behavior. In M. Fishbein (ed.), *Readings in attitude theory and measurement* (pp. 477–492). New York: Wiley.

Fishbein, M. (1980). A theory of reasoned action: Some applications and implications. In H. Howe and M. Page (Eds.), Nebraska symposium on motivation, 1979. Lincoln: University of Nebraska Press, 65–116.

Fishbein, M. (2000). The role of theory in HIV prevention. *AIDS Care, 12*(3), 273–278.

Fishbein, M., and Ajzen, I. (1975). *Belief, attitude, intention and behavior: An introduction to theory and research*. Reading, MA: Addison-Wesley.

Fishbein, M., Triandis, H. C., Kanfer, F. H., Becker, M. H., and Middlestadt, S. E. and Eichler, A. (2001). Factors influencing behavior and behavior change. In A.Baum, T.R. Revenson and J.E. Singer (eds.), *Handbook of health psychology*. NJ: Lawrence Erlbaum Associates, 3–17.

Gerrard, M. Gibbons, F. X. Stock, M. L., Vande Lune, L. S., Cleveland, M. J. (2005). Images of smokers and willingness to smoke among African American pre-adolescents: An application of the prototype/willingness model of adolescent health risk behavior to smoking initiation. *Journal of Pediatric Psychology. 30*(4), 305–318.

Gibbons, F. X., Gerrard, M., Blanton, H., and Russell, D. W. (1998). Reasoned action and social reaction. Willingness and intention as independent predictors of health risk. *Journal of Personality and Social Psychology*; 74(5), 1164–1180.

Gibbons, F. X., Gerrard, M., Cleveland, M. J., Wills, T. A., and Brody, G. (2004). Perceived discrimination and substance use in African American parents and their children: A panel study. *Journal of Personality and Social Psychology*; 86(4), 517–529.

Gibbons, F. X., Godin, G. and Kok, G. (1996). The theory of planned behavior: A review of its applications to health-related behaviors. *American Journal of Health Promotion, 11*, 87–98.

Hausenblas, H. A., Carron, A. V., and Mack, D. E., (1997). Application of the theories of reasoned action and planned behavior to exercise behavior: A meta-analysis. *Journal of Sport and Exercise Psychology, 19*, 36–51.

Hornik, R., Jacobsohn, L., Orwin, R., Plesse, A., and Kalton, G. (in press). Effects of the National Youth Anti-Drug Media Campaign on youth. *American Journal of Public Health.*

Hornik, R., and Woolf, K. D. (1999). Using cross-sectional surveys to plan message strategies. *Social Marketing Quarterly, 5*, 34–41.

Ingham, R. (1994). Some speculations on the concept of rationality. *Advances in Medical Sociology, 4*, 89–111.

IOM committee on communication for behavior change in the 21st century: Improving the health of diverse populations (2002). *Speaking of health: Assessing health communication strategies for diverse populations.* Washington, DC: National Academy Press.

Morojele, N. K., and Stephenson, G. M. (1994). Addictive behaviors: Predictors of abstinence intentions and expectations in the theory of planned behavior. In D. R. Rutter and L. Quine (eds.). *Social Psychology and Health*: European Perspectives. Aldershot, UK: Avebury/Ashgate, 47–70.

NAS Committee on the Youth Population and Military Recruitment (2002): Attitudes, aptitudes, and aspirations of American youth: Implicatons for military recruitment. Washington, DC: National Academy Press.

Niederdeppe, J., Hornik, R., Kelly, B., Frosch, D., Romantan, A., Stevens, R., Barg, F., Weiner, J., and Schwarz, S. (in press). Examining the dimensions of cancer-related information scanning and seeking behavior. *Health Communication, 22*(2), 153–167.

Notani, A. S. (1998). Moderators of perceived behavioral control's predictiveness in the theory of planned behavior: A meta-analysis. *Journal of Consumer Behavior, 7*(3), 247–271.

Randall, D. M., and Wolff, J. A. (1994). The time interval in the intention-behaviour relationship: Meta-analysis. *British Journal of Social Psychology, 33*(4), 405–418.

Reyna, V. F., and Farley, F. (2006). Risk and rationality in adolescent decision-making: Implications for theory, practice, and public policy. *Psychological Science in the Public Interest, 7*(1), 1–44.

Rosenstock, I. M. (1974). Historical origins of the health belief model. *Health Education Monographs, 2*, 328–335.

Sheeran, P. (2002). Intention-behavior relations: A conceptual and empirical review. In W. Stroebe and M. Hewstone (eds.), *European review of social psychology*, (Vol. 12, pp 1–36). Chicester, UK: Wiley.

Sheeran, P., and Orbell, S. (1998). Do intentions predict condom use? Meta-Analysis and examination of six moderator variables. *British Journal of Social Psychology*; *37*(2), 231–250.

Sheppard, B. H., Hartwick, J., and Washsaw, P. R. (1988). The theory of reasoned action: A meta-analysis of past research with recommendations for modifications and future research. *Journal of Consumer Research*; *15*(3), 325–343.

Smith-McLallen, A., and Fishbein, M. (2008). Predictors of intentions to perform six cancer-related behaviors: Roles for injunctive and descriptive norms. *Psychology, Health and Medicine*, *13*(4), 389–401.

van den Putte, B. (1993). On the theory of reasoned action. Unpublished doctoral dissertation. University of Amsterdam, The Netherlands.

van der Pligt, J., and de Vries, N. K. (1998). Expectancy-value models of health behavior: The role of salience and anticipated regret. *Psychology and Health*, *13*, 289–305.

Warshaw, P. R., and Davis, F. D. (1985). Disentangling behavioral intention and behavioral expectation. Journal of Experimental Social Psychology; 21(3), 213–228.

PART

2

COMMUNITY-BASED APPROACHES

CHAPTER

9

THE COMMUNITY COALITION ACTION THEORY

Frances D. Butterfoss
Michelle C. Kegler

COMMUNITY COALITIONS AND PUBLIC HEALTH

Communities, organizations, businesses, and even nations today form alliances, joint ventures, and public-private partnerships. One type of strategic relationship, a coalition, develops when different sectors of the community, state, or nation join together to create opportunities that will benefit all of the partners. Community coalitions are a specific type of coalition defined as a group of individuals representing diverse organizations, factions, or constituencies *within the community* who agree to work together to achieve a common goal (Feighery and Rogers, 1990).

The development of coalitions escalated rapidly over the past twenty-five years. Thousands of coalitions anchored by government or community-based organizations formed to support community-based, health-related activities across the United States. For example, coalitions of health-related agencies, schools, and community-based action groups have formed to prevent tobacco use and promote healthy weight and physical activity among youth. Advocates for environmental issues such as asthma and lead contamination have rallied to highlight their issue or enable favorable policy and legislation. Civic and faith-based groups developed coalitions to ensure adequate housing for the elderly and health insurance for low-income populations. The best of these coalitions have been vehicles to bring people together, expand available resources, focus on a problem of community concern, and achieve better results than any single group or agency could have achieved alone.

Coalitions, however, are not a panacea. Although coalitions are usually built from unselfish motives to improve communities, they still may experience difficulties that are common to many types of organizations, as well as some that are unique to collaborative efforts (Dowling, O'Donnell, and Wellington Consulting Group, Ltd., 2000; Wolff, 2001). With the initiation of a coalition, frustrations can arise. Promised resources may not be made available; conflicting interests may prevent the coalition from having its desired effect in the community; and recognition for accomplishments may be slow in coming. Because coalition building involves a long-term investment of time and resources, a coalition should not be established if a simpler, less complex structure will get the job done or if the community does not embrace this approach.

The premise of this chapter is that public health professionals have eagerly embraced the practice of coalitionbuilding. They have looked for an effective, inclusive approach to complex health issues, and coalitions fit the bill. Coalitions are now commonplace in community based efforts to improve health. With the development of the community coalition action theory (CCAT), we have committed ourselves to step back from the widespread *practice* of building coalitions, and continue to forge and refine a comprehensive *theory* of community coalitions. We believe that this theory, complete with constructs and propositions, will lead to an increased understanding of how community coalitions work in practice.

Origins and/or Roots of the Theory

The underlying theoretical basis for the development and maintenance of community coalitions borrows from many arenas, including community development, citizen participation, political science, interorganizational relations, and group process. Community development and related approaches such as community organization, community empowerment, and citizen participation, provide much of the philosophy that underlies community coalition approaches. Coined by the United Nations in 1955, community development was designed to create conditions of economic and social progress for the whole community, with its active participation and the fullest possible reliance on the community's initiative. (Brager, Sprecht, and Torczyner, 1987). This approach is based on several assumptions, namely that: (1) communities can develop capacity to deal with their own problems; (2) people should participate in making, adjusting, or controlling the major changes taking place in their communities; and (3) changes in community living that are self-imposed or self-developed have a meaning and permanence that changes imposed from outside do not have. Additional assumptions underlying community approaches to problem solving are that: (1) holistic approaches can deal successfully with problems where fragmented approaches cannot; (2) democracy requires cooperative participation and action in the affairs of the community; and (3) people must learn the skills that make this possible.

In a similar vein, *community participation* is the process of involving people in the institutions or decisions that affect their lives (Checkoway, 1989). *Citizen participation* is the mobilization of citizens for the purpose of undertaking activities to improve conditions in the community. Much of the initial coalition research in the 1990s was based on two significant research efforts in the area of citizen participation. The Neighborhood Participation Project examined the process of citizen participation through a systematic study of block organizations in a Nashville neighborhood (Florin and Wandersman, 1990; Prestby, Wandersman, et al., 1990; Prestby and Wandersman, 1985; Giamartino and Wandersman, 1983). Researchers posed questions similar to those posed in coalition research: who participates, who doesn't, and why? What are the effects of citizen participation in block organizations? What are the characteristics of organizations that are active and successful versus those that are inactive (Florin and Wandersman, 1990)? Research questions asked in the Block Booster Project in New York City also helped shape the coalition research agenda (Perkins, Florin, Rich, Wandersman, and Chavis, 1990). Community-based coalitions differ from block organizations, however. Although some coalition members can be characterized as "interested citizens" (or volunteers), many of the members represent organizations. Thus, research and conceptual work done in the field of interorganizational relations also is relevant to coalition theory. Much of the early research on interorganizational relations focused on the formation of collaborative relationships in an effort to

> Community development and related approaches such as community organization, community empowerment, and citizen participation, provide much of the philosophy that underlies community coalition approaches. Coined by the United Nations in 1955, community development was designed to create conditions of economic and social progress for the whole community, with its active participation and the fullest possible reliance on the community's initiative.

understand why organizations join collaborative alliances (Gray and Wood, 1991; Berlin, Barnett, Mischke, and Ocasio, 2000; Provan and Milward, 1995).

Gray and Wood (1991) discuss several theoretical perspectives that help to inform interorganizational collaboration. For example, resource dependence theory posits that acquiring resources and reducing uncertainty are the primary forces underlying collaboration (Sharfman et al., 1991; Mizruchi and Galaskiewicz, 1994). Institutional theory suggests that organizations adjust to institutional directives and norms in an attempt to achieve legitimacy (Gray and Wood, 1991; Gulati, 1995). Political science emphasizes the negotiation of potential conflict through coalitions and power distribution within coalitions (Bazzoli et al., 1997).

Each of these perspectives sheds insight into the formation of community coalitions. For example, community coalitions often form in response to an opportunity, such as new funding, exemplified by the tobacco settlement funds made available for coalition building around tobacco control and prevention. They may form because of a threat such as a national story about rising asthma prevalence, or a local event such as an outbreak of meningitis on a college campus. Local health organizations may voluntarily form or join coalitions to augment their limited resources of staff, time, talent, equipment, supplies, materials, contacts, and influence. Joining with other agencies and individuals can benefit an organization, giving it expanded access to printing and postage services, media coverage, marketing services, meeting space, community residents, influential people, personnel, community and professional networks, and expertise (Whitt, 1993). Additionally, coalitions may be mandatory or required by a funding source, such as the Robert Wood Johnson Allies Against Asthma initiative, or the Centers for Disease Control and Prevention's (CDC) Community Coalition Partnership for the Prevention of Teen Pregnancy (Cassell et al., 2005).

Another major contribution of the field of interorganizational relations to coalition theory is the fact that organizations decide to join collaborative relationships when the benefits outweigh the costs (Gray, 1989; Prestby et al., 1990; Roberts-DeGennaro, 1986, 1987; Whetten, 1981). Ultimately, collaboration is possible when a perceived need exists and an organization anticipates deriving a benefit that is contingent on mutual action (Wood and Gray, 1991). Coalitions offer such benefits by serving as effective and efficient vehicles for the exchange of knowledge, ideas, and strategies. Through coalitions, individuals and organizations can become involved in new, broader issues without assuming sole responsibility. Coalitions can also demonstrate and develop community support or concern for issues, maximize the power of individuals and groups through collective action, improve trust and communication among community agencies and sectors, mobilize diverse talents, resources, and strategies, build strength and cohesiveness by connecting individual activists, build a constituency for a given issue, reduce the social acceptability of health risk behaviors, and change community norms and standards (Whitt, 1993). Additional benefits include: the potential to minimize duplication and use resources efficiently; the opportunity to gain access to new information, ideas, materials, and other resources; the opportunity to reduce uncertainty in the environment; and the sharing of costs and associated risks (Alter and Hage, 1993; Gray, 1989; Whetten, 1981; Zapka et al., 1992; Wandersman and Alderman, 1993; Butterfoss, Goodman, and Wandersman, 1993; Penner, 1995).

The costs associated with coalition membership may include: loss of autonomy and the ability to unilaterally control outcomes, conflict over goals and methods, loss of resources (time, money, information, and status), risk of losing competitive position, and possible delays in solving problems (Alter and Hage, 1993). Community coalitions that survive over time must provide ongoing benefits that outweigh the costs of membership.

The field of interorganizational relations also contributes to our understanding of the stages of collaboration. Gray (1989), for example, proposes three stages: *problem setting, direction setting*, and *implementation*. Similarly, Alter and Hage (1993) suggest a model of network development, with networks evolving from exchange networks through action networks to fully developed systemic networks. According to their model, action networks result when organizations can no longer meet a goal alone due to environmental conditions. A network shifts from an exchange to an action network when members: (1) contribute private resources for access to collective output, (2) depend on the collective output, and (3) feel a normative obligation to comply with the coordinating mechanism. An action network shifts to a *systemic* network when it begins to produce together, with specialized roles.

Although clear and definite theoretical underpinnings exist for community coalitions, the practice of coalition building has outpaced the development of coalition theory. Practically speaking, the rise of coalitions as a prominent health promotion strategy parallels the growth of community-wide health promotion over the past several decades. This growth is partially due to the widespread dissemination of strategies employed in the National Heart, Lung and Blood Institutes' community demonstration projects (Mittelmark, 1999). These projects, which include the Stanford Three Community and Five City Projects, and the Minnesota and Pawtucket Heart Health Programs, used community advisory boards to plan and implement community-wide cardiovascular disease prevention strategies (Shea and Basch, 1990; Carlaw, Mittelmark, Bracht, and Luepker, 1984; Mittelmark, Luepker, Jacobs et al., 1986; Lefebvre, Lasater, Carleton, and Peterson, 1987; Farquhar, Fortmann, Flora, et al., 1990). Additionally, the Centers for Disease Control and Prevention (CDC) advocated forming community coalitions in the Planned Approach to Community Health (PATCH) which was widely adopted by state and local health departments in the late 1980s and early 1990s (Kreuter, 1992; Green and Kreuter, 1992). Major tobacco initiatives also required coalitions, including ASSIST and Smokeless States, as did CSAP's community partnership and community coalition programs (Yin et al., 1997; Crowley, Yu, and Kaftarian, 2000; Moon et al., 2005).

In contrast to traditional behavior change efforts focused on the individual, community approaches—including those that build coalitions—attempt to alleviate community problems by organizing the community to bring about change. These community-wide approaches recognize that behaviors are inextricably tied to the environment (Milio, 1989; Thompson and Kinne, 1990; Stokols, 1992; Tesh, 1988). In theory, no single approach for community change is as effective as a broad-based coalition effort that provides the means for multiple strategies and involves key community members (McLeroy et al., 1994). The general focus of community organizing for health promotion is on changing systems, rules, social norms, or laws, in order to ultimately change the social acceptability of certain behaviors. The venue for community organizing is often the policy arena, and can often involve community elected officials, businesses, community groups, media, and local and state legislatures to create positive community change.

Community coalitions have the potential to involve multiple sectors of the community and to conduct multiple interventions that focus on both individuals and their environments. The pooling of resources and the mobilization of talents and diverse approaches inherent in a successful coalition approach make it a logical strategy for disease prevention, based on a social ecological model that acknowledges the significance of the environment on health. The fact that individuals and organizations apply their skills and resources in collective efforts to meet their own needs is also the basis of *community empowerment*. Community empowerment enjoyed a resurgence of interest and also fueled the formation of community coalitions in the early 1990s (Israel et al., 1994; Labonte, 1994; Minkler, 1994; Perkins, 1995; Rappaport, 1987; Robertson and Minkler, 1994; Wallerstein, 1992; Zimmerman and Rappaport, 1988).

Finally, interest in how well community coalitions develop the *capacity* of communities to address future critical health issues is growing. Community coalitions are a promising strategy for building capacity and competence among member organizations and, ultimately, in the communities they serve (Clark, Friedman, and LaChance, 2006; Chavis, 2001; Garza, 2005; Kegler, Steckler, McLeroy, and Malek, 1998a; Zakocs and Guckenburg, 2007). Associated increases in community participation and leadership, skills, resources, social and interorganizational networks, sense of community, and community power should contribute to future successful community problem-solving efforts (Goodman, Spears, McLeroy, Fawcett, Kegler, Parker, Smith, Sterling, and Wallerstein, 1998).

> Community coalitions have the potential to involve multiple sectors of the community and to conduct multiple interventions that focus on both individuals and their environments.

We should mention that our theory is consistent with several other models for partnership building, some of which were published after the CCAT Theory. Two of these focus on community building and community development (Braithwaite, Murphy, Lythcott, and Blumenthal, 1989; Habana-Hafner, Reed, and Associates, 1989) and others focus on the development and structure of collaborative organizational relationships within communities (Minkler and Wallerstein, 2005; Katz and Kahn, 1978; Prestby and Wandersman, 1985; Butterfoss, Goodman, and Wandersman, 1993; Francisco, Paine, and Fawcett, 1993; Francisco, Fawcett, Schultz, and Paine-Andrews, 2000; National Network for Collaboration, 1996; Lasker and Weiss, 2003). New models continue to be developed (Clark et al., 2006). Each of these organizational models emphasizes important variables, but individually does not provide as complete a contextual understanding of interorganizational collaboration in a community health promotion context as our comprehensive Community Coalition Action Theory (CCAT).

To summarize, coalitions are excellent vehicles for consensus building and active involvement of diverse organizations and constituencies in addressing community problem(s). They enable communities to build capacity and to intervene using a social ecological approach. By involving community members, coalitions help to ensure that interventions meet the needs of the community and are culturally sensitive. Community participation through coalitions also facilitates ownership, which, in turn, is thought to increase the chances of successful institutionalization into the community (Bracht, 1990). These advantages of community coalition approaches are widely accepted by government agencies and foundations and, as a result, the majority of prevention initiatives over the past two decades required the formation of community coalitions. The next section describes the theory, constructs, and assumptions developed to further our understanding of community coalitions.

Description of Theory, Constructs, Assumptions

Certain theoretical underpinnings and assumptions form the framework upon which most community coalitions are, or should be, built. First, we have developed a set of constructs and *practice-proven propositions* based on sound public health practice that provide the foundation for a grounded theory about the development and maintenance of coalitions, as well as how they result in successful actions and health outcomes. The major theoretical constructs are defined in Table 9.1. They were used to develop the twenty-one propositions presented in Table 9.2, reduced from twenty-three in our original version. Together, the constructs and propositions build a rationale for the Community Coalition Action Theory. Figure 9.1 depicts the entire theory visually, while Figures 9.2 through 9.6 relate groups of constructs to corresponding parts of the theoretical model. The theory applies primarily to community coalitions.

A community coalition is different from other types of community entities in that a structured arrangement for collaboration between organizations exists in which all members work together toward a common purpose. If a group is composed solely of individuals and not organizations, then it is not a "coalition" in its truest form. As an action-oriented partnership, a coalition usually focuses on preventing or ameliorating a community problem by: (1) analyzing the problem; (2) gathering data and assessing need; (3) developing an action plan with identified solutions; (4) implementing those solutions; (5) reaching community-level outcomes, such as health behavior changes; and (6) creating social change (Whitt, 1993). This theory does not apply to short-term grassroots coalitions that form for a specific purpose, such as opposing a landfill, and then disband when the goal is achieved.

In addition, community coalitions are characterized as formal, multipurpose and long-term alliances (Butterfoss, Goodman, and Wandersman, 1993). The scope of community coalition work tends to be local or regional, and coalitions usually have some paid staff whose time is dedicated to coalition efforts. The size of membership varies, as

TABLE 9.1 Definition of Constructs, Community Coalition Action Theory.

Constructs	Definition
Stages of Development	The specific stages or phases that a coalition progresses through from formation to implementation to maintenance to institutionalization. Coalitions may recycle through stages more than once or as new members are recruited, plans are renewed, and/or new issues are added.
Community Context	The specific factors in the community that may enhance or inhibit coalition function and influence how the coalition moves through its stages of development. These factors include: history of collaboration, politics, social capital, trust between community sectors and organizations, geography, and community readiness.
Lead Agency or Convening Group	The organization that responds to an opportunity, threat or mandate by agreeing to convene the coalition; provide technical assistance, financial or material support; lend its credibility and reputation to the coalition; and provide valuable networks/contacts.
Coalition Membership	The core group of people who represent diverse interest groups, agencies, organizations, and institutions and are committed to resolving a health or social issue by becoming coalition members.
Processes	The means by which business is conducted in the coalition setting by developing clear processes that facilitate staff and member communication, problem solving, decision making, conflict management, orientation, training, planning, evaluation, and resource allocation. These processes help create a positive organizational climate in which the benefits of participation outweigh the costs.
Leadership and Staffing	The volunteer leaders and paid staff with the interpersonal and organizational skills to facilitate the collaborative process and improve coalition functioning.

Structures	The formalized organizational arrangement, rules, roles, and procedures that are developed in a coalition to maximize its effectiveness. These include: vision and mission statements, goals and objectives, an organizational chart, steering committee and work groups, job descriptions, and meeting schedules.
Pooled Member and External Resources	The resources that are contributed or elicited as in-kind contributions, grants, donations, fund-raisers, or dues from member organizations or external sources that ensure effective coalition assessment, planning, and implementation of strategies.
Member Engagement	The satisfaction, commitment, and participation of members in the work of the coalition.
Collaborative Synergy	The mechanism through which coalitions gain a collaborative advantage by engaging diverse members and pooling member, community, and external resources.
Assessment and Planning	The comprehensive assessment and planning activities that make successful implementation of effective strategies more likely.
Implementation of Strategies	The strategic actions that a coalition implements across multiple ecological levels that make changes in community policies, practices and environments more likely.
Community Change Outcomes	The measurable changes in community policies, practices, and environments that may increase community capacity and improve health or social outcomes.
Health/Social Outcomes	The measurable changes in health status and social conditions of a community that are the ultimate indicators of coalition effectiveness.
Community Capacity	The characteristics of communities that affect their ability to identify, mobilize, and address social and public health problems. Participation in a coalition may enhance these characteristics, which include: citizen participation and leadership, skills, resources, social and interorganizational networks, sense of community, and power.

TABLE 9.2   Constructs and Related Propositions, Community Coalition Action Theory.

Constructs		Propositions
Stages of Development	1.	Coalitions develop in specific stages and recycle through these stages as new members are recruited, plans are renewed, and/or new issues are added.
	2.	At each stage, specific factors enhance coalition function and progression to the next stage.
Community Context	3.	Coalitions are heavily influenced by contextual factors in the community throughout all stages of development.
Lead Agency or Convening Group	4.	Coalitions form when a lead agency or convening group responds to an opportunity, threat, or mandate.
	5.	Coalition formation is more likely when the lead agency or convening group provides technical assistance, financial or material support, credibility, and valuable networks/contacts.
	6.	Coalition formation is likely to be more successful when the lead agency or convening group enlists community gatekeepers to help develop credibility and trust with others in the community.
Coalition Membership	7.	Coalition formation usually begins by recruiting a core group of people who are committed to resolving the health or social issue.
	8.	More effective coalitions result when the core group expands to include a broad constituency of participants who represent diverse interest groups and organizations.
Processes	9.	Open and frequent communication among staff and members helps make collaborative synergy more likely by engaging members and pooling resources.
	10.	Shared and formalized decision making helps make collaborative synergy more likely by engaging members and pooling resources.
	11.	Conflict management helps make collaborative synergy more likely by engaging members and pooling resources.

Leadership and Staffing	12.	Strong leadership from a team of staff and members improves coalition functioning and makes collaborative synergy more likely by engaging members and pooling resources.
	13.	Paid staff make collaborative synergy more likely by engaging members and pooling resources.
Structures	14.	Formalized rules, roles, structures, and procedures improve collaborative functioning and make collaborative synergy more likely by engaging members and pooling resources.
Member Engagement	15.	Satisfied and committed members will participate more fully in the work of the coalition.
Pooled Member and External Resources	16.	The synergistic pooling of member and external resources prompts comprehensive assessment, planning, and implementation of strategies.
Assessment and Planning	17.	Successful implementation of effective strategies is more likely when comprehensive assessment and planning occur.
Implementation of Strategies	18.	Coalitions are more likely to create change in community policies, practices, and environments when they direct interventions at multiple levels.
Community Change Outcomes	19.	Coalitions that are able to change community policies, practices, and environments are more likely to increase capacity and improve health/social outcomes.
Health/Social Outcomes	20.	The ultimate indicator of coalition effectiveness is the improvement in health and social outcomes.
Community Capacity	21.	By participating in successful coalitions, community members and organizations develop capacity and build social capital that can be applied to other health and social issues.

FIGURE 9.1 *The Community Coalition Action Theory (CCAT)*

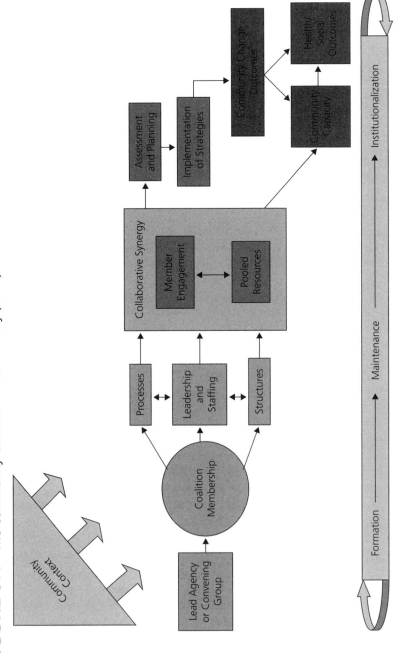

does the diversity of professional and grass-roots organizations, and the balance of organizational and individual members. The degree of formalization of working relationships and role expectations ranges from very formal, with strict adherence to bylaws and contractual relationships, to rather informal.

According to the theory, coalitions progress through stages from formation to institutionalization, with frequent loops back to earlier stages as new issues arise or as planning cycles are repeated (Propositions 1 and 2). The theory also acknowledges contextual factors of the community, such as the sociopolitical climate, geography, history, and norms surrounding collaborative efforts that will impact each stage (Proposition 3). Figure 9.2 shows the details of how Propositions 1 through 3 relate to the model of coalition development from formation to institutionalization.

In the formation stage depicted in Figure 9.3, a convening group or lead agency with given strengths and linkages to the community brings together core organizations that recruit an initial group of community partners to initiate a coalition effort focusing on a health or social issue of concern (Propositions 4 through 8). The coalition identifies key leaders and staff, who then develop structures (for example, committees, rules) and operating procedures (processes) that promote coalition effectiveness.

Structural and process elements in the coalition (Propositions 9 through 14), illustrated in Figure 9.4, can help to ensure a positive organizational climate, an engaged coalition membership, and the pooling of member and external resources. This stage also requires balancing benefits associated with membership to ensure they outweigh any costs of participation.

The maintenance stage, shown in Figure 9.5, involves sustaining member involvement and creating collaborative synergy (Proposition 15). Success in this stage also depends on the mobilization and pooling of member and external resources (Proposition 16). The coalition relies on resources from members and external sources to design creative and comprehensive strategies and/or to identify and adapt evidence-based interventions that are appropriate for the local context and have the greatest chance of leading to the desired health or social outcomes. Acquisition of resources, combined with engaged coalition members and a comprehensive and multilevel planning and implementation process, lead to changes in community policies, practices, and environments (Propositions 17 and 18). Successful implementation is also a precursor to the institutionalization stage of coalition development.

In Figure 9.6, we see that by implementing multilevel strategies of sufficient duration and intensity according to an action plan, shorter-term outcomes such as changes in individual knowledge, beliefs, self-efficacy, and behavior may occur, as well as changes in community systems, policies, practices, and environments (Proposition 19). These intermediate changes should lead to long-term outcomes, such as reductions in morbidity and mortality or substantive progress toward other social goals (Proposition 20).

In the institutionalization stage, shown in Figure 9.6, successful strategies result in outcomes. If resources have been adequately mobilized and strategies effectively address an ongoing need, coalition strategies may become institutionalized in a community as

FIGURE 9.2 *Community Coalition Action Theory Propositions 1 Through 3*

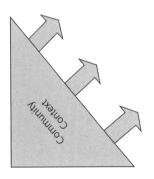

Community Context

Stages of Development

1. Coalitions develop in specific stages and recycle through these stages as new members are recruited, plans are renewed, and/or new issues are added.

2. At each stage, specific factors enhance coalition function and progression to the next stage.

Community Context

3. Coalitions are heavily influenced by contextual factors in the community throughout all stages of coalition development.

Formation → Maintenance → Institutionalization

FIGURE 9.3   *Community Coalition Action Theory Propositions 4 Through 8*

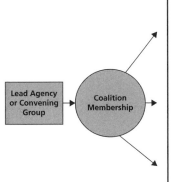

Lead Agency or Convening Group
4. Coalitions form when a lead agency or convening group responds to an opportunity, threat, or mandate.
5. Coalition formation is more likely when the convening group provides technical assistance, financial or material support, credibility and valuable networks/contacts.
6. Coalition formation is more likely to be successful when the convening group enlists community gatekeepers who thoroughly understand the community to help develop credibility and trust with others in the community.

Coalition Membership
7. Coalition formation usually begins by recruiting a core group of people who are committed to resolve the health or social issue.
8. More effective coalitions result when the core group expands to include a broad constituency of participants who represent diverse interest groups and organizations.

FIGURE 9.4   *Community Coalition Action Theory Propositions 9 Through 14*

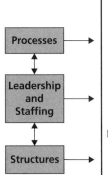

Processes
9. Open and frequent communication among staff and members helps to create a positive climate, to ensure that benefits outweigh costs, and to make collaborative synergy more likely.

10. Shared and formalized decision making helps to create a positive climate, to ensure that benefits outweigh costs, and to make collaborative synergy more likely.

11. Conflict management helps to create a positive climate, to ensure that benefits outweigh costs, and to make collaborative synergy more likely.

Leadership and Staffing
12. Strong leadership from a team of staff and members improves coalition functioning and makes collaborative synergy more likely.

13. Paid staff who have the interpersonal and organizational skills to facilitate the collaborative process, improve coalition functioning, and make collaborative synergy more likely.

Structures
14. Formalized rules, roles, structures, and procedures make collaborative synergy more likely.

FIGURE 9.5 *Community Coalition Action Theory Propositions 15 Through 18*

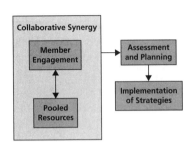

Member Engagement

15. Satisfied and committed members will participate more fully in the work of the coalition.

Pooled Member and External Resources

16. The synergistic pooling of member and external resources prompts comprehensive assessment, planning and implementation of strategies.

Assessment and Planning

17. Successful implementation of effective strategies is more likely when comprehensive assessment and planning occur.

Implementation of Strategies

18. Coalitions are more likely to create change in community policies, practices, and environments when they direct interventions at multiple levels.

FIGURE 9.6 *Community Coalition Action Theory Propositions 19 Through 21*

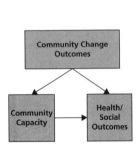

Community Change Outcomes

19. Coalitions that are able to change community policies, practices, and environments are more likely to increase capacity and improve health/social outcomes.

Health/Social Outcomes

20. The ultimate indicator of coalition effectiveness is the improvement in health and social outcomes.

Community Capacity

21. By participating in successful coalitions, community members and organizations develop capacity and build social capital that can be applied to other health and social issues.

part of a long-term coalition, or be adopted by organizations in the community. The coalition itself may or may not be institutionalized in a community. Both maintenance and institutionalization stages have the potential to increase community capacity to solve problems. Progress in ameliorating one community problem can potentially increase the capacity of local organizations to apply these skills and resources to address additional issues that resonate with the community (Proposition 21).

Empirical Support for the Theory

The CCAT debuted in the 2002 edition of this text. Although CCAT has not yet been tested in its entirety, in part due to its complexity, research continues to accumulate on specific factors outlined in the theory. Several researchers have noted its potential utility in providing a unifying framework for guiding future coalition research and coalition practice (Zakocs and Edwards, 2006; Bartholomew et al., 2006). So far, CCAT has been used most often to aid in selecting coalition factors for evaluation, rather than as a theory to be tested (Lengerich et al., 2005).

The following section describes the practice-proven propositions that accompany the model presented in Figure 9.1 and the empirical evidence that supports these propositions. Each box in the model is sustained by one or more propositions (Table 9.2), which in turn are supported by empirical evidence and material from the wisdom literature when empirical evidence is still limited. The studies cited in this chapter are not meant to be a comprehensive review of the coalition literature on each construct in the model. Several reviews offer a more comprehensive summary of recent coalition and community partnership research (Roussos and Fawcett, 2000; Foster-Fishman, 2001; Holden, Pendergast, and Austin, 2000; Lasker, Weiss, and Miller, 2000; Zakocs and Edwards, 2006). Rather, the selected studies are those that most heavily influenced development of CCAT or examined associations between constructs as outlined in the theory.

Stages of Development

Researchers and practitioners agree that the following tasks must occur at some stage to assure coalition effectiveness: recruiting and mobilizing coalition members, establishing organizational structure, building capacity and planning for action, selecting and implementing strategies, evaluating outcomes, refining strategies and approaches, and institutionalizing those strategies and/or the coalition itself.

Researchers and practitioners agree that effective coalitions develop over a period of time. Proposition 1 states that coalitions develop in stages and recycle through these stages as new members are recruited, plans are renewed and/or new issues are added. Thus, the process of building and maintaining coalitions is not linear, but rather cyclical, with coalitions returning to earlier stages as community situations dictate (McLeroy, Kegler, Steckler, Burdine, and Wisotzky, 1994). The naming of those stages and the specific tasks that should be accomplished at each stage, however, differ. Several different series of stages have been proposed, including: formation, implementation, maintenance, and outcomes (Butterfoss, Goodman, and Wandersman, 1993); planning, intervention and outcomes (Fawcett, Paine, Francisco, and Vliet, 1993); and mobilizing, establishing structure and function, building capacity for action, planning for action, implementation, refinement, and institutionalization (Florin, Mitchell, and Stevenson, 1993).

Researchers and practitioners agree that the following tasks must occur at some stage to assure coalition effectiveness: recruiting and mobilizing coalition members, establishing organizational structure, building capacity and planning for action, selecting and implementing strategies, evaluating outcomes, refining strategies and approaches, and institutionalizing those strategies and/or the coalition itself (McLeroy, Kegler, Steckler, Burdine and Wisotzky, 1994). The same authors agree that at each stage, certain factors enhance coalition function and progression to the next stage (Proposition 2). Finally, those who study or work in coalition settings concur that to accomplish their objectives, attention must be paid to maintaining coalitions and constantly recruiting new organizations (Kreuter, Lezin, and Young, 2000; Kaye and Wolff, 1995; Dowling et al., 2000; Butterfoss et al., 1998). Much of the research to date has focused on the earlier stages of coalition development; consequently, less is known about the factors related to coalition success in the later stages of development. One of the few studies that looked at sustainability over time showed that factors known to be important in the formation and maintenance stage, such as staff competence and coalition functioning, were not associated with institutionalization of coalitions into the community (Kegler et al., 2005). This finding raises the possibility that factors external to a coalition may be more critical at this stage of coalition development.

Community Context

Coalitions are embedded in communities, and as a result, factors in the environment can have a significant impact on a coalition (Butterfoss et al., 1993; McLeroy et al., 1994; Lasker et al., 2000). Proposition 3 asserts that coalitions are heavily influenced by contextual factors throughout all stages of development. Several studies support this proposition. For example, Reininger and colleagues (1999) discuss tension and mistrust between groups and how the lack of trust affected a coalition. Others have documented the impact of political and administrative contexts on coalitions (Dill, 1994; Clark et al., 1993; Nelson, 1994). Kegler, Steckler, Malek, and McLeroy et al. (1998b) noted the impact of tobacco-related politics on tobacco control coalitions in several stages of coalition development, from recruitment in the formation stage to types of activities conducted in the maintenance stage. History of collaboration is widely cited in the wisdom and theoretical literature as another contextual factor that can affect the formation of collaborative relationships, including coalitions (Gray, 1989; Butterfoss, LaChance, and Orians, 2006), with experience and positive norms for collaboration increasing the likelihood of future successful collaboration. Feinberg and colleagues (2004) observed strong correlations between community readiness and both internal functioning and perceived coalition effectiveness. Additional contextual factors that affect coalitions include social capital, trust between segments of a community and geography (Wolff, 2001).

> Coalitions are embedded in communities, and as a result, factors in the environment can have a significant impact on a coalition.

Lead Agency or Convening Group

Proposition 4 states that coalitions usually form when a lead agency or convening group responds to an opportunity, threat, or mandate. Propositions 5 and 6 state that a lead agency or convening group begins coalition formation by recruiting a core group of community leaders and providing initial support for the coalition. The lead agency or convening is the organization that has the vision or mandate to initially mobilize community members to form a coalition focused on a specific issue of concern. This organization may or may not have written a grant or otherwise procured funds for coalition operation. The convener does, however, accept responsibility to host an initial meeting and recruit prospective partners. The lead agency or convening group may also provide physical space for coalition operation and a part- or full-time staff person to manage the initiative.

Although the practice literature acknowledges that the lead agency or convening group must have sufficient organizational capacity, commitment, leadership and vision to build an effective coalition, research on these and other factors that lead agencies or convening groups should possess is limited (Butterfoss et al., 1993). In one of a handful of studies comparing coalitions with differing reasons for initiation, Mansergh and colleagues (1996) found that researcher and community-initiated coalitions were similar in terms of perceived coalition efficiency, outcome efficacy, benefits of involvement, and interagency collaboration. The only difference between the two was that action committee effectiveness ranked higher in the researcher-initiated coalition. The researchers concluded that factors other than the impetus for initiation may be more critical for coalition effectiveness. In a study of teen pregnancy prevention coalitions, Kramer and colleagues (2005) reported that coalitions with community-based organizations for lead agencies were viewed by members as less effective than governmental and academic lead agencies. The authors speculated that this may be related to a lead agency's or convening group's level of experience in leading collaborative efforts. A related issue that requires further study is whether coalitions develop anew or simply evolve from other preexisting coalitions and networks in a community (Butterfoss, LaChance, and Orians, 2006; Herman, Wolfson, and Forster, 1993; Nezlek and Galano, 1993).

Coalition Membership

Limited research has focused on the defining characteristics of the *founding members* of community coalitions. Common wisdom holds that previous experience with the health issue or experience with coalitions increases the commitment of these core members. Experience shows that members participate in coalitions with varying levels of intensity, what Brager et al. (1987) describe as "active, occasional and supporting participants." Flexible participation is essential when working with volunteers.

Composition of the core group may affect its ability to engage a broad spectrum of the community. Propositions 6, 7, and 8 state that the core group must recruit community gatekeepers, those committed to the issue, and a broad constituency of diverse groups and organizations. This pooling of diverse views, perspectives, and resources is one of the hallmarks of coalitions and gives them the potential to solve problems that individual agencies could not address alone. As such, effective coalitions make concerted efforts to recruit diverse memberships, in terms of expertise, constituencies, sectors, perspectives, and backgrounds. Additionally, funders are often concerned about increasing the diversity of coalition members as evidenced by the continued focus on reducing health disparities in such efforts as CDC's REACH initiative.

Several studies have examined the influence of diverse coalition membership on intermediate outcomes of effectiveness. Hays and colleagues (2000) found that greater representation of community sectors was associated with action plan quality and perceptions of policy change. Diversity, measured by the percentage of nonwhite members, was not associated with action plan quality or policy change, but was associated with perceived impact on local prevention systems. Jasuja et al. (2005) found that breadth of representation and size were not associated with progress in adopting evidence-based programs. Interestingly, Florin et al. (2000), in one of the few longitudinal studies of coalitions, reported that coalition size was correlated with action plan quality, but not with perceived accomplishments. These findings highlight one of the challenges in coalition research, that is, inconsistency in what is measured.

Coalition Processes

Coalitions must fulfill certain basic functions, such as making decisions, communicating, and managing conflict (Propositions 9–11). Indeed, much of the research on coalitions has focused on internal processes and operations, with the assumption that effective internal functioning is necessary for progress in achieving goals. The quality of interactions among member networks is demonstrated by the frequency and intensity of contacts, and the benefits that members receive from them, such as emotional or tangible support, and access to social contacts (Israel, 1982). Research demonstrates that the extent of regular contacts among community members can foster cooperation (Putnam, 1993). Similarly, members can be empowered by building networks and experiencing positive social relationships (Kumpher et al., 1993). Research has shown that frequent and productive communication and networking among members increases satisfaction, commitment, implementation of strategies and perceived accomplishments (Rogers et al., 1993; Kegler et al., 1998a; Kegler et al., 2005). Similarly, staff are most satisfied and committed when good communication exists between members and themselves (Rogers et al., 1993). Coalition studies have also examined decision making and shown that the influence that participants have in making decisions is vital to a partnership. Influence in decisionmaking is related to increased satisfaction and participation and reporting of more positive benefits (Butterfoss et al., 1996; Butterfoss et al., 2006; Mayer et al., 1998; Kegler et al., 2005). A task-focused organizational climate is also beneficial, and has been linked to member engagement and perceived accomplishments (Florin et al., 2000; Kegler et al., 1998a).

Another internal process that must be initiated to ensure smooth internal functioning is conflict management. Mizrahi and Rosenthal (1992) argue that conflict is an inherent characteristic of partnerships. Conflict may arise between the partnership and its priorities for social change or among partners concerning issues such as loyalty, leadership, goals, benefits, contributions, and representation. Conflict has been shown to lead to staff turnover, avoidance of certain activities and difficulty in recruiting members (Kegler et al., 1998b). Conflict transformation is the process whereby resolution of conflict strengthens the coalition and builds capacity. Research shows that it results from effective coalition planning and contributes to coalition goal attainment (Mayer et al., 1998).

Leadership and Staffing

Propositions 12 and 13 emphasize the importance of leadership and staffing in coalitions. Without these, coalitions are unlikely to move beyond the initial steps in the formation stage of development. Coalition leaders and staff organize the structures through which coalitions accomplish their work and are responsible for coalition processes, such as communication and decision making, that keep members satisfied and committed to coalition efforts. Effective coalition leadership requires a collection of qualities and skills that are typically not found in one individual, but rather in a team of committed leaders. A common approach to leadership in coalitions is the formation of steering committees composed of leaders from action-focused work groups. Empirical research on coalitions shows a consistent relationship between leader competence and satisfaction.

Leadership is complex and researchers have examined many facets in addition to member perceptions of leader competence (Glidewell, Kelly, Bagby, and Dickerson, 1998). For example, Kumpher et al. (1993) studied leadership style and found that an empowering style was related to action plan quality. Butterfoss and colleagues (1996) found that leader support and control were related to several member-related outcomes, but not to plan quality. Reininger et al. (1999) explored how leaders being indigenous or not affected coalitions. In a study of ten rural coalitions formed to prevent drug abuse, Braithwaite and colleagues (2000) noted that the most successful coalitions had strong leadership and a commitment to a common goal. Others have found that the ability of a coalition to develop a clear and shared vision, a likely result of good leadership, is associated with success (Kegler et al., 1998b; CSAP, 1998).

In many coalitions, leadership and staffing are intertwined, with paid staff fulfilling many leadership functions, such as setting agendas and facilitating meetings. Staff often support the coalition, encourage membership involvement, and build community capacity (Sanchez, 2000). Some research suggests that coalitions with staff who play a supportive role for the coalition, rather than a visible leadership role, have higher levels of implementation (Kegler et al., 1998b).

Several studies of coalitions have examined how staffing is related to intermediate indicators of effectiveness, including member-related outcomes, plan quality, resource mobilization, and implementation of planned activities. Several of these studies demonstrate relationships between staff competence and member satisfaction (Rogers et al., 1993; Kegler et al., 1998a; Kegler et al., 2005). Butterfoss and colleagues (1996) found an association between staff competence and member benefits. Kegler and colleagues (2005) found associations between staff competence, member participation, and perceived accomplishments. Kegler et al. (1998a) also found a relationship between staff time devoted to coalition efforts and the amount of resources mobilized and level of implementation of planned activities, thereby lending support to the need for paid staff with sufficient time to devote to the coalition. Florin et al. (2000) reported an association between paid staff hours and plan quality. Minimal or nondisruptive staff turnover has also been linked to positive outcomes (CSAP, 1998; Kegler et al., 1998b).

Coalition Structures

Proposition 14 asserts that coalitions are more likely to engage members, pool resources, and assess and plan well when they have formalized rules, roles, structures, and procedures. Formalization is the degree to which rules, roles, and procedures are precisely defined. Examples of formal structures include committees, written memoranda of understanding, bylaws, policy and procedures manuals; clearly defined roles; mission statements, goals, and objectives; and regular reorientation to the purposes, goals, roles, and procedures of collaboration (Butterfoss et al., 1993; Goodman and Steckler, 1989). Formal structures often result in the routinization or persistent implementation of the partnership's operations. The more routinized operations become, the more likely it is that they will be sustained (Goodman and Steckler, 1989). Research on the importance of formalization is mixed. One study shows that the existence of formal structural elements such as bylaws, agendas, and minutes is related to organizational commitment (Rogers et al., 1993). However, another indicates no association between formalization, plan quality, scope of strategies, or perceived accomplishments (Florin et al., 2000). A second dimension of structure, organizing a coalition to focus on action by creating task forces or action teams, is associated with increased resource mobilization, implementation of strategies, and progress in adopting evidence-based programs (Kegler et al., 1998a; Jasuja et al., 2005).

Member Engagement

Collaborative synergy is generated through successful engagement of diverse coalition members. Member engagement is best defined as the process by which members are empowered and develop a sense of belonging to the coalition. Positive engagement is evidenced by commitment to the mission and goals of the coalition, high levels of participation both in and outside of coalition meetings and activities, and satisfaction with the work of the coalition. Several factors enhance engagement, namely, that the benefits of membership outweigh the costs, and that members experience a positive coalition environment (Butterfoss et al., 1996).

Members who experience more benefits than costs participate more fully and are more satisfied with the work of the coalition. Proposition 15 asserts that satisfied and committed members will have higher levels of participation than less satisfied members. Research supports this assertion and consistently demonstrates that satisfied and committed members will also participate more in the work of the coalition (Butterfoss et al., 1996; Kumpher et al., 1993; Roberts-DeGennaro, 1986; Rogers et al., 1993; Mayer et al., 1998). Although, satisfied and highly participating members are valued, the same studies did not demonstrate that these factors lead to desired intermediate outcomes (for example, producing high-quality action plans) or long-term outcomes (reducing alcohol, tobacco, and other drug use). However, case examples of coalitions exist where practitioners attribute their intermediate and long-range successes to the commitment and satisfaction of their members (Butterfoss et al., 1998).

> Collaborative synergy is generated through successful engagement of diverse coalition members.

Pooled Member and External Resources

A major premise underlying the widespread adoption of coalitions to address community problems is that working together creates a synergy that enables individuals and organizations to accomplish more than they could achieve independently (McLeroy et al., 1994). Proposition 16 asserts that this pooling of resources ensures more effective assessment, planning, and implementation of strategies. Resource sharing also gives coalitions unique advantages over less collaborative problem-solving approaches. Lasker and colleagues (2001) correctly point out that much of the research on coalitions focuses on internal functioning, but does not explicate the pathways through which collaboration increases the likelihood of achieving outcomes over traditional single-agency interventions. They, and we, propose that "synergy" is the mechanism through which partnerships gain advantage over more traditional, less collaborative approaches.

Resources, defined broadly, are one of the major determinants of synergy as conceptualized by Lasker and colleagues. Coalition members are the greatest asset in a coalition-based initiative. They bring energy, knowledge, skills, expertise, perspectives, connections, and tangible resources to the table. The pooling of these diverse resources enables coalition members to achieve together what they could not accomplish alone. Successful resource mobilization, in theory, allows for more creative solutions and more practical, comprehensive approaches (Lasker et al., 2000). Research has shown that staffing and structure of coalitions are related to resource mobilization, which in turn is related to effective implementation of coalition strategies (Kegler et al., 1998a).

Resources from outside the membership, and even the community, are also helpful, as they often fund staff and pay costs associated with implementing planned activities. Such resources relieve some of the burden faced by communities with limited financial resources. External resources may also provide additional expertise, meeting facilities, mailing lists, referrals, additional personnel for special projects, grant funding, loans or donations, equipment, supplies, and cosponsorship of events (Chavis, Florin, Rich, and Wandersman 1987; Prestby and Wandersman 1985; Braithwaite et al., 2000).

Despite compelling logic that synergy is a proximal outcome that links coalition functioning to achievement of outcomes, this has yet to be proven. Weiss, Anderson, and Lasker (2002) documented associations between coalition functioning variables, such as leadership and synergy, but did not examine whether synergy leads to improved outcomes. Several studies have examined pieces of this puzzle, but no clear pattern has yet emerged. If scope and comprehensiveness of planned and implemented activities are indicators of successful synergy, which is consistent with the theory, then scope and/or comprehensiveness of intervention strategies may be reasonable pathways through which synergy leads to outcomes. Hallfors (2002), however, found that coalitions with more comprehensive sets of intervention strategies did not lead to improvements in outcomes (that is, drug use and treatment indicators). Similarly, Florin and colleagues (2000) found no association between scope, operationalized as the number of types of prevention strategies, and plan quality or perceived accomplishments. Interestingly, none of the coalition factors measured by Florin et al. were related to scope.

Assessment and Planning

Achieving a coalition's goals involves assessing the situation and deciding on what action to take. A coalition-based initiative—such as one that is a part of a state or national program—usually engages in an extensive assessment and planning process. This process, lasting as long as two years in some initiatives, is typically followed by a three- to five-year implementation phase. Several coalition studies have examined the quality of the action plans produced by these types of coalition efforts. Analyses of activities selected by coalitions have shown a tendency toward activities that promote changes in awareness (Florin et al., 1993). Kreuter and colleagues (2000) note that despite a strong emphasis on needs assessment, written objectives and logic models that depict cause-effect relationships between interventions and outcomes, many collaborative efforts fail to produce rigorous plans. Quality plans, associated with competent and adequate staffing, leadership, and resource mobilization in several studies, contribute to successful implementation (Butterfoss, 1996; Kumpher 1993; Kegler et al., 1998a; Florin et al., 2000). Proposition 17 states that successful implementation of strategies is more likely when comprehensive planning and assessment occur. Few studies have examined this widely accepted assumption.

Implementation of Strategies

Successful implementation depends on numerous factors such as sufficient resources, completion of tasks on schedule, fidelity to the planned intervention strategies, and supportive, or nonturbulent, organizational and community environments. Assuming the interventions link logically to planned outcomes, the likelihood of achieving these outcomes depends on the extent to which the strategies are implemented and reach the priority populations. Adaptations of interventions that have been previously evaluated (evidence-based) or are commonly accepted as best practices increase the likelihood that interventions will result in community change, and ultimately, desired health and social outcomes.

Using best practices or evidence-based interventions should minimize the tendency of coalitions to focus so heavily on building community awareness. This tendency to focus on quick wins may help to maintain member interest, but is unlikely to lead to more valued outcomes, and may help explain why some coalition-based efforts are not able to achieve systems and/or health outcomes change (Kreuter et al., 2000). Most researchers and practitioners agree that effective health promotion efforts require change at multiple levels, including environmental and policy change (McLeroy, 1988). Goodman and colleagues (1996) further suggest that as coalition interventions become more complex and focus less on individual behavior change, the assessments of such coalitions should focus across multiple levels and take community readiness into account. Proposition 18 emphasizes the importance of implementing interventions at multiple levels in order to create change in community policies, practices, and environments. Crowley and colleagues (2000) tested a coalition model similar to CCAT and found that implementation of programs and community actions were related to community outcomes, such as substance abuse behavior change, but that coalition characteristics were not associated with implementation.

> Successful implementation depends on numerous factors such as sufficient resources, completion of tasks on schedule, fidelity to the planned intervention strategies, and supportive, or nonturbulent, organizational and community environments.

Community Change Outcomes

By implementing interventions at multiple levels, coalitions are able to create change in communities that can reduce risk factors and increase protective factors. Fawcett and colleagues (1997) categorize these into changes in programs, changes in policies, and changes in practices of community agencies, businesses, and government entities.

By implementing inter-ventions at multiple levels, coalitions are able to create change in com-munities that can reduce risk factors and increase protective factors.

Zakocs and Guckenburg (2007) reported that coalitions contributing to greater changes in programs, policies, and services across multiple community sectors were characterized by stable staffing, supportive lead agencies, democratic decision making, and collaborative leader-ship. In CCAT, these factors are hypothesized as mediated through syn-ergy and related constructs such as member engagement. Studies of interorganizational collaboration have used social network analysis to document increased referrals and information exchange associated with membership in a coalition (Provan et al., 2003; Foster-Fishman et al., 2001). The community coa-lition action theory posits that coalitions that are able to create these types of commu-nity change are more likely to increase community capacity to address other issues of concern and to realize their long-term goals (Proposition 19).

Health and Social Outcomes

Proposition 20 states that the ultimate indicator of coalition effectiveness is improve-ment in health and/or social outcomes.

Several recent reviews have been published documenting only modest evidence of effective collaborative partnerships. Roussos and Fawcett (2000) reviewed thirty-four studies that represented 252 collaborative partnerships. The authors categorized the stud-ies into those that provided evidence for more distant population-level outcomes, commu-nity-wide behavior change, and environmental change. The review stated that research is insufficient to make strong conclusions about the impact of partnerships on population-level outcomes largely due to design issues (most of the research consists of case studies).

The ultimate indicator of coalition effectiveness is improvement in health and/or social outcomes.

With respect to community-wide behavior change, Roussos and Fawcett concluded that partnerships can make modest contributions. Strongest evidence existed for the contribution of partnership to environmental change, broadly defined to include changes in programs, services, and practices (conceptualized as community change in CCAT).

A more recent review by Zakocs and Edwards (2006) noted only three studies that reported behavior change. Most studies used coalition member perceptions of change or accomplishments as the primary outcomes. Similarly, Kreuter and colleagues (2000) reviewed sixty-eight published descriptions of coalitions and consortia with evaluation protocols in place, and found only six examples of documented health status or systems change. Numerous reasons have been discussed in the literature as possible explanations for the disappointing findings associated with collaborative initi-atives (Roussos and Fawcett, 2000; Mittelmark, 1999; Kreuter et al., 2000; Berkowitz, 2001; Green and Kreuter, 2002). In addition to design issues and secular trends that make detecting community-level change challenging, some note that coalitions tend to focus on "quick wins" and awareness activities (Florin et al., 2000; Hallfors et al., 2002). These strategies alone will not lead to significant changes in systems or health status. Proposition 20 states that the ultimate indicator of coalition effectiveness is the improvement in health and social outcomes.

Community Capacity

In addition to coalition outcomes associated with health or social issues, another set of outcomes is associated with increases in a community's capacity to solve problems. Proposition 21 asserts that coalitions can enhance community capacity. Coalitions can also create change in communities by enhancing the skills of individuals, increasing the sense of community, and providing new perspectives on community problem solving for residents. At other levels, coalitions can create changes in opportunities for civic participation, linkages between organizations, and the physical and social environment of a community (Kegler et al., 2000). Community capacity has been discussed both as a possible prerequisite to community problem solving and as an outcome of community health promotion efforts (Goodman et al., 1998). Community capacity includes dimensions that coalitions can theoretically impact (either positively or negatively), such as participation and leadership, networks of individuals and organizations, skills and resources, and sense of community. Crisp and colleagues (2000) identify the development of partnerships as one of four distinct approaches to building capacity, arguing that two-way communication between groups not previously working together can result in more resources for planning and implementation. Coalition research focused on community capacity outcomes is just beginning to accumulate. Kegler and colleagues reported skill increases among coalition members as a result of participation in a coalition-based healthy cities and communities initiative (Kegler, Norton, and Aronson, 2007). They also documented the ways in which coalitions contribute to new leadership opportunities within communities (Kegler, Norton, and Aronson, in press). Figure 9.1 shows that community capacity can be strengthened directly as a result of member engagement and pooling of resources, or through an assessment, planning, and implementation process that results in community change.

APPLICATION OF THE MODEL: CONSORTIUM FOR INFANT AND CHILD HEALTH (CINCH)

In 1992, the CDC National Immunization Program established Norfolk, Virginia as a site to demonstrate how a community coalition could improve immunization rates for children under two years of age. Norfolk was selected due to its low immunization rates (49 percent of two-year-olds in 1993), ethnic diversity, and public, private, and military health care systems. By helping citizens develop and implement comprehensive, effective strategies, the Consortium for the Immunization of Norfolk's Children (CINCH) realized its goals and increased childhood immunization rates by 17 percent. This case example shows how CINCH followed the community coalition model presented in Figure 9.1.

Stages of Development

CINCH was in the formation stage for approximately six months. During this time, under-immunization was defined as a community problem, coalition members were recruited and trained and mission, and rules and roles were specified. During the next stage, maintenance, coalition membership was sustained and actual work began. Coalition members assessed needs and assets, collected and analyzed data, developed a plan, initiated and monitored strategies, and supported and evaluated their group process. After three years, the coalition expanded geographically to include the Hampton Roads region and was renamed the Consortium for Infant and Child Health (thus keeping the same acronym). CINCH subsequently recycled through formation and maintenance stages as it engaged in a new recruitment and assessment process. In February 1997, CINCH released the Report on the Health of Children in Hampton Roads. After engaging in a priority-setting process, the coalition decided to focus on immunization and add perinatal issues (for example, low birth weight, teen pregnancy, and infant mortality) to its mission. CINCH collaborated with and reenergized an existing perinatal council and eventually relinquished responsibility for this health issue (institutionalization stage).

While continuing to emphasize immunizations with its "Stay on Track" program for daycare centers and the Annual Vaccine Issues Update Conference for medical providers and advocates, CINCH expanded rapidly from 2001–2006 to focus on children living below 200 percent of poverty with disparities in health. During this period of expansion, the second and third *Reports on the Health of Children in Hampton Roads* provided comprehensive data on children's health that guided CINCH's direction and led to new work groups:

- Allies Against Asthma Work Group (AAA) recruited members with asthma expertise, conducted a comprehensive assessment, and was funded to develop community-based interventions.

- Covering Kids and Families Work Group (CKF) was created from a smaller community coalition and secured funds to identify and enroll over eighteen thousand uninsured children in a health insurance program. CKF provides feedback to the state departments of Medical Assistance Services and Social Services to reduce barriers and improve the program for all families.

- Obesity Prevention Work Group developed a regional agenda for childhood obesity, hosted annual obesity summits for local advocates, and created Healthy Kid Kits for Food and Fitness to build community awareness and capacity. The kits are used to train school nurses and physical education teachers by the Department of Education. CINCH recently collaborated with local media to produce a documentary on obesity in children and helped the YMCA sponsor an *Activate America* walk.

- Injury Prevention Work Group focuses on oceanfront injury, playground safety, child passenger seat safety and installation, and poison prevention.

- Children with Special Health Care Needs Work Group, like CKF, was formed in 2007 from an existing group to galvanize the community around this population.

CINCH has recycled through developmental stages three times during the past fourteen years as new issues arose, strategies were revised, or new members were recruited. Today, the region's children still have health concerns that need to be addressed, and they continue to benefit by having one of the country's oldest and most active children's health coalitions.

Lead Agency or Convening Group

The Center for Pediatric Research, a joint program of a children's hospital and a medical school, convened CINCH and served as the original lead agency or convening group until 2006. Although the Center was new, the region valued collaborative efforts and embraced the concept of coalition building as proposed by the Center staff who were experienced with this strategy. The staff recruited a core group of organizations, who then recruited fifty-five service agencies, academic, civic, and faith-based institutions, health care providers, and parents.

In 2006, the medical school assumed full responsibility as lead agency or convening for CINCH, housing the coalition in a redesigned division of the department of pediatrics that focused on community health and research. The lead agency or convening group continues to fund the office space and infrastructure for CINCH. The school has expanded its coverage for staff salaries that are unfunded by grants. In turn, CINCH demonstrates its value by the community service and positive press that it brings to the school.

Coalition Membership Members from various grassroots and professional organizations provide diversity in age, occupation, race, and ethnicity. They willingly put aside differences in order to share responsibility for all of the community's children. Relying on new knowledge and core values, the coalition developed its earlier mission "to improve immunization rates for children under two years of age", as well as its current mission "to promote health and prevent disease among all children in Hampton Roads, Virginia." This common mission and commitment to community improvement helps members overcome barriers that often stall coalitions, such as lack of direction or turf battles (Kaye and Wolff, 1995; Butterfoss, Goodman or convening group and Wandersman, 1996).

Coalition Processes CINCH surveys report that members either have a great degree of influence or some influence in determining policies and actions of the consortium. When conflict arises, the majority of members report that they are able to resolve it effectively. Content analysis of meetings shows that activities are balanced among tasks of orienting members, assessing needs and assets, planning/revising coalition structure and functions, sharing information, and developing/evaluating products or services. Members evaluate meetings to identify successful elements (Goodman and Wandersman, 1994), and the overwhelming majority rate work group and general meetings as effective. Leaders and staff debrief about barriers to effective meetings and recommend improving agendas, attendance, tardiness, participation, leadership, and diverse representation.

Leadership and Staffing From the onset, CINCH had a full-time director and part-time administrative assistant. This latter position was expanded to full-time, and an assistant director was added in 2006. The leaders of the coalition are community members who are elected by the membership. The steering committee, which consists of coalition and work group chairs and vice-chairs, as well as staff and other nonvoting honorary members, prepared the job description, advertised, interviewed, and hired the past two coalition directors.

Leaders are sensitive to member needs by allowing varying levels of participation during each coalition stage. They reduce burnout and maximize resources by recognizing that some members are better *planners*, while others are better *doers*. Staff members support members by preparing draft documents, minutes, rosters, meeting reminders, and mailings. They help leaders set agendas, run effective meetings, and plan strategies to promote member retention. To engage members, lead agency or convening group staff members provide regular training on a variety of health and leadership issues.

Membership and commitment may waiver when a coalition realizes that it takes time to accomplish its goals. To keep members involved, CINCH participates in health fairs, walks, and other community health efforts. Leaders work to maximize member participation. Meetings provide opportunities to cultivate and renew relationships and to celebrate incremental achievements. Members receive email reminders and phone calls about meetings, and follow-up when absent. Member surveys measure satisfaction and participation and define areas for improvement.

Coalition Structures Members develop written rules of operation, criteria for membership, and roles for members, leaders, and staff. CINCH also develops work groups focused on specific tasks and populations that complement each other. Chairs and vice-chairs are elected for work groups and the coalition at large.

Member Engagement Training, defined roles, and ongoing contact with participating institutions are essential for member retention. Member involvement is bolstered by achievement of objectives and positive results. A clear vision of leadership and commitment to quality processes keeps members interested. CINCH also makes good use of each member's linkage with others. Members constantly recruit others who provide resources or represent the priority population. New recruits stimulate creativity and renewed effort among founding members. Early and subsequent member surveys showed that most were satisfied with the work of the coalition (Butterfoss, et al., 1998). Attendance at meetings averages more than 50 percent, considered acceptable by coalition research (Prestby and Wandersman, 1985).

Pooled Member and External Resources Each member brings individual skills to the coalition, but also represents an organization that commits its resources. Member organizations contribute financially or in-kind to implement strategies, since grant funds are usually earmarked for research. When personal agendas are put aside, resources may be effectively pooled. Work group members invite health departments, hospitals, professional and voluntary agencies from neighboring cities to join them at the table. As previously competitive organizations learn the value of collaborating to accomplish tasks, the level of trust improves.

CINCH relies on community support for its activities in order to increase the likelihood of sustaining its efforts beyond grant funding cycles. Foundation funding has enabled the coalition to hire outreach workers, conduct media campaigns, and implement key strategies. In-kind contributions from CINCH members included printing of posters, flyers, and brochures, arranging satellite teleconferences, and contributing parent incentives. In this way, resources from grants, contracts, and member organizations complement each other and create synergy.

Assessment and Planning Following formation, CINCH's major tasks focused on assessment, data collection, analysis, feedback, and plan development. Work group members continue to participate in assessments to diagnose causes of under-immunization, under-insurance, asthma, and obesity. Parent focus groups, patient exit interviews, household and health care provider surveys are planned and conducted (Houseman, Butterfoss, Morrow, and Rosenthal, 1997; Butterfoss, Morrow, Rosenthal, Dini, Crews, Webster, and Louis, 1998; Taylor-Fishwick, Major, Kelly, Butterfoss, Clarke, and Cardenas, 2004; Butterfoss, Kelly, and Taylor-Fishwick, 2005).

Staff regularly conduct workshops to train work group members to develop quality action plans. Once trained, each work group uses data to identify a prioritized set of issues related to their priority group (for example, parents, nurses, physicians). Goals, objectives, and strategies are developed, and the groups consider the strengths of their community and the resources they can draw on to implement various strategies. Linkages among community agencies are identified, and evaluation of strategies is planned. Work group leaders combine individual plans into overall strategic plans that focus on parent and provider education, support for at-risk families, access to quality health care, and advocacy efforts. The intrinsic negotiation involved in this process cements relationships among group leaders and strengthens internal support for the plan. The planning process for immunization led to the creation of a steering committee that still meets regularly to plan and share successes and challenges. Members have learned that planning is a continuous process that involves time lines, management plans, and budgets.

Implementation of Strategies As CINCH evolves, new strategies are initiated and others are maintained and monitored. Work groups collaborate on strategies and responsibilities and, sometimes, merge to streamline operations. Some activities are initiated and finish quickly, while others are not achieved until after funding ends. Originally, CINCH had an impact on the Norfolk community by effectively implementing sixty-one of seventy-nine planned immunization strategies (77 percent). Currently, many strategies are developed to test a promising practice or replicate an intervention that has worked elsewhere. An evaluation component for each strategy helps members decide whether it is based on need, implemented as planned, and can be improved. Action plans for each work group are revised annually. CINCH is an organization that builds awareness and education about child health, trains providers and parents, and advocates for a healthy community. The coalition is intentionally not an established service provider, so that it does not compete with its partners and cause distrust and conflict (Butterfoss, Gilmore, Krieger, LaChance, Lara, Meurer et al., 2006).

Community Change and Health Outcomes CINCH has accomplished many difficult objectives, such as WIC linkage, physician practice assessment and feedback, hospital birth reminder systems, health insurance enrollment and maintenance, and policy and legislative action. Members not only direct the course of community events, but also wield power to influence larger institutions such as hospitals and the state legislature. Although any change in immunization levels for two-year-olds could not be attributed to CINCH alone, rates rose from 48 percent in 1993 to 66 percent in 1996, with higher rates reported among hospital and military clinics (Morrow et al., 1998). AAA's Asthma Action Plan and Authorization for Medication was adopted by all regional school systems and medical providers and by the Virginia Asthma Coalition (Lara, Cabana, Houle, Krieger, LaChance, Meurer, et al., 2006). CINCH's Injury Prevention Work Group's interventions led to safety revisions in forty-four city playgrounds.

Community Capacity Through training and practice in leadership, meeting facilitation, needs assessment, and planning, coalition members develop skills that improve their participation and can be generalized to other civic areas. Members and staff provide technical assistance to other local partnerships that deal with asthma, tobacco use, child safety, and school health. CINCH collaborates with projects focused on case management, community policing, and neighborhood improvement. Additionally, CINCH fosters new state contracts and federal grants that promote environmental change. A contract between CINCH's lead agency or convening group and the state health department was forged to develop and manage a state immunization coalition, Project Immunize Virginia (PIV). PIV used the "CINCH model" to help other localities develop community partnerships to advocate for immunizing children across the state. Under an Association of Teachers of Preventive Medicine grant, the Coalition Training Institute was established in Norfolk to train key health agency staff that coordinated immunization coalitions in eighty-eight urban, state, and territorial sites (Butterfoss, Morrow, Webster, and Crews, 2003).

STRENGTHS AND LIMITATIONS OF THE THEORY

Any theory as young as CCAT is bound to have strengths and limitations, and must be open to constructive criticism from practitioners and researchers who have a stake in the related work. The CCAT was long overdue. The benefit of its delayed appearance, however, is that it is grounded in almost two decades of practice and research. Perhaps one reason that this theory was not developed earlier is that the complexity of community coalitions and the multifaceted nature of their work overwhelm researchers and practitioners alike. The model that describes our theory is likewise complex and takes into account the diverse factors that influence the formation, implementation, and maintenance of coalitions.

Although community coalitions are found in a variety of settings that range from urban to rural, the empirical research and subsequent findings have focused mostly in the area of alcohol, tobacco, and other drug abuse prevention. This is not surprising, when one considers that the highest level of foundation and governmental agency funding for coalition work has centered on this health issue. Although coalitions exist for many other health issues to include cardiovascular disease, HIV/AIDS, unintentional injury prevention, and immunization, large-scale evaluative research findings have not yet been reported for these issues. Furthermore, much of the research that forms the basis of the CCAT is from studies conducted in the 1990s and tends to focus on coalition functioning and intermediate indicators of effectiveness, such as satisfaction, participation, action plan quality, implementation, and perceived accomplishments. Because of the widely acknowledged difficulty in attributing health outcome change to community collaborative efforts, much of the more recent research uses case study methodology. While informative, case study findings are difficult to generalize and focus less often on associations among constructs.

The constructs used in the Community Coalition Action Theory are informed by research, yet we have speculated on how they interrelate with one another. We have used a set of propositions to help us order the constructs in a logical sequence and develop reciprocal or directional linkages among them. But the research evidence does not assure that these assumptions are correct. Since the theory was introduced, evidence that supports specific bivariate relationships continues to accumulate, but research on the pathways as outlined in the theory is rare. Synergy, and the components we have listed as its dimensions—member engagement, member, community, and external resources—are rarely assessed as mediating variables. Testing of the full CCAT model would require more sophisticated analyses than are typically done, such as structural equation modeling. A few coalition studies have employed such techniques, but given that the proper unit of analysis is often the coalition, this type of research requires a large number of coalitions. Qualitative approaches, such as multiple case studies, may be more feasible, but causal relationships would remain uncertain.

In addition, we have not weighted each variable in our model—how important are coalition processes, for example, as compared to coalition structures? The model does not quantify the resources needed to implement successful strategies, nor the level of member engagement that leads to effective assessment and planning. Further research should help clarify the constructs, their importance to the whole, linkage patterns, and directionality.

The model is further complicated by the complexity of each of the constructs. For example, the processes construct includes communication, decision making, and conflict management. All of these are likely related to organizational climate, but which are more important and in what situations and stages? Similarly, we identify several dimensions of community context and assert that context affects each construct in the model and each stage in coalition development. Yet, much research remains to be done to understand how distribution of power in a community, for example, affects what organization serves as the lead agency or convening group, who makes up the core group, and whose "needs" are assessed.

Additional issues in the coalition literature have implications for testing the CCAT. Zakocs and Edwards (2006) note the large number of factors and indicators of effectiveness used in coalition research. Even when similar factors are studied, measurement methods vary considerably (Granner and Sharpe, 2004; Zakocs and Edwards, 2006). For example, Zakocs and Edwards (2006) observed five different ways leadership has been measured, and Butterfoss (2006) notes numerous ways in which participation is measured in coalition research. A further methodological complication is that much of the coalition research is cross-sectional. Even when a relationship between constructs is observed, knowing if it is causal as specified in the CCAT is often impossible.

Numerous types of collaborative relationships exist. We focused on community coalitions and defined them as long-term community structures that enable organizations and individuals to work collaboratively to address community problems. We also were careful not to cite research done with other types of collaborative initiatives because, in the past, careful distinctions have not been made when summarizing "coalition" findings. Different types of collaborative partnerships (state-level, grassroots, mandated, voluntary, etc.) may function differently and be influenced by different factors in each stage of coalition development. Stages of development may also need to be conceptualized differently for different types of coalitions. For example, a grassroots coalition formed to keep a landfill out of a neighborhood may not need to institutionalize anything once the landfill is sited elsewhere.

FUTURE DIRECTIONS

We need to be careful lest we "throw the baby out with the bathwater" by criticizing coalitions for not achieving measurable outcomes. Future research efforts should focus on what coalitions contribute to community-based interventions above and beyond more traditional approaches.

With the advent of evidence-based medicine and outcomes-based interventions, coalitions have been criticized as not meeting expectations for success (Green, 2000; Hallfors, Cho, Livert, and Kadushin, 2003). Given the tremendous infusion of resources, both monetary and in donated volunteer time, some feel this criticism is well deserved. In truth, the overall evidence for positive coalition outcomes is lacking. Traditional scientific methodology may not be adequate to capture the outcomes of these complex collaborative organizations (Berkowitz, 2000; Gabriel, 2000; Merzel and D'Afflitti, 2003). We cannot underestimate the amount of time that it takes to create and sustain viable coalitions, the difficulty in identifying and implementing promising practices, the reluctance of accepting qualitative methods of evaluation, the identification of realistic intermediate- and long-term outcomes, and, finally, the understanding of long-term benefits and unintended positive outcomes for communities. However, we need to be careful lest we "throw the baby out with the bathwater" by criticizing coalitions for not achieving measurable outcomes.

Future research efforts should focus on what coalitions contribute to community-based interventions above and beyond more traditional approaches. (Lasker et al., 2001; Berkowitz et al., 2001; Butterfoss et al., 2001). For example, do coalition approaches develop more innovative strategies due to the pooling of expertise and resources? Do they reach previously untapped community assets? Are they better able to implement certain types of interventions than traditional public health and social service agencies, such as policy or media advocacy efforts? Although initial research has been done on what Lasker and colleagues term partnership "synergy," it focuses on coalition functioning and self-reported synergy, is cross-sectional, and has not been linked to outcomes (Weiss et al., 2002).

For better or worse, community coalitions are in the same situation as almost all community-level initiatives that are challenged to document intermediate and long-term outcomes and attribute resulting changes to the initiative (Florin, Mitchell, Stevenson, and Klein, 2000; Gabriel, 2000). In their commentary on community coalitions, Green and Kreuter (2002) question why coalitions are identified as the primary independent variables in complex, collaborative community interventions. Our contention is that by strengthening the theoretical base and developing a model of action for community coalitions, we will advance this area of scientific inquiry. We encourage theoreticians to test the logic of this model. We challenge researchers and evaluators with access to large numbers of coalitions to use the model to field test our assumptions and advance the understanding of which coalition characteristics and interactions are most likely to fuel goal attainment. Finally, we ask practitioners, the front-line coalition pioneers, to determine whether this model is useful to increase local support and capacity for further coalition development. This theoretical model is still simply a starting point—we welcome all contributions that improve its validity, reliability, and utility.

SUMMARY

Coalitions provide an important mechanism for building consensus and actively involving diverse organizations and constituencies in addressing community problems. Coalitions form when a lead agency or convening group responds to a threat, opportunity, or mandate. The CCAT offers a series of practice-proven propositions that explain how coalitions evolve through stages, with different factors and tasks more or less important at various stages. The theory builds upon past work in the areas of community development, political science, inter-organizational relations, and group process. Research to date tends to be descriptive or focus on associations between major constructs rather than on the causal pathways predicted by the theory.

REFERENCES

Alter, and Hage CA (1993). *Organizations working together: Coordination in interorganizational networks.* Newbury Park: Sage.

Bartholomew, L, Parcel, G, Kok, G, Gottlieb, N. *Planning health promotion programs: An intervention mapping approach.* 2nd ed. San Francisco: Jossey-Bass, 2006.

Bazzoli, G., Stein, R., Alexander, J., Conrad, D., Sofaer, S., and Shortell, S. (1997). Public-private collaboration in health and human service delivery: Evidence from community partnerships. *The Milbank Quarterly, 75*(4), 533–561.

Berkowitz B. (2001). Studying the outcomes of community-based coalitions. *American Journal of Community Psychology, 29*(2):213–27.

Berlin, X., Barnett, W., Mischke, G., and Ocasio W. (2000). The evolution of collective strategies among organizations. *Organization Studies*, *21*(2), 325–354.

Bracht, N (Ed.). (1990). *Health promotion at the community level*. Newbury Park, CA: Sage.

Brager, G. A., Sprecht, H., and Torczyner, J. L. (1987). *Community organizing*. 2nd ed. New York: Columbia University Press.

Braithwaite, R., Taylor, S., and Austin, J. (2000). *Building health coalitions in the black community*. Thousand Oaks, CA: Sage.

Butterfoss, F. (2006). Process evaluation for community participation. *Annual Review of Public Health*, 27, 323–40.

Butterfoss, F., Cashman, S., Foster-Fishman, P., and Kegler, M. (2001). Roundtable discussion of Berkowitz's paper. *American Journal of Community Psychology*, *29*(2), 229–240.

Butterfoss, F., Goodman R., and Wandersman, A. (1996). Community coalitions for prevention and health promotion: Factors predicting satisfaction, participation and planning. *Health Education Quarterly*, *23*(1), 65–79.

Butterfoss, F., Goodman, R., and Wandersman, A. (1993). Community coalitions for prevention and health promotion. *Health Education Research, 8*(3), 315–330.

Butterfoss, F. D., Kelly, C. K., and Taylor-Fishwick, J. (2005). Community planning that magnifies the community's voice: Allies Against Asthma. *Health Education and Behavior*, *32*(1), 113–128.

Butterfoss, F. D, LaChance, L. L., and Orians, C. E. (2006). Building Allies coalitions: Why formation matters. *Health Promotion Practice*, *7,* 23–33S.

Butterfoss, F. D., Gilmore, L. A., Krieger, J. W., LaChance, L. L., Lara. M., Meurer, J. R., Nichols, E. A., (2006). From formation to action: How Allies Against Asthma coalitions are getting the job done. *Health Promotion Practice*, *7,* 34–43S.

Butterfoss, F. D., Morrow, A. L., Rosenthal, J., Dini, E., Crews, R. C., Webster, J. D., and Louis, P. A. (1998). CINCH: An urban coalition for empowerment and action. *Health Education and Behavior*, *25*(2), 213–225.

Butterfoss, F. D., Morrow, A. L., Webster, J. D., and Crews, C. (2003). The Coalition Training Institute: Training for the long haul. *Journal of Public Health Management and Practice*, *9*(6), 522–529.

Carlaw, R., Mittelmark, M., Bracht, N., and Luepker, R. (1984). Organization for a community cardiovascular health program: Experiences from the Minnesota Heart Health Program. *Health Education Quarterly*, *11*(2), 243–252.

Cassell, C., Santelli, J., Gilbert, B., Dalmat, M., Mezoff, J., and Schauer, M. (2005). Mobilizing communities: An overview of the Community Coalition Partnership Programs for the Prevention of Teen Pregnancy. *Journal of Adolescent Health*, *37*(3S), S3–S10.

Center for Substance Abuse and Prevention. (1998). *National evaluation of the Community Partnership Demonstration Program. final report,1997.* Substance Abuse and Mental Health Services Administration, U.S. Department of Health and Human Services.

Chavis, D.M. (2001). The paradoxes and promise of community coalitions. *American Journal of Community Psychology 29*(2), 309–320.

Chavis, D. M., Florin, P., Rich, R., and Wandersman, A. (1987). The role of block associations in crime control and community development: The Block Booster Project. *Report to the Ford Foundation*.

Checkoway, B. (1989). Community participation for health promotion: Prescription for public policy. *Wellness Perspectives: Research, Theory and Practice*, *6*(1), 18–26.

Chinman, M., Anderson, C., Imm, P., Wandersman, A., and Goodman R. (1996). The perceptions of costs and benefits of high active versus low active groups in community coalitions at different stages in coalition development. *Journal of Community Psychology, 24, 263–274.*

Clark, N., Baker, E., and Chawla, A. (1993). Sustaining collaborative problem-solving: Strategies from a study in six Asian countries. *Health Education Research, 8*(3), 385–402.

Clark, N. M, Friedman, A. R., and LaChance, L. L. (2006). Summing it up: Collective lessons from the experience of seven coalitions. *Health Promotion Practice*, Supplement, *7*(2), 149–52S.

Crisp, B., Swerissen, H., and Duckett, S. (2000). Four approaches to capacity building in health: consequences for measurement and accountability. *Health Promotion International*, *15*(2), 99–107.

Crowley, K., Yu, P., and Kaftarian, S. (2000). Prevention actions and activities make a difference: a structural equation model of coalition building. *Evaluation and Program Planning*, 23, 381–388.

Dill, A. (1994). Institutional environments and organizational responses to AIDS. *Journal of Health and Social Behavior, 35,* 349–369.

Dowling, J., O'Donnell, H. J., and Wellington Consulting Group (2000). *A development manual for asthma coalitions*. Northbrook, IL: The CHEST Foundation and the American College of Chest Physicians.

Farquhar, J., Fortmann, S., Flora, J., Taylor, C., Haskell, W., Williams, P., Maccoby, N., and Wood, P. (1990). Effects of community-wide education on cardiovascular disease risk factors: The Five-City Project. *Journal of the American Medical Association, 264*(3), 359–365.

Fawcett, S., Lewis, R., Paine-Andrews, A., Francisco, V., Richer, K., Williams, E., and Copple, B. (1997). Evaluating community coalitions for prevention of substance abuse: The case of Project Freedom. *Health Education and Behavior, 24*(6), 812–828.

Fawcett. S., Paine, A., Francisco, V., and Vliet, M. (1993). Promotion health through community development. In Glenwick, D., and Jason, L.A. (eds.), *Promoting Health and Mental Health in Children, Youth and Families*. New York, Springer, 233–255.

Feighery, E., and Rogers, T. (1990). *Building and maintaining effective coalitions*. Palo Alto, CA: Health Promotion Resource Center, Stanford Center for Research in Disease Prevention.

Feinberg, M., Greenberg, M., and Osgood, D. (2004). Readiness, functioning and perceived effectiveness in community prevention coalitions: A study of Communities That Care. *American Journal of Community Psychology, 33*(3/4), 163–176.

Florin, P., and Wandersman A. (1990). An introduction to citizen participation, voluntary organizations, and community development: Insights for empowerment research. *American Journal of Community Psychology, 18*(1), 41–54.

Florin, P., Mitchell, R., and Stevenson, J. (1993). Identifying training and technical assistance needs in community coalitions: A developmental approach. *Health Education Research, 8*(3), 417–432.

Florin, P., Mitchell, R., Stevenson, J., and Klein, I. (2000). Predicting intermediate outcomes for prevention coalitions: A Developmental Perspective. *Evaluation and Program Planning, 23,* 341–346.

Foster-Fishman, P., Berkowitz, S., Lounsbury, D., Jacobson, S., and Allen, N. (2001). Building collaborative capacity in community coalitions: A review and integrative framework. *American Journal of Community Psychology, 29*(2), 241–261.

Foster-Fishman, P., Salem. D., Allen, N., and Fahrbach, K. (2001). Facilitating interorganizational collaboration: The contributions of interorganizational alliances. *American Journal of Community Psychology, 29*(6), 875–905.

Gabriel, R. (2000). Methodological challenges in evaluating community partnerships and coalitions: Still crazy after all these years. *Journal of Community Psychology, 28*(3), 339–352.

Garza, H. (2005). Evaluating partnerships: Seven success factors. *The Evaluation Exchange, 10*(1), 18–19.

Giamartino, G., and Wandersman, A. (1983) Organizational climate correlates of viable urban block organizations. *American Journal of Community Psychology, 11*(5), 529–541.

Glidewell, J., Kelly, J., Bagby, M., and Dickerson, A. (1998). Natural development of community leadership. In: R.S. Tindale et al., *Theory and research on small groups*, New York: Plenum Press.

Goodman, R. M., Speers, M., McLeroy, K., Fawcett, S., Kegler, M., Parker, E., Smith, S., Sterling, T. and Wallerstein, N. (1998). Identifying and defining the dimensions of community capacity to provide a basis for measurement. *Health Education and Behavior, 25*(3), 258–278.

Goodman, R. M., and Steckler, A. (1989). A model for institutionalization of health promotion programs. *Family and Community Health, 11,* 63–78.

Goodman, R. M., and Wandersman, A. (1994). FORECAST: A formative approach to evaluating community coalitions and community-based initiatives. *Journal of Community Psychology*, CSAP Special Issue, 6–25.

Goodman, R. M., Wandersman, A., Chinman, M, Imm, P., and Morrisey, E. (1996). An ecological assessment of community-based interventions for prevention and health promotion: Approaches to measuring community coalitions. *American Journal of Community Psychology, 24*(1), 33–61.

Granner, M., and Sharpe, P. (2004). Evaluating community coalition characteristics and functioning: a summary of measurement tools. *Health Education and Behavior*, *19*(5), 514–32.

Gray, B., and Wood, D. (1991). Collaborative alliances: Moving from practice to theory. *Journal of Applied Behavioral Science*, *27*(1), 3–22.

Gray, B. (1989). *Collaboration: Finding common ground for multiparty problems*. San Francisco: Jossey-Bass.

Green, L. (2000). Caveats on coalitions: In praise of partnerships. *Health Promotion Practice*, *1*(1), 64–65.

Green, L., and Kreuter, M. (1992). CDC's planned approach to community health as an application of PRECEDE and an inspiration for PROCEED. *Journal of Health Education*, *23*(3), 140–147.

Green, L., and Kreuter, M. (2002). Fighting back or fighting themselves? Community coalitions against substance abuse and their use of best practices. *American Journal of Preventive Medicine*, *23*(4), 303–306.

Gulati, R. (1995). Social structure and alliance formation patterns: A longitudinal analysis. *Administrative Science Quarterly*, *40,* 619–652.

Hallfors, D., Cho, H., Livert, D., and Kadushin, C. (2003). 'Fighting back' against substance abuse: Are community coalitions winning? *American Journal of Preventive Medicine*, *23*(4), 237–245.

Hays, C., Hays, S., DeVille, J., Mulhall, P. (2000). Capacity for effectiveness: the relationship between coalition structure and community impact. *Evaluation and Program Planning*, *23,* 373–379.

Herman, K., Wolfson, M., and Forster J. (1993). The evolution, operation, and future of Minnesota SAFEPLAN: A coalition for family planning. *Health Education Research*, 8(3), 331–344.

Holden, D., Pendergast, K. and Austin, D. (2000) *Literature review for American Legacy Foundation's statewide youth movement against tobacco use—draft report*. Research Triangle Park, NC: Research Triangle Institute.

Houseman, C., Butterfoss, F. D., Morrow, A. L., and Rosenthal, J. (1997). Focus groups among public, military and private sector mothers: Insights to improve the immunization process. *Journal of Public Health Nursing*, *14*(4), 235–243.

Israel, B. A. (1982). Special networks and health status: Linking theory, research and practice. *Patient Counseling and Health Education*, *4*(2), 65–79.

Israel, B.A., Checkoway, B., Schultz, A., Zimmerman, M. (1994). Health education and community empowerment: Conceptualizing and measuring perceptions of individual, organizational and community control. *Health Education Quarterly*, *21*(2), 149–170.

Jasuja, G., Chou, C., Bernstein, K., Wang, E., McClure, M., Pentz, M. (2005). Using structural characteristics of community coalitions to predict progress in adopting evidence-based prevention programs. *Evaluation and Program Planning*, *28*, 173–184.

Kaye G. and Wolff T. (1995). *From the ground up: A workbook on coalition building and community development*. Amherst, MA: AHEC/Community Partners, 1995.

Kegler M., Norton B., and Aronson R. (2007) Skill improvement among coalition members in the California Healthy Cities and Communities Program, *Health Education Research*, 22(3), 450–457.

Kegler M., Norton B., Aronson R. Strengthening community leadership: Evaluation findings from the California Healthy Cities and Communities Program. *Health Promotion Practice*, in press.

Kegler, M., Steckler, A., McLeroy, K., and Malek, S. (1998a). Factors that contribute to effective community health promotion coalitions: A study of 10 Project ASSIST coalitions in North Carolina. *Health Education and Behavior*, *25*(3), 338–353.

Kegler, M., Steckler, A., Malek, S., and McLeroy, K. (1998b). A multiple case study of implementation in 10 local Project ASSIST coalitions in North Carolina. *Health Education Research*, *13*(2), 225–238.

Kegler, M., Twiss, J., and Look, V. (2000). Assessing community change at multiple levels: The genesis of an evaluation framework for the California Healthy Cities and Communities Project. *Health Education and Behavior*, *27*(6), 760–779.

Kegler, M., Williams, C., Cassell, C., Santelli, J., Kegler, S. Montgomery, S., et al. (2005). Mobilizing communities for teen pregnancy prevention: Associations between coalition characteristics and perceived accomplishments. *Journal of Adolescent Health*, *37* (3S), S31–S41.

Kramer, J., Philliber, S., Brindis, C., Kamin, S., Chadwick, A., Revels, M., et al. (2005). Coalition models: Lessons learned from the CDC's Community Coalition Partnership Programs for the Prevention of Teen Pregnancy. *Journal of Adolescent Health, 37* (3S), S20–S30.

Kreuter, M. (1992). PATCH: Its origins, basic concepts, and links to contemporary public health policy. *Journal of Health Education, 23*(3), 135–139.

Kreuter, M., Lezin, N., and Young, L. (2000). Evaluating community-based collaborative mechanisms: Implications for practitioners. *Health Promotion Practice, 1*(1), 49–63.

Kumpher, K., Turner, C., Hopkins, R. and Librett, J. (1993). Leadership and team effectiveness in community coalitions for the prevention of alcohol and other drug abuse. *Health Education Research, 8*(3), 359–374.

Labonte, R. (1994). Health promotion and empowerment: Reflections on professional practice. *Health Education Quarterly, 21*(2), 253–268.

Lara, M., Cabana, M. D., Houle, C. R., Krieger, J. W., LaChance, L. L., Meurer, J. R., Rosenthal, M. P., and Vega, I. (2006) Improving quality of care and promoting health care system change: The role of community-based coalitions. *Health Promotion Practice, 7,* 87–95S.

Lasker, R., Weiss, E., and Miller R. (2001a). Partnership synergy: a practical framework for studying and strengthening the collaborative advantage. *The Milbank Quarterly, 79*(2),179–205.

Lasker, R., Weiss, E., and Miller, R. (2000b). Promoting collaborations that improve health. Paper Commissioned for the 4th Annual Community-Campus Partnerships for Health Conference, April 29, 2000-May 2, 2000, Arlington, VA.

Lefebvre, R., Lasater, T., Carleton, R., and Petersen, G. (1987). Theory and delivery of health programming in the community: The Pawtucket Heart Health Program. *Preventive Medicine, 16,* 80–95.

Lengerich, E. J., Rucker, T. C., Powell, R. K., Colsher, P., Lehman, E., Ward, A. J., et al. Cancer incidence in Kentucky, Pennsylvania, and West Virginia: Disparities in Appalachia. *Journal of Rural Health, 21*(1), 39–47, 2005.

Mansergh, G., Rohrbach, L., Montgomery, S., Pentz, M., and Johnson, C. (1996). Process evaluation of community coalitions for alcohol and other drug abuse: A case study comparison of researcher- and community-initiated models. *Journal of Community Psychology, 24,* 118–135.

Mayer, J., Soweid, R., Dabney, S., Brownson, C., Goodman, R., and Brownson R. (1998). Practices of successful community coalitions: A multiple case study. *American Journal of Health Behavior, 22*(5), 368–377.

McLeroy, K., Bibeau, D., Steckler A., and Glanz, K. (1988). An ecological perspective on health promotion programs. *Health Education Quarterly, 15*(4), 351–377.

McLeroy, K., Kegler, M., Steckler, A., Burdine, J., and Wisotzky, M. (1994). Editorial. Community coalitions for health promotion: Summary and further reflections. *Health Education Research, 9*(1), 1–11.

McMillan, B., Florin, P., Stevenson, J., Kerman, B., and Mitchell, R. (1995). Empowerment praxis in community coalitions. *American Journal of Community Psychology, 23*(5), 699–727.

Merzel, C., and D'Afflitti, J. (2003). Reconsidering community-based health promotion: promise, performance and potential. *American Journal of Public Health, 93*(4), 557–74.

Milio, N. (1989). *Promoting health through public policy*. Ottawa: Canadian Public Health Association.

Minkler, M. (1994). Ten commitments for community health education. *Health Education Research, 9*(4), 527–534.

Mittelmark, M. (1999). Health promotion at the communitywide level: Lessons from diverse perspectives. In: Bracht N. (ed.). *Health Promotion at the Community Level*. Thousand Oaks CA: Sage.

Mittelmark, M., Luepker, R., Jacobs, D., Bracht, N., Carlaw, R., Crow, R., Finnegan, J., Grimm, R., Jeffery, R., Kline, F., Mullis, R., Murray, D., Pechacek, T., Perry, C., Pirie, P. and Blackburn H. (1986). Community-wide prevention of cardiovascular disease: Education strategies of the Minnesota Heart Health Program. *Preventive Medicine, 15*(1), 1–17.

Mizrahi, T., and Rosenthal, B. (1992). Managing dynamic tensions in social change coalitions. In Mizrahi, T. and Morrison, J. (eds.). *Community Organization and Social Administration*, Haworth Press.

Mizruchi, M., and Galaskiewicz, J. (1994). Networks of interorganizational relations, Chapter 9. In S. Wasserman and J. Galaskiewicz J. (eds*). Advances in social network analysis: Research in the social and behavioral sciences*. Thousand Oaks, CA: Sage.

Moon, R., Havlicek, D., Garcia, J., Vollinger, R., and Motsinger, B. Chapter 2. *The conceptual framework. ASSIST: Shaping the future of tobacco prevention and control.* Tobacco Control Monograph No. 16. Bethesda, MD: U.S. Dept of HHS, NIH, NCI, NIH Pub. No. 05–5645, 2005.

Morrow, A. L., Rosenthal, J., Lakkis, H., Bowers, J. C., Butterfoss, F. D., Crews, R. C., and Sirotkin, B. (1998). A population-based study of risk factors for under-immunization among urban Virginia children served by public, private and military health care systems. *Pediatrics*, 101(2), E5.

Nelson, G. (1994). The development of a mental health coalition: A case study. *American Journal of Community Psychology*, 22(2), 229–255.

Nezlek, J., and Galano, J. (1993). Developing and maintaining state-wide adolescent pregnancy prevention coalitions: A preliminary investigation. *Health Education Research*, 8(3), 433–447.

Penner, S. A study of coalitions among HIV/AIDS service organizations. (1995). *Sociological Perspectives*, 38(2), 217–239.

Perkins, D. (1995). Speaking truth to power: Empowerment ideology as social intervention and policy. *American Journal of Community Psychology*, 23(5), 765–794.

Perkins, D., Florin, P., Rich, R., Wandersman, A. and Chavis, D. (1990). Participation and the social and physical environment of residential blocks: Crime and community context. *American Journal of Community Psychology*, 18(1), 83–115.

Perkins, D., Florin, P., Rich, R., Wandersman, A., and Chavis, D., (1990). Six strategies of community change (1995). *Community Development Journal* 30, 2–20.

Prestby, J., and Wandersman, A. (1985). An empirical exploration of a framework of organizational viability: maintaining block organizations. *The Journal of Applied Behavioral Science*, 21(3), 287–305.

Prestby, J., Wandersman, A., Florin, P., Rich, R., and Chavis, C. (1990). Benefits, costs, incentive management and participation in voluntary organizations: A means to understanding and promoting empowerment. *American Journal of Community Psychology*, 18(1), 117–149.

Provan, K., and Milward, H. (1995). A preliminary theory of interorganizational network effectiveness: A comparative study of four community mental health systems. *Administrative Science Quarterly*, 40, 1–33.

Provan, K., Nakama, L., Veazie, M., Teufel-Shone, N., and Huddleston, C. (2003). Building community capacity around chronic disease services through a collaborative interorganizational network. *Health Education and Behavior*, 30(6), 646–62.

Putnam, R. (1993). *Making democracy work*. Princeton, NJ: Princeton University Press.

Rappaport, J. (1987). Terms of empowerment/exemplars of prevention: Toward a theory for community psychology. *American Journal of Community Psychology*, 15, 121–144.

Reininger, B., Dinh-Zarr, T., Sinicrope, P., and Martin, D. (1999). Dimensions of participation and leadership: Implications for community-based health promotion for youth. *Family and Community Health*, 22(2), 72–82.

Roberts-DeGennaro, M. (1986). Factors contributing to coalition maintenance. *Journal of Sociology and Social Welfare*, 248–264.

Robertson, A., and Minkler, M. (1994). New health promotion movement: A critical examination. *Health Education Quarterly*, 23(3), 295–312.

Rogers, T., Howard-Pitney, B., Feighery, E., Altman, D., Endres, J., and Roeseler, A. (1993). Characteristics and participant perceptions of tobacco control coalitions in California. *Health Education Research*, 8(3), 345–357.

Roussos, S., and Fawcett, S. (2000). A review of collaborative partnerships as a strategy for improving community health. *Annual Review of Public Health*, 21, 369–402.

Sanchez, V. (2000). Reflections on community coalition staff: Research directions from practice. *Health Promotion Practice*, 1(4), 320–322.

Sharfman, M., Gray, B., and Yan, A. (1991). The context of interorganizational collaboration in the garment industry: An institutional perspective. *Journal of Applied Behavioral Science*, 27(2), 181–208.

Shea, S., and Basch, C. (1990). A review of five major community-based cardiovascular disease prevention programs. Part 1: rationale, design and theoretical framework. *American Journal of Health Promotion*, 4(3), 203–213.

Stokols, D. (1992). Establishing and maintaining healthy environments: Toward a social ecology of health promotion. *American Psychologist, 47*(1), 6–22.

Taylor-Fishwick, J., Major, D. A., Kelly, C. K., Butterfoss, F. D., Clarke, S. M., and Cardenas, R. A. (2004) Community focus groups for Allies Against Asthma. *Pediatric Asthma, Allergy and Immunology, 17*(1).

Tesh, S. (1988). *Hidden arguments: Political ideology and disease prevention policy.* New Brunswick: Rutgers University Press.

Thompson, B., and Kinne, S. (1990). Social change theory: Applications to community health. In: Bracht N. (ed.). *Health promotion at the community level.* Newbury Park CA: Sage.

Wallerstein, N. (1992). Powerlessness, empowerment and health: Implications for health promotion programs. *American Journal of Health Promotion, 6*(3), 197–205.

Wandersman, A., and Alderman, J. (1993). Incentives, barriers and training of volunteers for the American Cancer Society: A staff perspective. *Review of Public Personnel Administration, 13*(1), 67–76.

Wandersman, A., Florin, P., Friedmann, R., and Meier, R. (1987). Who participates, who does not and why? An analysis of voluntary neighborhood associations in the United States and Israel. *Sociological Forum, 2,* 534–555.

Weiss, E., Anderson, R., and Lasker, R. (2002). Making the most of collaboration: exploring the relationship between partnership synergy and partnership functioning. *Health Education and Behavior, 29*(6), 683–698.

Whetten, D. (1981). Interorganizational relations: A review of the field. *Journal of Higher Education, 52*(1), 1–28.

Whitt, M. (1993). *Fighting tobacco: A coalition approach to improving your community's health.* Lansing, MI: Michigan Department of Public Health.

Wolff, T. (2001). Community coalition building—Contemporary practice and research. *American Journal of Community Psychology, 29*(2), 165–172.

Wood, D., and Gray, B. (1991). Toward a comprehensive theory of collaboration. *Journal of Applied Behavioral Science, 27*(2), 139–162.

Yin, R., Kaftarian, S., Yu, P., and Jansen, M. (1997). Outcomes from CSAP's Community Partnership Program: Findings from the national cross-site evaluation. *Evaluation and Program Planning, 20*(3), 345–355.

Zakocs, R. C., and Edwards, E. M. (2006). What explains community coalition effectiveness? A review of the literature. *American Journal of Preventive Medicine, 30*(4), 351–361.

Zakocs, R., and Guckenburg, S. (2007). What coalition factors foster community capacity? Lessons learned from the Fighting Back Initiative. *Health Education and Behavior, 34*(2), 354–75.

Zapka, J., Marrocco, G., Lewis, B., McCusker, J., Sullivan, J., McCarthy, J., and Birth, F. (1992). Interorganizational responses to AIDS: A case study of the Worcester AIDS consortium. *Health Education Research, 7*(1), 31–46.

Zimmerman, M. A., and Rappaport, J. (1988). Citizen participation, perceived control, and psychological empowerment. *American Journal of Community, 16,* 725–750.

COMMUNITY CAPACITY: THEORY AND APPLICATION

Monica L. Wendel

James N. Burdine

Kenneth R. McLeroy

Angela Alaniz

Barbara Norton

Michael R. J. Felix

COMMUNITY-BASED APPROACHES TO PUBLIC HEALTH

Over the past three decades, there has been a dramatic increase in the interest of public health researchers and practitioners in community-based approaches to improving the health of the public, particularly in the areas of health promotion and disease prevention. This increased emphasis on community approaches is due to a variety of factors, including an understanding of the complex etiology of contemporary health problems (Florin and Chavis, 1990; Krieger, 2008; Adler and Rehkopf, 2008); an appreciation for the importance of the interplay between humans and their environments (McLaren and Hawe, 2005; DiClemente, Salazar, and Crosby, 2007); and a recognition among public health professionals of limits to fostering individually oriented strategies for behavior change (Udehn, 2002).

Despite this increased attention, there is considerable variation in the extent to which "community" is incorporated in interventions. McLeroy and colleagues (2003) provide a useful typology for contrasting perspectives in community focus: community as *setting*, community as *target*, community as *resource*, and community as *agent*. In practice, the application of these perspectives results in a continuum of "community-based" interventions. Interventions may range from those that take place in a community setting and target community members to those that acknowledge and utilize the community's assets, including community-based participatory research models (CBPR) that have the community itself set the agenda for health interventions and research (McLeroy et al., 2003; Minkler and Wallerstein, 1997).

Advocates for more intensive community involvement in public health programming suggest that the results of efforts to significantly change individual health behaviors within communities, when community is treated as setting, have been disappointing (Merzel and D'Afflitti, 2003). Moreover, while characteristics of communities may inhibit action in addressing social problems, the nature of community relationships may also be part of the solution (Chavis et al., 1993; Davis, Cohen, and Mikkelsen, 2003). For example, it has been noted that community has a powerful influence on individuals, symbolically and tangibly, by shaping identity and meaning, communicating norms, and offering and limiting opportunities for behavior (Sites, Chaskin, and Parks, 2007; Liburd and Sniezek, 2007). Communities offer a resource for change because communities can be mobilized to identify and channel resources and undertake effective action for health promotion and health enhancing social change.

The 1988 Institute of Medicine report, *The Future of Public Health*, issued a call for public health organizations to reorient their activities to assure conditions for health and to give prominence to the community as not only the logical setting, but also as the catalyst for health-promoting change. Building on the concept of community as problem and solution, a number of researchers have urged an ecological approach to public health interventions (McLeroy et al., 1988; Stokols, 1992; IOM, 2003). An ecological framework utilizes a systemic perspective regarding the interdependence of people, institutions, services, and the broader social and political environment. When used to examine the nature and extent of social relationships that exist within communities and the presence of community factors that may affect the ability of communities to mobilize to address systemic problems, this approach is based upon a theoretical concept known as **community capacity**. As will be discussed, community capacity has fostered inquiry by foundations, government agencies, and a wide array of nonprofits and academic institutions to identify and measure its associated factors.

Building capacity is seen by funding organizations as an untapped resource for improving health status and has become an integral goal of numerous grant initiatives. Grant-making institutions are keenly interested in improving their tools for identifying communities with the capacity to effect positive change, and community capacity may provide useful criteria for the awarding of grants or tailoring of interventions (Easterling et al., 1998a; MacLellan-Wright et al., 2007). If community capacity is found lacking, it may be possible to adapt health-related interventions or to develop antecedent capacity-building activities prior to implementation of health enhancing programs. Unfortunately, rating community capacity as part of a funding process could also potentially result in victim-blaming and decisions that ultimately leave some communities worse off (Burdine et al., 2003). If funding decisions are made based upon an assessment of a community's existing capacity, those with low measures of capacity may be refused funding, which may actually reduce their ability (or perceived ability) to address local issues.

In addition to community capacity as a means for achieving community health improvement, it can also be viewed as an important outcome of public health interventions (Burdine, Felix, and Wendel, 2007; MacLellan-Wright et al., 2007). Many public health interventions have as desired outcomes strengthening the capacity of individuals, families, social networks, organizations, communities, public policy, and the broader social environment (McLeroy et al., 1994). Foundations view capacity-building as an essential strategy for sustaining programs and health improvements long after grant funding periods have ended, because organizational infrastructure and the community commitment for continuation are created in the process.

Interest in community capacity touches many disciplines, including organizational development, community development, sociology and social work, criminal justice, political science, and public health. Some of this inquiry focuses on civic infrastructure, social service reform, and urban revitalization. While the end goals of interventions in these various fields differ, they share a common interest in drawing upon and building the capacity of communities to effectively address their problems. This has involved a fundamental shift away from a focus exclusively on deficit and scarcity to an *assets* perspective, embodying a dynamic and positive understanding of human, material, power, and social resources.

Despite the current interest, effective application is limited because measurement of community capacity is still in its infancy. We would like to believe that public health interventions always have positive and lasting outcomes. However, without a metric for measurement, it will remain a matter of conjecture whether community health interventions result in increased sustainability and capacity for future problem solving.

Thus, the identification and assessment of community capacity, as both an input and an outcome, is important to those striving to develop healthy communities.

This chapter will provide an overview of the concepts of community, community capacity, and its theoretical perspectives, followed by a comparison of the work of various researchers who have attempted to identify the dimensions of community capacity as a first step in the development of indices. The chapter concludes with a case study and discussion of measurement and ethical issues critical to future research. Our aim is to provide a clearer conceptual understanding of community capacity, which will contribute to the development of measurable indices and greater practical application of the construct in the field of public health.

Background

It would be difficult to discuss the concept of community capacity without first briefly discussing the concept of community. How we think about community affects how we think about the concept of community capacity, including the resources that may exist within communities to address common problems. The concept of community has a history that places it squarely in opposition to the idea of individualism and traditional liberalism (Reynolds and Norman, 1988). The essence of this tension is captured by Keller (1988):

> American society confronts a paradox. Historically, the culture has emphasized the language of individualism, laissez faire, and private property; it has valued the idea of . . . a do-it-yourself, do-your-own-thing philosophy. These ideals go against the idea of a collective destiny, of community that speaks of wholeness, interdependence, mutual trust, cooperation. (pp. 167–168)

Beginning with Thomas Jefferson's vision of democratic ideals and notions about "public work" to Tocqueville's astute observations about America's vibrant associational life (Tocqueville, 2000), the importance of communal bonds in providing essential ballast for grounding the country's moral and social fabric was established. It may be argued that historically, these community bonds represented kinship and close neighborly ties; however, it appears that perceptions of community have gradually shifted to more disperse "social kinship" relationships, yielding the ability of community to exist in less geographically bounded contexts (Keller, 1988; Macionis, 1978). This shift is illustrated in the concepts of **gemeinschaft** and **gesellschaft**, initially explored by Tönnies (1967).

As Tönnies conceived it, *gemeinschaft* was defined by bonds among individuals, rooted in kinship, tradition, affinity, and solidarity. Several definitions of community to date echo these characteristics (Hillery, 1955; Wellman and Leighton, 1979). Historically, these communities were required to be geographically bounded, because people were not as mobile. In contrast, *gesellschaft* represented the broader society, less familiar and more impersonal, but also the locus of structures (that is, government, corporations, media) upon which community members were dependent to meet their more global needs. While some interpreted and applied these distinctions as a binary pair, with *gesellschaft* ultimately positioned to overcome and replace *gemeinschaft*, more thoughtful perspectives recognized them as dialectic, needed in balance (Brint, 2001; Keller, 1988).

These concepts of community are significant in the ongoing U.S. dialogue regarding health care, as the argument has traditionally been one of "right" versus "privilege." In their volume *Medicine and the Market: Equity v. Choice*, Callahan and Wasunna (2006) argue that the adoption of a perspective of solidarity makes the current argument obsolete—the dialogue should be about in what type of society we all want to live, and subsequently what obligations we have to each other as members of the same society.

Community is most commonly described in geographically or relationally bounded terms (Hillery, 1955; Hawe, 1994). Within a geographic or political boundary, however, it is important to attend to the social dynamics of membership—who is included, or more importantly excluded, from a community bears significant weight in understanding the nature of that community.

With the rise of technologically mediated communication and relationships, the boundedness of some communities is becoming less relevant. Wellman has written extensively on distributed communities, social networks that exist based upon shared interests or experiences but may never share a face-to-face meeting (Wellman et al., 2000). Regardless of the boundaries, communities typically share values and institutions. A shared identity and interdependency are extremely important, as highlighted in this definition: "a sense of membership; common symbol systems; common values; reciprocal influence; common needs and a commitment to meeting them; and a shared history" (Israel et al., 1994). As Wellman points out, these characteristics of community can be manifested in a variety of contexts: rural village, urban neighborhood, or cyber network (Wellman et al., 2000).

While many perspectives exist, it is useful to acknowledge "that meanings of *community* in the health promotion or public health context must be seen as representations used for specific purposes in particular situations" (Stephens, 2007, p. 103).

Perspectives on Community Capacity

The concept of community capacity is consistent with Kretzmann and McKnight's conception of functional communities being defined by human and material resources that are the building blocks for assets; these assets can be identified, mobilized, and used to address issues of concern and bring about change (1993; see also Raeburn et al., 2007; Smith et al., 2001). While not inherently a health construct in the narrow or traditional sense, community capacity is tightly bound to the World Health Organization's expanded definition of health, which emphasizes the importance of control over health determinants and the inclusion of "social and personal resources, as well as physical capacities" (WHO, 1984). Community capacity is linked to quality of life and public health's goal of fostering conditions conducive to health for all, as outlined in the Ottawa Charter (WHO, 1986). However, there are real differences in conceptions of just how community capacity contributes to health.

Theoretical Perspectives

Because it is an evolving construct, it is important to examine some of the fundamental assumptions and variations in assumptions about community capacity. These assumptions are portrayed in Table 10.1 below. Each assumption stands on its own, and is not necessarily vertically linked to others. Although each of these assumptions is described as a pair of dichotomous terms, and examples or references are offered to illustrate these extremes, it is important to stress that no theory of community capacity is represented in such absolute terms. Rather, perspectives on community capacity are oriented, either explicitly or implicitly, toward one side or the other of each continuum.

Value System

Community capacity has been presented by many as a value-free concept, something that assists communities in accomplishing their purposes as they choose (Jackson et al., 2003; Labonte and Laverack, 2001b). However, a value-free approach must allow for the possibility that a community may engage in capacity-building activities that enhance the well-being of one particular community or segments within it, but are harmful to those outside it. Carried to its logical end, rapacious communities can appropriate and dominate resources to the exclusion of others, such as weaker communities or disenfranchised groups.

TABLE 10.1 Contrasting Theoretical Perspectives on Community Capacity.

Value-free	**Value System**	Value-based
Individual	**Level of Analysis**	Social organization
Harmonious and consensus-driven	**Approach**	Open to conflict and risk-driven
Homogenous	**Community Composition**	Heterogenous
Locational	**Definition of Boundaries**	Relational
Fixed	**Stability of Social System**	Dynamic
Emic	**Point of View**	Etic
Specific	**Issue Focus**	Generalized

Level of Analysis

Community capacity may be described as an underlying framework for understanding human behavior, interaction, and organization. The level of analysis may range from an individual orientation that emphasizes concepts from social psychology, such as trust, identity, self-efficacy, or the psychological sense of community, to those prominent in social organization theory, such as ties that exist among community organizations and the extent to which individual social networks share members or network ties. When community capacity is examined through an individual or psychological lens, it is viewed primarily as a set of belief systems and resources that can be measured on an individual basis and then aggregated for approximation of a community-level phenomenon.

In contrast, a more structural view of capacity would focus on the availability and accessibility of mediating structures, interorganizational relationships, distribution of power and authority.

Approach

Perspectives on community capacity are based on seeking a common ground in developing community solutions. Processes that accommodate and integrate different perspectives through use of a consensus-based, collaborative process are highly valued. Central principles include equity, participation, and self-determination (Raeburn et al., 2007).

Conflict is inherent in the nature of community life, and under some circumstances conflict may play an important role in building capacity, since it may serve as a catalyst for action (Labonte, 1997; Chaskin et al., 2001). In communities with large disenfranchised populations and community norms that mitigate political and social participation of significant minorities, consensus-based approaches may not be the only solution to building capacity, or even the most appropriate.

Definition of Boundaries

Definition of a community and its subsequent community capacity may be dramatically affected by the boundaries through which the community is defined. At one extreme, a locational perspective defines a community by geographic boundaries, such as streets, freeways, or other man-made or natural features. At the other extreme, a relational perspective defines a community by social networks or associational patterns.

In defining community capacity, then, it is important to focus not only on geographic or geopolitical boundaries, but also on the nature of ties or connections that exist within communities, including network connections among individuals and interorganizational relationships.

Community Composition

With relational communities defined, at least in part, by shared social norms, the extent of homogeneity in a community will have considerable influence on the ease or challenge of fostering greater connectedness among community members and on the strengthening of community capacity. More homogeneous communities may find it easier to build a sense of trust and sense of belonging. However, homogeneous communities may lack the variety of different perspectives inherent in more heterogeneous settings, hampering the long-term development of a civil society (O'Connell, 1999). Granovetter (1973) highlights the importance of weak ties that bridge social distance between different sectors or social groupings. Bridging ties have value in diffusion of innovations, access to mobility opportunities for individuals, and in enhancing cohesion for community building.

Stability of Social Systems

A critical issue in using this construct to strengthen community is the extent to which community interaction patterns, social norms, and organizational structures are malleable. On the one hand, we may regard community capacity as resulting from an evolutionary process that has historical foundations in the development of solidarity and social institutions over time. While some aspects of capacity are more challenging to modify, others may be more sensitive to change. On the other hand, even if this latter assumption is made, respect for the stability, longevity, and functional role of existing social systems is paramount. Dimensions of social systems are fragile and more vulnerable to erosion than to fortification.

Insider vs. Outsider Point of View

Although used primarily within the field of anthropology to describe the two principal approaches to the study of native peoples (Lett, 1990), the constructs of *emic* and *etic* points of view are useful in the discussion of community capacity. An emic view represents concepts and categories that are meaningful and appropriate from the perspective of the people being studied, while an etic view presents constructs that are meaningful and appropriate to those conducting the analysis. The importance of this distinction is more than simple semantics. A lack of sensitivity to "native" wisdom or view of community members about what constitutes community and capacity may threaten the validity of findings and conclusions, may threaten our ability to work productively with communities, and may threaten our capacity to inform broader audiences.

Issue Focus

A very practical and theoretical issue with community capacity is whether or not it is a generalized state or condition in communities or a specific response to a given problem or concern. The extent to which capacity is mobilized to address a specific problem may be contingent upon the extent to which a social issue is on the public agenda, and the extent to which individuals or organizations are available to serve a catalytic or leadership role.

Theoretically, community capacity consists of characteristics that affect a community's mobilization of resources, the extent to which communities are open to new problem definitions, and their ability to disseminate information and develop consensus.

However, communities, like individuals, may have a limited span of attention. Too many items on the public agenda may lead to a less effective allocation of resources and reduced capacity around specific concerns.

Definitions of Community Capacity

Chaskin and colleagues (2001) drew upon their experiences with comprehensive community initiatives to develop a definition of community capacity that also addresses ways to build capacity, and incorporates the influence of community context and desired outcomes.

> Community capacity is the interaction of human capital, organization resources, and social capital existing within a given community that can be leveraged to solve collective problems and improve or maintain the well-being of that community. It may operate through informal social processes and/or organized efforts by individuals, organizations, and social networks that exist among them and between them and the larger systems of which the community is a part. (p. 7)

The Aspen Institute calls community capacity "the ability of individuals, organizations, businesses, and governments in their community to come together, learn, make well-reasoned decisions about the community's present and future, *and* to work together to carry out those decisions" (1996). Within a public health context, Speers and colleagues (1996) provide a definition of community capacity as: "characteristics of communities that affect their ability to identify, mobilize, and address social and public health problems." Jackson and colleagues (2003) emphasize the role of broader environmental forces on the manifestation of existing capacity. They argue that community capacity is "a combination of (i) talents and capabilities, and (ii) the socioenvironmental conditions . . . that enable or disable the expression of the existing talents" (p. 340).

Building upon Chaskin's definition, community capacity is regarded as *a set of dynamic community traits, resources, and associational patterns that can be brought to bear for community building and community health improvement.* Captured within the definition are structural networks and the processes to cultivate and maintain them, as well as the perceptions, skills, and resources of individuals that are channeled through these social structures. This definition makes clear a theoretical position of community capacity as a value-laden concept focused upon the attributes of both individuals and social structures.

DIMENSIONS OF COMMUNITY CAPACITY

A number of researchers have attempted to develop a set of dimensions or characteristics for the construct of community capacity. Table 10.2, which follows, provides a sense of the dimensions various researchers view as most important; this comparison

TABLE 10.2 Dimensions of Community Capacity and Cognate Constructs.

	Cottrell, 1976 (community competence)	Goodman et al., 1998 (community capacity)	Easterling et al., 1998 (community capacity)	Chaskin et al., 2001 (community capacity)	Laverack, 2001 (community capacity)
Skills and Resources	Articulateness Management of relations with the larger society	Skills Resources (financial, technological, other material, etc.)	Skills and knowledge	Access to resources	Ability to mobilize internal resources and access external resources
Nature of Social Relations	Commitment Conflict containment and accommodation	Sense of community Social capital/ trust (listed as type of "resource")	Trusting relationships and norms of reciprocity Sense of efficacy and confidence among residence	Commitment among community members Sense of community	Links with others Role of outside agents (facilitators/ organizers, consultants)
Structures and Mechanisms for Community Dialogue	Communication Machinery for facilitating participant interaction and decision making	Social and interorganizational networks Mechanisms for communication across the community and for citizen input (listed as type of "resource")		Mechanisms of problem solving	Organizational (mediating) structures Program management (includes community control)

Leadership	Leadership	Leadership		Strong leadership
Civic Participation	Participation	Participation	Participation	Participation
	Awareness of self and others and clarity of situational definitions	Community power (distribution)		Problem assessment (identification of problems and action to resolve are carried out by the community; self-determination)
Value System		Community values		
Learning Culture	Understanding of community history	Culture of learning		"Asking why"
	Critical reflection			

Notes: a. The Harwood Group's model of public capital defines categories of dimensions: (1) tangible dimensions; (2) links between the tangible dimensions; (3) underlying values. b. Certain dimensions of the models above have been split into more than one category. The way that the researcher originally classified the dimension is shown in parentheses.

is not intended to be comprehensive, but rather to provide a sense of the similarities and variations in existing conceptualizations of community capacity. A total of five research models and their dimensions are presented in order of the year in which they were published.

Four models describe dimensions of what the researchers call "community capacity." These include: Goodman et al. (1998) from the field of public health; Easterling et al. (1998b) writing on behalf of a Colorado-based philanthropic organization; Chaskin et al. (2001) from the field of social work and urban policy; and Laverack (2005) also from public health. The other research model and its dimensions are displayed to both highlight the similarities and illustrate a few areas of departure from the construct of community capacity, as we describe it. The cognate constructs of this model are characterized in terms of "community competence" (Cottrell, 1976).

Cottrell (1976) described "community competence" as the ability of a community to draw together its parts to collaborate effectively in identifying its problems and needs, developing a consensus on solutions and implementing their planned actions. He outlined eight dimensions that he saw as critical to community competence. A community psychologist by training, he placed his greatest emphasis on individual perceptions, skills, and consciousness. Among the elements, he included a mechanism for facilitating interaction, but made no mention of social networks or leadership, two essential dimensions of community capacity.

A set of seven dimensions defining the community capacity construct are distilled from this analysis. These dimensions are constructed to represent the highest degree of consensus among researchers, while preserving the particular character and emphasis of each model. The categories are labeled to avoid jargon, and any explicit terms used for the various constructs themselves (for example, social capital). Because of the variability in the way that researchers characterize different dimensions of these models, the placement of any dimension within a given model is open to debate. However, this display represents one attempt at illustrating both the similarities and the differences among these cognate constructs and their various interpretations of community capacity.

Level of Skills, Knowledge, and Resources

Skills and knowledge are identified as critical to community capacity by many researchers. This dimension includes skills for strategic planning and those related to interpersonal communication and group process. Chaskin et al. (2001) discussed this in terms of **human capital** and leadership. He linked human capital and leadership by explaining that the use of skills, knowledge, and resources by residents through participation in community improvement activities entails the exercise of leadership.

Although the most common emphasis is placed upon internal community resources—a community's gifts and assets (Kretzmann and McKnight, 1993)—access to resources external to the community may be equally vital. An excessive or deficient level of resources available to a community can impair the process of building capacity. External resources are not viewed as capacity enhancing unless they reduce dependency through the transfer of skills from external to internal sources. A reliance on externally imported skills and expertise is viewed as counter to capacity-building goals. Interventions typically stress the benefits of expanding a community's information base—data and knowledge. Technical assistance has been the principle vehicle for achieving this purpose, but asset mapping and skill/resource inventories are increasingly used (Raeburn et al., 2007).

Nature of Social Relationships

The concept of social relationships builds upon the idea of communities as social networks and social ties, and is integral to the construct of social capital, as it is defined in most of the scholarly literature. The notion of **social connectedness** highlights the quality of ties that exist among community members and the type and strength of sentiments embodied within those relationships. Included in this dimension is the belief that one matters to the community; that there is sufficient strength of social ties to work through serious differences; and that one's actions, on both an individual and collective basis, will have desired results. For this reason it includes a sense of community, a sense of commitment and harmony, social trust, norms of reciprocity, and positive intergroup relations.

Structures, Mechanisms, and Spaces for Community Dialogue and Collective Action

This dimension represents a collection of tangible assets that provide the structural framework for community capacity. Included are social and interorganizational networks, especially voluntary associations; mechanisms for prompting and conducting community planning and action; "safe" community spaces for socializing and for problem solving; and systems for community-wide communication.

Social networks refer to the extent to which individuals are connected to each other through formal and informal networks of relationships, and the extent to which social networks in the community share linkages or members. Since social resources—including instrumental assistance, emotional support, social identity, access to new social contacts, and information—flow across network ties, the distribution of social resources will be affected by the nature and extent of connectedness that exist in a community (Israel, 1985).

Social networks, such as friendship groups, are frequently developed within the context of the workplace, neighborhood, church, school, or other informal and formal organizations to which individuals belong. Thus, an important part of a community's capacity is its voluntary associational life.

In addition to social networks and collaborative interorganizational structures, mechanisms for community dialogue may include catalytic organizations within communities and gathering spaces for interaction and public debate. Catalytic organizations can provide the impetus for changing the status quo by making the gap between what is and what could be visible to leaders and community members.

Quality of Leadership and Its Development

Leadership is critical in identifying problems, fostering community change activities, and providing opportunities for citizen participation. Effective leadership, then, requires qualities of communication, analysis and judgment, coaching, visioning, trust building, teamwork, reflection, learning, and partnering (Human Resources Development Canada, 2000). Several issues are important for this dimension: the types of community leaders utilized, the development of leadership roles and new leaders, and the process for transitioning from old to new leadership.

Communities with greater capacity draw upon the skills of not only those in positions of office, supervision or management, but also tap the talents of those who are extensively connected within and across diverse community constituencies. In addition, new leaders are needed as new leadership positions develop and as "older" leaders retire, step down, or move onto other interests. With the rapid changes in the demographic composition of many communities—including the rapid growth in populations from other cultures and ethnic backgrounds, the aging of society, and changes in gender, age, and marital status roles—the development of new community leaders is critical. New leadership, however, must represent the increasing diversity of groups, cultures, and orientations present in many of our communities.

Extent of Civic Participation

The importance of **civic participation** as an essential element in community capacity is inconsistently addressed by researchers who have defined community capacity and similar constructs (although it may be implied within other dimensions by those who fail to specify it explicitly). It is maintained here, as an explicit and distinct dimension, to emphasize its significance, and because it serves as an important area of capacity-building leverage for health improvement interventions. This dimension describes the extent to which individuals within a community concern themselves with issues of broad public concern, including those relating to governance. It encompasses everything from PTA membership to voting behavior, from volunteering rates to participation in small groups that provide input from specific constituencies, to groups and institutions at higher organizational or community levels.

Attributes of participation relate to breadth, depth, and intensity. A broad and representative base of citizen involvement is made possible when there is continuous conversation with all community segments. This requires constant outreach efforts and communication on the part of community leaders and members. It also requires vigilance in the cultivation of mutual trust and a vitality of neighborhood and social networks that link with each other, not simply within themselves. Mediating structures play a critical role in defining the nature, extent, and intensity of civic participation, since they provide the primary vehicle for its expression.

Value System

Community capacity is not value free, and must encompass the norms, standards, expectations, and desires of particular communities. What is essential to capacity is not only that a community be able to articulate a clear and shared set of values, but that these values reflect a public moral philosophy (Elshtain, 1999). Many researchers agree that core values for capacity-building include: equity, democratic participation, collaboration, inclusion, and social responsibility (Goodman et al., 1998).

Learning Culture

This dimension defines a community's ability to think critically and reflect upon assumptions underlying one's ideas and actions, to consider alternative ways of thinking and doing, and to mine lessons from one's actions. This reflects a high degree of self-awareness about a community's values and interests and a strong institutional memory. The community culture must be one in which errors and failures are viewed as resources for learning instead of excuses for nonaction or instruments of blame. Communities that can reflect upon the outcomes of their actions and upon new options available to them may be more effective in maintaining change and improvements in social and health-related conditions.

Application

Labonte and Laverack (2001a; 2001b) describe community capacity as simultaneously the means and end of community-based health promotion. Building community capacity should be a "parallel track" to improving the target issue of an intervention. Thus, in working with communities to implement programs, capacity is both an outcome and an enabling factor (Laverack, 2005; Smith et al., 2001). Organizing community partnerships or local collaboratives to improve health status is not a new idea. The Partnership Approach, for example, was first implemented in the late 1970s in Lycoming County, Pennsylvania, and later adopted by the Kaiser Family Foundation. It is an example that incorporates community capacity-building as an outcome equal to population health status improvement (Felix, 1993). Efforts by the United Nation's World Health Organization date back to at least the 1980s.

Other examples of specific interventions that emphasize community capacity-building as a key component of health status improvement efforts are found in WISEWOMAN (Yancey, 2004), the American Indian Oncology Program (Coe et al., 2006), Center for Substance Abuse Treatment projects (Maxwell and Husain, 2005), and others.

International examples allow us to appreciate the importance of understanding context, and that fundamental processes and principles translate from setting to setting. Yuasa et al. emphasize the importance of attending to skills and relationship networks in their discussion of building social capital along with financial and physical capital in health promotion infrastructure development (Yuasa et al., 2007). Studies from Africa (Chilaka, 2005), China (Tang et al., 2005), and Canada (Dressendorfer et al, 2005), among others, demonstrate the effectiveness of community capacity-building initiatives.

Although the contexts and approaches to building community capacity vary widely, several common themes emerge:

- The need to recognize community capacity-building as a parallel outcome of health improvement initiatives;

- The need for facilitators trained to focus on building community capacity for health improvement, as well as more traditional health outcomes;

- The need to recognize that the participatory nature of communities varies with culture and economic settings;

- The need to firmly establish the role and impact of the social determinants of health in community capacity-oriented initiatives; and

- The need to recognize that capacity-building has both skill and knowledge as well as relational aspects.

CASE STUDY: THE BRAZOS VALLEY, TEXAS

Two related models of capacity-building are offered in the recent literature: the community action model (Lavery et al., 2005) and the community health development model (Burdine, Felix, and Wendel, 2007). Community health development, guided by the Partnership Approach, emphasizes community capacity-building; this model is the basis of the activities described in the case study (Wendel, Burdine, and McLeroy, 2007). The Brazos Valley example is one that provides illustrations from a geographically defined community consisting of numerous smaller communities. The region is unique in that its rurality and size contribute to dense, local networks, while at the same time the presence of a large university within the region brings more cosmopolitan residents with external ties—a good example of the balance of *gemeinschaft* and *gesellschaft*. The case study also provides perspective on examining the nature of capacity—particularly how capacity may be manifested in different ways and be applied diversely to address similar issues.

Background

In the fall of 2001, the School of Rural Public Health at the Texas A&M Health Science Center made a commitment to establishing relationships with communities in the Brazos Valley, where it is located. The region consists of a small urban center, Brazos County, with an estimated population of slightly more than 170,000, and six surrounding rural counties ranging in population from approximately 13,500 to just over 32,000, for a regional total of about 275,000.

To initiate collaboration with the community, the School of Rural Public Health (SRPH) arranged a meeting in June 2001 for regional leaders representing health care, local government, social services, private business, education, and faith-based organizations, among others, to learn about the newly established Center for Community Health Development (CCHD). At this meeting, the Center director introduced the concept of community health development and offered the school's resources to initiate a region-wide, population-based health status assessment and the creation of a local health partnership focused on building capacity for regional health improvement.

The objectives of the assessment were to identify factors influencing health status, to recognize issues and needs of the local community, to inventory resources within the region, and to produce a source of reliable information that could be utilized in developing effective solutions. This assessment consisted of three components: community discussion groups, mailed household surveys, and secondary data analysis. From the discussion groups, perceptions, attitudes, and concerns of community members were obtained. In addition, the resources available to address problems and advice about how to go about solving problems were identified.

The findings of the 2002 assessment were released as part of a two-day regional health summit in July of that year. The key issues identified included limited access to care and disparities in health resources and health status for residents of the rural communities of the region. At the conclusion of the summit, the attendees organized themselves as the Brazos Valley Health Partnership (BVHP), with the mission "to improve health status and access to care in the seven-county region of the Brazos Valley through the collaboration of services and the creation of local partnerships." At its inception, BVHP membership consisted of representatives from thirty health, social services, community-based, and local government organizations.

Over the next few months, the partnership worked through task groups that would develop plans for their regional health improvement strategy: creation of local health partnerships in the rural communities that would oversee and manage new health resource centers to expand access to care for rural residents. A health resource center, as designed by the partnership, is a single facility where various providers can simultaneously offer services either on a regular or itinerant basis and share the administrative costs associated with providing a "satellite office" in a rural community. The colocation of providers is also intended to provide a natural setting for the collaboration and coordination of services. Each center would be unique based upon each county's capacity to leverage local resources to develop the center, and upon their community's specific needs and local characteristics. However, all health resource centers would have five basic service components: (1) information and referral provided by the local United Way's 2–1–1 service; (2) case management provided by a local nonprofit; (3) transportation offered through local volunteers; (4) medication assistance; and (5) access to remote care via telehealth through an existing regional telehealth system.

Staffed by the Center for Community Health Development, the BVHP worked with rural communities to forge county-level health partnerships that would plan for, develop, monitor, and sustain their community's health resource center. Between 2003 and 2006, four counties—Burleson, Madison, Grimes, and Leon—developed local health partnerships that were all subsequently given formal appointments as county health resource commissions. Each of the four counties planned, financed, and opened health resource centers to serve their local residents. We will draw on specific experiences from those communities to illustrate the seven overarching dimensions of community capacity as outlined in Table 10.2.

Level of Skills, Knowledge, and Resources

When the communities began organizing their local health partnerships, they largely deferred to staff from CCHD. In addition, a large grant to the region provided seed funding to each community to launch their health resource centers. Initially, CCHD personnel were developing agendas, planning meetings, taking and distributing meeting minutes, identifying resources, and facilitating strategic planning. Over time, the community members engaged in the process gradually assumed those responsibilities. In Burleson County, for example, the commission appointed an executive director and charged him with managing the administrative responsibilities.

Another interesting change among community members was the adoption of a broader definition of health. Encouraged through discussions with center staff, they began to recognize that "broader" issues, such as transportation and family stability affected their overall well-being and prioritize them in their strategic plans.

In addition, the startup funding from the regional grant provided a unique opportunity for local organizations in the rural communities to attempt to leverage their resources at relatively low risk. In Madison and Burleson counties, the local hospital committed space and utilities to potential service providers. Seeing the hospitals' commitment, the City, County, and school districts also committed funding. As the health resource commissions planned for the grant to end, they actively reaffirmed with each contributor their intentions of continuing their support, and both communities to date are locally sustaining the activities begun with grant funding. Leon County had a similar experience, but in addition to local resources, they were subsequently able to obtain a federal grant to expand their local initiative to improve access to mental health services.

Nature of Social Relationships

Because many families in the four rural counties have lived on their family land for multiple generations and know their fellow residents very well, capacity-building efforts can take advantage of these dense social networks. Capitalizing on these close ties and the ties among government leaders with their counterparts in other Brazos Valley communities, CCHD staff were able to facilitate the organization of partnerships and activities relatively quickly. In addition, new ties were fostered among individuals not directly related to health services and those who were not previously in positions of community leadership, as will be discussed. The county judges from Leon and Burleson counties began consulting with each other about the strategies in their respective communities, as did the public health nurses and the commission chairpersons.

The health resource commissions in each community consist of residents from various perspectives, not all inherently health-focused. Representatives from public education, private farmers and ranchers, business owners, retired military and law enforcement personnel all realized their ability to influence what health priorities were pursued in their community, and became active in their local commissions.

Forum for Community Dialogue and Collective Action

Texas counties are governed by an elected county judge and four elected commissioners; the judge serves as the CEO of the county, while the commissioners are equivalent to the board. Most of the cities are governed by a city council, headed by a mayor (and sometimes a city manager). In rural communities, the meetings of these bodies provide a regular forum for dialogue and action for issues related to the city or county agenda.

In recognition of the lack of opportunities to promote dialogue and action specifically around community health-related issues, the BVHP's regional plan was to help establish informal county health partnerships, leading to formal resource commissions that would include a broad cross-section of community stakeholders. The commissions in each county developed bylaws containing specific processes and mechanisms for assessment, planning, evaluation, and negotiation with external agents.

To overcome the mixed results of previous efforts to help establish local services provided by regional organizations, Burleson, Leon, and Madison counties each created a process for service providers to present their proposals to the health resource commission at an open meeting. The commission then discusses the proposal privately and solicits feedback from other community members before giving an answer to the service provider. If the commission elects to support the service provider, a formal agreement is executed, specifying the expectations of both parties. This process illustrates the key philosophical underpinnings of community capacity-building—including participation and self-determination.

Leadership

As the BVHP's regional health initiative was begun in each new county, the primary focus at the outset was to identify local leaders who could "champion" health initiatives. Leaders in each community came from different sectors—a county judge, a hospital CEO, a retired Army colonel, the local mayor. Because the nature of leadership in rural communities is often for one leader to "wear multiple hats," CCHD's efforts were twofold: (1) identify existing leadership that could assist in organizing a partnership, and (2) determine the best way to develop new leadership in the community to expand their ability to implement and manage health initiatives.

In Grimes County, many of the local residents reminisced about days past when strong leadership provided solid direction for their community. Now, they reported, the old leaders had moved on and there was no one to take their place. Filling this void had been problematic. After two false starts in organizing a local partnership, the executive director of a local foundation finally realized that she could take charge of the health resource commission's activities, although she had not been placed in a formal position of community leadership in Grimes County. With the blessing of the mayor, she has been able to mobilize the human, social, and material capital necessary to open their health resource center.

In Madison County, developing new leadership was also a challenge. Historically, the same eight men served on every local board and were seen as the leaders. Without their support, efforts in the community were unlikely to succeed. Unfortunately, as is often the case in rural communities, these men were already overcommitted and unwilling to take on an additional responsibility. Working through the networks they had identified, CCHD found the owner of a local home health agency about to retire; she was recruited to become the leader of Madison's health resource commission. Mentored both by CCHD staff and by the executive director of the Burleson Health Resource Commission, this woman has taken on the responsibilities of leadership in her community at a level she had not previously experienced.

Civic Participation

Civic participation is perhaps the characteristic that connects community capacity to related constructs like social capital, community competence, and civic engagement. In the rural counties of the Brazos Valley, a norm of civic participation already existed. Parents are generally active in school activities, businesses are active in giving back to their communities, and leaders volunteer their time. Most residents read their local paper when it is published each week, and most residents attend church regularly. These dense social networks also facilitate communication and dissemination of information that allow residents to identify opportunities to get involved in activities of interest.

Given the existing level of civic participation, creating a forum specific to health issues provided an avenue for residents to engage and, as anticipated, they did. As a result, CCHD staff were able to focus on the residents who were typically not represented in these forums—the low-income, minority, and geographically isolated. Finding the venues to access these populations—mostly through local intermediaries and churches or faith-based organizations—was challenging, but the response was consistently, "We've never been asked." Given this feedback, Burleson County acknowledged the lack of effort to communicate with and engage those residents, and subsequently began developing mechanisms to include underrepresented populations in the broader community dialogue.

Community Values

A source of pride for many Texas communities is their strong "rugged individualism," pulling themselves "up by their bootstraps." In attempting to facilitate collaboration, CCHD staff were initially challenged by this staunch independence, forced to wonder if nurturing relationships within and among these communities would ever yield results. Staff identified an effective strategy building on this sense of independence. Once the community representatives understood that the counties—and even the region—could not count on the state capital or Washington, D.C. to deliver solutions, they realized that coming together and doing it "on their own" fit their philosophy very well.

Burleson, Leon, and Madison counties have since achieved enough success that they routinely refer to that success as an indicator of their local ability to address issues. Grimes County, while not as far along in the process, is beginning to demonstrate similar appreciation of their growing local problem-solving capacity.

Learning Culture

Goodman et al. (1998) characterize this dimension as critical reflexivity; others describe it simply as a community "asking why" (MacLellan-Wright et al., 2007; Laverack, 2005). In each of the communities, their newness to health planning allowed them a lot of latitude in considering multiple perspectives. In Leon County, the twenty-three-member health resource commission wrestled with the pros and cons of collaborating with other communities, as opposed to "going it alone." Their experiences with previous regional collaborations addressing local issues encouraged them to be independent and not rely on anyone outside their community. But as they began to appreciate and value the resources available to them through this collaboration, they began to reevaluate their "go it alone" attitude. This ongoing process of evaluation and planning has led them to engage very actively in the regional partnership.

Grimes County is a community deeply rooted in their historical traditions, with a very strong sense of insiders versus outsiders. Consequently, there exists a strong undercurrent of resistance to change, even if it would mean progress and development for the county's residents. Initiated by a county commissioner who had been exposed to the successes of the other counties, community members began asking why Grimes County could not establish its own health resource commission and health resource center. CCHD staff worked with potential commission members over many months to assist them in identifying their opportunities for collaboration, as well as the barriers they faced. Once the commission members were able to achieve consensus about what they believed would fit their community, they have aggressively pursued development of their resource center and expansion of services.

FUTURE DIRECTIONS

The experiences of the Brazos Valley Health Partnership and its constituent communities over the past several years provide rich examples of the struggles and successes of capacity-building efforts that touch on the domains of community capacity to varying degrees. It also highlights the parallel track perspective—that building capacity can be both the means and outcome of health promotion efforts.

In addition to the multidimensional models presented in Table 10.2, it is important to note an emerging perspective on community capacity that is less well defined, but insightful and promising. Foster-Fishman and colleagues (2001) and Merzel and

Moon-Howard (2003) both present a social ecological perspective on community capacity that acknowledges component capacities within community members and their relationships, organizations, and programs, community systems, policies, and the broader environment. This systems perspective, while inherently complex, is valuable to understanding the dynamics and interplay among the myriad factors affecting communities' ability to access and use existing resources to enhance their capacity.

As the identified dimensions of community capacity have begun to converge, several researchers have undertaken the task of measurement. Some approaches to measurement are intended to provide a way to visualize changes over time, such as the "spider-gram," which provides a "leg" to each dimension, with a scale of one to four (Laverack, 2005). Connecting the corresponding markers on each leg yields a polygon whose area denotes the measure of overall community capacity. Others have focused on validating measurement of one of the dimensions, such as leadership (Granner and Sharpe, 2004), interorganizational networks (Singer and Kegler, 2004), or social capital (Putnam, 2000). Jackson and colleagues (2003) emphasize the interplay of internal and external forces that either enable or constrain a community's ability to use its capacity. Through work with residents of four neighborhoods in Toronto, they developed a capacity model and proposed a set of comprehensive indicators and measures. Although they did not attempt to test or validate their measures, MacLellan-Wright and colleagues (2007) synthesized items from four validated instruments and expanded on those measures, developing a new scale covering nine domains of community capacity consonant with the models outlined in Table 10.2.

Researchers involved in the Brazos Valley Health Partnership routinely wrestle with selecting the best way to capture changes in capacity over time, given the limitations of existing mechanisms for measurement. The partnership has formally measured various dimensions of capacity, such as participation, leadership, and interorganizational networks. More informal measures are used to evaluate skills/resources, values, and reflexivity. While these measures seem to indicate positive changes in capacity, the measures were developed independently of each other, not specifically focused on capacity, and it is unclear how the data from each dimension should be used in relation to the other dimensions.

The experience of researchers working with the Brazos Valley Health Partnership is indicative of the challenges that face others interested in understanding a measuring community capacity. In spite of the varying perspectives and applications of both community and capacity, it seems that three themes are emerging in the research agenda related to community capacity. First, there is a need to narrow the gap between theory and practice; that is, research should be designed in a way to capture and disseminate what many practitioners already know.

Second, we must consider the possibility that by distilling community capacity into distinct components to more clearly explain the concept, we may have actually weakened our understanding by not adequately reflecting the relationships among those components. Perhaps it would be useful to apply a systems perspective to the study of community capacity, focusing on the dynamics of the ways in which the components are connected, and viewing capacity, like community, as an emergent property rather than merely a sum of the parts.

Finally, to enhance our understanding of the dynamics of community capacity, we need to synthesize the measures. Fortunately, the constructs of capacity are inherently measurable, and we know how to capture most of them. The problem in measurement in this case is not the lack of tools or instruments, but that community capacity as a concept is complex; it is cumbersome to attempt to use measures of the different dimensions simultaneously, and even if we did, we do not have a strong enough understanding of how they fit together to make sense of the results. Utilizing more qualitative, contextual measures to facilitate synthesis of community information may provide additional insight.

As the principles of capacity-building continue to be applied in communities throughout the world, researchers will continue to have ample opportunity to continue in developing our collective understanding.

SUMMARY

Community capacity refers to the characteristics of a community that enable it to identify and address issues of community concern. Community capacity can be thought of as both a means and an end for community-based health promotion efforts. A certain level of community capacity is needed for a community to successfully mount an effective community health improvement initiative. At the same time, individuals, social groups, and community institutions can be strengthened through involvement in a health promotion effort with these new skills, resources, relationships, norms, and practices applied to future community issues and concerns. Key dimensions of capacity, identified across several models, include: level of skills, knowledge, and resources, the nature of social relationships, quality of leadership and its development, extent of civic participation, value systems, community boundaries, and community composition. Community capacity is challenging to measure, and distillation of capacity into a set of dimensions, while an important measurement task, may mask important relationships between components unless a systems perspective is taken.

REFERENCES

Adler, N. E., and Rehkopf, D. H. (2008). U.S. disparities in health: Descriptions, causes, and mechanisms. *Annual Review of Public Health*, *29*, 10.1–10.18.

Aspen Institute. (1996). *Measuring community capacity: A workbook-in-progress for rural communities.* Washington, D.C.: Aspen Institute Rural Economic Development Policy Program.

Brint, S. (2001). *Gemeinschaft* revisited: A critique and reconstruction of the community concept. *Sociological Theory*, *19*(1), 1–23.

Burdine, J. N., Felix, M.R.J., and Wendel, M. L. (2007). The basics of community health development. *Texas Public Health Association Journal*, *59*(1), 10–11.

Burdine, J. N., Felix, M.R.J., Wendel, M. L., and Somachandran, S. (2003). A discussion of the political and policy implications of a rating system of community capacity to improve population health. *Family and Community Health Journal, 26,* 254–267.

Callahan, D., and Wasunna, A. A. (2006). *Medicine and the market: Equity v. choice.* Baltimore, MD: Johns Hopkins University Press.

Chaskin, R. J., Brown, P., Venkatesh, S., and Vidal, A. (2001). *Building community capacity.* New York: Aldine de Gruyter.

Chavis, D. M., Speer, P. W., Resnick, I., and Zippay, A. (1993). Building community capacity to address alcohol and drug abuse: Getting to the heart of the problem. In R. C. Davis, A. J. Lurigio and D.P. Rosenbaum, *Drugs and the community.* Springfield, IL: Charles C. Thomas.

Chilaka, M. A. (2005). Ascribing quantitative value to community participation: A case study of the Roll Back Malaria (RBM) initiative in five African countries. *Public Health, 119*(11), 987–994.

Coe, K., Wilson, C., Eisenberg, M., Attakai, A., and Lobell, M. (2006). Creating the environment for a successful community partnership. *Cancer, 107*(8 Supplement), 1980–1986.

Cottrell, L. (1976). "The competent community." In B. Kaplan, R. Wilson and A. Leighton (eds.). *Further explorations in social psychiatry.* New York: Basic Books.

Davis, R., Cohen, L., and Mikkelsen, L. (2003). *Strengthening communities: A prevention framework for reducing health disparities.* Oakland, CA: Prevention Institute.

DiClemente, R. J., Salazar, L. F., and Crosby, R. A. (2007). A review of STD/HIV preventive interventions for adolescents: Sustaining effects using an ecological approach. *Journal of Pediatric Psychology, 32*(8), 888–906.

Dressendorfer, R. H., Raine, K., Dyck, R. J., Plotnikoff, R. C., Collins-Nakai, R. L., McLaughlin, W. K., and Ness, K. (2005). A conceptual model of community capacity development for health promotion in the Alberta Heart Health Project. *Health Promotion Practice, 6*(1), 31–36.

Easterling, D., Gallagher, K., Drisko, J., and Johnson, T. (1998a). *Promoting health by building community capacity: Evidence and implications for grantmakers.* Denver: The Colorado Trust.

Easterling, D., Gallagher, K., Drisko, J., and Johnson, T. (1998b). *Promoting health by building community capacity: Summary.* Denver: The Colorado Trust.

Elshtain, J. B. (1999). Civil society and the American family: A call to civil society. *Society, 36*(5), 11–19.

Felix, M.R.J. (1993). The partnership approach for sustaining heart health. *Canadian Journal of Cardiology, 9,* Supplement D.

Florin, P., and Chavis, D. (1990). Community development and substance abuse prevention." In *Community development, community participation and substance abuse prevention.* Bureau of Drug Abuse Services, Santa Clara, CA.

Foster-Fishman, P. G., Berkowitz, S. L., Lounsbury, D.W.; Jacobson, S., and Allen. N. A. (2001). Building collaborative capacity in community coalitions: A review and integrative framework. *American Journal of Community Psychology, 29*(2), 241–261.

Goodman, R. M., Speers, M. A., McLeroy, K. L., Fawcett, S., Kegler, M., Parker, E., Smith, S., Sterling, I. T., and Wallerstein, N. (1998). An attempt to identify and define the dimensions of community capacity to provide a basis for measurement. *Health Education and Behavior, 25*(3), 258–278.

Granner, M. L., and Sharpe, P. A. (2004). Evaluating community coalition characteristics and functioning: A summary of measurement tools. *Health Education Research, 19*(5), 514–532.

Granovetter, M. (1973). The strength of weak ties. *American Journal of Sociology, 78*(6), 1360–1379.

Hawe, P. (1994). Capturing the meaning of "community" in community intervention evaluation: Some contributions from community psychology. *Health Promotion International, 9*(3), 199–210.

Hillery, G. A. (1955). Definitions of community: Areas of agreement. *Rural Sociology, 20,* 111–123.

Human Resources Development Canada. (2000). *Community capacity building toolkit.* © Her Majesty the Queen in Right of Canada. Available at http://www.participation.net/english/ccbgoc.htm

Institute of Medicine. (1988). *The future of public health.* Washington, DC: National Academy Press.

Institute of Medicine. (2003). *Who will keep the public healthy?* Washington, DC: National Academy Press.

Israel, B. A. (1985). Social networks and social support: Implications for natural helper and community-level interventions. *Health Education Quarterly*, *12*(1), 65–80.

Israel, B. A., Checkoway, B. Schulz, A., and Zimmerman, M. (1994). Health education and community empowerment: Conceptualizing and measuring perceptions of individual, organizational, and community control, *Health Education Quarterly*, *21*(2), 149–170.

Jackson, S. F., Cleverly, S., Poland, B., Burman, D., Edwards, R., and Robertson, A. (2003). Working with Toronto neighborhoods toward developing indicators of community capacity. *Health Promotion International*, *18*(4), 339–350.

Keller, S. (1988). The American dream of community: An unfinished agenda. *Sociological Forum*, *3*(2), 167–183.

Kretzmann, J., and McKnight, J. (1993). *Building Communities from the inside out*. Evanston, IL: Center for Urban Affairs, Northwestern University.

Krieger, N. (2008). Proximal, distal, and the politics of causation: What's level got to do with it? *American Journal of Public Health*, *98*, 221–230.

Labonte, R., and Laverack, G. (2001a). Capacity building in promotion, Part 1: for whom? And for what purpose? *Critical Public Health*, *11*(2), 111–127.

Labonte, R., and Laverack, G. (2001b). Capacity building in promotion, Part 2: Whose use? And with what measurement? *Critical Public Health*, *11*(2), 129–138.

Labonte, R. (1997). Community, community development, and the forming of authentic partnerships. In M. Minkler (ed.), *Community organizing and community building for health*. New Brunswick, NJ: Rutgers University Press.

Laverack, G., and Labonte, R. (2000). A planning framework for community empowerment goals within health promotion. *Health Policy and Planning*, *15*(3), 255–262.

Laverack, G. (2005). Evaluating community capacity: Visual representation and interpretation. *Community Development Journal, 41*(3), 266–276.

Lavery, S., Smith, M., Esparza, A., Hrushow, A., Moore, M., and Reed, D.F. (2005). The community action model: A community-driven model designed to address disparities in health. *American Journal of Public Health*, *95*(4), 611–616.

Lett, J. (1990). Emics and etics: Notes on epistemology of anthropology. In Thomas N. Headland, K. L. Pike and M. Harris, *Emics and etics: The insider/outsider debate*. Newbury Park, CA: Sage.

Liburd, L. C., and Sniezek, J. E. (2007). Changing times: new possibilities for community health and well-being. *Preventing chronic disease* [serial online]. Available at http://www.cdc.gov/pcd/issues/2007/jul/07_0048.htm

Macionis, J. J. (1978). The search for community in modern society: An interpretation. *Qualitative Sociology*, *1*(2), 130–143.

MacLellan-Wright, M. F., Anderson, D., Barber, S., Smith, N., Cantin, B., Felix, R., and Raine, K. (2007). The development of measures of community capacity for community-based funding programs in Canada. *Health Promotion International*, *22*(4), 299–306.

Maxwell, K., and Husain, T. (2005). Public private partnerships: building capacity while effecting change. *Evaluation and Program Planning*, *28*, 349–353.

McLaren, L., and Hawe, P. (2005). Ecological perspectives in health research. *Journal of Epidemiology Community Health*, *59*, 6–14.

McLeroy, K. L., Bibeau, D., Steckler, A., and Glanz, K. (1988). An ecological perspective on health promotion programs. *Health Education Quarterly*, *15*(4), 351–377.

McLeroy, K. R., Kegler, M., Steckler, A., Burdine, J., and Wisotsky, M. (1994). Editorial: Community coalitions for health promotion: Summary and further reflections. *Health Education Research*, *9*(1), 1–11.

McLeroy, K. R., Norton, B. L., Kegler, M. C., Burdine, J. N., and Sumaya, C. V. (2003). Community-based interventions. *American Journal of Public Health*, *93*(4), 529–533.

Merzel, C., and D'Afflitti, J. (2003). Reconsidering community-based health promotion: Promise, performance, and potential. *American Journal of Public Health*, *93*, 557–574.

Merzel, C., and Moon-Howard, J. (2003). Building community capacity: An ecological perspective on the impact of community health promotion collaborations. Unpublished manuscript, used with permission.

Minkler, M., and Wallerstein, N. (1997). Improving health through community organization and community building: A health education perspective. In M. Minkler (ed.). *Community organizing and community building*. New Brunswick, NJ: Princeton University Press.

O'Connell, B. (1999). *Civil society*. Hanover, NH: University Press of New England.

Putnam, R. D. (2000). *Bowling alone*. New York: Simon and Schuster.

Raeburn, J., Akerman, M., Chuengsatiansup, K., Mejia, F., and Oladepo, O. (2007). Community capacity building and health promotion in a globalized world. *Health Promotion International, 21*(S1), 84–90.

Reynolds, C. H., and Norman, R.V. (eds.). (1988). *Community in America: The challenge of habits of the heart*. Berkeley: University of California Press.

Singer, H. H., and Kegler, M. C. (2004). Assessing interorganizational networks as a dimension of community capacity: Illustrations from a community intervention to prevent lead poisoning. *Health Education and Behavior, 31*(6), 808–821.

Sites, W., Chaskin, R. J., and Parks, V. (2007). Reframing community practice for the 21st Century: Multiple traditions, multiple challenges. *Journal of Urban Affairs, 29*(5), 519–541.

Smith, N., Littlejohns, L., and Thompson, D. (2001). Shaking out the cobwebs: Insights into community capacity and its relation to health outcomes. *Community Development Journal, 36*(1), 30–41.

Speers, M., Goodman, R., McLeroy, K., Kegler, M., and Rogers, T. (1996). *Community capacity building*. Presentation at the Society for Public Health Education Annual Meeting, New York: December.

Stephens, C. (2007). Community as practice: Social representations of community and their implications for health promotion. *Journal of Community and Applied Social Psychology, 17*, 103–114.

Stokols, D. (1992). Establishing and maintaining healthy environments: Toward a social ecology of health promotion. *American Psychologist, 47*(1), 6–22.

Tang, K., Nutbeam, D., Kong, L., Wang, R., and Yan, J. (2005). Building capacity for health promotion- a case study from China. *Health Promotion International, 20*(3), 285–295.

Tocqueville, A. (2000). *Democracy in America*. Translation by Harvey Mansfield. Chicago: University of Chicago Press.

Tönnies, F. (1967). *Community and society*. Lansing, MI: Michigan State University Press.

Udehn, L. (2002). The changing face of methodological individualism. *Annual Review of Sociology, 28*, 479–507.

Wellman, B., and Leighton, B. (1979). Networks, neighborhoods, and communities: Approaches to the study of the community question. *Urban Affairs Quarterly, 14*(3), 363–390.

Wellman, B., Salaff, J., Dimitrova, D., Garton, L., Gulia, M., and Haythornthwaite, C. (2000). Computer networks as social networks: Collaborative work, telework, and virtual community. In: E. Lesser, M. Fontaine and J. Slusher, eds., *Knowledge and communities*. Burlington, MA: Butterworth-Heinemann.

Wendel, M. L., Burdine, J. N., and McLeroy, K. R. (2007). CDC's Prevention Research Centers and community health development. *Texas Public Health Association Journal, 59*(2), 5–7.

World Health Organization. (1986). *Ottawa charter for health promotion*. Ottawa, Ontario.

World Health Organization. (1984). *Health promotion: A discussion document on the concepts and principles*. Copenhagen, Denmark: WHO Regional Office for Europe.

Yancey, A. K. (2004). Building capacity to prevent and control chronic disease in underserved communities: Expanding the wisdom of WISEWOMAN in intervening at the environmental level. *Journal of Women's Health, 13*(5), 644–649.

Yuasa, M., de Sá, R., Pincovsky, S., and Shimanouchi, N. (2007). Emergence model of social and human capital and its application to the Healthy Municipalities project in Northeast Brazil. *Health Promotion International, 22*(4), 292–298.

NATURAL HELPER MODELS TO ENHANCE A COMMUNITY'S HEALTH AND COMPETENCE

Eugenia Eng
Scott D. Rhodes
Edith Parker

NATURAL HELPERS AND LAY HEALTH ADVISORS

The quotation came from an evaluation of a health promotion project that applied a natural helper model to improve community competence and health (Eng and Parker, 1994). Mrs. Smith and Mrs. Jones did "what they had always done" in their communities because they were "natural helpers." They were trusted, and others within their familial and social networks often turned to them for informal guidance and advice; however, in this project they were trained to improve the accessibility and coordination of health and nutrition services that were available but underutilized.

Natural helpers are particular individuals to whom others naturally turn for advice, emotional support, and tangible aid. They provide informal, spontaneous assistance, which is embedded in everyday life—so much so that its value is often not recognized (Israel, 1985). Consequently, their contributions to community health and well-being may be invisible to others, and frequently to the community health advisors themselves. Being unobtrusive, natural helping can be difficult to demonstrate, operationalize, and capture empirically.

> The folks down in my area . . . may not know that Mrs. Smith and Jones are "health advisors." They may not know to call them that . . . But if you got a problem, you call Mrs. Smith and you call Mrs. Jones, and they are going to help you. You can call it whatever you want, but they get the job done. They meet the needs.
> —A Community Health Advisor in the Mississippi Delta, 1992

Natural helpers are effective because they are part of the communities in which they work, ethnically, socioeconomically, and experientially. They possess an intimate understanding of community social networks, strengths, and health needs. Such understanding comes from their "insider's" knowledge of what is meaningful to members of their communities; how to communicate in a similar language, and recognize and incorporate culture (for example, cultural identity, spiritual coping, traditional health practices) to promote health and improve health outcomes within their communities.

In the last fifteen years, public health professionals have introduced a number of approaches, loosely referred to as "lay health advisor" (LHA) interventions, which include a parallel but separate line of work with natural helpers. The United States (U.S.) Centers for Disease Control and Prevention (CDC; USDHHS, 1994) compiled a two-volume directory of LHA projects and programs in the United States, as well as a computerized database that is regularly updated. The following are a few examples that illustrate the wide range of settings, health issues, and populations involving natural helpers and other types of LHAs.

> Natural helpers are particular individuals to whom others naturally turn for advice, emotional support, and tangible aid.

Barbers (Wilkinson, 1992) and church members nominated by their pastors in North Carolina (Eng and Hatch, 1992) served as LHAs to improve hypertension screening, management, and control among African Americans. Migrant farmworker women served as *promotores* to address the maternal and child health needs of families traveling in the Midwest (Booker et al., 1997) and East Coast Migrant Streams (Watkins et al., 1994). A program known as Save Our Sisters with 160 LHAs was established across five rural counties in eastern North Carolina to assist older African American women in breaking the silence about breast cancer screening (Eng and Smith, 1995; Earp et al., 1997). Lay Health Advisors known as "Village Health Workers" in Detroit have undertaken activities in their neighborhoods to improve the health of women and children (Parker et al., 1998). In a suburban Midwestern high school, the Peer Helping Program (PHP) was implemented for students to receive confidential health counseling in a designated room during specified class periods from peer educators, who had been nominated by the student body and the adults they trust (Berkley-Patton et al., 1997). These adolescent LHAs provided support; information relevant to their peers, including substance use, violence, and pregnancy; and referrals to appropriate services. Evaluation found the importance of "being there" as peer resources and making linkages to existing services that were not being utilized by the students previously. A health coalition in rural Massachusetts selected and hired local residents to work as community health advisors, resulting in increased health care access, increased medical compliance, and better problem solving (Baker et al., 1997).

Approaches by LHAs may be especially appropriate for sexual health promotion and sexually transmitted diseases (STDs) and HIV prevention, because LHAs can reach populations not easily accessed by health professionals, including individuals with asymptomatic infections, and people who encounter barriers to or avoid care for STDs and HIV. In a small southern town with "big city" STD rates, a community group identified twenty-five natural helpers willing to serve as Respect and Protect Advisors and help people they know to use condoms with their main partners and seek screening when they had unprotected sex (Thomas et al., 1998). Furthermore, LHAs have been used online in chat rooms designed for social and sexual networking among men who have sex with men (MSM). Trained LHAs, known as CyBER educators, provided information about HIV, offered referrals, addressed chat-room norms around sexual health and risk behavior, and fed important information back to the local providers to improve systems of care (Rhodes, Hergenrather, Duncan, Ramsey, Yee, Wilkin, 2007).

In short, LHA interventions have emerged as an important approach in health promotion, spanning all health topics and within various types of communities. Implicit in this approach is the exchange of social support, such as information, advice, tangible aid, and referrals to external resources (House, 1981). From a public health perspective, the associations found between social support and health (Nuckolls et al., 1972; Cassel, 1976; Kaplan et al., 1977; Broadhead et al., 1983) hold substantial potential for translating the health-enhancing effects into social support interventions (Heaney and Israel, 1997). The common feature of LHA interventions is to enlist indigenous members of a given population in channeling health-enhancing social support to individuals and groups (Eng and Young, 1992; Israel, 1985; Service and Salber, 1979). At the same time, important conceptual and methodological distinctions among LHA interventions have been viewed as falling along a continuum (Eng, Parker, and Harlan, 1997). On one end of the continuum are interventions in which LHAs serve as paid employees of an agency, such as a paraprofessional or outreach worker, and seek to deliver social support, such as information and assistance to individuals to protect the health of those individuals. At the other end are interventions for which LHAs are natural helpers with expertise and knowledge that enhance the health and competence of their community through information distribution, assistance and organization of community-building activities within their social networks. This emphasis on natural helpers working within their own social network, defined as person-centered webs of relationships that connect individuals to other individuals or groups (Israel, 1982; Israel and Rounds, 1987), differs from the LHA, such as an outreach worker, who provides social support to individuals who may or may not be in his or her social network.

Interventions by LHAs that explicitly collaborate with natural helpers to enhance a community's health and competence are the focus of this chapter. The key principles and methods are examined for their relevance to the fields of health education, community development, and social epidemiology. Following an overview of the historical emergence of natural helper models as a specific line of LHA intervention research and practice, the underlying concepts and principles in public health practice are explored. Evidence is presented from empirical studies that applied natural helping models with different communities to respond to different health needs, and one case study will be described in detail. Future directions are proposed on further work that remains to be done to demonstrate, operationalize, and empirically capture the health-enhancing effects from a community's natural helping system. The goal is to translate the health-enhancing effects into effective interventions.

THE GENESIS AND EMERGENCE OF NATURAL HELPER INTERVENTIONS IN PUBLIC HEALTH

With this observation, a group of South African researchers began their pioneering work of uncovering the structure and function of a community's natural helping system, examining associations between social relationships and health, and recognizing that health is a social concern. Their initial studies were conducted in communities of various incomes and ethnicities in South Africa, which were served by seven primary health care centers from 1945 to 1959. Their methodology and broad inclusion of social factors as determinants of health have been acknowledged as the fundamental work of the twentieth century in social epidemiology (Trostle, 1986).

> In lesser degree than the family, but with similar dynamics, the primary friendship group may prove to be an epidemiological unit of some significance.
> —Steuart and Kark, 1962, p.41

Sidney Kark, the group's leader, credited Guy Steuart, the psychologist in the group, with calling their attention to the importance of social networks and primary groups for their work in community health education (Israel et al., 1993). Steuart developed a unique procedure for recording the structure and functions of a community's natural helping system. His findings revealed sophisticated and complex skill sets and expertise on how to manage with life, deal with its frustrations, and strive to ensure the conditions for good health for its members (Steuart, 1978). Natural helping was a part of everyday living—even for communities where life conditions, such as apartheid policy or rural poverty, would be expected to exert an undeniably harmful influence on health.

The staff for the seven health centers in South Africa was trained at the Institute of Family and Community Health to conduct research on the connection between social relationships and health. The significant feature of their work was that they developed techniques that incorporated the findings into the daily practice of the health centers (Kark, 1951). Staff began working with social groupings of people as a natural extension of their interviews with individuals receiving medical care and guidance. That is, by entering into a functional relationship with the presumed *natural helpers* in a social group, health center staff facilitated a two-way flow of communication and influence that would be mutually beneficial. For example, they found that by engaging natural helpers and their social networks in a ten-week mutual exchange of discussion-decision, changes in infant feeding practices were achieved in the desired direction (Steuart and Kark, 1962). Of equal significance, health center staff increased their own understanding of individuals in terms of their family situation, of families in their life situation within a community, and of what it is like to live in a community in relation to the social structure of South Africa (Kark, 1951).

The experience of working through natural helpers' social networks, ranging from formalized groups to only two or three intimate friends gathered together in a home, was considered by this group of South African researchers to be among the Institute's most important (Steuart and Kark, 1962). Their experiment, however, came to an abrupt end in South Africa in 1959, when the new government began to apply apartheid policy to the medical professions. Individual members of the group dispersed to Israel, Kenya, and the United States, where they continued to develop their methods and ideas on the social determinants of health.

Those who relocated to North Carolina refined their ideas and methods for engaging a community's natural helping system in behavioral and social change interventions. Steuart (1969b, 1977) introduced the procedure, *action-oriented community diagnosis*, into the MPH degree curriculum in the Department of Health Education at the University of North Carolina (Eng and Blanchard, 1991). He used the term *diagnosis* to indicate that the purpose of the analysis is to result in action, change, and improvement that meet a community's needs (Steuart, 1969). The procedure drew on methods of inquiry from the disciplines of epidemiology and anthropology to reveal:

- The nature of a community's power structure and the lay groups who might participate in both planning and implementing an intervention.
- The appropriate unit of practice, such as the individual, family, social groups, neighborhood.
- The interpersonal and nonpersonal methods most appropriate to the tasks of behavior and social change.

■   The informal opinion leaders and "influentials" in social networks through whom influence may be brought to bear on a health issue.

Eva Salber, a colleague of Steuart's in South Africa, conducted such a diagnosis in a rural community of North Carolina while at Duke University's Department of Family and Community Medicine. She and a small team of health educators documented the detailed procedures they used to identify social networks and their natural helpers, and recruited these particular individuals to complete training sessions on the needs and issues that had emerged from the community diagnosis (Salber, Beery, and Jackson, 1976; Service and Salber 1979; Jackson and Parks, 1997). They linked these natural helpers to the resources of the local health care system. For many public health scholars, Salber's systematic application of the principles and methods developed in South Africa to a rural community in the United States marks the beginning of our field's conceptualization of natural helper interventions (Eng and Young, 1992; Jackson and Parks, 1997; Earp et al., 1997; Watkins et al., 1994, Parker et al., 1998).

At the University of North Carolina, John Hatch designed and implemented the first church-based LHA intervention by building on the skills and expertise of natural helpers in congregations of rural Black churches (Hatch and Lovelace, 1980). Before joining Steuart's faculty, Hatch had been applying the principles and methods developed in South Africa with rural, African American communities in the Mississippi Delta. His collaborator in Mississippi was Jack Geiger, who, when a medical student at Case Western Reserve University, had completed a clerkship with Steuart and his colleagues at the South African Institute for Family and Community Health (Geiger, 1984; Trostle, 1986). Geiger and Hatch had received "War on Poverty" federal funding to establish in Mississippi the first rural community health center in the United States, for which they have clearly acknowledged the work of the South African Institute for Family and Community Health (Hatch and Eng, 1983; Geiger, 1971; Israel et al., 1993).

The focal point of Hatch's body of work is the Black church as a community-based institution with structures and functions that nurture leadership, accord rewards and recognition, mobilize social action, and ensure mutual aid for its members (Hatch and Lovelace, 1980; Eng, Hatch, and Callan, 1985; Eng and Hatch, 1992). His research on the health-enhancing effects of natural helping in the Black church opened up new space for developing LHA interventions that are relevant and authentic to the everyday lives of African Americans. Hatch is recognized nationally and internationally for promoting collaborative methods of inquiry and planning between health service delivery systems and African American communities' natural helping systems (Hatch et al., 1993).

CONCEPTS OF NATURAL HELPER INTERVENTIONS IN PUBLIC HEALTH PRACTICE

To recognize the relevance of natural helping to public health practice, it is essential to understand the following concepts: *community support system*, *neighborhood attachment*, *informal helping networks*, and *community competence*. Understanding these concepts and their relationship to public health practice is key to understanding the public health natural helper interventions.

Community Support System

The President's Commission on Mental Health (1978, Vol. II) defined a *community support system* as: (1) natural helping networks to which people belong, (2) worksite relationships, and (3) self-help or mutual aid groups. This Commission's Community Support Systems Task Panel, chaired by June Jackson Christmas and directed by Marie Killilea, marked the first time that a prestigious nationwide study group afforded such prominence to the role of community and its support systems in mental health (HEW, 1979; Biegel and Naparstek, 1982). In addition, the Commission devoted a separate section of their report to disease prevention and health promotion, and its role in improving coping and enabling people to realize their full potential. The Surgeon General's (USDHEW, 1979) Report, *Healthy People*, provided further impetus for the field of public health to recognize the importance of life circumstances, such as housing or employment, life events, such as immigrant status or divorce, and lifestyles that may affect people's vulnerability to a wide range of disorders and disease (Cassel, 1976; Jessor and Jessor, 1981; Bloom, 1979).

The emphasis of these two national reports on community support systems and conditions of community life that enable people to be healthy signified a distinct departure from medical models and theories (Biegel and Naparstek, 1982). First, these reports suggested that health promotion interventions do not need to stress the role of identifiable factors in the etiology of a particular class of disorders. Second, these reports suggested that health promotion interventions can have non-specific preventive consequences. Moreover, as observed by Caplan (1982), routine intervention by health professionals, if not done with recognition of natural support systems, may weaken instead of strengthen the operation of a community's natural support systems and mutual-help organizations. This recognition of the existence and power of community support systems to reduce people's vulnerability to disease and illness has continued to increase among public health professionals as is reflected in the recent popularity of concepts, such as social capital, in the field of public health.

> This recognition of the existence and power of community support systems to reduce people's vulnerability to disease and illness has continued to increase among public health professionals as is reflected in the recent popularity of concepts, such as social capital, in the field of public health.

The professional fields of public health and social work have drawn heavily from Roland Warren's (1963) conceptualization of community as a social system with structures and functions that help its members adjust to social, political, and economic change. Donald Warren (1971) delineated the following five functions of a community: center for interpersonal influence, source of mutual aid, base for formal and informal organizations, reference group and social context, and an arena for according status. In the context of these functions, community members' adjustment to social, political, and economic change is viewed as a process of help-seeking and help-giving, as opposed to a discrete event or behavioral occurrence. Similarly, problems do not just happen, but are manifest through an accumulation of events, behaviors, and symptoms during a period of time. The point at which a problem begins is as indeterminate as the point at which help becomes effective, and the course between these two vague points is often a long one. This view that most people are engaged in help-seeking and help-giving processes opened up new space for health and human service professionals to examine how their programs could strengthen the natural helping networks of communities, workplaces, and associations (Gottlieb, 1982).

Neighborhood Attachment

The body of work on natural helping networks has offered evidence for the important role of *neighborhood attachment* to place, groups, and other individuals. These attachments, viewed as a proxy for adjustment to one's environment (Nuckolls et al., 1972; Lin et al., 1979), have been found to improve people's adaptive competence at times of life stress (Killilea, 1976; Caplan, 1974, 1976). Neighborhood attachment has been shown to provide a sense of belonging, reduce alienation, and offer a reason for overcoming the frustrations of a changing world (Warren, 1977). Explanations have been attributed to communality of experience, collective willpower, sharing of information, constructive activity, and receiving help through giving it (Riessman, 1965; Plaut, 1982; Shanas, 1978; Cantor, 1979; Guttman, 1979).

Scholars have emphasized, therefore, taking into account communities' social and cultural backgrounds (Hamburg and Killilea, 1979; Biegel et al., 1982; Lin et al., 1979) when developing health promotion programs aimed at strengthening natural helping networks.

Furthermore, natural helping has been found to flourish when the issues were either of little interest to professionals or involved considerable numbers of people who did not have access to services of professionals (Tracy and Gussow, 1976). Ethnic communities, for example, with disproportionately more members who were elderly and low income, showed stronger neighborhood attachment and patterns of natural helping than that of the general population (Mann, 1965; Gans, 1961; Lee, 1968; Biegel et al., 1982; Stack, 1974). Scholars have emphasized, therefore, taking into account communities' social and cultural backgrounds (Hamburg and Killilea, 1979; Biegel et al., 1982; Lin et al., 1979) when developing health promotion programs aimed at strengthening natural helping networks.

Informal Helping Networks

Informal helping networks are those indirect ties to resources that one may have access to through the different social groupings to which one belongs (family, neighborhood, work, voluntary associations). Through interactions with persons in one's social groupings, one may gain access to information, resources, people, and pathways for help that are outside of one's intimate circles (Warren, 1963b). The social groupings may themselves be linked, and thereby can tie people indirectly to a variety of helping networks simultaneously. For example, a woman confides a recent concern to her daughter-in-law, who mentions relevant information she had gained from one of her coworkers. Although the woman never needs to be in contact with the coworker, she is part of a viable helping network through a helping transaction with one person. Furthermore, being a part of a helping network can direct her attention to the needs of others in her community (Warren, 1982).

These informal helping transactions are relatively spontaneous and mutual exchanges of support for a variety of large and small stresses of everyday life, when compared to the more formally organized services provided by paid staff in agencies. Health and human service professionals have long recognized that for most people, their principal sources of help for a wide range of problems are family, friends, neighbors, coworkers, and other personal relationships (Gourash, 1978; Litwak and Szelenyi, 1969; Pancoast and Chapman, 1982). The focus of agency services on delivering care to an identified patient or client population represents only a small proportion of the support, crisis intervention, and problem solving that occurs in communities. Agencies have consequently recognized the potential of forming partnerships with informal helpers, and have developed different intervention strategies for cooperating with and reinforcing a community support system's natural helping networks.

The body of work by Froland and colleagues (1980) on the interface between formal and informal helping systems generated a valuable typology of informal helping network interventions they observed to be the most relevant and accessible to health and human service professionals (Table 11.1). The interventions are based on six types of relationships found in informal helping networks of communities:

■ *Family and Friends*: These are the most intimate of helping relationships and are characterized as being long standing through preexisting ties and involve equality of exchange over the long term. In informal helper interventions involving family and friends, agencies usually only ask for commitment to help, without requiring special skills or knowledge, and the intervention is short-term.

■ *Neighbors*: Those who live next door or very close are the most likely to be involved in helping, but when encouraged by an agency, they may live in an area beyond the geographic boundaries of a neighborhood. Their helping relationship is characterized as being long standing through preexisting ties, involves equality of exchange over the long term, and is locality-based. Informal interventions involving helping from neighbors need to consider that the forms of helping from neighbors are not based on obligation of kinship or friendship, but have defined limits on level of involvement and what is appropriate to ask for and offer.

■ *Natural Helpers:* These are particular individuals to whom people naturally turn for advice, emotional support, and tangible aid. They may be known in a neighborhood context or in a wider network. Their helping relationship is characterized as being long standing through preexisting ties, locality-based, and a central part of their activities. Helping from natural helpers is based on personal motivation to help others and skills that have earned them respect and confidence. Although they share many of the same sociodemographic characteristics as those they help, their coping abilities are superior. In interventions involving natural helpers, agencies usually link natural helpers to appropriate formal services and provide them with social, emotional, and material resources.

■ *Role-Related Helpers*: These are individuals in such positions as hair stylists, shopkeepers, and ministers who come in contact with a large number of people

TABLE 11.1 Typology of Informal Helper Interventions.

Type of Informal Helper	Examples of Activities Conducted by Agencies
Family and Friends	• Elicit commitment from clients' personal networks to share tasks during clients' short-term limitation in functioning • Reinforce preexisting helping relationships by providing counseling or training on how to be more supportive to clients • Identify and train focal person to mobilize and maintain helping relationships
Neighbors	• Broker help for individual clients from their neighbors • Create helping relationships by creating opportunities for neighbors to interact, such as by organizing block groups to help residents-in-need or reviving old acquaintances
Natural Helpers	• Identify natural helpers by conducting reputational method • Reinforce preexisting helping relationships to provide improved advice, assistance, material resources, and referrals • Link appropriate formal agency services to informal helping network • Support natural helpers in implementing short- and long-term self-help action in response to local needs
Role-Related Helpers	• Make contact with individuals who are influential and visibly located at a crossroads, such as storekeepers, pharmacists • Create helping relationships in which they can be a source of information and referral to people they encounter in their positions • Encourage them to make their institutions and businesses more responsive to needs of agency clients
People with Same Problems	• Legitimate groups' learning from one another using experiential rather than professional knowledge • Create helping relationships by facilitating groups meeting each other • Mobilize agency resources • Share skills in group dynamics and group process
Volunteers	• Recruit willing individuals by advertisement, referral, or from client group • Create, initiate, and sustain helping relationships for isolated people • Heavy investment of agency resources for more specialized problem-solving

Source: Based on Pancoast and Chapman, 1982.

through the positions they hold. Their helping relationship is characterized as being long standing through preexisting ties and locality-based. In addition, they are often active on agency-sponsored task forces, boards, and committees to improve services. For their agency-defined role as informal helpers, they are more likely to be a source of information and referral and to work to make the agency more responsive than to provide friendship and emotional support.

- *People with Similar Problems*: These are helping relationships that are usually fostered by an agency or program that brings together people with similar problems to share their experiences and support one another. The help involves equality of exchange over time, but seldom occurs in the homes of participants. Helping usually takes place within a self-help group and short-term returns are often expected. The role of agencies varies from being proactive by taking the initiative in establishing a mutual-aid program to being responsive when approached by one or more persons with similar problems requesting resources.

- *Volunteers*: These individuals are the most familiar informal helpers to most professionals because volunteers require heavy input from professionals. They are usually recruited, trained, and channeled through a formal organization's programs to offer help, on a stranger-to-stranger basis, to persons who do not have a helping network of their own. The volunteer is clearly defined as "the helper" and therefore, the helping relationship is most likely to involve inequality in social status and coping ability.

Acknowledging that informal helping network interventions do not all engage the natural helping networks of a community's support system has important implications for public health practice (Eng et al., 1997). It is important to distinguish between interventions that are embedded within ongoing networks of relationships, such as interventions working with family and friends, neighbors or natural helpers, and those helping relationships that are *created* by an agency, such as volunteers and people with similar problems (Pancoast and Chapman, 1982). Although the latter type of interventions are formed to meet a specific need on a short-term basis, helping relationships based on kinship, friendship, residential proximity, and natural helping are long-term, highly individualized, flexible, and are likely to be meeting some basic needs. Agencies that want to interface with embedded helping relationships such as these must, therefore, be willing to be flexible and spend time in the beginning to identify natural helpers, analyze their networks, and understand the particular culture of their community support system. Interventions that create helping relationships, such as those that use volunteers or people with similar problems, will require a heavy investment of agency resources to sustain them.

Recruitment methods of programs that intend to certify and employ local residents as LHA, but without consideration of the origin of helping relationships, may use eligibility criteria according to qualifications set by personnel policies. The natural helpers to whom people in a community turn, therefore, may not necessarily be among the local residents recruited, because they are not seeking employment or do not fit the agency's qualifications for an LHA. In contrast, the qualifications for a natural helper have been set by his or her community. Other programs, which intend to accept all willing volunteers, may cast as wide a recruitment net as possible through posters, windshield leaflets, and media ads. Natural helpers, however, may not respond because they are already too busy helping people and groups in their communities, or do not self-identify as natural helpers

The nature and level of influence or impact that can be expected from natural helper interventions may also differ from those based on agency-created helping relationships. Although all informal helper interventions are generally aimed at enhancing the health and well-being of individuals through peer-to-peer dynamics, natural helper interventions operate through a community's political dynamics and neighborhood attachment. Because natural helping networks are part of a community support system, natural helper interventions can bring people together and set a political dynamic in motion to transform and secure improved quality of community life (Labonte, 1989; McKnight, 1991; Heller, 1989). Hence, in addition to securing well-being for members of a community, natural helper interventions also give attention to changing policies and practices of organizations and act upon environmental factors that impede the health and development of a community (Ketterer et al., 1980; Plaut, 1982; Eng and Parker, 1994). One important outcome from natural helper interventions, therefore, is a more competent community.

Community Competence The term *community competence* was first codified in social psychiatry by Cottrell (1976). His conceptualization of a community being competent was strongly influenced by George Herbert Mead's body of work on the process of social interaction (Cottrell, 1980). Cottrell's description of a competent community is one in which its various component parts are able to: (1) collaborate effectively in identifying collective problems and needs; (2) achieve a working consensus on goals and priorities; (3) agree on ways and means to implement the agreed-upon goals, and (4) collaborate effectively in the required actions. He observed that the more competent a community, the more mentally healthy its members. From these observations, he defined eight dimensions of community competence that represent social interactions among community members, as well as between a community and the larger society (Table 11.2).

A few empirical studies of community competence have attempted to operationalize its dimensions (Denham and Quinn, 1998) and develop measures to evaluate community development programs (Hurley et al., 1981; Gatz et al., 1982) and health promotion programs (Goeppinger and Baglioni, 1985; Knight et al., 1991). With regard to applying the concept to natural helper interventions, only one study evaluated changes in community competence as an outcome, and will be described later in this chapter (Eng and Parker, 1994).

The next section presents a natural helper intervention model and how it has been applied by several health promotion programs. This is followed by a more detailed case study.

TABLE 11.2 Community Competence Dimensions.

Dimensions	Definitions	Illustrative Quotes from a Natural Helper
Participation in Community Life	Process by which a community member commits him or herself to a community and contributes to the definition of goals as well as to ways and means for their implementation	I always been the type to want to help, but just didn't know how to go about doing it. So, that way, this health advisor program has helped me to do things I always wanted to do.
Commitment to the Collective	Commitment to a community as a relationship worth enhancing and keeping	One of the things is the pulling together of the community to get things done. And we found out that we had to do that in order to get things done. We were not going to get things done apart. The more of us that come together and shared ideas, we realized the problems we were having were about the same.
Self-Other Awareness and Clarity of Situational Definitions	Clarity with which each part of a community can perceive its own identity and position on issues in relationship to other parts of a community	And the people are now beginning to realize who the power brokers are . . . Well, they were aware before, but they didn't know how it impacts their lives. They didn't realize the role an election plays in getting things done.
Articulateness Communication	Ability of a community to articulate involvement in community collective views, attitudes, needs, and intentions. Process by which information is exchanged in a community and ability to amass common meanings among different parts of a community	Health advisors talked to people to tell people that might need some of the things that they could do . . . In fact, that very day, just in conversation, they learned about somebody that needed some food. They didn't have any food in their house. And health advisors were able to make a contact there.

TABLE 11.2 *(Continued)*

Conflict Containment and Accommodation	Ability to establish procedures by which open conflicts may be accommodated and interaction between different parts of a community will continue	I think the health advisor program as a whole is probably our best bet to get a racial community effort. An interracial, biracial. [And] since the program has been here, I say I could see greater unity with people working together to try to improve their conditions.
Management of Relations with the Wider Society	Ability to use resources and supports that the larger society makes available and to act to reduce the threats to community life posed by a larger social pressure	As far as actual person-to-person contact . . . one of the strongest points of the health advisor program was this working together and knowing where services can be provided and people willing. And people will channel things to us now that would not have ever been addressed.
Machinery for Facilitating Participant Interaction and Decision Making	Ability of a community to establish more formal means for ways to ensure representative input in decision making as size of community increases	The health advisors have gone to the [county board of] supervisors and their representatives to talk about housing. They are now building two new housing projects.
Social Support	Community members know and care about neighbors; show willingness to lend a hand in cognitive, instrumental, and emotional support	Health advisors have helped in terms of going into the patient's home to teach or render some kind of care, if it's nothing other than companionship.

Source: Based on Cottrell, 1976; Eng and Parker, 1994.

THE NATURAL HELPER INTERVENTION MODEL AND APPLICATIONS

The field of health promotion has realized that a partnership with natural helpers can interweave formal services with the help provided by a community support system and result in a more appropriate response to the needs of clients and communities (Pancoast and Chapman, 1982; Service and Salber, 1979; Eng and Hatch, 1991; Eng and Young, 1992). Natural helpers provide a community-based system of care and social support that complements, but does not extend or serve as a replacement for, the more specialized services of health professionals (Eng and Smith, 1995). Through a wide spectrum of associations in a community, as formal as a church or guild (Eng et al., 1985) or as informal as a neighbor's kitchen (Heaney and Israel, 1997), natural helpers are linked to individuals, groups, and the wider society that no health professional could begin to reach by him or herself.

The outcomes and intermediate benefits from the various roles and social action arenas through which natural helpers and health professionals can collaborate are presented in Figure 11.1. Professionals can form a partnership with natural helpers to achieve three levels of outcomes: improved health practices, improved coordination of agency services, and improved community competence.

Improved Health Practices

Health professionals can offer training to natural helpers to assist individuals, who are already part of a natural helper's social networks, with needs, such as information, and referrals that are difficult for professionals to provide directly. A natural helper intervention to reduce transmission of sexually transmitted diseases (STDs) in a small southern town, for example, conducted in-depth interviews with young, African American women. The findings revealed that the principal barriers to seeking STD screening and care were confusion about the services offered by local health agencies and apprehension about interacting with the predominantly white staff at the local health department (Schuster et al., 1995). To overcome these barriers, staff from the STD clinic and local health department was invited to participate in training natural helpers. Staff listened to their concerns, explained how their respective agencies operated, and offered to be a contact person for referrals from the natural helpers (Thomas et al., 2000). In turn, the natural helpers could demystify the agencies for members within their helping networks. After eighteen months, the evaluation showed an increase of 60 percent in seeking STD care within three days of symptoms among African American women who reported experiencing symptoms. An increase of 26 percent was found for those who said they sought care when they thought they had an STD but no symptoms (Thomas et al., 2000).

A natural helper intervention implemented with Latino migrant farmworker families reported that between 50 percent and 82 percent of maternal and child health patients at two migrant health centers interacted with a trained natural helper (Watkins et al., 1994). Mothers who had contact with a trained natural helper were significantly more likely to bring their children for sick care and had significantly greater knowledge of health practices. Moreover, a significantly higher proportion of pregnant migrant farmworker women, who had contact with a trained natural helper, reported completing the recommended number of prenatal visits. These findings indicate that Latina women in this migrant farmworker population were connected to one another through natural helping relationships that can bridge cultural diversity in language and health beliefs between farmworkers and health providers.

Improved Coordination of Agency Services

A second partnership opportunity is for health professionals to link their formal service delivery system with the informal helping networks of natural helpers, with the benefit being that agencies can become more aware and responsive to community needs. A statewide program in North Carolina, for example, offered subsidized breast cancer screening to income-eligible women. The number of forms to be completed and the number of documents required to determine eligibility proved to be a barrier for older African American women, particularly for those with low literacy and who were embarrassed by demographic questions about family income and sensitive questions about the onset of menopause. Natural helpers, who were recruited and trained through an intervention, negotiated with the clinic to cosponsor two breast cancer screening days and organize a campaign, called "Days of Our Lives," in which they assisted women with the paperwork in the privacy of their homes before going to the clinic.

Improved Community Competence

A third opportunity for health professionals to collaborate with natural helpers is to mobilize the resources of associations in their community to implement self-help action that responds to local health needs. The benefit is to increase a community's social unity and problem-solving capacity. For example, older African American women in rural North Carolina who participated in focus group interviews, revealed that they delayed or avoided annual breast cancer screenings largely due to their memories of a segregated health care system (Tessaro et al., 1994). In addition, the stigma of the fatal and hereditary nature of cancer imposed a prevailing silence in their communities about discussing cancer. Given older African American women's sense of modesty about their bodies, they would discuss concerns and questions about breast cancer only with women they knew. Natural helpers, recruited and trained as "Save Our Sisters" LHAs, share this same history, placing them in a position of trust. They are able to help overcome the barriers to mammography screening faced by older African Americans (Eng and Smith, 1995).

To break this silence, natural helpers used their existing channels of influence and communication to show an educational video they had produced, as well as to raise funds from churches to cover the cost of bringing a mobile mammography unit to housing projects (Eng and Smith, 1995). The intervention appears to have had an impact on reducing disparity between African Americans and whites in mammography use, particularly among lower-income women, among whom the racial gap has been nearly eliminated (Earp et al., 2000). In the first two and one-half years of the project period, mammography use in the past two years increased by 42 percent (from 41 percent to

58 percent) among African American women, compared to a rise of 11 percent in white women (67 percent to 74 percent). Among lower-income women (those with family incomes below $12,000 a year), African American women's use increased from just 37 percent to 59 percent, nearly overtaking white women, whose mammography use rose from 54 percent to 60 percent.

Gaining Entry to Natural Helping Networks

The intervention inputs of training natural helpers, linking them to service providers, and supporting their actions in a community are typically coordinated by a Community Outreach Coordinator. Hiring a Coordinator, who is active in a range of local social groups and associations of the participating community, is the critical first step toward identifying and gaining entry to the various natural helping networks. The Coordinator's initial task is to form a Community Advisory Group (CAG) with contacts to additional groups and organizations, such as churches, community-based organizations, and so on. to increase the intervention's reach to natural helping networks. The CAG offers entry to these groups and guidance on collecting and interpreting data during the formative phase of the intervention. For the breast cancer intervention, for example, the focus group interviews with older African American women were arranged through CAG members (Tessaro et al., 1994). The CAG also provided technical assistance in interpreting the findings and using them to: develop the learning objectives for training natural helpers; determine the characteristics of natural helpers; develop strategies for recruiting natural helpers; and identify potential trainers (Eng and Smith, 1995).

Natural helpers can do much more than counsel and assist individuals to change their behaviors. They can build a partnership with the formal service delivery system that acknowledges the community natural helping system's difference, and which would enable both systems to develop.

In sum, natural helpers can do much more than counsel and assist individuals to change their behaviors. They can build a partnership with the formal service delivery system that acknowledges the community natural helping system's difference, and which would enable both systems to develop. Natural helpers can also work as a group with the Coordinator and CAG members to recognize a problem, plan a solution, and take action that strives for structural change in the health system and social change in their communities.

CASE STUDY: MAN FOR HEALTH AND *HOMBRES*

This case study illustrates how the natural helper intervention model and concepts have been applied in a CDC-funded health promotion project in rural North Carolina. Pseudonyms are used to assure the privacy of participating communities. With initial funding from the W. K. Kellogg Foundation through the North Carolina Community-Based Public Health Initiative, members of Carolina Communities in Action (CCIA) have been conducting research that adheres to the principles of community-based participatory research (CBPR) since 1991. CCIA's original members were the local public health department, community action agency, several religious organizations, and two academic institutions; it grew to include representatives from local Latino-serving community-based organizations, an AIDS service organization, and a Latino soccer league of eighteen hundred men.

Background

Given a rapidly growing Latino population in the county since the mid-1990s, CCIA members were concerned about the capacity of the local service delivery system to elicit and respond to Latino health priorities, and wanted to reach out to this community to explore health-related needs and identify strategies to support Latino health. The health agenda was not predetermined by a funding agency; rather, the partners convened and collected, analyzed, and interpreted data.

Using multiple sources of data including focus group interviews with members of a Latino soccer league and extant data from action-oriented community diagnoses that had been recently completed (Rhodes, Eng, et al., 2007), CCIA partners identified the following five primary themes.

■ Sexual health is a priority for Latino men.

■ Misinformation and myths about HIV and STDs exist.

■ Several barriers to accessing health care in the United States exist, including:
  – Lack of knowledge about service provision and eligibility
  – Fear that confidentiality will not be maintained
  – Need for qualitative interpretative services
  – Need for male providers.

■ Sociocultural norms and expectations of masculinity promote sexual risk, including:
  – A man continually must prove his manhood
  – A man must be independent and strong
  – Immigration threatens a man's masculinity
  – Providing for others is a double-edged sword.

■ Intervention approaches to reach Latino men should be:
  – Community based
  – Male centered
  – Built upon existing community social structures.

Carolina Communities in Action joined two other CBPR partnerships in applying for funding to develop, implement, and evaluate a male natural helper intervention to improve cardiovascular health among urban African American men, prostate health among rural African American men, and sexual health among rural Latino men. The Latino component of this CBPR project, titled HoMBReS (*Hombres Manteniendo Bienestar y Relaciones Saludables*), was funded by CDC to:

■ Develop and implement an LHA intervention based in the natural helping model that recruits and trains *Navegantes* (Navigators) through an adult male Latino soccer league in central North Carolina, to assist other Latino men (*Confidantes*) in reducing STD/HIV risk behaviors.

- Evaluate the efficacy of the intervention using self-reported sexual risk behaviors and utilization of STD/HIV counseling, testing, and treatment services; and important psychosocial correlates (perceived racism, attitude toward health, masculinity, behavioral empowerment, and coping style).

- Monitor changes experienced by the *Navegantes* from being trained and serving as male LHAs.

The Intervention

Through a collaborative partnership approach led by a steering committee, the Project Coordinator recruited and trained a total of twenty-one male *Navegantes* to serve as: (1) health advisors to offer information, referrals, and health-promoting materials (for example, condoms); (2) opinion leaders to reframe negative and bolster positive sociocultural perspectives of what it means to be a man; (3) community advocates; and (4) co-investigators. Each *Navegante* recruited an average of seven other Latino soccer league members as their *Confidantes* to participate for twelve months in MAN (Men as Navigators) activities and three waves of data collection. Being among only a few LHA interventions focused on Latino men, MAN's start-up phase required six months to design and translate the intervention protocols and evaluation instruments, recruit and hire the bilingual Project Coordinator, and enroll the first group of *Navegantes* and *Confidantes*. MAN generated the following innovations and products:

- Application of the *Triple Quandary Model* (Boykin, 1986) to address *male gender socialization*, which promotes men's high-risk attitudes and behaviors, and local health departments' *organizational culture of institutionalized racism* that limits services to men of color. This model defines three realities that people of color in the United States deal with on a daily basis: Mainstream reality shaped by public policies, institutions, and organizations usually encountered by all members of U.S. society; minority reality shaped by the unequal treatment and racism experienced by the minority community in the United States, which has an impact on community structure and norms; and cultural reality rooted in traditional culture by which members interpret and negotiate social reality in their own social relationships.

- Use of the empowerment education technique of *learning circles* as a men's health promotion tool. *Learning circles* used scenarios developed by a subgroup of the MAN Steering Committee (informed by focus group findings) to trigger discussion and encourage practice of collaborative activities within social groups that relieve men of the expectations of masculinity.

- Developed, pretested, and revised *Project Coordinator Training Manual* and *Navigator Training Manual*.

- Adding the role of co-investigator to the responsibilities of an LHA. A specific three-hour session on evaluation was included in the twelve-hour training for *Navegantes* so that they could review and discuss expected outcomes and data collection methods with the evaluators.

- Pretested and IRB-approved research ethics training for non-traditional investigators, Protecting People Who Participate in Research. The Project Coordinator and *Navegantes* were trained and certified in research ethics prior to data collection.

- Application of *Navegante* Activity Logs for process evaluation. An Activity Log was a written monthly record submitted by each *Navegante* to the Project Coordinator on **who** he had reached (number and characteristics) and **how** (individually or in a group). Given low literacy in Spanish among the *Navegantes*, their Activity Log used pictures and required them to enter only checks and numbers.

In sum, project staff, the steering committee, and the *Navegantes* worked shoulder-to-shoulder to articulate and frame their respective definitions of "effective" in ways that could be assessed during the three-year funding period.

The Project Coordinator was a native of Mexico and fourteen-year resident of North Carolina who had completed his GED and an associate's degree in psychology. He was employed full-time and supervised by the AIDS Service organization through a subcontract with MAN. During the twelve-month implementation period, the Project Coordinator met with his twenty-one *Navegantes* as a group every month, usually before or after a soccer practice, to plan collaborative activities that would emerge from Learning Circles and other discussions. Examples of collaborative activities included: sponsoring and staffing displays at health fairs sponsored by local CBOs and agencies; condom distribution and HIV rapid testing during soccer games; and accompanying *Confidantes* to the public health department to navigate the system for HIV and STD counseling and testing.

At the end of each monthly meeting, each *Navegante* turned in his Activity Log to the Project Coordinator. The Logs provided insight into the activities that the *Navegantes* conducted between their meetings with the Project Coordinator, including types of interactions (for example, one-on-one discussions, group discussions, condom distribution or skills building), and with whom (for example, soccer league members, neighbors of coworkers). Simple descriptive analysis of Activity Log entries found that 94 percent of their interactions were with men, and 54 percent were with soccer league teammates. The most common types of interaction were: distributing condoms (46 percent); discussing sexual health and risks (15 percent); discussing individual sexual problems (13 percent); and discussing health in general (13 percent).

Analysis of qualitative process evaluation data from the *Navegantes* indicated that they felt appreciated by community members and filled an important gap as the "only" resources for Latino men in the community. They described the local commercial sex work industry; how they used condom distribution as a way to initiate discussions with other men and commercial sex workers; and how they personally "grew" through the process of being trained and serving as *Navegantes*: increased confidence, public speaking skills, and assertiveness. The suggested changes to help them in their roles as *Navegantes* included: more locally produced, lower Spanish literacy materials, more information on gay issues, and formalizing the structure of the network of *Navegantes*.

For the outcome evaluation, three waves of data were collected from *Navegantes* and *Confidantes*: at baseline, at six months, and at twelve months. Surveys were self-administered in a group setting and took thirty to sixty minutes to complete, depending in part on the skip pattern for each participant. The survey items and response categories were read aloud by the *Navegante* to his group of *Confidantes*, or by the Project Coordinator to his group of *Navegantes*. Findings from the outcome evaluation, using a pre-post-test longitudinal approach to data analysis, indicated that both condom use and HIV testing rates significantly increased ($p < 0.05$).

FUTURE DIRECTIONS FOR RESEARCH AND PRACTICE

The natural helper intervention model presented in Figure 11.1 is a distillation of concepts, theories, and findings from descriptive and applied studies in social epidemiology, mental health, community psychology, social work, and organization development.

Although the intervention model represents a *planned* attempt to induce behavioral, organizational, and social changes, the actual design and implementation of natural helper interventions almost always depend on *unplanned* or *natural* determinants of stability and change (Steuart, 1969a; Parker et al., 1999). A growing body of research on the social ecology of health promotion (McLeroy et al., 1988; Stokols, 1992), community assessments (CDC, 1992), social diagnosis (Green and Kreuter, 1991), and action-oriented community diagnosis (Eng and Blanchard, 1991; Eng et al., 2005) highlights the importance of uncovering the range of natural determinants of stability and change that exist in each community's social and physical environment.

The challenge for natural helper interventions is to enable the structure and functions of community support systems and their natural helping networks to understand and respond to unplanned determinants of stability and change. At the same time, a fair number of examples, including the MAN/ HoMBReS case study described in this chapter, suggest that a generic natural helper intervention model is unlikely to exist. Comprehensive recruitment and training of natural helpers is necessary but not sufficient for an intervention to engage them in multiple arenas of social action and achieve multiple levels of outcomes (Blumenthal et al., 1999; Altpeter et al., 1999). Instead, natural helper interventions that deserve the greatest attention for future research and practice are those for which: (1) the natural helpers and health educators are equally active in designing and adapting the intervention and the evaluation to unplanned determinants; (2) defining and monitoring intervention effects on community competence is as important to the evaluation as monitoring the effects on health practices;

FIGURE 11.1 *Natural Helper Intervention Model*

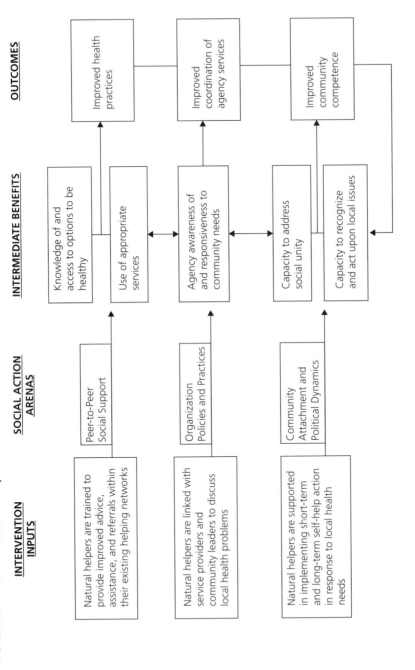

and (3) intervention activities to recognize and address power differentials between the formal and informal helping systems are carefully described.

A key asset of a natural helper intervention is that it builds upon and is responsive to the particular characteristics and resources of a local community support system. The features that make a natural helper intervention effective in one community may be different in another. Such variations in natural helper interventions will likely require evaluation measures and study designs that differ. For example, there has been increased recognition in recent years that embedded support systems are moving beyond geographically defined neighborhoods and communities to locations, such as worksites, special interest clubs, or even the Internet. Given these evolving sources of social support, future research will need to explore the feasibility of newly emerging informal helping networks, such as chat rooms at a Web site, for possible natural helping interventions. The research and practice reviewed in this chapter suggest that although the challenges are substantial, the potential health benefits are considerable from a natural helper intervention model that is structured around people who are trusted, addresses organizational change, and builds community competence.

SUMMARY

Lay Health Advisor interventions have emerged as an important approach in health promotion, spanning all health topics and within various types of communities. Implicit in this approach is the exchange of social support, such as information, advice, tangible aid, and referrals to external resources. From a public health perspective, the associations found between social support and health suggest that lay health advisor interventions can positively affect health. The common feature of LHA interventions is to enlist indigenous members of a given population in channeling health-enhancing social support to individuals and groups (Eng and Young, 1992; Israel, 1985; Service and Salber, 1979). At the same time, important conceptual and methodological distinctions among LHA interventions fall along a continuum (Eng, Parker, and Harlan, 1997). On one end of the continuum are interventions in which LHAs serve as paid employees of an agency, such as a paraprofessional or outreach worker, and seek to deliver social support, such as information and assistance to individuals that protect their health. At the other end are interventions for which LHAs are natural helpers with expertise and knowledge that enhance the health and competence of their community through information distribution, assistance, and organization of community-building activities within their social networks. This emphasis on natural helpers working within their own social network, defined as person-centered webs of relationships that connect individuals to other individuals or groups (Israel, 1982; Israel and Rounds, 1987), differs from the LHA, such as an outreach worker, who provides social support to individuals who may or may not be in his or her social network. LHA interventions that explicitly collaborate with natural helpers to enhance a community's health and competence are the focus of this chapter. The key principles and methods are examined for their relevance to the fields of health education, community development, and social epidemiology. Following an overview of the historical emergence of natural helper models as a specific line of LHA intervention research and practice, the underlying concepts and principles in public health practice are explored. Evidence is presented from empirical studies that applied natural helping models in different communities to respond to different health needs, and one case study is described in detail. Future directions are proposed on work that remains to be done to demonstrate, operationalize, and empirically capture the health-enhancing effects from a community's natural helping system. The goal is to translate the health-enhancing effects into effective interventions.

REFERENCES

Altpeter, M., E., J. A., Bishop, C., and Eng, E. (1999). Lay health advisor activity levels: Definitions from the field. *Health Education and Behavior 26*, 495–512.

Baker, E. A., Bouldin, N., Durham, M., Lowell, M. E., Gonzalez, M., Jodaitis, N., and Cruz, L. N. (1997). The Latino health advocacy program: A collaborative lay health advisor approach. *Health Education and Behavior 4*(4), 495–509.

Berkley-Patton, J., Fawcett, S. B., Paine-Andrews, A., and Johns, L. (1997). Developing capacities of youth as lay health advisors: A case study with high school students. *Health Education and Behavior 24*(4), 481–494.

Biegel, D. E., and Naparstek, A. J. (eds). (1982). *Community support systems and mental health*. New York, Springer.

Biegel, D. E., Naparstek, A. J., and Khan, M. M. (1982). Social support and mental health in urban ethnic neighborhoods, in Biegel, D.E., Naparstek, A. J. (eds.) *Community support systems and mental health*. New York, Springer.

Bloom, B. L. (1979). Prevention of mental disorders: Recent advances in theory and practice. *Community Mental Health J 15*(3), 179–191.

Blumenthal C., Eng, E., and Thomas, J. C. (1999). STEP sisters, sex, and STDs: A process evaluation of the recruitment of lay health advisors. *Am J Health Promotion 14*, 4–6.

Booker, V. K., Robinson, J. G., Kya, B. J., Najera, L. G., and Stewart, G. (1997). Changes in empowerment: Effects of participation in a lay health promotion program. *Health Education and Behavior 4*(4), 452–464.

Boykin, A. W. (1986). The triple quandary and the schooling of Afro-American children. In U. Neisser (Ed.), *The school achievement of minority children: New perspectives*. Hillsdale, NJ: Erlbaum.

Broadhead, W. E., Kaplan, B. H., James, S. A., Wagner, E. H., Schoenbach, V. J., Grimson, R., Heyden, S., Tibblin, G., and Gehlbech, S. H. (1983). The epidemiologic evidence for a relationship between social support and health. *Am J Epid 117*, 521–537.

Cantor, M. H. (1979). The informal support system of New York's inner city elderly: Is ethnicity a factor?, in Gelfand, D. E., Kutzik, A. J. (eds) *Ethnicity and aging: Theory, research, and policy*. New York: Springer.

Caplan, G. (1974). *Support systems and community mental health: Lectures on concept development*. New York: Behavioral Publications.

Caplan, G. (1976). *Support systems and mutual help*. New York: Grune and Stratton.

Caplan, G. Foreword, in Biegel, D. E., Naparstek, A. J. (eds.) (1982). *Community support systems and mental health*. New York: Springer.

Cassel, J. C. (1976). The contribution of the social environment to host resistance. *Am J Epid 104*, 107–123.

Centers for Disease Control and Prevention, National Center for Chronic Disease Prevention and Health Promotion. (1992). Patch: Planned approach to community health. *Journal of Health Education 23*(3), 129–192.

Cottrell, L. S. (1976). The competent community, in B. H. Kaplan, R. N. Wilson, A. H. Leighton, (eds) *Further explorations in social psychiatry*. New York: Basic Books.

Cottrell, L. S. (1980). George Herbert Mead, the legacy of social behaviorism, in R. K., Merton, M. W. Riley, (eds) *Sociological traditions from generation to generation*. Norwood, NJ: Ablex Publishing.

Denham, A., Quinn, S. C., and Gamble, D. (1998). Community organizing for health promotion in the rural south: An exploration of community competence. *Journal of Family and Community Health, 21*(1), 1–21.

Earp, J. A., Viadro, C., Vincus, A., Altpeter, M., Flax, V., Mayne, L., and Eng, E. (1997). Lay health advisors: A strategy for getting the word out about breast cancer, *Health Education and Behavior 24*(4), 432–451.

Earp, J. A., Rauscher, G., and O'Malley, M. S. (November 2000). *Closing the black-white gap in mammography use*. Paper presented at the 128th Annual Meeting of the American Public Health Association, Boston, MA.

Eng, E., Hatch, J. W., and Callan, A. (1985). Institutionalizing social support through the church and into the community. *Health Educ Q 12*(1), 81–92.

Eng, E., and Blanchard, L. (1991). Action-oriented community diagnosis: A health education tool. *International Quarterly of Community Health Education 11*(2), 93–110.

Eng, E., and Young, R. (1992). Lay health advisors as community change agents. *Family and Community Health 15*(1), 24–40.

Eng, E., and Hatch, J. W. (1992). Networking between agencies and Black churches: The lay health advisor model, in Pargament KI, Maton KI, Hess RE (eds.): *Religion and Prevention in Mental Health: Research, Vision, and Action*. New York: Haworth Press.

Eng, E. (1993). *Partners for improved nutrition and health: Did the partnership make a difference*. Final Evaluation Report, Davis, CA, Freedom from Hunger Foundation.

Eng, E., and Parker, E. A. (1994). Measuring community competence in the Mississippi Delta: The interface between program evaluation and empowerment. *Health Education Quarterly 21*(2), 199–220.

Eng, E., and Smith, J. (1995). Natural helping functions of lay health advisors in breast cancer education. *Breast Cancer Res Treatment 35*, 23–29.

Eng, E., Parker, E. A., and Harlan, C. (1997). Lay health advisor intervention strategies: A continuum from natural helping to paraprofessional helping. *Health Education and Behavior 24*(4), 413–417.

Froland, C. (1980). Formal and informal care: Discontinuities in a continuum. *Social Service Review 54*(4), 572–587.

Gans, H. (1961). *The urban villagers*. New York: Free Press.

Gatz, M., Barbarin, O., Tyler, F., Mitchell, R., Moran, J., Wirzbicki, P., Crawford, J., and Engelman, A. (1982). Enhancement of individual and community competence: The older adult as community worker. *American Journal of Community Psychology 10*, 291–303.

Geiger, H. J. (1971). A health center in Mississippi—A case study in social medicine, in L. Corey, S. E. Saltman, M. F. Epstein (eds.) *Medicine in a changing society*. St. Louis, MO: Mosby.

Geiger, H. J. (1984). Community health centers: Health care as an instrument of social change, in V. W. Sidel, R. Sidel (eds.) *Reforming medicine: Lessons of the past quarter century*. New York: Pantheon Books.

Goeppinger, J., and Baglioni, A. J. (1985). Community competence: A positive approach to needs assessment. *American Journal of Community Psychology 13*, 507–523.

Gottlieb, B. H. (1982). Social support in the workplace, in D. E. Biegel, A. J. Naparstek, (eds.) *Community support systems and mental health*. New York: Springer.

Gourash, N. (1978). Help-seeking: A review of the literature. *American Journal of Community Psychology 6*, 413–423.

Green, L. W., and Kreuter, M. W. (1991). *Health promotion planning: An educational and environmental approach*. (2nd ed.) Mountain View, CA: Mayfield.

Guttman, D. (1979). Use of informal and formal supports by the ethnic aged, in D. E. Gelfand, A. J. Kutzik, (eds.) *Ethnicity and aging: Theory, research, and policy*. New York: Springer.

Hamburg, B., and Killilea, M. (1979). Relation of social support, stress, illness and use of health services, in *Surgeon General's report: Background papers*. Washington DC, U.S. Government Printing Office.

Hatch, J. W., and Lovelace, K. (1980). Involving the southern rural church and students of the health professions in health education. *Public Health Reports 95*, 23–25.

Hatch, J. W., and Eng, E. (1983). Health worker role in community oriented primary care, in E. Connor, F. Mullan, (eds.) *Community oriented primary care*. Washington, DC: National Academy Press.

Hatch, J. W., and Moss, N., Saran, A., Presley-Cantrell, L. and Mallory, C. (1993). Community research: Partnerships in Black communities. *American Journal of Preventive Medicine 9*, 27–31.

Health, Education, and Welfare Task Force. (1979). *Report to the President from the President's Commission on Mental Health*. Washington DC, U.S. Goverrnment Printing Office.

House, J. (1981). *Work stress and social support*. Reading, MA: Addison-Wesley.

Heaney, C. A., and Israel, B. A. (1997). Social networks and social support, in K. Glanz, F. M. Lewis, B. K. Rimer, (eds.) *Health behavior and health education: Theory, research, and practice*, San Francisco: Jossey-Bass.

Heller, K. (1989). The return to community. *American Journal of Community Psychology. 17*, 1–15.

Hurley, D., Barbarin, O., and Mitchell, R. (1981). An empirical study of racism in community functioning, in Barbarin, O., Good, P., Pharr, M., Suskind, J. (eds.) *Institutional racism and community competence*. Rockville, MD, National Institute of Mental Health.

Israel, B. A. (1982). Social network and health status: Linking theory, research, and practice. *Patient Counselling and Health Education 4*, 65–79.

Israel, B. A. (1985). Social networks and social support: Implications for natural helper and community level interventions. *Health Education Quarterly 1*(12), 65–80.

Israel, B. A., and Rounds, K. A. (1987). Social networks and social support: A synthesis for health educators. *Advances in Health Education and Promotion 2*, 311–351.

Israel, B. A., Dawson, L., Steckler, A. B., Eng, E., and Guy, W. (1993). Steuart: The person and his works. *Health Education Quarterly* Supplement *1*, S137–S146.

Jackson, E. J., and Parks, C. P. (1997). Recruitment and training issues from selected lay health advisor programs among African Americans: A 20-year perspective. *Health Education and Behavior 24*(4):418–431.

Jessor, R., and Jessor S. (1981). *Problem behavior and psycho-social development: A longitudinal study on youth*. New York: Plenum Press.

Kaplan, B. H., Cassel, J. C. and Gore, S. (1977). Social support and health. *Medical Care 15*(5), 47–58.

Kark, S. (1951). Health center service, in E. H. Cluver (ed) *Social medicine*, Johannesburg, South Africa, Central News Agency.

Ketterer, R. F., Bader, B. C., and Levy, M. R. (1980). Strategies and skills for promoting mental health, in R. H. Price, R. F. Ketterer, B. C. Bader, J. Monahann (eds.) *Prevention in mental health*, Beverly Hills, CA: Sage.

Killilea, M. (1976). Mutual help organizations: Interpretations in the literatures, in G. Caplan, M. Killilea, (eds) *Prevention in mental health*, Beverly Hills, CA: Sage.

Knight, E., Johnson, H. H., and Holbert, D. (1991). Analysis of the competent community: Support for the community. *International Quarterly Community Health Education 11*, 145–154.

Labonte, R. (1989). Community empowerment: The need for political analysis. *Canadian Journal of Public Health 80*, 87–88.

Lee, T. (1968). Urban neighborhood as a socio-spatial schema. *Human Relations 21*(3), 241–268.

Lin, N., Simeone, R., Ensel, W., and Kuo, W. (1979). Social support, stressful life events and illness: A model and an empirical test. *Journal of Health and Social Behavior 20*, 108–119.

Litwak, E., and Szelenyi, I. (1969). Primary group structures and their functions: Kin, neighbors, and friends. *American Sociological Review 34*, 465–481.

Mann, P. (1965). *An approach to urban sociology*. London: Routledge and Kegan Paul.

McLeroy, K. R., Bibeau, D., Steckler, A., and Glanz, K. (1988). An ecological perspective on health promotion programs. *Health Education Quarterly 15*, 351–377.

McKnight, J. (1991). *Comments made at Leadership and Model Development Meeting for Community-Based Public Health Initiative*. Chicago: W. K. Kellogg Foundation.

Nuckolls, K. B., Cassel, J. C., and Kaplan, B. H., (1972). Psycho-social assets, life crisis and the prognosis of pregnancy. *Americsn Journal of Epidemiology 95*, 431–441.

Pancoast, D. L., and Chapman, N. J. (1982). Roles for informal helpers in the delivery of human services, in D. E. Biegel, A. J. Naparstek, (eds.) *Community support systems and mental health.* New York: Springer.

Parker, E. A., Israel, B. A., Schulz, A. J., and Hollis, R. (1998). East Side Detroit village health worker partnership: Community-based lay health advisor intervention in an urban area. *Health Education and Behavior 25*(1), 24–45.

Parker, E. A., Eng, E., Laraia, B., Ammerman, A., Dodds, J., Margolis, L., et al. (1998). Coalition building for prevention: Lessons learned from the North Carolina community-based public health initiative. *Journal of Public Health Management Practice 4*(2), 25–36.

Parker, E. A., Eng, E., Schulz, A. J., and Israel, B. A. (1999). Evaluating community-based health programs that seek to increase community capacity. *New Directions for Evaluation 83*, 37–54.

Plaut, T. (1982). Primary prevention in the 80s: The interface with community support systems, in D. E. Biegel, A. J. Naparstek, (eds) *Community support systems and mental health.* New York: Springer.

President's Commission on Mental Health. (1978). *Report to the President from the President's Commission on Mental Health* (Vol. II). Washington, DC: U.S. Government Printing Office.

Rhodes, S. D., Eng, E., Arceo, R., Remnitz, I. A. (2007). Exploring Latino men's HIV risks using community-based participatory research. American Journal of Health Behavior, *31*(2), 146–158.

Rhodes, S. D., Hergenrather, K. C., Duncan, J., Ramsey, B., Yee, L. J., and Wilkin, A. (2007). Using community-based participatory research to develop a chat room-based HIV prevention intervention for gay men. *Progress in Community Health Partnerships: Research, Education, and Action 1*(2), 175–184.

Riessman, F. (1965). The "helper" therapy principle. *Social Work 10*, 27–32.

Salber, E. J., Beery, W. B., and Jackson, E. J. (1976). The role of the health facilitator in community health education. *Journal of Community Health 2*, 5–20.

Schuster, J., Thomas, J. C., and Eng, E. (1995). Bridging the culture gap in sexually transmitted disease clinics. *North Carolina Medical Journal 56*, 256–269.

Service, C., and Salber, E. J. (eds). (1979). *Community health education: The lay health advisor approach.* Durham, NC: Health Care Systems.

Shanas, E. (1978). The family as a social system in old age. *The Gerontologist 18*(4), 169–174.

Stack, C. B. (1974). *All our kin.* New York: Harper and Row.

Steuart, G. W., and Kark, S. L. (1993). Community health education. *Health Educ Q* Supplement *1*, S29–S47. (Originally published 1962 in Kark, S. L., Steuart, G. W. (eds.) *A practice of social medicine: A South African team's experiences in different African communities.* Edinburgh and London, E and S Livingstone).

Steuart, G. W. (1969a). Planning and evaluation in health education. *International Journal of Health Education 2*, 65–76.

Steuart, G. W. (1969b). Scientist and professional: The relations between research and action. *Health Education Monograms 29*, 1–10.

Steuart, G. W. (November 1977). *The world is not round: Innovation and the medical wheel.* Paper presented at the Annual Meeting of the American Public Health Association in Washington, DC.

Steuart, G. W. (February 1978). Social and cultural perspectives: Community intervention and mental health, in *Perspectives in primary prevention,* Proceedings of the Fourteenth Annual John W. Umstead Series of Distinguished Lectures, Raleigh, NC, North Carolina Division of Mental Health and Mental Retardation Services.

Stokols, D. (1992). Establishing and maintaining healthy environments: Toward a social ecology of health promotion. *American Psychologist 47*(1), 6–22.

Tessaro, I., Eng, E., and Smith, J. (1994). Breast cancer screening in older African-American women: Qualitative research findings. *American Journal of Health Promotion 8,* 286–293.

Thomas, J. C., Eng, E., Clark, M., Robinson, J., and Blumenthal, C. (1998). Lay health advisors: Sexually transmitted disease prevention through community involvement. *American Journal of Public Health, 88*, 1252–3.

Thomas, J. C., Earp, J. A., and Eng, E. (2000). Evaluation and lessons learned from a lay health advisor programme to prevent sexually transmitted diseases. *International Journal of STD and AIDS 11*, 812–818.

Tracy, G. S., and Gussow, Z. (1976). Self-help groups: A grassroots response to a need for services. *Journal of Applied Behavioral Science 12*, 381–396.

Trostle, J. (1986). Anthropology and epidemiology in the twentieth century: A selective history of collaborative projects and theoretical affinities, 1920 to 1970, in Janes, C. R., Stall, R., Gifford, S. M., (eds) *Anthropology and Epidemiology*. Boston: Reidel.

U.S. Department of Health, Education, and Welfare. (1979). *Healthy people: The Surgeon General's report on mental promotion and disease prevention*. Washington DC: U.S. Government Printing Office.

U.S. Department of Health and Human Services, Public Health Service, Centers for Disease Control and Prevention, National Center for Chronic Disease Prevention and Health Promotion, Division of Chronic Disease Control and Community Intervention. (1994) *Community health advisors: Models, research and practice selected annotations—United States* (Vol. 1). Atlanta, GA: Centers for Disease Control and Prevention.

U.S. Department of Health and Human Services, Public Health Service, Centers for Disease Control and Prevention, National Center for Chronic Disease Prevention and Health Promotion, Division of Chronic Disease Control and Community Intervention. (1994). *Community health advisors: Models, research and practice selected annotations—United States* (Vol. 2). Atlanta, GA: Centers for Disease Control and Prevention.

Warren, D. I. (1971). Neighborhoods in urban areas. *Encyclopedia of social work* (Vol. 1). New York: National Association of Social Workers.

Warren, D. I. (1977). Neighborhoods in urban areas. *Encyclopedia of social work* (Vol. 1). New York: National Association of Social Workers.

Warren, D. I. (1982). Using helping networks: A key social bond of urbanites, in D. E. Biegel, A. J. Naparstek, (eds) *Community support systems and mental health*. New York: Springer.

Warren, R. L. (1963a). *Social research consultation: An experiment in health and welfare planning*. New York: Russell Sage Foundation.

Warren, R. L. (1963b). *The community in America*. Skokie, IL: Rand McNally.

Watkins, E. L., Harlan, C., Eng, E., Gansky, S. A., Gehan, D., and Larson, K. (1994). Assessing the effectiveness of lay health advisors with migrant farmworkers. *Family and Community Health*, *16*(4), 72–87.

Wilkinson, D. Y. (1992). Indigenous community health workers in the 1960s and beyond, in R. L., Braithwaite, S. E. Taylor, (eds) *Health issues in the Black community*. San Francisco: Jossey-Bass.

CHAPTER

12

COMMUNITY-BASED PREVENTION MARKETING: A NEW FRAMEWORK FOR HEALTH PROMOTION INTERVENTIONS

Carol A. Bryant

Kelli R. McCormack Brown

Robert J. McDermott

Rita D. Debate

Moya L. Alfonso

Julie A. Baldwin

Paul Monaghan

Leah M. Phillips

ECONOMIC EQUALITY AND PUBLIC HEALTH

The overarching goal of public health programs is to decrease premature death, disease, and disability and increase the quality of life for each segment of society. Despite this aim, not all people enjoy equal health status or life quality. In the United States, low-income groups and persons in communities of color experience disproportionately poorer health outcomes across disease conditions (Prevention Institute, 2008a). Confounding the issue is the fact that not all Americans enjoy equivalent access to care. The gap in health status by socioeconomic, racial, and ethnic groups may be increasing. Furthermore, the combination of racism, poverty, and disparate environmental factors exacerbate the threats to health for these population segments (Prevention Institute, 2008b). Although these disparities are evident in the United States and are a major topic of health policy and politics, the differences between developed countries and economically disadvantaged ones are even more pronounced (World Health Organization, 2007).

Economics and oppression are fundamental causes of these disparities. They also are determinants of community environments, which, in turn, contribute to health. Even when community members know their health needs and priorities, they may not be in an advantageous position to influence improvement of the status quo. To advance health status and equity, attention needs to be focused on prevention initiatives by empowering the affected populations. Implementation of interventions, policies, and practices can make the environments in which people live and work better, and in turn enhance health-related outcomes (Prevention Institute, 2008b). The formation of a partnership between community members and university-based researchers may assist communities in identifying and prioritizing their health problems and in finding satisfactory ways to solve them. Whereas university-based researchers can carry out needs assessments and program interventions in communities *without* direct community support or participation, they risk ignoring existing local resources and failing to meet indigenous priorities. Consequently, research outcomes are less likely to be translated into action via programs, practices, or policies. Therefore, combining community assets, such as working coalitions with university researchers skilled in community-based participatory research methods, can produce a win-win situation. Unfortunately, such partnerships have not always been successful. According to Katz (2004):

> Part of the reason such a disconnect exists between research and advocacy is that partnership between these two groups isn't exactly the most natural thing. Community groups often distrust academics, and, it's only fair to say, with good reason. Historically, public health research has been conducted almost exclusively by academic investigators. This approach has been faulted for its exclusivity and arrogance in relying on people from outside a community to identify the community's "problems" and the likely means of fixing them. The approach has also resulted in some of biomedicine's most shameful abuses of human subjects. But even when no such transgressions occur, the

"for academics only" approach often leaves community members feeling used rather than involved.

Thus, strategies and frameworks are needed that bring together the strengths of community members and university-based researchers. The presentation that follows describes an innovative needs assessment and strategic program planning process—community-based prevention marketing (CBPM)—that assists communities in developing the capacity to address some of their most pressing health issues and to sustain improved health outcomes. CBPM is a program planning framework that blends social marketing techniques and community organization principles into a synergistic approach to design or tailor, implement, evaluate, translate, and disseminate public health interventions among selected audience segments (Bryant, Forthofer, McCormack Brown, Landis, and McDermott, 2000; Bryant, McCormack Brown, McDermott, Forthofer, Bumpus, Calkins, et al., 2007). Community and academic partners follow a nine-step process: (1) mobilize the community; (2) develop a profile of community problems and assets; (3) select target behaviors, audiences, and, when possible, interventions to tailor; (4) build community capacity to address the priority or target problem(s); (5) conduct formative research; (6) develop a marketing strategy; (7) develop or tailor program materials and tactics; (8) implement the new or tailored intervention; and (9) track and evaluate the program's impact. Of these nine steps, perhaps the most critical is Step Four, as "community capacity building" is an ongoing process that is operational throughout the CBPM process. Tasks that make up each step are outlined in Table 12.1; arrows indicate that the process is not necessarily a linear one and that many tasks are interconnected.

This chapter describes CBPM's theoretical constructs and then examines how it has been applied during the last decade. Two case studies are presented to illustrate how it can be used respectively to: (1) *design* a community-based extension of a national media campaign, and, (2) *tailor* an evidence-based intervention. Finally, the strengths and limitations of CBPM, as well as future directions for its use are discussed.

COMMUNITY-BASED PREVENTION MARKETING THEORETICAL CONSTRUCTS

Community Organization

Community organization, a cornerstone in CBPM, is the process by which community groups are helped to identify common problems, set goals, mobilize resources, and implement strategies for reaching those goals (Bond and Hauf, 2007; Minkler and Wallerstein, 1998). The principles of community participation and capacity-building are incorporated into all phases of the CBPM process, with the goal of empowering community members to make strategic planning decisions and be responsible for sustaining program activities.

Community participation is another central principle of the CBPM framework. Community members participate when they identify problems, mobilize resources,

TABLE 12.1 **Steps and Key Tasks in Community-Based Prevention Marketing.**

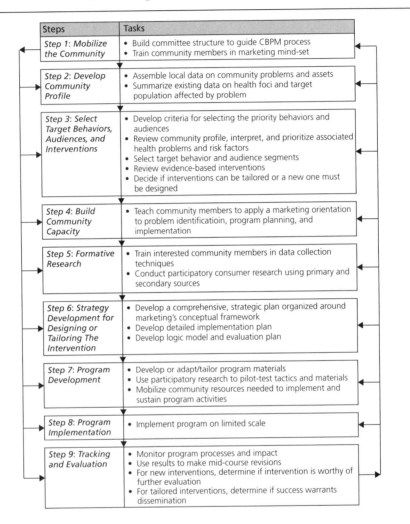

Steps	Tasks
Step 1: Mobilize the Community	• Build committee structure to guide CBPM process • Train community members in marketing mind-set
Step 2: Develop Community Profile	• Assemble local data on community problems and assets • Summarize existing data on health foci and target population affected by problem
Step 3: Select Target Behaviors, Audiences, and Interventions	• Develop criteria for selecting the priority behaviors and audiences • Review community profile, interpret, and prioritize associated health problems and risk factors • Select target behavior and audience segments • Review evidence-based interventions • Decide if interventions can be tailored or a new one must be designed
Step 4: Build Community Capacity	• Teach community members to apply a marketing orientation to problem identificatioin, program planning, and implementation
Step 5: Formative Research	• Train interested community members in data collection techniques • Conduct participatory consumer research using primary and secondary sources
Step 6: Strategy Development for Designing or Tailoring The Intervention	• Develop a comprehensive, strategic plan organized around marketing's conceptual framework • Develop detailed implementation plan • Develop logic model and evaluation plan
Step 7: Program Development	• Develop or adapt/tailor program materials • Use participatory research to pilot-test tactics and materials • Mobilize community resources needed to implement and sustain program activities
Step 8: Program Implementation	• Implement program on limited scale
Step 9: Tracking and Evaluation	• Monitor program processes and impact • Use results to make mid-course revisions • For new interventions, determine if intervention is worthy of further evaluation • For tailored interventions, determine if success warrants dissemination

and plan strategies to improve their lives (Bracht and Tsouros, 1990). In CBPM, community representatives "own" problem identification and program design and implementation. They also participate in all research activities, including problem definition, data collection, instrument design, sampling, and data interpretation (Israel, Schulz, Parker, and Becker, 1998). Social marketing experts from outside the community partner with community members (for example, professionals from varied backgrounds, lay leaders and activists, and representatives of local businesses, churches, voluntary organizations, and citizens) as they work through problem definition and prioritization of target behaviors and segments, formative research, and program design, implementation and evaluation of interventions.

Building community capacity is a critical element of CBPM and includes "the characteristics of communities that affect their ability to identify, mobilize, and address social and public health problems" (Goodman, Speers, McLeroy, Fawcett, Kegler, Parker, et al., 1998). When mobilizing a community, local capacity or readiness to act is assessed. Some communities already possess the resources to address identified problems; however, most community groups need basic training or technical assistance to effectively use a marketing orientation.

Community empowerment and enhanced competence are desired outcomes of CBPM. Empowerment is the process by which community members acquire the skills needed to improve their lives (Minkler and Wallerstein, 1998), including application of a "marketing mind-set" to set goals and develop strategies for achieving them. In CBPM, experts teach interested citizens the marketing skills, including participatory research techniques for designing, tailoring, and implementing behavior change strategies. As community members collaborate to influence decisions in the larger social system, *collective efficacy* is established and a more equitable share of resources is obtained (Israel, Checkoway, Schulz, and Zimmerman, 1994; Robertson and Minkler, 1994).

Social Marketing

Social marketing gives CBPM its strategic planning tool. Social marketing is distinguished from other health promotion approaches by its conceptual framework (a commitment to create satisfying exchanges and create an integrated strategy based on marketing's four *P*s—*p*roduct, *p*rice, *p*lace, and *p*romotion), competitive analysis, audience segmentation, use of formative research to make strategic decisions, and ongoing monitoring and evaluation (Grier and Bryant, 2005; Hastings, 2007).

Social marketing is committed to creating satisfying exchanges. Approaching the task with a marketing mind-set teaches community members that people act largely out of self-interest. Consequently, health promotion interventions must optimize the benefits people gain and minimize the "costs" they "pay" when they change their behavior. This commitment to creating satisfying exchanges is quintessential in CBPM because it reminds program planners that they must understand people's *wants* and not just meet their public health *needs*. The *VERB™ Summer Scorecard* case study at the end of this chapter exemplifies the importance of promising the consumer (the people you hope to change) what they really want instead of what you want for them.

Marketing's four *P*s, also known as the *marketing mix*, direct program planners to consider the relationships among the product, price, place, and promotion. *Product* refers to the benefits consumers gain by adopting the proposed behavior or practice. Many social marketers distinguish among the core, actual, and augmented product (Kotler and Lee, 2008; McCormack Brown, 2006). In this scheme, the *actual product* is the practice being promoted (for example, being physically active for sixty minutes or more on most days); the *core product* is the benefit gained by adopting the actual product (for example, having fun with friends and trying new things while being physically active); and the *augmented product* is special features or tangible goods or services that facilitate adoption (for example, a means for monitoring activity) (Grier and Bryant, 2005).

The other side of the exchange, *price*, refers to the costs or sacrifices people exchange for product benefits. In most public health offerings, price includes non-monetary costs (for example, embarrassment, diminished pleasure, time, the hassle of changing established habits, and having financial outlays for transportation or child care costs).

In social marketing, *place* has several referents: the location where sales and service encounters take place (including service hours, parking arrangements, and physical attributes of the locale), distribution networks or channels, and the partners or intermediaries that support the exchange. A good placement strategy ensures that the product is accessible, convenient, and adequately supported at the right times and places in the consumer's life.

The *promotion* refers to the variety of activities employed to facilitate product adoption. Promotional activities may include printed materials, direct marketing, public relations, promotional items, signage, media, special events and displays, and face-to-face selling. For effectiveness, the promotion is integrated with other components of the marketing mix, so that activities reinforce product benefits, costs that must be lowered, and placement considerations.

CBPM necessitates that a *competitive analysis* is performed. Competition refers to the risk behaviors people currently practice—what they are doing instead of the desired health behavior. CBPM asks that program planners understand the competition when designing an intervention, to ensure that the product offers a more satisfying exchange (Clay-Wayman, Beall, Thackeray, and McCormack Brown, 2007; Hastings, 2007). Thus, a marketer whose product is increased physical activity is going to have to understand the appeal of its competition—coming home after a hard day at work or school, and watching television, playing video games, or engaging in some other sedentary endeavor. The marketer's *product* must have a desirable benefit as well as a *price* that is equal to or lower in cost than the competition. To this end, program planners conduct consumer research to identify the behaviors or services competing with those being promoted and the benefits they offer consumers. Findings are then used to develop a sustainable competitive advantage or position that optimizes the product's appeal.

Historically, public health interventions often have a "one size fits all" appearance, a possible result of which is that the intervention appeals to no one. CBPM incorporates *audience segmentation*, the process of dividing a potential audience into distinct segments based on characteristics that influence their responsiveness to interventions. It is rare for one product to meet everyone's needs equally well; therefore, audiences are segmented to identify subgroups to give greatest priority in planning program interventions and design the most effective marketing mix for each (Slater, Kelly, and Thackeray, 2006). A variety of variables are used to segment a population. Frequently used variables include current behavior, desired benefits, other factors that affect adoption, psychographics, and demographics (Forthofer and Bryant, 2000).

All marketing decisions are made with the *consumer's viewpoint* in mind, and *formative* (or consumer) *research* is used to understand how they perceive product benefits, costs, placement, and promotional activities (Parsons and McCormack Brown, 2004). In CBPM, community members are taught how to collect qualitative and quantitative data and use findings to create a marketing plan. Whereas using community participatory research to make informed decisions is not unique, using marketing's conceptual framework to guide the formative research is a hallmark of CBPM.

As CBPM program interventions are implemented, *monitoring* of their components is carried out to assess their effectiveness in influencing the desired behavior change. Monitoring identifies activities that are worthy of being sustained, as well as those requiring revision. Program *tracking* also serves as a documentation process for process *evaluation* (for example, documenting program fidelity in effectiveness trials) as well as mediating factors (McDermott, 2004).

GENESIS AND NEED FOR THE MODEL

CBPM's development was conceptualized after years of observing social marketing conducted *in* communities rather than *with* communities. Community organizing principles were expected to optimize the long-range impact of social marketing interventions and make the planning process more consistent with public health's ethical commitment to community empowerment. Working with a variety of community groups highlighted the power of local wisdom in understanding public health problems, as well as the difficulties groups have in designing strategies to address them. In these failed circumstances, community members likely could have been more successful if they had used a marketing orientation to select priority behaviors and audiences, and used consumer research to guide planning decisions.

These experiences and convictions led to formalizing CBPM as part of an application to the Centers for Disease Control and Prevention (CDC) for designation as a center for excellence in prevention research. The Florida Prevention Research Center (FPRC) was established in 1998 and initiated a series of CBPM demonstration projects. A few of these are described below.

COMMUNITY-BASED PREVENTION MARKETING APPLICATIONS

CBPM has been applied successfully in four settings. Whereas three demonstration projects have been coordinated and partially funded by the FPRC, the fourth was conducted by the University of South Carolina Prevention Research Center (USCPRC). As shown in Table 12.2, these applications have differed by audience, community context, and health problem focus.

The FPRC's first CBPM demonstration project examined the feasibility of teaching a community group to use marketing principles and techniques to promote preventive behaviors. Of special interest were questions such as: "Will community members embrace audience segmentation and other marketing techniques?" and "Will they rely on formative research results to make strategic decisions around marketing's four Ps?" The first project was based in Sarasota County, Florida, because of the strong leadership and overall level of community readiness. The Director of Health Promotion and

TABLE 12.2 Overview of Four Community-Based Prevention Marketing Projects.

Site		Sarasota, FL	PCWH (Immokalee, FL)	Kentucky Tweens Nutrition and Fitness Project (Lexington, KY)	Step Up, Step Out!, Central South Carolina
Target Audience		Middle school youth	Florida citrus pickers	Tweens	Sedentary or insufficiently active middle-aged women
Health Focus		Healthy youth behaviors	Eye injuries	Obesity prevention	Chronic disease prevention
Product Strategy	Actual (behavior)	Do not initiate smoking and/or drinking	Use of safety glasses	Physical activity	Physical activity
	Core (benefits)	Improved health; approval by mothers	Pick rapidly without fear of injury or daily irritation	Have fun, spend time with friends, explore new and adventurous activities, and master new skills	Meet and spend time with others; toning and overall health
	Augmented (tangible service/ product)	n/a	Use Revelations by Radians	Scorecard to monitor activity events	Trail guide; buddy system; special exercise events

	Perceived Costs			
Pricing Strategy	Loss of driver's license; looking stupid; getting caught	Discomfort; fogging; impedes picking by getting tangled in tree branches or falling to the ground; slows picking by making it hard to see the fruit; increases chance of falling off ladder	Fear of embarrassment	Lack of time and competing demands, fear due to safety concerns

	Other *Deterrents* *Partners* *Distribution*			
Placement-Strategy	Schools and school board; Health Department; Sheriff's Department School health liaisons; community youth organizations	Lack of role models; mistrust of employers and supervisors Community health workers; crew leaders; company policy makers Community health workers	Fears about children's safety, and monetary cost of equipment or participation fees Community organizations, businesses that offer opportunities to be active Libraries, schools, businesses willing to distribute Scorecards	Physical limitations Organize group walks for trails and malls Work with recreation department Community partners distribute flyers and brochures

	Believe in All Your Possibilities campaign Web site, print materials, teen SOURCE Theatre, and public relations activities			
Promotional Strategy	Use community health workers to model, encourage, and educate peers; use crew leaders to encourage and support injury reports	Free and paid media were used to promote the program	Newspaper, radio, television and outdoor advertising; promotional events and incentives; e-mail reminders	

Planning at the Sarasota County Health Department had organized one of the nation's oldest operating Planned Approach to Community Health (PATCH) coalitions (Alfonso, Lopez, Bryant, and Bumpus, 2001), which followed community development principles similar to ones described in the CBPM framework (Bryant et al., 2007). The community had formed a coalition, developed a community profile, and selected youth smoking and drinking as priority problems. Building on their successful capacity to work together, FPRC researchers were able to proceed quickly to steps Three, Four, and Five of the CBPM process—selecting specific behaviors and audience segments, enhancing the community's capacity to use a marketing mind-set, and conducting formative research.

The project culminated in the development of a comprehensive social marketing plan and intervention to prevent middle school youth from starting to smoke cigarettes and drink alcohol, called *Believe in All Your Possibilities* (Bryant et al., 2007). For more information on *Believe* or to download program materials, visit the *Believe* Web site at http://www.believe-in-all-your-possibilities.org/index.html. This coalition has continued to function since its 1998 inception, using the *Believe* intervention as a platform for preventing multiple risk behaviors among youth. Some activities, such as an annual theater-as-education production performed in middle schools by high school students, have been institutionalized; others, such as issuance of smoking citations, have been sustained using local funds.

The Sarasota County project provided many lessons (Bryant et al., 2007). The most critical issue confronted was the community's impatience with the protracted time line required to develop an intervention based on participatory research. In response to the community's desire to accelerate the time to launch an intervention, the CBPM framework was modified to make greater use of existing literature to identify findings not requiring replication. For more information on lessons learned from this project, see Bryant et al., (2007). Whenever possible, community groups are encouraged to tailor evidence-based projects, and pilot-test existing materials and tactics concurrently with collection of primary consumer data (Bryant et al., 2007). Subsequent projects have examined the feasibility of using CBPM to: (1) tailor evidence-based interventions for local use; and (2) develop a community extension of a national social marketing campaign.

The second demonstration project, the *Partnership for Citrus Worker Health*, focused on the initial steps of the CBPM framework as well as the feasibility of modifying evidence-based interventions for local use. For this application, an underserved occupational community, Florida's citrus harvesters, was selected, making it possible to examine questions, such as: "Will research guided by marketing's conceptual framework reveal the insights needed to address an occupational community's unique needs?" and "Can marketing principles be used to design an intervention to modify the safety culture of a disenfranchised occupational community?"

Working with a migrant worker advocacy group, the Farmworker Association of Florida (FWAF), FPRC researchers organized a community board, developed a profile of community problems and assets, and taught board members to use marketing principles to select a health problem. After the board selected eye injuries as the project's focus, and use of safety glasses as the target behavior, a literature review identified an eye injury prevention program designed for agricultural workers in the Midwest (Forst, Lacey, Chen, Jimenez, Bauer, Alvarado, et al., 2004) that could be tailored for this population. Although this project demonstrated CBPM's utility in tailoring existing evidence-based interventions for unique settings, it also revealed new insights, challenges, and the time required to mobilize a disenfranchised population with few organizational assets.

The third demonstration project examined a different way to accelerate the planning process—the use of CBPM to create a community extension of a national media campaign. FPRC researchers worked with a community coalition in Lexington, Kentucky that selected childhood obesity as its health focus. Using a marketing orientation, it selected physical activity as a target behavior and moderately active tweens (youth nine to thirteen years old) as the priority population. Relying heavily on existing data to minimize the time and cost of conducting formative research, the coalition discovered the CDC's physical activity promotion campaign, *VERB™—It's What You Do*. Guided by the *VERB* program's audience research (Aeffect Inc., 2000; Aeffect Inc., 2001), the coalition created a program to offer local tweens opportunities to be physically active. Because the community-based program was compatible with the national media campaign's underlying marketing plan, it was able to capitalize on *VERB's* brand equity and extensive media coverage (Bretthauer-Mueller, Berkowitz, Thomas, McCarthy, Green, Melancon, et al., 2008). In contrast to the previous demonstration projects that required years to come to fruition, the coalition launched the *VERB Summer Scorecard* program in less than a year.

Galvanized by rapid success, the Lexington Tweens Nutrition and Fitness coalition has used CBPM to tailor another evidence-based program, *We Can!*, for teaching parents how to reduce children's risks for obesity. They also have advocated successfully for policy changes in the state legislature and local public school district. Information about their activities is available at http://www.fitky.org/Default.aspx?id=25 and http://health.usf.edu/publichealht/prc/downloads.html.

Concurrently, USCPRC researchers worked with a South Carolina coalition to promote physical activity. The Sumter County Active Lifestyles Coalition and Recreation and Parks Department, which was already active in promoting physical activity, responded to the USCPRC's invitation for community partners. After training the coalition in marketing principles, USCPRC researchers worked with coalition members to conduct research and design an intervention known as *The Step Up, Step Out!* (Burroughs, Peck, Sharpe, Granner, Bryant, and Fields, 2006; Peck, Sharpe, Burroughs, and Granner, 2008)

VERB™ SUMMER SCORECARD CASE STUDY

The *VERB Summer Scorecard* project illustrates how a youth obesity prevention coalition in Lexington, Kentucky used CBPM to design a community-based physical activity promotion program to capitalize on the national media campaign *VERB—It's What You Do*. (For more information on the campaign, visit their Web site at http://www.cdc.gov/youthcampaign/.

Step One: Mobilize the Community

In 2003, the FPRC and the Lexington-Fayette County Health Department (LFCHD) agreed to collaborate on a CBPM demonstration project targeting childhood obesity. The health promotion director of the LFCHD had extensive network ties with local organizations interested in the problem and skills with coordinating complex projects. Her supervisors understood and valued social marketing and agreed to serve as the fiscal agent for the project. External funds were provided by the FPRC and the Kentucky Department for Public Health's CDC obesity planning grant.

The first task was to recruit persons to serve on the coalition that would direct the project. Original members included representatives from the YMCA, Parks and Recreation Department, school food service personnel, physical education teachers, youth advocates, local government representatives, cooperative extension agents, business and media representatives, Latino community members, children's museum administrators, pediatricians, faith-based group leaders, and nutrition, physical activity, and family experts from local universities. Most members were already committed to helping youth or fighting obesity. However, a few joined because they wanted to learn more about social marketing. The coalition grew to more than fifty people.

Step Two: Develop Community Profile

As the coalition was assembled, health department and FPRC personnel assembled body mass index (BMI) data collected from students entering middle school and conducted a literature review. About 22 percent of sixth-graders were overweight, and an additional 19 percent were at risk of becoming overweight, demonstrating a need for intervention. The literature identified behaviors that showed the most promise for combating childhood obesity (Center for Weight and Health, 2001). Audience research conducted by CDC's youth media campaign, later called *VERB* (Aeffect Inc., 2000; Aeffect Inc,, 2001), provided valuable insights into the audiences at greatest risk of obesity, and factors that influenced lifestyle decisions.

Step Three: Select Target Behaviors and Audiences

As previously mentioned, CBPM is not necessarily a linear process. Capacity-building takes place throughout the planning cycle, overlapping with many other steps. In Kentucky, coalition meetings were structured to teach community members to use marketing principles to select target behaviors and audiences, and to tailor evidence-based interventions. Each meeting began with a short presentation of relevant marketing principles and techniques (for example, criteria marketers use to select the audience segments they will give the highest priority in their planning efforts). Next, coalition members were given a summary of information related to that marketing decision (for example, potential segmentation schemes) and encouraged to apply the principles and methods they had just learned (for example, to select a target audience segment).

During the first meeting, coalition members prioritized target behaviors based on two criteria—the behavior's impact on childhood obesity and the likelihood that the coalition could change it. Physical activity in community settings was one of several target behaviors the coalition decided to address. (The other priorities were improving physical activity and nutrition in schools and increasing parental influence on good nutrition habits.) In the next meeting, coalition members reviewed local information on obesity rates from preschool through high school and selected tweens (youth ages nine to thirteen) as the priority audience segment. In the third meeting, the group reviewed information about interventions implemented in other community settings and decided to invite the national *VERB* program director to explain the campaign's rationale and key components. The next month, the *VERB* director described the program's underlying marketing strategy, and the coalition decided to capitalize on the campaign's brand equity (Huhman, Potter, Wong, Banspach, Duke, and Heitzler, 2005) by creating opportunities for tweens to be active around the community throughout the summer. Several coalition members had been part of local projects that encouraged youth to track the number of books they had read or cultural sites they had attended, and suggested a similar monitoring device be used for tracking physical activity. Familiar with marketing principles, coalition members were well-prepared to make the local program compatible with the national campaign's marketing strategy, encouraging tweens to have fun with friends as they tracked their activities.

Step Four: Build Community Capacity

In addition to short training sessions incorporated into monthly coalition meetings, the FPRC held a two-day social marketing training session for approximately thirty interested coalition members. Five members, including the Health Promotion Director and two of her staff, subsequently enrolled in the University of South Florida social marketing field school courses, and seven coalition members attended the Social Marketing in Public Health conference the following June. The additional training enabled these coalition members to use social marketing techniques to tailor other evidence-based interventions (for example, *We Can!*) and promote policy changes.

Step Five: Conduct Formative Research

Community capacity building activities also were an essential ingredient in the formative research. Consistent with community participatory research principles, the FPRC trained youth board and coalition members to conduct focus groups. During spring 2004, community members conducted four focus groups with tweens and two with their parents. Results confirmed *VERB's* strategy of promoting physical activity as a way to have fun, try new things, and spend time with friends. Findings supported the monitoring idea, but suggested that the program needed to offer a variety of free or low-cost activities that were easily accessible and safe. Prizes and other incentives also were recommended.

Step Six: Develop Marketing Strategy

During the strategy development phase, health department staff and FPRC researchers prepared a strategy workbook (http://health.usf.edu/NR/rdonlyres/24FB1973-AA10-470C-B1CD-AD32B63A2BA4/0/physicalactivitycommunity.pdf) to guide coalition members in translating research findings into a comprehensive marketing plan. During a special six-hour meeting, coalition members further segmented the target audience and developed the marketing plan (summarized in Table 12.2). The monitoring idea was transformed into the *VERB Summer Scorecard* program to help tweens track their activity. Each time a tween was active for a designated period of time (typically an hour) at a *Scorecard* site or at home, an adult would sign one of twenty-four squares on the back. When the card was filled, it could be redeemed for physical activity-related prizes (for example, karate lessons, YMCA memberships, skate boards, and so on).

After developing the marketing plan, a coalition subcommittee developed a more detailed implementation plan outlining each organization's responsibilities for specific activities, and a timeline for completion. FPRC researchers created a logic model and an evaluation plan for the coalition's review and approval.

Step Seven: Program Development

In this phase, the marketing plan served as the blueprint for developing program materials and tactics. A graphic artist, who served on the coalition and worked for the health department, designed the *VERB Summer Scorecard* (Figure 12.1) and related promotional materials.

FIGURE 12.1 VERB *Summer Scorecard*

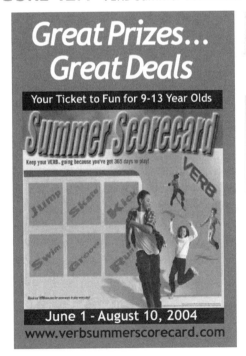

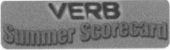

Get your Scorecard stamped each time you do an activity at any Scorecard site. You can get your card stamped at the same place over and over. Or, mix it up and try different places.

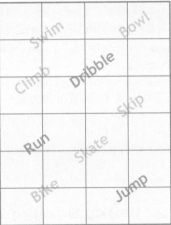

Parents can initial one of your squares each time you play an hour on up to 12 squares. If all 24 squares are stamped or initialed by August 10, you're eligible for prizes.

Program materials and tactics were pilot tested with youth, their parents, and potential program partners (for example, businesses that offered activity-related services to tweens). Feedback suggested the *Scorecard* should be small for easy handling; the program should offer a variety of free and affordable physical activity options; and activity-related prizes should be offered as incentives for card completion.

Step Eight: Program Implementation

The coalition then mobilized resources needed to pilot test the *Scorecard* intervention. Health department staff managed numerous logistical program details, such as *Scorecard* distribution and recruitment of activity sponsors and prize donors. Fourteen businesses and twelve community groups offered the activities for free or at a reduced price. Eighteen organizations sponsored activities for tweens on the summer solstice, June 21st, promoted as the *Longest Day of Play*. Approximately 950 youth attended the event to partake in games, tennis lessons, whiffle ball, dance, aerobics, and relay and sack races.

The *VERB Summer Scorecard* program ended with a Grand Finale event, a two-hour gathering at a minor league baseball park in August. More than a thousand tweens and their families were able to try new activities at twenty-five activity stations and register for fall activities, such as scouting, karate, dancing, and sports teams. At the end of the evening, everyone was invited into the bleachers for the grand prize drawing, and tweens were given a chance to run the bases and take home a backpack of smaller prizes.

Since its initial rollout in 2004, the *VERB Summer Scorecard* program has been implemented annually in Lexington and tailored for use in sixteen additional communities around the United States. Whereas most communities have implemented the program during the summer, others have tailored the program for use during the winter school break or school year. More information and program materials are found at http://hsc.usf.edu/publichealth/prc/downloads.htm.

Step Nine: Program Tracking and Evaluation

Beginning with the program's launch in 2004, FPRC researchers and coalition members have tracked program activities to identify program strengths and weaknesses. Youth board members have taken field notes at swimming pools and skating rinks, providing feedback about program perceptions of tweens, parents, and community partners. Health department employees visited *Scorecard* sites to verify program material availability and detect implementation problems. During fall 2004, colleagues at the University of Kentucky Prevention Research Center interviewed parents of tweens who had submitted cards to identify program components that should be retained and those that needed revision. Their recommendations led to improvements in the 2005 program—development of a calendar to help parents track sponsored events, expansion of the proportion of squares that could be signed by parents for home play, and other changes. Interviews with parents whose tweens did not

TABLE 12.3   **History of Scorecard Program Awareness and Participation.**

	2004 N = 4049	2006 N = 2623	2007 N = 2966
Awareness of VERB Summer Scorecard	35%	62%	79%
Receipt of Scorecard[a]	44%	59%	53%
Number of Scorecards submitted	355	878	1720
Completion of Scorecard[a]	25%	37%	30%
Intention to complete again	NA	20%[b]	NA

[a]Among those who had heard of VERB Summer Scorecard.

[b]Among those who had completed at least part of a VERB™ Summer Scorecard.

participate also yielded valuable information. For example, to help parents overcome transportation barriers, a partnership was established with the local public transportation agency, LexTran, allowing the *Scorecard* to serve as a bus pass for tweens and an accompanying adult traveling to *Scorecard* events.

FPRC researchers and coalition members also have conducted surveys in Lexington-Fayette County middle schools to assess tweens' program exposure, program participation, physical activity levels, and, in 2006, their intentions to participate the following summer. As summarized in Table 12.3, program awareness and participation have increased annually. Program awareness increased from 35 percent to almost 80 percent, and the number of cards submitted for inclusion in the grand finale drawing rose from 355 to 1,720 over a four-year period.

Whereas the cross-sectional nature of the data prevents a cause-and-effect conclusion between program participation and higher activity levels, elements analyzed to date suggest the program offers great promise—for each increase in participation level, there was a 16 percent increase in the odds that a child was active for sixty minutes or more on each of the previous seven days.

Next Steps

FPRC researchers will examine further the various permutations of the *Scorecard* interventions in the numerous communities that have implemented it. In addition, a small-scale efficacy trial is planned for the state of Florida.

PARTNERSHIP FOR CITRUS WORKER HEALTH (PCWH) CASE STUDY

This case study describes how an occupational community used CBPM to tailor an eye injury prevention program adapted from one designed for Midwestern agricultural workers to fit the unique demands of workers harvesting Florida's citrus crop.

Step One: Mobilize the Community

FPRC researchers invited the Farmworkers Association of Florida (FWAF) to partner on this project because of its ability to work with migrant agricultural workers. Florida's citrus harvesting community was selected as the target population because it had not been previously organized or assisted by governmental or academic projects, making it possible to focus on the initial steps in the CBPM framework.

The first task was to establish a board of citrus workers and other members who served or represented the industry. As anticipated, the FWAF had relatively little difficulty recruiting citrus workers, and the FPRC was able to recruit representatives from the local health department and social service agencies. It was more difficult, however, to recruit members from other ranks within the citrus industry because of their concerns that the FWAF would leverage access to the groves to unionize workers. Fortunately, one occupational safety manager received permission from his supervisor to attend a board meeting, and after learning more about program goals and the planning framework, endorsed the program and recruited other industry representatives.

Board meetings were held during the evenings after workers returned from the groves. To build familiarity and trust among board members, each meeting began with dinner and time to socialize. PCWH board members assigned the project its name and mission statement, established guidelines for various partners to work together, and made key project decisions described below.

Step Two: Develop Community Profile

When the project began, citrus workers were not identified in existing data sets, and few studies had examined problems in this community. To create a community profile, FPRC researchers trained some FWAF staff and board members to collect data from citrus workers, industry representatives, and community organization representatives. These community researchers conducted participant observation, individual interviews, and brief surveys of citrus workers waiting for a free eye examination.

Step Three: Select Target Behaviors and Audiences

This step was especially difficult because of the stark differences in perceptions of community problems and their priorities between workers and managers. The harvesters, most of whom were members of the FWAF, wanted to focus the project on pesticide exposure—a problem they had targeted with nursery workers and fern harvesters. Citrus industry managers strongly opposed this topic because of their belief that pesticides created little risk to citrus workers, and if selected as a target problem, would attract unwanted attention.

Before making a final decision, the board determined the criteria and process for selecting the project's health focus. Over time, board members became more comfortable working together, and agreed upon a voting method that enabled consensus development. Called *fist to five*, this method required each member to vote publicly on each problem area, raising five fingers for issues they were willing to give their greatest support, fewer fingers to indicate declining levels of support, and a fist to indicate active opposition to the issue. This method allowed the group to determine which issues had widespread support and avoid those that would be alienating to one or more board members. Unsurprisingly, the pesticide proposal was eliminated by citrus industry managers early in the process. Fortunately, citrus workers and community advocates were not deterred by their veto, and quickly reached a consensus that eye injuries were the most important issue to address in their work together.

Step Four: Build Community Capacity

Partly due to the diversity of members on the PCWH board (which included large citrus companies and community activists), and because of the poverty and lack of resources in the migrant farmworker community, board members' adoption of social marketing has been more limited than in other CBPM projects. However, because of the synergy from the project, the partners have taken steps to work together on a variety of interventions, and have created capacity in the community to address health and safety interventions in the future. The companies involved have increased health screenings in partnership with the county health department, and the FWAF has partnered with the health department to do outreach on diabetes, hypertension, and sexually transmitted diseases. The FWAF also hired a community organizer with extensive health research experience to work with FPRC-based researchers and develop future grants on issues of farmworker safety. The sustainability of the PCWH efforts will also be aided by the chartering of a Lions Club, formed by members of the PCWH board. This largely Hispanic group has chosen to address the chronic disease issues prevalent in the immigrant community, and will perhaps adopt a social marketing mindset. So, whereas social marketing has yet to institutionalize, there is consensus that the project has taught important skills needed to work together to identify and solve community problems.

Step Five: Conduct Formative Research

Despite the paucity of data available on Florida's citrus harvesting community, a literature review on other migrant agricultural workers was useful. Particularly valuable was the identification of an eye injury prevention program—the Great Lakes Partnership for Agricultural Safety and Health, or GLPASH (Forst et al., 2004). This program used peers as community health workers (CHWs) to promote use of safety glasses among agricultural harvesters and nursery workers in the Midwest. CHWs modeled the use of safety glasses, educated workers about preventive measures, and provided first aid to injured workers.

The GLPASH was pilot tested to determine how it should be tailored for the citrus worker community. Six citrus harvesters were trained to be CHWs for their respective crews. CHWs were paid for ten hours a week to: (1) attend training sessions; (2) wear safety glasses during harvesting; (3) distribute safety glasses to crew mates; (4) encourage crew mates to wear glasses; (5) conduct four health education sessions with crew members; (6) train crew members about eye safety; (7) meet weekly with the project coordinator; (8) administer eye wash or other first aid to injured crew members; and (9) document their activities.

FPRC researchers also worked with the CHWs to test commercially available safety glasses and identify features that affected their compatibility with the demands of citrus harvesting. Workers identified a specific style—Revelation by Radians™—as the most comfortable and least likely to fog. They also recommended use of a sports-style headband to keep the glasses from getting entangled in tree branches or falling to the ground.

Concurrently, FPRC and community researchers conducted formative research to understand citrus workers' experience with eye injuries and perceptions of safety eyewear use. It included participant observation with ten crews, six focus groups, fifteen in-depth interviews with citrus managers and industry researchers, and a survey of 105 citrus workers. Results revealed that workers had detailed knowledge of eye injuries and were aware of the injury risk, but rarely reported injuries or sought medical treatment. Most workers realized safety glasses could protect them from the dangers of foreign objects and more traumatic injury, and many reported having been given safety glasses by their employers. However, most workers had lost the glasses without wearing them because they considered safety wear incompatible with the demands of harvesting fruit in a hot, humid climate. Those who had tried them briefly in other jobs or when harvesting citrus reported the lenses required frequent cleaning to remove dirt, sweat, and condensation. Perceiving a work slowdown, workers believed safety glasses use would reduce their piece-rate productivity, and therefore, their income. Almost all workers expected glasses to be uncomfortable.

Step Six: Develop Marketing Strategy

Drawing on results of the GLPASH pilot test and formative research, FPRC personnel worked with the PCWH board to tailor the program for eye injury reduction among citrus harvesters. The marketing plan is summarized in Table 12.2.

Step Seven: Program Development

Training materials for the CHW intervention were modified to reinforce the marketing strategy and address problems identified in the pilot test. The training curriculum was expanded and made more interactive. A training manual was produced to improve consistency in how materials were used, and the program was implemented (Luque, Monaghan, Contreras, August, Baldwin, Bryant, et al., 2007). Training materials are available at http://publichealth.usf.edu/prc/citrus_worker.

Step Eight: Program Implementation

The CHW intervention was pilot tested in 2004 with six harvesting crews employed by three citrus companies. FPRC researchers worked with community members to ensure the data collected provided necessary feedback to revise materials and strategies. Six CHWs distributed over three hundred pairs of safety eyewear and provided first aid to ninety workers.

Step Nine: Tracking and Evaluation

A process evaluation was conducted by the field supervisor, community researchers, and CHWs. Results refined program elements for subsequent years. To assess whether the program increased the proportion of workers using safety eyewear, eight unannounced visits to the groves were made by observers as workers harvested. In contrast to pre-intervention rates (below 2 percent), after the pilot phase, 28 percent of harvesters on the crews with CHWs were observed wearing glasses at all times of the day, and 37 percent wore them later in the day when dew and humidity declined.

Two other important findings had implications for the marketing plan. Workers who wore the glasses no longer believed safety eyewear reduced productivity and earning capacity. Moreover, they reported that their eyes were less irritated by dust, sand, insects, and chemicals. As a result, the product strategy (core benefits offered) was modified from the original promise to *pick without fear of injury* to the more competitively attractive position of *pick rapidly without fear of injury or daily irritation*. Company policies and incentives also were recommended to persuade workers to wear glasses during a trial period.

With these encouraging results, FPRC researchers and members of the community designed a small-scale efficacy trial to measure program impact on using safety glasses. FPRC partners provided the methodological expertise, and community members offered the necessary practical experience for identifying problems that could threaten the program's implementation fidelity and eventual adoption. Thirteen crews from two large citrus companies were recruited. Nine crews received the CHW intervention and four crews acted as controls. The control groups were provided with glasses, following a widespread industry practice, but were unexposed to the CHW intervention.

Observations occurred at intervals throughout the 2007–2008 harvest season by FPRC researchers, beginning two months before the CHW intervention began through the end of the season in May. During unannounced visits, researchers walked through each row in the grove where the crew was picking and counted workers wearing safety glasses. Each crew member was observed two or more times during the day, because climatic conditions (for example, humidity, temperature) still affected use. During the baseline observations, overall use of safety glasses was 2.4 percent among control and 11 percent among intervention crews. After the intervention, use remained at 2.6 percent among controls but increased significantly to 35.5 percent among those working on crews with CHWs.

Next Steps

Plans call for recruiting more citrus companies to adopt and fund the CHW intervention as part of a statewide effectiveness trial. In keeping with the CBPM framework, FPRC partners will provide methodological guidance in selecting the research design for the effectiveness trial and oversee its implementation. PCWH board members will identify potential problems that could threaten the program's adoption and implementation, and assist with recruitment of trial participants. As FPRC researchers coordinate the effectiveness trial, they and their community-based partners will conduct in-depth interviews with local leaders, other program partners, and other community members to identify potential incompatibilities and other factors that threaten implementation fidelity. Working in conjunction with FPRC researchers, board members will review research findings to determine if the intervention's effectiveness justifies dissemination on a larger scale, and to identify factors that may affect local adoption and implementation (for example, modifications in protocols, ideas, and supporting materials, and other features to "fit" local preferences). Researchers also will use results of the trial to identify core program elements that affect fidelity and outcomes, and develop strategies that optimize them. Company injury records will be analyzed to estimate the cost versus benefit associated with the program, and develop a dissemination plan.

SUMMARY

CBPM is a promising and emerging community-based participatory research and strategic planning framework, and offers its adopters numerous strengths. Experience in the FPRC's four demonstration projects suggests that community board members find value in marketing principles and can use marketing techniques to design interventions that result in behavior change (for example, Bryant et al., 2007). These projects also have demonstrated that CBPM can enhance community capacity to use marketing approaches for policy advocacy, service delivery improvement, and other activities launched without external funding or assistance.

CBPM gains much of its synergism from its blending of community organiza-

tion and social marketing, and on the rich community-campus partnership. CBPM's use of community organizing principles gives it a similarity to other widely used and emerging models that leverage the wisdom and power of local groups, and nurtures ownership of a process for identifying, prioritizing, and identifying responsive solutions to health related problems. Through this community direction, there is an increased likelihood that change efforts will succeed (Green and Kreuter, 1991; Minkler and Wallerstein, 1998). In addition, research conducted *with* community members increases the validity of results and fosters the translation of evidence into practice (Israel et al., 1998). Community organizing also influences health through strengthening social networks and enhancing participants' sense of social connectedness, control over their lives, and ability to change (Minkler and Wallerstein, 1998). Moreover, it improves the chance of sustained program success, because citizens participated in its design and implementation (Bracht, 1990).

CBPM's uniqueness as a planning model, however, is in its consumer orientation, its reliance on marketing data, and its cultivation of a marketing mind-set among community decision makers. Its framework also provides a systematic and sequential strategy for applying behavioral and social change theories appropriate for specific problems and populations. Careful evidence-based development of the marketing mix—that is, clear delineation of the four *Ps*—optimizes the program's focus and use of resources on the intended audience segment(s).

Moreover, individuals who participate in community coalitions may not represent the community at large or be familiar with the community's assets, culture, and power structure (Eisen, 1994). CBPM's reliance on formative research gathered from a more representative sample provides the coalition with a truer understanding of the community's issues and concerns, making it possible to design interventions that better meet audience needs and cultural preferences. Evaluation is currently underway to assess the value added by blending marketing and community organization.

CBPM is not without its challenges. Implementing the principles of community self-determination and relevance can be difficult and time-consuming. Community organization requires unique and practiced skills that some social marketers lack. Trust and cooperation between "outsiders" (for example, social marketing experts) and community members can be difficult to establish.

The absence of a large and available cadre of individuals with *formal social marketing education* and *skills acquired through multiple professional experiences* may make it difficult for communities to access high quality social marketing technical assistance to pursue CBPM. A further limitation is the ability of community members to differentiate between persons who can "speak the language" of social marketers and persons who have actually carried out projects and programs with these skills—and who can teach the marketing mind-set. Moreover, social marketing itself is sometimes misunderstood as being *only* carrying out formative research through focus groups, creating advertisements, or developing clever media messages. Good social marketing is rarely a quick and easy process, and many novices underestimate its sophistication and the time required to pursue it systematically. CBPM may not be appropriate for all communities and problems. Some communities may not be in a state of readiness, possess the resources, or identify an agency or individual to "champion" the process.

PREVENTION RESEARCH, TRANSLATION TO PRACTICE, AND THE FUTURE OF CBPM

Developers of the CBPM framework believe its role in prevention research can be expanded in the future as experience with its use and adaptability increase. *Prevention research* focuses the CBPM program planner on an ecological view of behavior change and provides the framework with a natural linkage to the five-phase Prevention Services Development Model (Sandler, Ostrom, Bitner, Ayers, Wolchik, and Daniels, 2005).The prevention research cycle is a logical sequence of steps with multiple feedback loops among steps that involve the following phases: (1) *Problem Analysis*: describing the problem and identifying the modifiable risk and protective factors; (2) *Intervention Design*: developing the intervention, including testing for acceptability, safety, and clinical quality; (3) *Efficacy Trial*: testing the intervention in a controlled environment; (4) *Effectiveness Trial*: testing the intervention in the actual setting; and (5) *Dissemination*: adoption, implementation, and ongoing evaluation of the intervention (Sandler et al., 2005).

Unfortunately, many concerns have been voiced regarding the feasibility of the prevention research cycle in research-to-practice interventions. For example, less than one percent of programs that have undergone efficacy trials are actually implemented in real world settings (Ginexi and Hilton, 2006; Glasgow, 2003; Jensen, 2003). Programs that are efficacious in controlled settings often cannot be implemented and replicated on a wider scale. In contrast, when evidence-based programs are disseminated in real world settings, concerns exist with fidelity of program implementation (Gottfredson and Gottfredson, 2002). Secondly, other programs that have demonstrated little efficacy are often readily adopted and disseminated in communities (for example, DARE) (Wandersman and Florin, 2003). Finally, a lack of fit between evidence-based prevention research interventions and community capacity has been observed (Sandler et al., 2005). Thus, there are often major gaps between evidence-based prevention programs and actual prevention services (Altman, 1995).

CBPM can address these concerns because it incorporates elements of the Prevention Services Development Model (Sandler et al., 2005) by applying a marketing orientation across the scope of the prevention research cycle. In the CBPM framework, "prevention" is the application of the prevention research cycle to the design of interventions involving health-promoting and risk-reducing behaviors. CBPM builds upon the position that adoption of a marketing mind-set is critical in helping prevention researchers partner with communities to develop, implement, evaluate, translate, and disseminate effective interventions. CBPM's inclusion of a consumer-orientation in each phase of the research cycle enhances the adoption of prevention interventions and their effectiveness in promoting health and preventing disease.

Historically, prevention science has been focused mostly on behavioral change at the individual level because many lifestyle practices (for example, smoking, heavy alcohol and other substance use, unsafe sexual activity, physical inactivity, and poor nutrition) are known to lead to poor health status. Whereas CBPM is designed to change individual behavior, its comprehensive marketing mix incorporates a social ecological perspective and acknowledges the interaction of the individual and the environment. Thus, program planners recognize the interplay of factors across multiple levels and stay focused on the need for multiple intervention levels to address intrapersonal, interpersonal, organizational, and broader societal factors. When intervention strategies are available at each level of influence, access and support are provided for people at many different points (for example, schools, clinics, worksites), thereby expanding their reach (Sallis and Owen, 2002; Ockene, Edgerton, Teutsch, Marion, Miller, Genevro, et al., 2007). CBPM's ecological perspective also avoids a dependence on education, communications, and other strategies criticized for "blaming the victim" (Ling, Franklin, Lindsteadt, and Gearon, 1992; Rothschild, 1997).

The failure of research-to-practice translation extends beyond U.S. borders as public health professionals have found it difficult to adapt, implement, and sustain evidence-based interventions around the globe (Madon, Hofman, Kupfer, and Glass, 2007). Theoretical frameworks such as CBPM may be effective in translation of evidence-based interventions to communities outside of the U.S. because it provides a strategy for enabling public health professionals to work with existing social networks and organizational, infrastructural, and resource constraints.

ACKNOWLEDGMENTS

This project was supported by: *CDC/Health Promotion and Disease Prevention Centers U48/CCU415803-05) (Cooperative Agreement Number 1-U48-DP-000062). Community Based Prevention Marketing: Building Local Capacity for Disease Prevention and Health Promotion.

This chapter was supported by Cooperative Agreement Number 5U48DP000062-05 from the Centers for Disease Control and Prevention. The findings and conclusions in this chapter are those of the authors and do not necessarily represent the official position of the Centers for Disease Control and Prevention.

REFERENCES

Aeffect, Inc. (2000). *Review of literature to support development of the Youth Media Campaign: Exploring how to motivate behavior change among tweens in America.* Lake Forest, IL: Department of Health and Human Services' Centers for Disease Control and Prevention.

Aeffect, Inc. (2001). *Message strategy research to support development of the Youth Media Campaign: Exploring how to motivate behavior change among tweens in America.* Lake Forest, IL: Department of Health and Human Services' Centers for Disease Control and Prevention.

Alfonso, M., Lopez, I., Bryant, C., and Bumpus, L. (2001). Planned Approach to Community Health (PATCH): A review and discussion of PATCH in Sarasota County, FL. *Florida Journal of Public Health, 12*(1–2), 19–26.

Altman, D. (1995). Sustaining interventions in community systems: On the relationship between researchers and communities. *Health Psychology, 14*(6), 526–536.

Bond, L., and Hauf, A. (2007). Community-based collaboration: An overarching best practice in prevention. *The Counseling Psychologist, 35,* 567–575.

Bracht, N. (1990). *Health promotion at the community level.* Newbury Park, CA: Sage.

Bracht, N., and Tsouros, N. (1990). Principles and strategies of effective community participation. *Health Promotion International, 5*(3), 199–208.

Bretthauer-Mueller, R., Berkowitz, J., Thomas, M., McCarthy, S., Green, L., Melancon, H., et al. (2008). Catalyzing community action within a national media campaign: VERB™ community and national partnerships. *American Journal of Preventive Medicine, 6S,* S210–S221.

Bryant, C., Forthofer, M., McCormack Brown, K., Landis, D., and McDermott, R. J. (2000). Community-based prevention marketing: The next steps in disseminating behavior change. *American Journal of Health Behavior, 24*(1), 61–68.

Bryant, C., McCormack Brown, K., McDermott, R. J., Forthofer, M., Bumpus, E., Calkins, S., et al. (2007). Community-based prevention marketing: A framework for facilitating health behavior change. *Health Promotion Practice, 8*, 154–163.

Burroughs, E., Peck, L., Sharpe, P., Granner, M., Bryant, C., and Fields, R. (2006). Using focus groups in the consumer research phase of a social marketing program to promote moderate intensity physical activity. *Preventing Chronic Disease, 3*(1), 1–13.

Center for Weight and Health. (2001). Pediatric overweight: A review of the literature. Berkeley: The Center for Weight and Health, College of Natural Resources, University of California.

Clay-Wayman, J., Beall, T., Thackeray, R., and McCormack Brown, K. (2007). Competition: A social marketer's friend or foe? *Health Promotion Practice, 8*(2), 134–139.

Eisen, A. (1994). Survey of neighborhood-based, comprehensive community empowerment initiatives. *Health Education Quarterly, 21*, 235–252.

Forst, L., Lacey, S., Chen, H., Jimenez, R., Bauer, S., Alvarado, S. S. R., et al. (2004). Effectiveness of community health workers for promoting use of safety eyewear by Latino farm workers. *American Journal of Industrial Medicine, 46*, 607–613.

Forthofer, M., and Bryant, C. (2000). Using audience-segmentation techniques to tailor health behavior change strategies. *American Journal of Health Behavior, 24*(1), 36–43.

Ginexi, E., and Hilton, T. (2006). What's next for translation research? *Evaluation and the Health Professions, 29*(3), 334–347.

Glasgow, R. (2003). Translating research to practice: Lessons learned, areas for improvement, and future directions. *Diabetes Care, 26*(8), 2451–2456.

Goodman, R., Speers, M., McLeroy, K., Fawcett, S., Kegler, M., Parker, E., et al. (1998). Identifying and defining the dimensions of community capacity to provide a basis for measurement. *Health Education and Behavior, 25*(3), 258–278.

Gottfredson, D., and Gottfredson, G. (2002). Quality of school based prevention programs: Results from a national survey. *Journal of Research on Crime and Delinquency, 39*, 3–35.

Green, L., and Kreuter, M. (Eds.). (1991). *Health promotion planning: An educational and environmental approach* (2nd ed.). Mountain View, CA: Mayfield.

Grier, S., and Bryant, C. (2005). Social marketing in public health. *Annual Review of Public Health, 26*, 319–339.

Hastings, G. (2007). *The potential of social marketing: Why should the devil have all the best tunes?* Oxford, UK: Elsevier.

Huhman, M., Potter, L., Wong, F., Banspach, S., Duke, J., and Heitzler, C. (2005). Effects of a mass media campaign to increase physical activity among children: Year-1 results of the VERB campaign. *Pediatrics, 116*, e277–e284.

Israel, B., Checkoway, B., Schulz, A., and Zimmerman, M. (1994). Health education and community empowerment: Conceptualizing and measuring perceptions of individual, organizational, and community control. *Health Education Quarterly, 21*(2), 149–170.

Israel, B., Schulz, A., Parker, E., and Becker, A. (1998). Key principles of community-based research. *Annual Review of Public Health, 19*, 173–202.

Jensen, P. (2003). Commentary: The next generation is overdue. *Journal of the American Academy of Child and Adolescent Psychiatry, 42*(5), 527–530.

Katz, D. (2004). Representing your community in community-based participatory research: Differences made and measured. [Electronic Version]. *Preventing Chronic Disease, 1*. Retrieved March 21, 2008 from http://www.cdc.gov/pcd/issues/2004/jan/03_0024.htm.

Kotler, P., and Lee, N. (2008). *Social marketing: Influencing behaviors for good.* Thousand Oaks, CA: Sage.

Ling, J., Franklin, B., Lindsteadt, J., and Gearon, S. (1992). Social marketing: Its place in public health. *Annual Review of Public Health, 13*, 341–362.

Luque, J., Monaghan, P., Contreras, R., August, E., Baldwin, J., Bryant, C., et al. (2007). Implementation evaluation of a culturally competent eye injury prevention program for citrus workers in a Florida migrant community. *Progress in Community Health Partnerships, 1*(4), 359–369.

Madon, T., Hofman, K., Kupfer, L., and Glass, R. (2007). Implementation science. *Science*, *318*, 1728–1729.

McCormack Brown, K. (2006). Defining the product in a social marketing effort. *Health Promotion Practice*, *7*(4), 384–387.

McDermott, R. J. (2004). Essentials of evaluating social marketing campaigns for health behavior change. *The Health Education Monograph Series*, *21*(1), 13–20.

Minkler, M., and Wallerstein, N. (1998). Community organizing and community building for health. In M. Minkler (ed.), *Improving health through community organization and community building: A health education perspective* (pp. 30–52). Gaithersburg, MD: Aspen Publishers, Inc.

Ockene, J., Edgerton, E., Teutsch, S., Marion, L., Miller, T., Genevro, J., et al. (2007). Integrating evidence-based clinical and community strategies to improve health. *American Journal of Preventive Medicine*, *32*(3), 244–252.

Parsons, N., and McCormack Brown, K. (2004). Formative research: The bedrock of social marketing. *Health Education Monograph Series*, *21*(1), 1–5.

Peck, L., Sharpe, P., Burroughs, E., and Granner, M. (2008). Recruitment strategies and costs for a community-based physical activity program. *Health Promotion Practice*, *9*(2), 191–198.

Prevention Institute. (2008a). Strengthening communities: A prevention framework for eliminating health disparities. Retrieved March 26, 2008, from http://www.preventioninstitute.org/strength_draft.html.

Prevention Institute. (2008b). Health equity and community health. Retrieved March 20, 2008, from http://www.preventioninstitute.org/healthdis.html.

Robertson, A., and Minkler, M. (1994). New health promotion movement: A critical examination. *Health Education and Behavior*, *21*(3), 295–312.

Rothschild, M. (1997). A historic perspective of social marketing. *Journal of Communication*, *2*, 308–309.

Sallis, J., and Owen, N. (2002). Ecological models of health behavior. In K. Glanz, F. Lewis, and B. Rimer (eds.), *Health behavior and health education: Theory, research, and practice* (3rd ed.). San Francisco: Jossey-Bass.

Sandler, I., Ostrom, A., Bitner, M., Ayers, T., Wolchik, S., and Daniels, V. (2005). Developing effective prevention services for the real world: a prevention service development model. *American Journal of Community Psychology*, *35*(3–4), 127–142.

Slater, M., Kelly, K., and Thackeray, R. (2006). Segmentation on a shoestring: Health audience segmentation in limited-budget and local social marketing interventions. *Health Promotion Practice*, *7*(2), 170–173.

Wandersman, A., and Florin, P. (2003). Community interventions and effective prevention. *American Psychologist*, *58*(6–7), 441–448.

World Health Organization. (2007). The top 10 causes of death. Retrieved March 20, 2008, from http://www.who.int/mediacentre/factsheets/fs310/en/.

PART

3

ECOLOGICAL APPROACHES

13

CHANGING OUR UNHEALTHY WAYS: EMERGING PERSPECTIVES FROM SOCIAL ACTION THEORY

Craig K. Ewart

CHANGING HARMFUL HEALTH BEHAVIORS

A daunting challenge facing public health today is to help people alter health-damaging habits that they perform daily with little or no thought. Habitual activities such as eating, drinking, or smoking are harder to modify than are health-related actions performed less frequently, such as getting a flu shot or a mammogram, or installing a smoke detector in one's home (Ewart, 1991). Habits have properties that make them highly resistant to change: They are performed frequently, they run off automatically, and they usually generate powerful reinforcers (Wood and Neal, 2007). What is more, health habits are woven into a fabric of daily settings and routines that cue the habits, routines which the habits help to sustain, for example, by serving as self-rewards for completing an odious task, or as a means to renew energy, or to relieve emotional stress.

Most models of health behavior long in vogue explain how to predict health habits but not how to change them. Models derived from expectancy-value theory, such as the health belief model (Becker, 1974), theory of reasoned action (Fishbein, 1980), or stage theories of change (Prochaska, DiClemente, and Norcross, 1992) do not offer highly specific (and thus useful) accounts of how people actually translate health-related expectancies, values, goals, or intentions into appropriate actions and, more important, into sustainable habits. To explain how behavior change attempts succeed or fail, it is necessary to understand how people develop self-regulatory action goals, how they modify these goals in light of ongoing experience, and how they deliberately construct patterns of habitual activity (for example, eating, exercising) that run off automatically, with little or no reasoning or reflective thought.

A major step toward understanding change mechanisms was taken by social-cognitive theory, which highlights ways in which peoples' beliefs about their personal capabilities, or self-efficacy, influence their attempts to alter ingrained habits (Bandura, 1986). Yet much more than an analysis of efficacy enhancement is required. Self-efficacy is regulated by a host of psychological and social factors that also combine with efficacy appraisals to shape behavior. A more broadly synthetic process analysis of human action is needed to identify those other mechanisms, to clarify how they both affect each other and work together, and to prescribe how to manipulate them to generate change.

Health behavior change models typically emphasize subjective beliefs and expectations (Fishbein et al., 2001). But barriers to habit change do not reside solely within the mind. A major problem now facing public health is the challenge of explaining the "socioeconomic gradient," or the observation that health tends to decline with each step-wise descent in socioeconomic status (SES) (Adler, Epel, Castellazzo, and Ickovics, 2000; Kawachi and Kennedy, 2002; Siegrist and Marmot, 2004). Although this gradient appears to have a variety of causes, it is worth noting that the prevalence of health-damaging habits also increases as one moves down the SES ladder (Sidanius and Pratto, 1999). Cross-cultural studies in industrial and developing nations have found that, in all societies studied, people at the lower end of the economic scale are more likely to exhibit patterns of self-debilitating behavior that tend to exacerbate and perpetuate their disadvantaged status (Marmot et al., 1991; Matthews, Kelsey, Meilahn, Kuller, and Wing, 1989). Discovering how physical and social environments foster and sustain debilitating habits poses a vital challenge to health psychology.

Social action theory (SAT) was developed to address these needs. SAT proposes that people's personal goals and characteristic problem-solving strategies in everyday contexts generate habitual action patterns that persist over time (Ewart, 1991). Health habit change involves detecting these patterns, identifying the goals and strategies that create them, and then systematically developing new goals, strategies, and action sequences that are compatible with good health. **Self-change** is accomplished through goal-directed action, which involves envisaging a desired habit or "**action state**," devising a strategy to attain it, and continually revising the strategy in light of experienced outcomes until one achieves one's aim. This analysis builds upon and extends a well-established functionalist tradition in psychology grounded in the Law of Effect, including applied behavior analysis, cognitive information processing models, and social-cognitive theories, to name some prominent examples (Leahey, 2001; Woodward, 1982).

Yet SAT moves beyond individually focused functionalist approaches to health behavior. First, SAT offers a more specific contextual model of how personal goals influence health. Goals can assume many forms, ranging from broad aspirations to highly specific objectives. SAT focuses on core self-goals that give rise to persisting daily routines, and proposes that a person's core goals and the routines that serve them can pose significant obstacles to self-change. In this analysis, health goals and habits are embedded in a larger matrix of aims that humans in all cultures pursue daily; they include striving to maintain basic biological functions, to build and nurture social connections, and to accumulate and preserve material assets that serve adaptive ends. Stated simply, our most vital routines serve universal human pursuits of "health," "love," and "wealth." Efforts to change health habits are apt to founder if they thwart—or fail to serve—these central aims.

SAT also expands the familiar social-cognitive frame by specifying how our important goals and routines are shaped by our physical and social environments. SAT identifies ways in which environmental structures shape self-regulatory resources in the form of social-emotional competence, material assets, and social power, and thereby foster the expectations, emotions, self-goals, and routines that enhance or threaten health. SAT thus offers an ecological analysis to guide our quest to understand how physical and social environments influence health.

Finally, by synthesizing individual self-processes within a larger ecological perspective, SAT generates a practical, programmatic approach to health habit change. This approach identifies interventions that can be used to enhance health by altering self-goals, strategies, and environments.

During the interval since SAT was introduced (Ewart, 1991), the theory has undergone further development in community-based studies of psychological stress, health behavior, and disease risk in low-income urban youth and young adults. This work investigated how social-emotional competence, social power, and neighborhood environments contribute to debilitating behavior patterns that increase vulnerability to cardiovascular disease and HIV (Curbow et al., 2005; Ewart, 1995, 2004c; Ewart and Jorgensen, 2004; Ewart, Jorgensen, and Kolodner, 1998; Ewart, Jorgensen, Suchday, Chen, and Matthews, 2002; Ewart and Kolodner, 1991, 1994; Ewart and Suchday, 2002; Fitzgerald, Brown, Sonnega, and Ewart, 2005). Socioemotional competence and social power have emerged as important self-regulatory resources that enable personal agency and resilience, which are needed to support self-change. These discoveries suggested a further elaboration of the contextual dimension of the SAT behavior change model, which now specifies the competence and power constructs and indicates how they act together to support the development of health-protective habits. This chapter will offer a brief overview of the emerging SAT analysis as it applies to health habit change.

OUR MISCARRIED ENDEAVORS

SAT proposes that we pursue our strivings for health, love, and wealth by organizing our various goals and daily activities into adaptive "self-endeavors" that let us exercise personal agency with a minimum of disruption. Self-endeavors are action systems composed of focal goals that drive and guide an endeavor, behavioral strategies that serve one's aims, anticipatory or "proactive" thoughts and emotions aroused by goal pursuit, and the patterns of social engagement and mutual interdependence that one's actions generate. Familiar examples are found in work and commuting routines, child care, and educational and recreational pursuits. Behavioral routines give rise to habits, which usually—but not always—facilitate goal attainment. Many health-damaging habits support cherished routines by offering a means to modulate arousal, connect with others, or aid restorative coping. Because they serve critical adaptations, routines can be very difficult to change. A major shortcoming of health behavior models is a pervasive failure to consider habitual routines and the core self-goals they serve.

A social action analysis thus suggests that enduring health habit change cannot be achieved merely by altering a person's beliefs, expectancies, skills, or intentions. Much more is needed. SAT offers an integrative model to specify the critical microprocesses of change and show how they fit together as a larger action system (self-endeavor). This analysis suggests that interventions to create lasting habit change must target self-endeavor systems and the social-environmental influences that sustain or disrupt them.

A SOCIAL ACTION THEORY OF HEALTH BEHAVIOR CHANGE

SAT holds that behavior change involves restructuring self-endeavors, a process that unfolds in three distinct phases. Each phase addresses a different subcomponent of the SAT model. *Phase One* selects targets for change by defining habits as action sequences that should be increased or reduced, and then specifying how these sequences are (or might be) woven unobtrusively into important daily routines. The analysis considers how the routines are embedded in social interactions and material settings, thus suggesting contextual changes that may be needed to cue and support desired habits. Phase One analysis thus yields a set of behavioral and environmental targets for intervention.

Phase Two engages self-regulatory processes that must be activated to establish the action patterns, or habits, specified in Phase One. SAT offers a synthetic model of critical regulatory mechanisms in the form of *proactive awareness* (attention, evaluation, cognitive-affective construction) and *social engagement* (interpersonal orientation, engagement, control) that enable people to acquire and sustain the desired habits. Phase Two analysis suggests how to structure the intervention as an integrated and effectively sequenced set of tasks and roles.

Phase Three identifies critical regulatory resources that are needed to support the self-change processes activated in Phase Two. SAT offers a contextual analysis of regulatory resources that highlights the importance of *social-emotional competence* (mastery of the values, means, and proprieties of one's social milieu), objective *assets* (access to goods, information, services), and *social power* (relationships that let one influence others in desired ways). These three classes of resources represent a contextual architecture, or ecology, of health-protective action. Phase Three analysis suggests ways to support long-term change by enhancing social competence (for example, in self-activation and direction, proactive awareness, social engagement), increasing access to needed assets (for example, income, transportation, child care, health services), and restructuring the social environment to increase power (for example, by restructuring dyads, groups, hierarchies).

Phase One: Identifying Health Habits and Routines

SAT defines a "habit" as a highly routinized, automatic, and predictable sequence of anticipations, actions, and consequences that usually generates a desired outcome. Eating habits, for example, typically unfold in a series of steps that involve choosing and finding food, preparing a meal, and consuming it; each of these steps can be subdivided into sequences of component acts. Food finding, for example, can be broken down into the sequence of actions needed to prepare a grocery list, identify shopping places and arrange transportation, select grocery items at a market, and then store the groceries at home. Each act in the sequence is guided by anticipations, such as envisioning attractive fresh fruits at a familiar farmers market, and is rewarded or punished by the outcomes the act generates. Thus the anticipation of snacking on tasty seasonal fruit prompts the act of driving to a local farmers market, which is rewarded by the sight of fresh produce; the displays of fruits and vegetables conjure thoughts of meals that prompt and guide shopping choices, which then are rewarded by the sight, scent, and feel of ripe fruit placed gently in the shopping basket.

Habits are embedded in daily routines that are triggered by environmental cues, run along automatically with little conscious thought, and generate predictable rewards. The pleasing anticipation of coffee and a sweet snack is triggered by a familiar setting and activity, for example, such as completing a task at work, or seeing a friend during a break, or laboring late to meet a deadline. Or one's selection of breakfast follows a standard set of choices and preparations that are rewarded by being able to listen to the morning news while managing to arrive at work on time. Habitual action sequences are highly efficient because they allow us to do two things at once. Perhaps it is not surprising that experience sampling studies reveal that, in the course of a typical day, people report that 45 percent of their time is spent performing habitual activities (Wood and Neal, 2007; Wood, Quinn, and Kashy, 2002).

Our daily routines serve a vital social function; indeed, predictable shared routines facilitate social living by allowing us to coordinate our activities with those of important others such as family members, friends, or coworkers. Research suggests that predictable shared routines and habits are especially important for families and can be critical to child care and nurturance (Fiese, 2006). Regular routines appear to play an important protective function in vulnerable populations, such as low-income single African American mothers and their elementary school children (Brody and Flor, 1997). Regular routines also help buffer children against the stress of parental divorce; following divorce, the regularity of children's bedtime routines predicted their academic performance two years later (Guidubaldi, Cleminshaw, Perry, Nastasi, and Lightel, 1986) and was associated with fewer school absences and better overall health (Guidubaldi, Perry, and Nastasi, 1987). Children and adolescents raised in divorced households had fewer internalizing and externalizing symptoms when the custodial parent established regular family routines (Portes, Howell, Brown, Eichenberger, and Mas, 1992). These findings are consistent with evidence that predictable family routines may play an important role in protecting children from the negative effects of being raised under high-risk care-giving conditions, and may help explain why not all children raised in high-risk environments suffer psychological harm (Rutter and Sroufe, 2000; Sameroff and Chandler, 1975). SAT thus holds that the assessment and modification of shared routines—in couples, in families, in work or educational settings—is a critical objective in health habit change.

Within the SAT framework, intervention planning begins in Phase One by identifying habitual routines that threaten health and then specifying healthier routines that might replace them; in the previous example, a dieter might decide to replace snacking during a break by chewing sugarless gum while taking a brisk walk. As a stable behavioral system, a habit can be modeled as an "action state" composed of the elements shown in Figure 13.1. The action state model depicts the desired goal of health promotion, which strives to replace an existing health-damaging action state (habit) with a new action state designed to prevent, disrupt, or substitute for habits that undermine health. Figure 13.1 specifies the critical microprocesses that enable a desired action state to remain stable over time: A behavior pattern becomes habitual only if it produces desired effects (outcomes) that are experienced immediately, and often (that is, reliably), and if the behavior and its effects are compatible (congruent) with the habits and routines that one happens to share with others (social interdependence).

FIGURE 13.1 *An Action State Model for Habits*

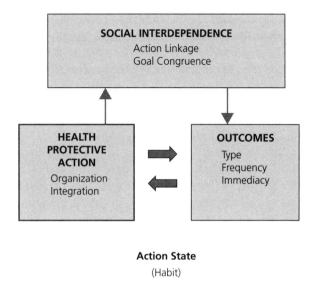

Action State
(Habit)

In Figure 13.1, the box labeled "Health Protective Action" specifies the sequence of actions needed to protect health, such as planning a healthy meal, and purchasing and preparing the needed items. To become an established routine, each act must be *organized* into a causally nested sequence of subroutines, each of which facilitates the next act in the series. It is not enough to master component acts; the full ensemble must be coordinated in a smoothly flowing script. This action script must be *integrated* with other scripts and routines that one performs regularly, including concurrent routines. I must learn to integrate into my dinner preparation routine the acts required to prepare a salad, for example, while simultaneously supervising my child's homework. Even if I master all of the essential actions, salads will not become a regular part of my diet if I fail to integrate vegetable chopping into my evening ritual.

The box labeled "Outcomes" specifies the consequences that my health-protective actions must generate if they are to become habitual. The outcome must be of a *type* I desire, whether biological gratification, or sensory, social, or intellectual stimulation, or some other desired outcome. The action must produce desired outcomes *frequently*, preferably every time I do the routine. And outcomes are more motivating if they are experienced *immediately* after performing the desired action, as opposed to being delayed.

Finally, the box labeled "Social Interdependence" highlights the fact that many of our health-protective routines are interconnected with the routines of important others. *Action Linkage* implies that my ability to perform a necessary step in an action sequence depends upon another's acts; for example, I can concentrate on slicing carrots for a salad only if my spouse is feeding our infant. *Goal Congruence* means that my actions must not thwart another's ability to attain a desired goal; for example, my morning exercise routine must not cause my partner to be late for work.

Guided by the organizational scheme in Figure 13.1, intervention begins by specifying goals for a new health-protective action system. Situations, settings, or conditions that cue the undesired habit can be avoided or changed; for example, outcomes that presently sustain the behavior can be targeted for reduction or elimination, and shared routines can be restructured. One builds a new habit by applying the same principles: one designs new contexts to trigger desired actions, arranges for the new behavior patterns to generate attractive outcomes, and integrates the novel action sequences, outcomes, and settings into shared routines.

The SAT analysis of habits as self-sustaining action states reveals principles that planners of health interventions are advised to bear in mind. First, unhealthy habits are *functional*: they reliably and quickly produce desired outcomes. The outcomes often are biological and social, and enable one to sustain important self-endeavors that serve strivings for health, love, and wealth. Snacking or smoking helps me cope with physical discomfort, for example, or enables me to connect with important others, or to work longer or harder. This analysis implies that replacing the unhealthy habit involves identifying and building healthier behaviors that can serve similar functions. Second, because unhealthy habits are functional, their disruption usually causes *frustration*. This means that strong positive rewards may be needed, early and often, during the training process. A third principle flows from viewing habits as action states composed of stable feedback loops established by performing the same action sequence in the same setting with the same results, over and over again. This means that habits can be set in motion, or "triggered," by *situational cues* and can operate with minimal external guidance or reflective thought. Changing a habit thus involves identifying and altering its contextual triggers, as well as disrupting the response sequence by inducing reflective self-awareness; that is, one must become aware of what one is doing. People must be able to monitor themselves, to learn to refocus their attention at critical moments, and to induce states of mental vigilance— all of which may require special training, facilitation, and reward. Finally, the notion that many habits exhibit *social interdependence* implies that many situational triggers and reinforcing outcomes are mediated via interpersonal exchanges. Altering cues, actions, and outcomes may involve restructuring or altering social interactions.

These principles have important practical implications for intervention design. First, the action state analysis encourages planners of health promotion programs to begin with the end in view by specifying the action system components identified in Figure 13.1. This useful exercise encourages planners to construe habits as interconnected sequences of events in concrete physical and social settings, rather than as isolated acts. Action state analysis also forces one to think carefully about the rewarding outcomes that will be needed to sustain a desired health routine. Unless it generates desired consequences that are experienced immediately, a novel behavior sequence that must be repeated frequently for many years will be difficult to establish. SAT's action state analysis thus poses health promotion's most daunting challenge: to ensure that those who try to adopt a recommended health behavior will experience rewarding outcomes—immediately, reliably, and often—whenever and wherever they perform the desired actions (Ewart, 2004a). All too often, a failure to solve this problem proves to be the Achilles heel of health promotion programs.

Second, whereas the importance of social relationships is widely acknowledged in models of health promotion, SAT specifies mechanisms by which interpersonal environments support or impede health habit change. The principle of action linkage implies that health-damaging habits often are embedded in shared routines; change on the part of one person can disrupt someone else's routine, spark frustration, and strain the relationship. Unhappy responses by one's friends or family members create undesired outcomes that punish habit change attempts instead of rewarding them. The degree to which two peoples' goals and routines are interconnected (that is, action linkage) determines how extensively habit change by one party is apt to affect the other. Social influence on habit change often is defined in terms of perceiving that important others "want me to change," or by assessing the level of emotional closeness or satisfaction in a dyadic relationship (Fishbein et al., 2001). But a partner who regularly urges me to lose weight may not be enthusiastic about a new weight loss plan that requires me to spend an hour jogging instead of performing needed household chores or assisting in child care at a demanding time of day. And a lack of emotional closeness in a relationship may pose no barrier to change if the partners' goals and valued routines are not densely interdependent.

Finally, an action state analysis highlights the importance of assessing action sequences in natural settings before trying to alter them. In population-level interventions where it may not be feasible to study everyone individually, intervention planning should be based on preliminary intensive studies of representative persons within carefully selected population subgroups. Intensive research is needed to identify who engages in behaviors that endanger health, when and where they do so, the environmental cues that trigger undesired habits, the outcomes people experience, and how soon and how often those outcomes are felt. The action state analysis also should try to identify social and structural influences that foster or support the undesired patterns; such investigation can reveal cultural factors that may create subgroup differences in behaviors, triggers, outcomes, and social action linkages. SAT proposes that the most effective way to conduct such studies is by observing people in situations that elicit the undesired behavior patterns, or in settings where desired behaviors might be encouraged by intervention. Self-observation using experience sampling methods, including electronic diaries, Internet, and telephone reports that capture events in real time can be very useful here (Smyth et al., 2001).

Self-Change Processes

Phase One analysis identifies objectives for preventive intervention. Phase Two specifies self-change mechanisms that must be activated and coordinated to reduce the unwanted habit and replace it with a desired one. An organizational scheme to guide these interventions is shown in Figure 13.2. The figure suggests that the self-change mechanisms

FIGURE 13.2 *Self-Change Processes*

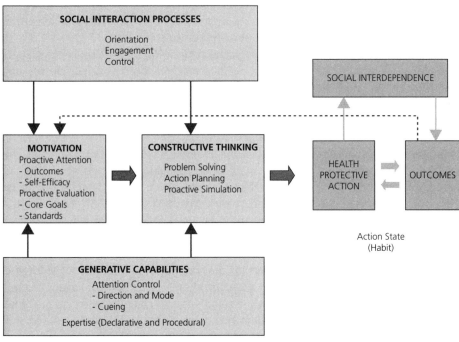

Self-Change Processes

and processes shown may interact in ways that have not been studied extensively in health behavior research. Processes of attentional focus, evaluation, and cognitive-affective problem solving play a central role in shaping people's motivation and ability to change.

As in the action state model of habits, self-change efforts are influenced by the effects they generate. The outcomes that people experience when performing new health protective action sequences and routines affect their desire to persevere in habit change. This feedback function is indicated by the broken line in Figure 13.2, which connects the Action State of Figure 13.1 to the box labeled "Motivation." Self-change processes that must be activated to alter health habits include motivational mechanisms, constructive problem-solving activities, generative capabilities, and social interaction processes.

Motivational Processes: Proactive Attention

People do not persist in trying to change unhealthy habits unless they anticipate positive benefits, believe themselves to be capable of taking the necessary actions, and find that the new habits are compatible with the personal goals, routines, and personal standards that serve valued self-endeavors. People motivate themselves by attending proactively to desired outcomes and the performances needed to attain them. *Outcomes* are the experiences that an action generates; anticipated outcomes motivate behavior by creating the expectation that "Action A in Situation B will produce desired Consequence C." The act of gauging one's ability to achieve a desired outcome generates expectations of *self-efficacy*: "If I attempt Action A in Situation B I'm likely to achieve Performance P" (Bandura, 1997). We combine these two types of expectations to generate anticipatory "if-then" rules of everyday action: "If I try to do A in situation B, I'm likely to achieve P, which will (or will not) produce C." We also proactively *evaluate* anticipated outcomes and actions; our if-then rules include evaluative appraisals that take the form, "In situation B, causing C by doing A is good/bad." Evaluative (good/bad) judgments involve comparing expected events with one's core self-goals and the routines that facilitate them, as well as with our personal self-standards. An action or outcome is judged favorably or negatively according to whether it enhances or conflicts with other important goals and self-aspirations.

Outcome expectancies have been a focus of extensive study in health behavior research; abundant evidence shows that they can be modified through social modeling and direct exposure (Bandura, 1986). In modeling interventions, attractive people who resemble the target audience are shown enjoying the rewards of healthy behavior or suffering the damaging effects of bad habits. Direct exposure involves letting target individuals experience a favorable outcome directly, as when patients with high blood cholesterol levels are introduced to a healthier diet by being served a delicious low-fat meal.

In addition to anticipating positive experiences, people must believe themselves to be capable of taking the steps that are needed to effect change. Self-efficacy can be increased by performing a new activity in gradually increasing doses, by watching others like oneself perform the behavior, by receiving verbal encouragement (persuasion) from persons whose opinion one respects, and by modulating one's level of arousal (for example, through relaxation) to lower internal anxiety cues (Bandura, 1997). Methods to measure outcome expectancies and self-efficacy appraisals have been developed for a wide variety of health behaviors; these scales have been used to predict health behavior change in a number of studies (for example, Ewart, 2004b). The evidence indicates that the relative predictive power of outcome expectancy and self-efficacy judgments varies with the type of behavior under investigation: When the health behavior is easy to perform (for example, selecting a high-fiber cereal instead of a low-fiber brand), self-efficacy is not a strong predictor of habit change. On the other hand, when the benefits of changing are evident but the behavior is difficult to perform (for example, weight loss), self-efficacy expectations predict behavior change better than outcome expectancies do.

Most health behavior research has failed to consider the implications of the fact that health habits compete with other self-goals and routines, and that the latter can influence the nature and power of outcome and efficacy expectancies. Health habits that disrupt valued routines will be judged to produce unwanted outcomes.

And habits that interfere with important self-endeavors by placing added demands on one's skills or energy will lower self-efficacy for habit change.

Figure 13.2 indicates that the influence of outcome and efficacy expectations is greatly affected by mechanisms of *focal attention*. Directing one's attention inward heightens awareness of internal cues and states; directing attention to one's environment heightens awareness of external outcomes. The mode of attention is important too: one can adopt a "synthetic" focus in which one perceives events as complete wholes, or one can adopt a detached "analytic" stance, in which one perceives events in terms of discrete subcomponents (Lambie and Marcel, 2002). The ability to induce a detached analytical view of tempting treats, for example, helps lower their arousing properties and increases one's ability to resist them (Mischel and Ayduk, 2004; Peake, Hebl, and Mischel, 2002).

Thus, by controlling the direction and mode of one's attentional focus, one can alter the power of experienced outcomes to influence one's motivation, as well as modulate one's level of self-efficacy (Ahles, Blanchard, and Leventhal, 1983; Dar and Leventhal, 1993).

Figure 13.2 implies that outcome expectancies and self-efficacy appraisals are *relative* and variable, rather than absolute. The benefit of changing a health habit is judged in relation to its effects on other goals and activities. The difficulty of adopting a new action pattern is judged in relation to the level of effort or skill it will require *over and above* the effort and skill needed to accomplish other important goals and routines. Thus it is important to assess people's competing endeavors, goals, and activities.

Self-endeavors can be measured by inviting people to examine their current routines and to consider how these might be affected, for good or ill, by adopting the recommended health habit (Ewart, 2004a). This involves offering examples of typical routines and goals in the domains of health (for example, trying to get in better physical shape, lose weight), love (for example, making friends, improving a relationship), and wealth (for example, sticking to a budget, saving money for a vacation), and then asking people to report their own current activities and preoccupations. The person is asked to envisage the sequence of actions that the new habit entails, the times and settings where it is to be performed, others who may be involved, and the immediate outcomes that the recommended actions are likely to produce. He or she then is asked to consider how those actions and outcomes might affect other valued activities. First, in what ways might the new habit disrupt or facilitate other important goal-directed pursuits, outcomes, or routines that one pursues individually, or that one shares with important others? Second, what might be the consequences for oneself, for others, and for one's relationships? For each current goal and routine, the individual is asked to indicate the expected degree of disruption, the likelihood of the anticipated consequences, and their desirability.

These responses can be used to predict adherence to the new habit and, more important, to help people reconsider their priorities and to identify ways to adjust their goals and routines in ways that might better accommodate the new behavior.

Intervention should seek to construct action routines that let important endeavors and recommended health habits support each other. For example, in the case where a new exercise program interferes with a need to stay abreast of new information by daily reading, one might arrange to read while pedaling a stationary bicycle. In this plan, reading is rewarded by the opportunity to exercise, while exercising is rewarded by the opportunity to keep up with new information.

Constructive Thinking: Problem Solving and Planning

Motivation accomplishes little without an effective plan of action. Whereas motivation involves anticipating and evaluating, planning entails thinking *constructively* by imagining appropriate action sequences and settings. When acting in a familiar domain, planning can be achieved almost instantly by following well-developed heuristics; for example, I quickly and effortlessly readjust my morning exercise routine to take account of the latest weather report. But when adopting a novel behavior, a guiding heuristic may not be available. In novel situations for which one lacks relevant expertise, constructive thinking involves imagining various options, selecting a promising course of action, and then formulating a workable strategy to attain one's goal. Such thinking requires much more than simply forming a behavioral intention or goal. One must be able to anticipate the various ways in which a chosen goal and strategy might interact with one's other important activities and social relationships, and then construct and revise a preferred strategy so as to minimize negative outcomes. Constructive thinking of this kind is facilitated by adopting a detached analytic attentional focus that lets one attend easily to self and world, a perspective that flexibly encompasses a broad array of possibilities while forestalling immersed goal-directed action. Thus interventions to foster constructive thinking often introduce techniques that help one alter, redirect, or widen attentional focus. A well-known example is the venerable technique of brainstorming, a procedure designed to expand attention by generating a highly diverse array of possible goals and strategies (D'Zurilla and Goldfried, 1971; D'Zurilla and Nezu, 1980; Parnes and Meadow, 1959; Weisskopf-Joelson and Eliseo, 1961). This is followed by evaluative exercises that help one select and refine an optimal goal and strategy (Nezu and D'Zurilla, 1979).

Yet creative problem solving, alone, is not enough. One also must remember to implement one's plan at the appropriate times and places. Forming a goal may not ensure timely and effective action if one gets distracted and forgets about the goal when the moment to act is at hand. SAT holds that goal selection must be bolstered by highly specific plans that prompt action through mechanisms of attentional cueing. For many years, behavior modification programs have taught people to prompt goal-directed behavior by placing physical cues in settings where a desired behavior is to be performed (Kazdin, 1975; Mahoney, 1975; Stuart, 1967; Watson and Tharp, 1972). Medication taking is prompted by placing a pill container on the breakfast table, for example, or reminders written on brightly colored sticky notes can be pasted in strategic locations. In settings where physical prompting is not practical, one can cue desired acts by mentally envisioning the situation in advance, and forming a cognitive cue by imagining that one is performing the desired act in that setting (Brownell, Marlatt, Lichtenstein, and Wilson, 1986; Mahoney, 1974; Richardson, 1967). Such "cognitive stimulus control" helps sensitize one's attention to the cue when the time for action arrives. It creates a link between an environmental cue (for example, walking through the dairy section of a grocery store) and a desired goal-directed act (for example, selecting a container of nonfat milk). By building mental links between a series of environmental cues and relevant goal-directed actions, we increase the probability that we will notice the cue when in that situation, and that our actions will be controlled by the cue.

Considering that changing an established habit can present a variety of novel challenges, interventions to promote adherence to new health routines are more effective if they help people develop action plans composed of a sequence of highly specific goals and actions that implement the plan, concrete descriptions of the situations in which the actions are to be performed, and, for each situation, environmental cues that can prompt the desired response (Baldwin and Baldwin, 1981; Kazdin, 1975). Such plans have been shown to help people follow through on intentions to alter their diets, stop smoking, control alcohol consumption, and exercise regularly (Marlatt and Gordon, 1985; Shiffman, 1982). Advance planning is especially helpful when one is tired, emotionally stressed, or feeling unsupported by others in one's social milieu. Having a prepared response, one that is ready to be triggered by an environmental stimulus, can allow me to perform competently when I'm not at my best (Gollwitzer, Fujita, and Oettingen, 2004).

Whereas constructive problem solving involves widening the focus of attention and adopting a detached analytical attentional mode, action planning narrows attention to specific situations and strives to focus attention on concrete cues in an immersed, synthetic way. Attentional immersion avoids distracting goal-irrelevant information while concentrating on the goal-relevant cues that prompt and guide one's action plan. By selectively focusing on the positive aspects of one's goal while ignoring potential negatives, one becomes more confident in one's ability to carry out the needed actions. An immersed focus helps one avoid considering other possibilities; this makes it easier to pursue a chosen objective even when other options are immediately in view. A certain degree of "narrow-mindedness" makes it easier to do what I need to do, when I need to do it, without endlessly debating the assorted pros and cons (Beckmann and Gollwitzer, 1987). A narrow action focus also allows me to perform needed tasks more effectively, thus raising my performance self-efficacy, and bolstering motivation.

When trying to enact a novel plan in an unfamiliar setting, mentally rehearsing the sequence of steps, envisioning environmental cues and relevant actions, can significantly enhance one's ability to implement the plan (Brownell et al., 1986), *Proactive simulation* involves the act of mentally picturing oneself doing the proposed action sequence, and experiencing the outcomes it produces (Kahneman and Miller, 1986; Taylor, Pham, Rivkin, and Armor, 1998). Research on mental simulation suggests that it is important to imagine, as vividly as one can, the actual performance, to picture oneself doing each step in the sequence, as opposed to focusing only on the final goal (Pham and Taylor, 1999). For example, it is more effective to picture myself exercising rather than to focus only on how much better my clothes will feel after I've lost weight. Detailed rehearsal helps one organize each act into a smoothly running script. By picturing the environments in which actions will be performed, one forges mental links between the desired acts and associated environmental cues. This makes it easier to notice the relevant cues and to remember to perform the desired routine when the moment to do so is at hand.

Thus, much of the work involved in replacing unhealthy habits with healthy ones involves anticipating potential problems and the situations in which they are likely to arise, formulating effective strategies, and then developing appropriate action plans to implement them (Hill-Briggs, 2003; Marlatt and Gordon, 1985; Perri et al., 2001; Perri, Nezu, and Viegener, 1992). To ensure that one is motivated to put the plan into practice at the right moment, it is helpful to focus one's attention on the positive outcomes one will experience, immediately and often, when implementing the plan. Thus SAT regards constructive problem solving and planning activities as the *fulcrum* of the habit change process (Ewart, 1991).

Generative Capabilities

The ability to anticipate outcomes, form goals, devise strategies, and engage in constructive problem solving and action planning for health behavior change requires an ability to control one's attention and to draw upon knowledge needed to evaluate outcomes, solve problems, form goals, and make action plans. One must acquire skill in controlling the direction and mode of one's attention, and in using mental and physical cues to prompt desired actions at the appropriate times and places. This calls for two basic forms of knowledge. *Declarative knowledge* consists of knowing what one should do and why; *procedural knowledge* consists of practical know-how, or the ability to perform a sequence of actions in order to produce a desired effect. Habit change requires *expertise* in the form of specific skills needed for a high level of mastery in a given performance domain (Sternberg, 2005); the domain and nature of the skill sets required may vary with the type of health behavior problem, although there is some degree of overlap. For example, skills in self-observation, monitoring, goal setting, and attentional cueing can be applied to a variety of problems, whereas skills needed to measure blood pressure differ from those needed to monitor blood glucose.

Attention control skills and high-level declarative and procedural expertise together constitute generative capabilities that allow one to understand, recall, organize, and apply the information one needs to anticipate events, evaluate outcomes, formulate appropriate strategies, construct novel solutions, and implement action plans. Figure 13.2 indicates that these capabilities undergird the motivational and constructive thinking components of the self-change model.

Health education approaches to behavior change often have been faulted for teaching health and illness facts without imparting procedural "how to" knowledge in the form of effective skills and action strategies. Behavior modification approaches sought to remedy this lack by identifying specific behavioral skills that could help one evade health threats or perform health-promoting activities. This typically involved assessing procedural knowledge by having target individuals role-play high-risk situations. But more is needed than skill training; one must be able to effectively apply the rules of constructive problem solving and planning mentioned above. This ability can be measured by means of open-middle narrative assessment tasks, in which the respondent is told the beginning of a story in which a protagonist confronts a problem, and is also told the story's successful ending, and then is asked to invent a narrative that connects the problematic beginning with the successful ending (Platt and Spivack, 1975; Spivack, Platt, and Shure, 1976). The respondent thus has to build a connecting story line. The ability to describe an effective course of action indexes one's ability to generate appropriate solutions to similar problems in daily living. In a recent study of childhood asthma management by families in low-income urban neighborhoods, for example, caretakers' asthma problem-solving skills, assessed by open-middle story narratives, proved superior to measures of asthma knowledge, outcome expectancies and self-efficacy ratings in predicting real-life asthma management practices and related emergency room visits (Wade, Holden, Lynn, Mitchell, and Ewart, 2000).

Social Interaction Processes

Changing habits that are embedded in shared routines can imperil one's relationships with others who may be affected by the change. Habit change often calls for more than individual generative capabilities. Successful self-motivation and problem solving depend also on the generative capabilities of the *relationship systems* of which one is a part, represented in Figure 13.2 by the box labeled "social interaction processes." This form of competence is constituted by the interactive capabilities of the relationship. Do those in the relationship have the ability to mutually generate patterns of interaction that enable them to avoid or accommodate the difficulties that may arise when a change by one party disrupts the goals and activities of the other? As with personal generative capabilities, social interaction capabilities and processes affect self-motivation, constructive problem solving, and action planning for habit change.

Interaction patterns that create relational competence can be characterized as processes of interpersonal *orientation, engagement*, and *shared control*. Orientation processes involve partners' attempts to ascertain and understand each others' needs, desires, and goals, and their ability to accommodate interpersonal conflicts by coordinating goals (for example, sequencing activities or taking turns), compromising (for example, ensuring that each person gets part of what he or she wants), or by agreeing to resolve the conflict by jointly pursuing a shared higher level goal (for example, a "win-win" solution). The ability to understand another's goals, to communicate one's own concerns, and to reach a mutually acceptable accommodation presupposes an ability to exchange information. This relational capability is represented in SAT by the notion of *engagement processes*, or the interaction patterns that partners generate when they try to understand and resolve goal conflicts. Positive engagement is exemplified by exchanges that facilitate mutual understanding, as in reflective listening, self-disclosure, and constructive problem solving, whereas negative engagement is exemplified by exchanges that prevent understanding by hurting or silencing the other person, as in interrupting, name-calling, use of put-downs, character assassination, and withdrawal (Ewart, 1993; Ewart, Taylor, Kraemer, and Agras, 1991; Gottman, 1994). A third relational capability consists of *control processes*, which represent forms of interaction that enable partners to specify behavioral objectives for each, to agree on an appropriate strategy and plan of action, and then to monitor the plan to make sure that it is working. Even when each partner understands the other's concerns, agrees on shared goals, and communicates effectively, the pair still may fail to support habit change by constructing an appropriate plan of action, and then monitoring the plan to ensure that it works.

More than half a century of research on marital and parent-child conflict resolution processes within diverse theoretical frameworks has achieved a notable degree of consensus in identifying basic dimensions of relationship styles that contribute to relational competence in families. Two dimensions have emerged repeatedly in factor analyses of family behaviors. One is a dimension of warmth versus hostility (often labeled acceptance/love versus rejection), whereas the other is a dimension of involvement versus detachment (often labeled dominance/control/restrictiveness versus submission/autonomy/permissiveness (Baldwin, 1955; Schaefer, 1959; Symonds, 1939). High levels of warmth and involvement in parent-child interactions have been found to predict child success in many domains; it is thought that a warm and involved relationship style enhances parents' ability to socialize their children (Darling and Steinberg, 1993). The SAT analysis of *orientation* processes identifies styles of interaction that support habit change by enhancing warmth and acceptance, whereas *engagement* processes support change by facilitating effective involvement. *Control* processes enable partners or families to reap the benefits of a warm and involved relational environment by implementing practical action plans to achieve habit change goals.

Although the importance of social support now is widely acknowledged in the health literature, support usually is defined as an individual difference variable (for example, subjective perceptions that various forms of emotional and practical aid are available), or as a structural property of a person's social network (for example, network size, frequency of contact, integration) (Uchino, 2004). SAT holds that such definitions, while useful, fail to address the relational processes that enable a social system to facilitate habit change. The ability to specify measurable processes of goal coordination (orientation), constructive communication, and problem solving (engagement), and joint action planning and monitoring (control) lets us move beyond conventions that define support only as a personality trait or a structural variable, and to examine specific forms of relational interaction that enable habit change to occur. Relational orientation, engagement, and control processes describe ways of interacting that can be measured reliably and enhanced through behavioral training techniques. Relational competence can be characterized and quantified by observing partners while they try to solve everyday problems, as well as by means of self-report questionnaires used in family research and counseling. SAT thus offers a practical framework for organizing research on family and relational problem-solving capabilities and processes that influence health habit change, and that could be targeted by preventive interventions. The theory identifies testable pathways through which interaction patterns generated by relational systems may influence self-motivation by shaping outcome and efficacy expectancies, self-goals, and personal problem solving for habit change. These causal pathways should be investigated. Along with this, methods developed in research on couples and parent-child interactions may be extended to other relational structures and cultures; research investigating this possibility is greatly needed.

CONTEXTUAL INFLUENCES

The self-change processes activated by Phase Two interventions draw upon self-regulatory resources in the form of social-emotional competence and the affordances of one's social and material environment. People need material resources in order to sustain life and health, attract mates, and nurture children. For primates that live in social groups, access to needed resources requires an ability to influence other group members. And exercising social influence and acquiring assets demands social competence. Assets, power, and competence thus form an interlocking architecture of resources that creates the ecology of action.

The contextual ecology of social action and human self-regulation is depicted in Figure 13.3. Self-regulatory resources needed to support self-change include objective *assets* in the form of goods, implements, information, and services that enable one to sustain life, move about, and understand and manipulate one's environment. One also needs *social power*, or the ability to affect other people in desired ways. But deploying assets and exerting social influence effectively is not easy to do. Effective action also demands *social-emotional competence*, which derives from accurate knowledge of oneself and one's world, supported by the biological capacity to act upon that knowledge. Social competence thus occupies a pivotal point in the ecology of adaptive self-endeavors.

Assets, power, and social-emotional competence refer to structural aspects of persons and environments that undergird or weaken self-change endeavors. Together, they constitute the regulatory resources needed to support our efforts to build new habits, yet they represent resources of very different kinds. Assets differ from the other resources in having an "objective" status, in that they exist independently of persons. Social competence, on the other hand, is a property of the individual alone. Social power differs from objective assets and competence in being relationally constituted by interactions among two or more people. The three resource classes thus represent qualitatively different kinds of resources whose effects on our self-endeavors are governed by very different principles.

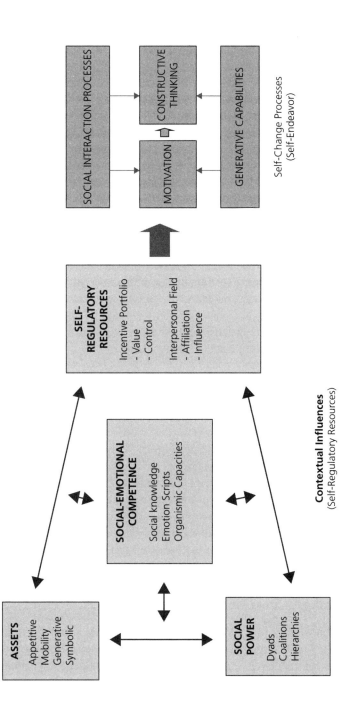

FIGURE 13.3 *Contextual Influences*

The arrows in Figure 13.3 indicate causal pathways through which resource structures shape self-regulatory activities, and regulatory activities affect resource structures. The double arrow connecting *assets* with *regulatory resources* shows that assets enable one to regulate one's acts, and self-regulation consumes assets. Also, ability to convert assets into action, and to conserve assets while pursuing goals, depends greatly upon the level of social competence; this is shown by an arrow pointing from *social-emotional competence* at the center of the figure to the double arrow of the *assets–self-regulation* axis. Thus, in the social action model of adjustment and stress, social competence moderates, or makes possible, the relationship between assets and regulatory resources for habit change. In the lower portion of Figure 13.3, another double arrow connecting *regulatory resources* to *power* depicts a similar bidirectional causal relationship between the ability to influence others and the capacity for effective self-regulation. Again, this relationship is moderated by social competence; the relevant social knowledge needed in order to deploy power effectively in action situations.

Finally, Figure 13.3 indicates that *power* and *assets* are causally interrelated. Assets may strengthen social influence, and greater influence may enable one to acquire and control assets. Again, social action theory proposes that the reciprocal relationship between *power* and *assets* is moderated by social competence. Accurate social knowledge and physical energy are needed to translate material assets into social influence, or to convert influence into needed assets. These relationships will become clearer as we examine each resource component in greater detail.

Social-Emotional Competence

Social-emotional competence, as noted earlier, consists of knowledge about one's social world, or mastery of the values, means, and proprieties of one's social milieu, which enables one to anticipate and evaluate outcomes, solve problems, and engage with others, and thus to motivate and direct one's behavior (Ewart and Jorgensen, 2004; Sternberg, 2005). Such knowledge includes an understanding of culturally based emotion categories and scripts, along with the ability to use them to regulate affect. Self- and social regulation depends, as well, on a biological capacity to act; this requires basic organismic capabilities in the form of neural-hormonal processes and psychomotor skills that enable effective behavior. Research on social competence shows that competence can be measured reliably with a semistructured behavioral interview (Curbow et al., 2005; Ewart et al., 2002; Ewart and Kolodner, 1991), and predicts behavioral and cardiovascular responses to social challenges in the laboratory (Ewart et al., 1998; Ewart, Jorgensen, Schroder, Suchday, and Sherwood, 2005) and in the natural environment (Ewart and Jorgensen, 2004). Together, social-emotional knowledge and organismic states determine our readiness to act in pursuit of our goals: quick, decisive action is facilitated by heuristic procedural knowledge in the form of mental short cuts and organismic states of hormonal, metabolic, and psychomotor activation. Social-emotional competence is a function of prior exposure to competent social models, as well as having adequate nutrition and rest, for example.

Objective Assets

Other self-regulatory resources are affordances of our environments. An *affordance* is defined as whatever the environment offers us, either for good or ill (Gibson, 1979, p.127). Desired asset affordances include a diverse array of objects and events that serve appetitive needs (for example, food, clothing, shelter), or let us move about (mobility), or enable us to create things we need (generative), or provide information (symbolic), to name some common examples (Reed, 1996). Access to assets lets us create an *incentive portfolio* of self-rewards and self-punishments that we can use to guide and motivate our acts. For example, I encourage myself to exercise by resolving not to enjoy a favorite snack until I complete my daily run.

SAT analysis of objective assets as self-regulatory resources offers useful insights into the well-documented negative relationship between health and poverty. Studies of families living in poverty have revealed the many challenges faced by those whose assets are limited. One way in which poverty undermines health is by making it very difficult for families to establish predictable routines. Objective resources contribute to flexible time management. Our personal timetables are embedded in social institutions that operate on public time (9:00 AM to 5:00 PM). But limited financial resources can make the task of commuting to and from work, arranging for child care, shopping for groceries, preparing meals, and making medical appointments extend across different timetables (Burton and Sorensen, 1993).

Roy et al. (2004) followed seventy-five low-income mothers for four years to learn about their daily schedules. Getting by on a low income makes complex demands on one's time. About half of the mothers were employed full-time and, of those, half worked a standard 9:00 AM to 5:00 PM shift. The other mothers, however, worked during second, third, or "off" shifts. The amount of time they had to spend using public transportation consumed at least two and up to five hours of each day. The long travel times and the poor quality of neighborhood grocery stores meant that the mothers were forced to relegate shopping trips to the weekend and sometimes had to arrange extra help with child care. Faced with multiple time demands, the mothers had to expend considerable effort coordinating their private and public schedules. The researchers noted that this made shifts from picking up children to preparing dinner, from waking, feeding, and grooming children in the morning to dropping them off on the way to work, uniquely demanding, as the burden of synchronizing these activities was born entirely by the mother. A child's illness that required a visit to the doctor could make matters much worse, for it could compromise the mother's ability to hold a job where there was little tolerance for her missing work to handle a medical emergency. For a parent in these circumstances, the ability to create an incentive portfolio of attractive outcomes that one might use to reward one's self-change efforts is severely limited.

Social Power

Our success in achieving lasting habit change is much affected by our ability to understand other people, to synchronize our actions with theirs, and to influence them in desired ways. Such influence constitutes one's *social power* (Keltner and Anderson, 2003).

Power is defined in SAT as the ability to affect other people in ways we wish to; including the ability to influence another's thoughts, feelings, or behavior. This definition envisages a continuum of influence, ranging from acts such as comforting a child, cheering a friend, seducing a lover, supervising an employee, disarming a critic, persuading an opponent, or defeating a bully. SAT proposes that power is created and exercised within *social frames*, or the relationship domains in which we typically interact with others. SAT emphasizes three power frames: (1) *reciprocal* power, as in a partnership between equals in which each person influences, and is influenced by, the other partner (dyadic relationships of this type usually involve a reciprocal exchange of resources); (2) *coalitional* power, as when people work together in a group of equals and coordinate their actions to exert influence collectively; (3) *hierarchical* power, as in relationships between persons of unequal status. A teacher can wield more influence over a student's thoughts, feelings, and actions than vice versa.

These three frames reflect basic social structures: dyads (for example, parent-child, parent-parent) are nested within family groups; which often are nested within communities of varying sizes (Blunt Bugenthal, 2000). Each level of structure creates its own distinctive power frame; dyads require balanced reciprocity, families demand loyalty and cohesion, and larger communities need to establish hierarchical structures (for example, leaders and subordinates) in order to function effectively. Some social relationships may blend different power frames. Two parents, for example, may exercise reciprocal power with each other as partners, hierarchical power over their young children, and coalitional power as members of a larger family group.

Within each relationship frame, principles of influence (power) specific to that frame typically apply (Blunt Bugenthal, 2000). In a reciprocal relationship, the governing principle is one of balance; each partner is expected to contribute equally. In marriage, for example, partners are expected to maintain a high ratio of positive to negative events; the occurrence of at least five positive relationship events for every negative event has been found to characterize successful relationships (Gottman, 1994). In coalitions, the governing principles emphasize the need to maintain clear in-group versus out-group boundaries, equality within the in-group, a shared goal, and group activities that reap rewards for all (McCauley, 2001). Within a hierarchical frame, rules of influence emphasize hierarchically ordered duties to those above one in the hierarchy, and responsibilities to those at lower levels. Those at the top are responsible for protecting and nurturing (and not abusing) those below; the latter, on their part, are expected to faithfully pursue goals and carry out tasks assigned by those above them.

Analysis of social power suggests contextual interventions to support health habit change by mobilizing dyads, support groups, and hierarchies. Typical examples include buddy systems (dyads), peer support groups (coalitions), and systems in which those with more experience in habit change help mentor novices (hierarchies). The effectiveness of such interventions depends on the degree to which they increase personal power by activating processes of dyadic reciprocity, group cohesion, and hierarchically ordered obligation (for example, nurturance, respect).

The affordances of our social frames create an *interpersonal field* composed of people to whom we can turn for aid and comfort. People within the social field are evaluated with respect to their attractiveness as partners, allies, mentors, or trusted supporters (affiliation), as well as our ability to influence them in ways we desire (power). Like the incentive portfolio generated by our access to objective affordances, the interpersonal field enables us to construct self-motivators to action by envisioning desirable or undesirable social outcomes of habit change, for example, by anticipating how changing might enhance valued relationships. Our interpersonal fields also affect health related concerns about personal identity. Many health problems challenge one's sense of self-identity by assigning an illness diagnosis, or by rendering salient one's gender, social class, or sexual orientation. SAT proposes that identity issues such as these can be analyzed as challenges to social power, and principles of dyadic, coalitional, or hierarchic relations can be used to design supportive interventions that bolster self-identities by enhancing power. Developing a desired health habit thus becomes part of a broader self-endeavor aimed at building a healthy self-identity (Johnson, Carrico, Chesney, and Morin, in press; Lightfoot, Rotheram-Borus, Milburn, and Swendeman, 2005).

Limits to social power and constricted interpersonal fields posed significant challenges for the low-income mothers studied by Roy and associates (Roy, Tubbs, and Burton, 2004). Although these highly capable women organized their days carefully, and tightly coordinated multiple schedules, their environments failed to afford them the social influence and interpersonal connections they needed to create stable routines. Many mothers depended on their own mothers for help in taking care of their children, and on their grandmothers for preparing meals. Mothers coped by harboring their scarce resources, and by trying to limit social obligations. These strategies enabled them to create a degree of predictability and order in their children's lives, yet also tended to isolate the mothers by making it difficult to form supportive connections with friends and groups. Establishing stable routines promotes health. Yet achieving this goal calls for a minimum of social resources. Poverty saps the interpersonal supports and social power needed to create and maintain health-protective routines.

Environmental affordances and social-emotional competencies interact to determine our ability to create attractive incentive portfolios and empowering interpersonal fields that make it possible to sustain self-change efforts over time. They thus can be viewed as contextual factors that must be present to sustain enduring habit change. Interventions to support change by increasing material resources (for example, income, child care) or to enhance social support by restructuring social frames (for example, buddy systems, changing group norms) are designed to enhance objective and social affordances.

PATHS TO SELF-DEBILITATION

Prevention accomplishes little without an accurate understanding of how health damaging habits develop. In SAT, an ecological analysis of goal-directed endeavors identifies two important causal pathways by which human environments may foster self-debilitating habits. Each pathway operates by adversely affecting goal-oriented striving, thus generating a "dysregulated" self-endeavor. The theory also specifies a more hopeful pathway by which people in stressful environments can build resilience and achieve greater control over their health.

Agonistic Striving (AS) describes a family of self-endeavors characterized by striving to manage, control, or dominate others in one's social milieu (Ewart and Jorgensen, 2004; Ewart et al., 2005). AS typically develops in environments where one is exposed to threats of social dominance (for example, in a hierarchy) or rejection (for example, exclusion from a group) (Ewart et al., 1998). Dominance and exclusion threats foster an attitude of wary vigilance, hostility, and aggressiveness in social interactions (Aldarondo and Sugarman, 1996; Hampton, 1987; Patterson, 1976, 1982; Sidanius and Pratto, 1999). One's relationships with others, including family members, become harsh and punitive with increased potential for child or spouse abuse. People often try to manage unpleasant cognitive and affective states associated with AS by using tobacco, alcohol, or other drugs that help lower arousal. Recurring interpersonal struggles sap self-regulatory resources and undermine self-change efforts.

Dissipated Striving (DS) describes a family of self-endeavors characterized by a tendency to disengage from long-term goals and a resulting "failure to strive." Frustrations and disappointments thwart goal-oriented striving by undermining self-efficacy (Ewart et al., 1998; Lyubomirsky and Nolen-Hoeksema, 1995; Lyubomirsky, Tucker, Caldwell, and Berg, 1999). Failure to achieve valued goals perpetuates anxiety, despondency, lethargy, and withdrawal from others. People often try to cope by resorting to activities that generate rapid surges in arousal or pleasant affect with little effort; alcohol, drugs, or calorie-rich foods may serve this need. Difficulty in identifying meaningful self-goals and devising appropriate ways to pursue them undermines self-change efforts.

AS and DS syndromes offer ways to link personal habits with physical and social environments. As one descends the SES-health gradient, exposure to dominance and exclusion (for example, discrimination), deprivation, violence, and uncertainty increases (Adler et al., 1994; Marmot et al., 1991; Matthews et al., 1989). These conditions foster AS and DS patterns, thereby increasing susceptibility to health damaging habits and rendering these habits more difficult to change. A social action analysis suggests structural changes that can be implemented to support people's efforts to protect their health by altering their behavior.

PATHWAYS TO HEALTH

Even in highly stressful environments, many people develop effective ways to pursue valued self-endeavors and to protect their health. These individuals remind us that it is a mistake to equate low SES with personal dysfunction. They also offer models of resilience, and provide clues to effective self-regulatory coping.

Transcendence Striving (TS) describes a family of self-endeavors characterized by striving to change oneself or one's life circumstances (Ewart and Jorgensen, 2004). TS is grounded in the basic evolutionary heuristic, "Maximize your value" as a mate, parent, partner, or group member. One responds to challenging circumstances by striving to improve oneself in ways that enhance one's personal capabilities. This boosts one's value by increasing one's ability to generate and control valued material or social resources. The result is greater personal agency and resilience. TS has three major aspects. First, one scans (explores) one's environment to discover attractive opportunities and form meaningful self-goals. Next, the quest to attain desired goals inspires a struggle to master the capabilities, or expertise, needed to realize them. Together, goal and skill orientations motivate efforts to direct, organize, and control one's actions. Goals encourage skill building, which, in turn, requires self-control. Social action theory proposes that fostering a TS orientation, by countering AS and DS syndromes is a powerful way to support health habit change.

The TS pattern suggests ways to link processes of positive self-change with physical and social environments. TS describes how people normally try to cope with stressful challenges. In a social action analysis, environments that afford a range of attractive goals, that support effective goal-attainment strategies, and that reward skill building and self-control tend to foster TS in place of the debilitating AS or DS patterns.

APPLICATIONS

The social action analysis outlined above offers highly specific guidelines for health behavior change interventions. In addition to the Three-Step Protocol for implementing habit change, the theory also specifies patterns of self-debilitation and transcendence that may impede or facilitate health habit modification, as well as social-environmental conditions that tend to foster the AS, DS, and TS patterns. These conditions can be targeted by structural and organizational interventions.

CASE EXAMPLE

Phase One

Failure in health promotion often results from a lack of appropriately selected and well-specified objectives. SAT thus encourages planners to begin by defining the desired health habit as an *action state*. It is helpful to approach this task as if writing a script for a documentary film about a person in the target population who is attempting to change. The script must describe in detail the settings, the actions to be performed by the protagonist and others, and the actors' thoughts and feelings. A series of scenes is constructed to portray a linear progression of events leading to and following the desired action. Using this script, the planner then identifies the discrete actions, outcomes, and interpersonal action linkages (for example, shared routines) that compose the desired action state. This state defines the intervention's behavioral objectives. In cases where the new health habit is meant to replace an existing unhealthy activity (for example, snacking on candy is to be replaced by snacking on fruit), the movie script exercise is performed to identify behaviors, outcomes, and action linkages that maintain the current undesired habit. These then can be targeted for disruption and replacement.

As noted earlier, the problem of arranging for rewarding outcomes to follow the new behavior every time it is performed often proves to be the Achilles heel of habit change interventions. To address this problem, it is helpful to construct an "outcome grid" consisting of four cells that are created by combining the dimensions of "outcome desirability" (desired versus undesired) and "outcome immediacy" (immediate versus delayed). The various outcomes identified in the action state analysis then are sorted into these four cells; it is important to include only those outcomes that the person who tries to change will *experience directly*. The analysis often discloses that the personally experienced rewards of attempting a new health behavior will be delayed, whereas the negative outcomes will be experienced immediately. This fact forces the planner to identify immediate positive outcomes that the intervention might introduce, and negative outcomes that might be removed or ameliorated, so as to strengthen motivation. Without this, the intervention is unlikely to succeed. A similar outcome grid analysis should be performed for existing unhealthy habits that will be targeted for reduction. Depending on the degree of action linkage, the analysis may reveal that many of the outcomes that must be changed are socially mediated, and therefore will involve encouraging others to change also.

Phase Two

Self-change is possible only if one becomes aware of what one is doing and experiencing before, during, and after the behavior one is trying to acquire or reduce. This involves learning that "doing X in situation Y causes Z." Self-monitoring techniques offer a powerful way to acquire such self-awareness, although simple questionnaires (Fishbein et al., 2001) can be helpful when direct self-monitoring is not feasible. Self-efficacy for habit change can be assessed by means of a standard scaling approach that must be tailored specifically to the target performances (Bandura, 1997). Self-expectations about behavioral outcomes and personal capabilities can be enhanced using social modeling and direct exposure methods that have been described in the extensive cognitive-behavioral literature (Bandura, 1986, 1997).

Often neglected in cognitive-behavioral approaches, however, is the degree to which outcome and self-efficacy expectations are affected by a new habit's impact on important daily routines, including activities shared with others. This impact can be assessed by helping target individuals identify their important routines during self-observational assessments or by using questionnaires. The objective is to specify regularly performed activities that serve goals of health, love, or wealth, and to estimate the extent to which a recommended habit change will support or impair these goals and routines. Routines then may be redesigned or adjusted to accommodate and support the new habit.

Even seemingly simple habit changes can generate a host of new problems, especially when they involve altering tightly interwoven routines in domains such as child care, commuting, or occupational activities. Flexibility in adjusting routines calls for constructive thinking in the form of problem solving and planning. Indeed, SAT holds problem solving to be the fulcrum of the habit change process, and suggests that ongoing engagement in constructive thinking should be regarded as a key behavioral objective for intervention. In addition to modeling basic techniques of brainstorming and decision making, it is important to ensure that those targeted by the intervention are encouraged to create detailed action plans that address behavioral goals, settings, cues, actions, outcomes, and resources. Those who strive to change themselves should be encouraged to view problem solving and action planning as a continuing process.

Phase Three

It is unrealistic to expect people to pursue a healthier lifestyle without building needed self-regulatory resources. Such resources include social-cognitive and organismic capabilities in the form of social-emotional competence, as well as environmental affordances in the form of objective assets and social power. Self-competencies and resources represent contextual influences that shape the long-term success of habit change interventions. Social-emotional competence is needed to act quickly and effectively in a wide range of social situations; such competence can be enhanced by modeling socially effective behavior in a variety of typical settings, by teaching self-management and affect regulation skills, and by providing opportunities for nourishment and rest.

The key objective resources needed to support desired health habits include transportation, help with child care, access to health services, education, employment, and nutrition, as well as physical settings where one can safely and easily engage in physical exercise. Health promotion programs must assess these assets, which may be available in neighborhoods, schools, or workplaces. Interventions to increase objective assets by redesigning settings or improving access to benefits and services may be needed.

SAT holds that social power is a vital self-regulatory resource that can be increased by contextual interventions (Keltner and Anderson, 2003; Uchino, Cacioppo, and Kiecolt-Glaser, 1996); increased power creates a rewarding sense of self-identity and expands one's base of social support, thus fostering adherence to an intervention program (Linden, 2005). But social interventions may accomplish little if they fail to apply the principles of power that govern a given social frame. Buddy systems based on principles of balanced dyadic reciprocity can create opportunities for mutual influence that are highly rewarding, because they allow a person both to give and to receive support. It is important, however, that the parties be matched appropriately on the basis of personalities and interests (Linden, Rutledge, and Con, 1998; Uchino et al., 1996). Groups can be an effective means of self-regulatory support if they adhere to well-established principles of group formation and cohesion. These include building a clear sense of group identity (for example, t-shirts, logo), collective goals and routines (for example, shared group activities), and working to win group-based rewards. Hierarchical frames can be designed to enhance social power of participants by having those who are more experienced in habit change mentor the novices. The latter benefit from access to effective coping models, whereas mentors benefit from a relationship that allows them to nurture new "recruits," while also creating an incentive to serve as a positive example by maintaining desired habits. SAT proposes that interventions designed to bolster social power may be especially helpful to those for whom health behavior change is part of an evolving personal quest to develop a robust sense of positive self-identity, a quest shared by many members of historically subordinated minority groups (Sidanius and Pratto, 1999).

SUMMARY

Strengths of Social Action Theory

For the last half century, theories of health promotion have treated health knowledge and outcome expectancies as the primary movers of health habit change. Although self-efficacy and, to a lesser extent, problem-solving processes, have lately joined the van, most research continues to test simple predictive models rather than to identify and evaluate causal mechanisms and pathways of change. Thus, despite the advent of social-cognitive theory, most research findings fail to yield practical information that intervention planners can use to foster health-protective habits. And although social-cognitive theory clarifies important cognitive regulatory mechanisms, further theoretical and empirical work is needed to identify social-contextual processes that shape cognition and thus create an ecology of action.

SAT addresses this need by specifying self-regulatory mechanisms that give rise to self-endeavors, and by indicating how these processes combine to promote habit change. Cognitive processes are shaped extensively by social interactions; action linkages within shared routines often govern the outcomes people experience when they try to acquire new habits. SAT also identifies personal and environmental self-regulatory resources that directly affect social interactions, problem solving, self-efficacy, and anticipated outcomes, and thereby facilitate or impede long-term habit change. These resources, which take the form of social-emotional competence, objective assets, and social power, represent measurable constructs that can be altered to support behavior change. Social-emotional competence represents a body of modifiable declarative and procedural knowledge structures; social power is governed by well-established principles that govern interpersonal transactions with dyads, groups, and hierarchies. These strengths have led public health planners to adopt SAT as basis for programs to lower heart disease risk, reduce drug abuse, and limit the spread of HIV, and have stimulated creative approaches to health promotion with under-studied groups (Johnson et al., in press; Lightfoot et al., 2005).

Limitations of Social Action Theory

As a theory intended to focus attention on promising new questions, SAT raises hypotheses that invite further study. The notion that increasing social power may bolster motivation for habit change, while plausibly derived from existing evidence, should be tested further in health habit research. The "goal congruence" hypothesis, that success in changing a habit is affected by the habit's compatibility with self-endeavors that serve goals of health, love, or wealth, should be tested, as should the notion that social-emotional competence is an important self-regulatory resource for sustaining behavior change. And SAT pathways to self-debilitation represented by AS and DS syndromes, as well as the TS pathway to health, need to be investigated as possible mediating chains linking stressful living environments to health-damaging or health-protective activities. It is hoped that these hypothesized causal linkages and frameworks will inspire more practically useful research into the processes and conditions of health habit change.

Ultimately, a theory's strengths and weaknesses depend upon the state of the discipline and its pressing needs. Theory building in science has advanced by following one of two alternative strategies (Kagan, 2007). One approach invents a simple but compelling idea and then devises a program of experiments to test it. This approach has worked best in highly developed disciplines such as physics, and is brilliantly exemplified by the work of Albert Einstein.

The other strategy begins by identifying a reliable phenomenon whose causes, consequences, and contextual limitations can be examined. One then gathers evidence and creates concepts to integrate the observed facts. This more empirical approach to theory building has worked best in new disciplines that are in the early stages of growth, and is beautifully exemplified by the work of Charles Darwin. But, as Darwin himself noted, a scientist does not get far simply by gathering lots of random facts, as if aimlessly collecting and describing the pebbles in a gravel pit. To work well, the empirical search needs a guiding framework to identify promising phenomena, to indicate how they might be interrelated, and to suggest where, beneath nature's gritty rubble, some patient digging might uncover robust patterns of relations among observations that are the skeletal foundation of a useful theory. For the yet-to-be-quarried field of health promotion, SAT offers a prospector's map to advance this quest.

REFERENCES

Adler, N. E., Boyce, T., Chesney, M. A., Cohen, S., Folkman, S., Kahn, R. L., and Syme, L. (1994). Socioeconomic status and health: The challenge of the gradient. *American Psychologist, 49*, 15–24.

Adler, N. E., Epel, E. S., Castellazzo, G., and Ickovicks, J. R. (2000). Relationship of subjective and objective social status with psychological and physiological functioning: Preliminary data in healthy white women. *Health Psychology, 19*, 586–592.

Ahles, T. A., Blanchard, E. B., and Leventhal, H. (1983). Cognitive control of pain: Attention to the sensory aspects of the cold pressor stimulus. *Cognitive Therapy and Research, 7*, 159–177.

Aldarondo, E., and Sugarman, D. B. (1996). Risk marker analysis of the cessation and persistence of wife assault. *Journal of Consulting and Clinical Psychology, 64*, 1010–1019.

Baldwin, A. L. (1955). *Behavior and development in childhood.* New York: Dryden Press.

Baldwin, J. D., and Baldwin, J. I. (1981). *Behavior principles in everyday life.* Englewood Cliffs, NJ: Prentice-Hall.

Bandura, A. (1986). *Social foundations of thought and action: A social cognitive theory.* Englewood Cliffs, NJ: Prentice Hall.

Bandura, A. (1997). *Self-efficacy: The exercise of control.* New York: Freeman.

Becker, M. H. (1974). The health belief model and personal health behavior. *Health Education Monographs, 2*, 324–508.

Beckmann, J., and Gollwitzer, P. M. (1987). Deliberative versus implementative states of mind: The issue of impartiality in predecisional and postdecisional information processing. *Social Cognition, 5*, 529–279.

Blunt Bugenthal, D. (2000). Acquisition of the algorithms of social life: A domain-based approach. *Psychological Bulletin, 126*, 187–219.

Brody, G. H., and Flor, D. L. (1997). Maternal psychological functioning, family processes, and child adjustment in rural, single-parent, African American families. *Developmental Psychology, 33*, 1000–1011.

Brownell, K. D., Marlatt, G. A., Lichtenstein, E., and Wilson, G. T. (1986). Understanding and preventing relapse. *American Psychologist, 41*, 765–782.

Burton, L. M., and Sorensen, S. (1993). Temporal dimensions of intergenerational caregiving in African-American multigeneration families. In S. H. Zarit and L. I. Pearlin and K. W. Schaie (eds.), *Caregiving systems: Informal and formal helpers* (pp. 47–66). Hillsdale, NJ: Erlbaum.

Curbow, B., McDonnell, K. A., Dreyling, E., Hall, A., Fitzgerald, S., and Ewart, C. K. (2005). Assessing cardiovascular reactivity in working women with the Social Competence Interview. *Women and Health, 41*, 51–68.

D'Zurilla, T. J., and Goldfried, M. R. (1971). Problem solving and behavior modification. *Journal of Abnormal Psychology, 78*, 107–126.

D'Zurilla, T. J., and Nezu, A. (1980). A study of the generation-of-alternatives process in social problem solving. *Cognitive Therapy and Research, 4*, 67–72.

Dar, R., and Leventhal, H. (1993). Schematic processes in pain perception. *Cognitive Therapy and Research, 17*, 341–357.

Darling, N., and Steinberg, L. (1993). Parenting style as context: An integrative model. *Psychological Bulletin, 113*, 487–496.

Ewart, C. K. (1991). Social action theory for a public health psychology. *American Psychologist, 46*, 931–946.

Ewart, C. K. (1993). Editorial comment: Marital interaction—The context for psychosomatic research. *Psychosomatic Medicine, 55*, 410–412.

Ewart, C. K. (1995). Social-cognitive origins of chronic stress in adolescents: Recent findings from school-based studies of urban youth. *Journal of Health Education, 26*(3), 132–138.

Ewart, C. K. (2004a). How integrative theory building can improve health promotion and disease prevention. In R. G. Frank and J. Wallander and A. Baum (Eds.), *Handbook of clinical health psychology, Vol. 3: Models and perspectives in health psychology* (pp. 249–289). Washington, DC: American Psychological Association.

Ewart, C. K. (2004b). Self-efficacy. In A. J. Christensen and R. Martin and J. M. Smyth (eds.), *Encyclopedia of health psychology* (pp. 260–262). New York: Plenum.

Ewart, C. K. (2004c). Social environments, agonistic stress, and elevated blood pressure in urban youth. In R. Portman and J. Sorof and J. Ingelfinger (eds.), *Pediatric hypertension*. Totowa, NJ: Humana Press.

Ewart, C. K., and Jorgensen, R. S. (2004). Agonistic interpersonal striving: Social-cognitive mechanism of cardiovascular risk in youth? *Health Psychology, 23*, 75–85.

Ewart, C. K., Jorgensen, R. S., and Kolodner, K. B. (1998). Sociotropic cognition moderates blood pressure response to interpersonal stress in high-risk adolescent girls. *International Journal of Psychophysiology, 28*, 131–142.

Ewart, C. K., Jorgensen, R. S., Schroder, K. E., Suchday, S., and Sherwood, A. (2005). Vigilance to a persisting personal threat: Unmasking cardiovascular consequences in adolescents with the Social Competence Interview. *Psychophysiology, 41*, 799–804.

Ewart, C. K., Jorgensen, R. S., Suchday, S., Chen, E., and Matthews, K. A. (2002). Measuring stress resilience and coping in vulnerable youth: The Social Competence Interview. *Psychological Assessment, 14*(3), 339–352.

Ewart, C. K., and Kolodner, K. B. (1991). Social Competence Interview for assessing physiological reactivity in adolescents. *Psychosomatic Medicine, 53*, 289–304.

Ewart, C. K., and Kolodner, K. B. (1994). Negative affect, gender, and expressive style predict ambulatory blood pressure in adolescents. *Journal of Personality and Social Psychology, 66*, 596–605.

Ewart, C. K., and Suchday, S. (2002). Discovering how urban poverty and violence affect health: Development and validation of a neighborhood stress index. *Health Psychology, 21*(3), 254–262.

Ewart, C. K., Taylor, C. B., Kraemer, C. H., and Agras, W. S. (1991). High blood pressure and marital discord: Not being nasty matters more than being nice. *Health Psychology, 10*, 155–163.

Fiese, B. H. (2006). *Family routines and rituals.* New Haven, CT: Yale University Press.

Fishbein, M. (1980). A theory of reasoned action: Some applications and implications. In H. Howe and M. Page (Eds.), *Nebraska symposium on motivation, 1979* (pp. 65–116). Lincoln: University of Nebraska Press.

Fishbein, M., Triandis, H. C., Kanfer, F. H., Becker, M., Middlestadt, S., and Eichler, A. (2001). Factors influencing behavior and behavior change. In A. Baum and T. A. Revenson and J. E. Singer (eds.), *Handbook of health psychology* (pp. 3–17). Mahwah, NJ: Erlbaum.

Fitzgerald, S. T., Brown, K. M., Sonnega, J. R., and Ewart, C. K. (2005). Early antecedents of adult work stress: Social emotional competence and anger in adolescence. *Journal of Behavioral Medicine, 28*, 223–230.

Gibson, J. J. (1979). *The ecological approach to visual perception.* Boston: Houghton-Mifflin.

Gollwitzer, P. M., Fujita, K., and Oettingen, G. (2004). Planning and the implementation of goals. In R. F. Baumeister and K. D. Vohs (eds.), *Handbook of self-regulation: Research, theory, and applications* (pp. 211–228). New York: Guilford Press.

Gottman, J. M. (1994). *What predicts divorce? The relationship between marital processes and marital outcomes.* Hillsdale, NJ: Erlbaum.

Guidubaldi, J., Cleminshaw, H. K., Perry, J. D., Nastasi, B. K., and Lightel, J. (1986). The role of selected family environment factors in children's post-divorce adjustment. *Family Relations, 35*, 141–151.

Guidubaldi, J., Perry, J. D., and Nastasi, B. K. (1987). Growing up in a divorced family: Initial and long-term perspectives on children's adjustment. In S. Oskamp (ed.), *Family processes and problems: Social psychological aspects* (pp. 202–237). Newbury Park, CA: Sage.

Hampton, R. L. (1987). Race, class and child maltreatment. *Journal of Comparative Family Studies, 18*, 113–126.

Hill-Briggs, F. (2003). Problem solving in diabetes self-management: A model of chronic illness self-management behavior. *Annals of Behavioral Medicine, 25*, 182–193.

Johnson, M. O., Carrico, A. W., Chesney, M. A., and Morin, S. F. (in press). Internalized heterosexism among HIV-positive gay-identified men: Implications for HIV prevention and care. *Consulting and Clinical Psychology.*

Kagan, J. (2007). *What is emotion? History, measures, meanings.* New Haven, CT: Yale University Press.

Kahneman, D., and Miller, D. T. (1986). Norm theory: Comparing reality to its alternatives. *Psychological Review, 93*, 126–153.

Kawachi, I., and Kennedy, B. (2002). *The health of nations: Why inequality is harmful to your health.* New York: New Press.

Kazdin, A. E. (1975). *Behavior modification in applied settings.* Homewood, IL: Dorsey Press.

Keltner, D. G., D. H., and Anderson, C. (2003). Power, approach, and inhibition. *Psychological Review, 110*, 265–284.

Lambie, J. A., and Marcel, A. J. (2002). Consciousness and the varieties of emotion experience: A theoretical framework. *Psychological Bulletin, 109*, 219–259.

Leahey, T. H. (2001). *A history of modern psychology* (3rd ed.). Upper Saddle River, NJ: Prentice Hall.

Lightfoot, M., Rotheram-Borus, M. J., Milburn, N. G., and Swendeman, D. (2005). Prevention for sero-positive persons: Successive approximation toward a new identity. *Behavior Modification, 29*, 227–255.

Linden, W. (2005). *Stress management: From basic science to better practice*. Thousand Oaks, CA: Sage.

Linden, W., Rutledge, T., and Con, A. (1998). A case for the usefulness of laboratory social stressors. *Annals of Behavioral Medicine, 20*(4), 310–316.

Lyubomirsky, S., and Nolen-Hoeksema, S. (1995). Effects of self-focused rumination on negative thinking and interpersonal problem solving. *Journal of Personality and Social Psychology, 69*, 176–190.

Lyubomirsky, S., Tucker, K. L., Caldwell, N. D., and Berg, K. (1999). Why ruminators are poor problem solvers: Clues from the phenomenology of dysphoric rumination. *Journal of Personality and Social Psychology, 77*, 1041–1060.

Mahoney, M. J. (1974). *Cognition and behavior modification*. Cambridge, MA: Ballinger.

Mahoney, M. J. (1975). The obese eating style: Bites, beliefs, and behavior modification. *Addictive Behaviors, 1*, 47–53.

Marlatt, G. A., and Gordon, J. R. (Eds.). (1985). *Relapse prevention: Maintenance strategies in the treatment of addictive behaviors*. New York: Guilford Press.

Marmot, M. G., Smith, G. D., Stansfeld, S., Patel, C., North, F., Head, J., White, I., Brunner, E., and Feeney, A. (1991). Health inequalities among British civil servants: The Whitehall II Study. *Lancet, 337*, 1387–1393.

Matthews, K. A., Kelsey, S., Meilahn, E., Kuller, L., and Wing, R. (1989). Educational attainment and behavioral and biologic risk factors for coronary heart disease in middle-aged women. *American Journal of Epidemiolgy, 129*, 1132–1144.

McCauley, C. (2001). The psychology of group identification and the power of ethnic nationalism. In D. Chirot and M.E.P. Seligman (eds.), *Ethnopolitical warfare: Causes, consequences, and possible solutions* (pp. 343–362). Washington, DC: American Psychological Association.

Mischel, W., and Ayduk, O. (2004). Willpower in a cognitive-affective processing system: The dynamics of delay of gratification. In R. F. Baumeister and K. D. Vohs (eds.), *Handbook of self-regulation: Research, theory, and applications* (pp. 99–129). New York: Guilford Press.

Nezu, A., and D'Zurilla, T. J. (1979). An experimental evaluation of the decision-making process in social problem solving. *Cognitive Therapy and Research, 3*, 269–277.

Parnes, S. J., and Meadow, A. (1959). Effects of "brainstorming" instructions on creative problem-solving by trained and untrained subjects. *Journal of Educational Psychology, 50*, 171–175.

Patterson, G. R. (1976). The aggressive child: Victim and architect of a coercive system. In L. A. Hamerlynck and L. C. Hardy and E. J. Mash (eds.), *Behavior modification and families: Vol.1. Theory and research*. New York: Brunner/Mazel.

Patterson, G. R. (1982). *Coercive family processes*. Eugene, OR: Castalia.

Peake, P., Hebl, M., and Mischel, W. (2002). Strategic attention deployment in waiting and working situations. *Developmental Psychology, 38*, 313–326.

Perri, M. G., Nezu, A., McKelvey, W. F., Shermer, R. L., Renjilian, D. A., and Viegener, B. J. (2001). Relapse prevention training and problem-solving therapy in the long-term management of obesity. *Journal of Consulting and Clinical Psychology, 69*, 722–726.

Perri, M. G., Nezu, A. M., and Viegener, B. J. (1992). *Improving the long-term management of obesity: Theory, research, and clinical guidelines*. New York: Wiley.

Pham, L. B., and Taylor, S. E. (1999). From thought to action: Effects of process- versus outcome-based mental simulations on performance. *Personality and Social Psychology Bulletin, 25*, 250–260.

Platt, J. J., and Spivack, G. (1975). *Measures of interpersonal cognitive problem solving for adults and adolescents* (Manual). Philadelphia.

Portes, P. R., Howell, S. C., Brown, J. H., Eichenberger, S., and Mas, C. A. (1992). Family functions in children's postdivorce adjustment. *American Journal of Orthopsychiatry, 62*, 613–617.

Prochaska, J. C., DiClemente, C. C., and Norcross, J. (1992). In search of how people change. *American Psychologist, 47*, 1102–1114.

Reed, E. S. (1996). *Encountering the world: Toward an ecological psychology*. New York: Oxford.

Richardson, A. (1967). Mental practice: A review and discussion. Part I. *Research Quarterly, 38*, 95–107.

Roy, K. M., Tubbs, C. Y., and Burton, L. M. (2004). Don't have no time: Daily rhythms and the organization of time for low-income families. *Family Relations, 53*, 168–178.

Rutter, M., and Sroufe, L. A. (2000). Developmental psychopathology: Concepts and challenges. *Development and Psychopathology, 12*, 265–296.

Sameroff, A. J., and Chandler, M. J. (1975). Reproductive risk and the continuum of caretaking causality. In F. D. Horowitz and M. Hetherington and S. Scarr-Salapetek and G. Siegel (eds.), *Review of child development research* (Vol. 4, pp. 187–244). Chicago: University of Chicago Press.

Schaefer, E. S. (1959). The circumplex model for maternal behavior. *Journal of Abnormal and Social Psychology, 59*, 226–235.

Shiffman, S. M. (1982). Relapse following smoking cessation: A situational analysis. *Journal of Consulting and Clinical Psychology, 50*, 71–86.

Sidanius, J., and Pratto, F. (1999). *Social dominance*. New York: Cambridge University Press.

Siegrist, J., and Marmot, M. (2004). Health inequalities and the psychosocial environment: Two scientific challenges. *Social Science and Medicine, 58*, 1463–1473.

Smyth, J., Wonderlich, S., Crosby, R., Miltenberger, R., Mitchell, J., and Rorty, M. (2001). The use of ecological momentary assessment approaches in eating disorder research. *International Journal of Eating Disorders, 30*, 83–95.

Spivack, G., Platt, J. J., and Shure, M. B. (1976). *The problem-solving approach to adjustment*. San Francisco: Jossey-Bass.

Sternberg, R. J. (2005). Intelligence, competence, and expertise. In A. J. Elliot and C. S. Dweck (eds.), *Handbook of competence and motivation* (pp. 15–30). New York: Guilford Press.

Stuart, R. B. (1967). Behavioral control of overeating. *Behavior Research and Therapy, 5*, 357–365.

Symonds, P. M. (1939). *The psychology of parent-child relationships*. New York: Appleton-Century-Crofts.

Taylor, S. E., Pham, L. B., Rivkin, I. D., and Armor, D. A. (1998). Harnessing the imagination: Mental simulation, self-regulation, and coping. *American Psychologist, 53*, 429–439.

Uchino, B. N. (2004). *Social support and physical health: Understanding the health consequences of relationships*. New Haven, CT: Yale University Press.

Uchino, B. N., Cacioppo, J. T., and Kiecolt-Glaser, J. K. (1996). The relationship between social support and physiological processes: A review with emphasis on underlying mechanisms and implications for health. *Psychological Bulletin, 119*, 488–531.

Wade, S. L., Holden, G., Lynn, H., Mitchell, H., and Ewart, C. (2000). Cognitive-behavioral predictors of asthma morbidity in inner-city children. *Journal of Developmental and Behavioral Pediatrics, 21*(5), 340–346.

Watson, D. L., and Tharp, R. G. (1972). *Self-directed behavior: Self-modification for personal adjustment*. Pacific Grove, CA: Brooks/Cole.

Weisskopf-Joelson, E., and Eliseo, S. (1961). An experimental study of the effectiveness of brainstorming. *Journal of Applied Psychology, 45*, 45–49.

Wood, W., and Neal, D. T. (2007). A new look at habits and the habit-goal interface. *Psychological Review, 114*, 843–863.

Wood, W., Quinn, J. M., and Kashy, D. (2002). Habits in everyday life: Thought emotion, and action. *Journal of Personality and Social Psychology, 88*, 918–933.

Woodward, W. R. (1982). The "discovery" of social behaviorism and social learning theory: 1870–1980. *American Psychologist, 37*, 396–410.

14

THE THEORY OF GENDER AND POWER: CONSTRUCTS, VARIABLES, AND IMPLICATIONS FOR DEVELOPING HIV INTERVENTIONS FOR WOMEN

Gina M. Wingood
Christina Camp
Kristin Dunkle
Hannah Cooper
Ralph J. DiClemente

GENDER, POWER, AND HIV PREVENTION

Early in the epidemic, HIV infection and AIDS were diagnosed among relatively few women and female adolescents. Currently, women account for more than 25 percent of all new HIV/AIDS diagnoses in the United States. Of the 126,694 women living with HIV, ethnic minority women account for over 80 percent of these cases, with African American women accounting for 64 percent of the women. Among African American women diagnosed with HIV/AIDS during 2001 to 2004, 78 percent contracted the infection via heterosexual contact (Centers for Disease Control and Prevention [CDC] 2006; Rangel, Gavin, Reed, Fowler, and Lee, 2006; CDC, 2005). Unfortunately African American women are being devastated by the HIV/AIDS epidemic. Thus, designing effective HIV prevention programs for this population is crucial. Theoretical frameworks are critical components of HIV prevention programs because they serve as guides for developing the core elements, vignettes, and activities of HIV prevention interventions.

Many theories have been used to design HIV prevention interventions, including social cognitive theory, the AIDS risk-reduction model, and the information-motivation-behavior model. One theoretical framework underlying several proven evidence-based HIV prevention efforts for African American women is the theory of gender and power (Wingood and DiClemente, 2000). In the first edition of *Emerging Theories in Health Promotion Practice and Research*, we described the theory of gender and power. In this second edition, we have six aims: (1) to discuss conceptualizing gender as a social structure; (2) to provide a brief overview of the theory of gender and power; (3) to discuss a research study, known as *SHAWL (the Social Health of African American Women)*, that describes the gender-related **risk factors** and exposures in the theory of gender and power; (4) to demonstrate how the theory of gender and power has been applied to HIV prevention interventions for African American women; (5) to describe future directions for the theory of gender and power; and (6) to conclude by exploring the implications for health education, action, and research.

CONCEPTUALIZING GENDER

Prior to describing the theory of gender and power, we introduce and discuss the concept of gender. Historical explanation of theories of gender socialization have been widely criticized (Connell, 1987; Connell, 1985; Kimmel, 1995; Courtenay, 2000; Connell, 1995) as they have implied that gender represents "two fixed, static and mutually exclusive role containers" (Kimmel, 1995). As opposed to conceptualizing gender as two static categories, social scientists have more recently conceptualized gender as a set of socially constructed relationships that are produced and reproduced through people's actions (Gerson and Peiss, 1995). Specifically, more novel approaches to conceptualizing gender have proposed viewing gender as something that one does, and does recurrently in interaction with others (West and Zimmerman, 1987). It is achieved or demonstrated and is better understood as a verb than as a noun (Bohan, 1993; Crawford, 1995). Gender does not reside in the person but rather in the social transactions defined as gendered. From this perspective gender is viewed as a dynamic social structure (Connell, 1987).

More recently gender has become constructed from cultural and subjective meanings that constantly shift and vary, depending on the generation and place (Bayne-Smith, 1996). Women from different cultures, races, ages, classes, and from different historical periods have often constructed gender differently, so there may not be one expression of gender that is found everywhere. Thus the expression of gender may look different when comparing African American women to Latina women, for example. The meaning of gender among working-class women may differ from the meaning of gender among women in a lower-class life. Moreover, all of the social experiences that women and men engage in inform their beliefs and behaviors (Kimmel, 1995). The numerous social transactions that are a result of these experiences occur in diverse institutions, at different developmental stages, and within an array of contexts in which women and men encounter. Subsequently, these social transactions often elicit gendered health beliefs and health behaviors. This is the primary reason that theories of gender relations, such as the theory of gender and power, can be used to understand health behaviors among women and can be used to design interventions that are tailored to women to reduce unhealthy behaviors.

THE THEORY OF GENDER AND POWER

Overview of the Theory of Gender and Power

The theory of gender and power, developed by Robert Connell (Connell, 1987), asserts that power relationships between genders and within genders arise from the global dominance of men over women. The theory of gender and power is a social structural model that attempts to understand women's risk as a function of three different interlinked structures (none of which can be independent of the others) that characterize the gendered relationships between men and women. These *three inseparable structures* are: (1) the sexual **division of labor**, which examines economic inequities that favor men; (2) the sexual **division of power**, which examines inequities and abuses of authority and control in relationships and institutions that favor men; and (3) the **structure of cathexis**, which examines social norms and affective attachments. Thus, in labor relations, evident in the structure of labor, men's position can yield a series of advantages (for example, higher incomes, easier access to education); what Connell has referred to as "patriarchal dividend." In terms of power relations, evident in the structure of power, men control the means of institutionalized power, such as the media and families. Finally, in terms of social relations, evident in the structure of cathexis, men's position is often characterized by male superiority rather than reciprocity and intimacy. The three structures exist at two levels, the societal and the institutional level. The *societal level* is the highest level in which the three social structures are embedded. The three structures are rooted in society through numerous abstract, historical and sociopolitical forces that consistently segregate power and ascribe norms on the basis of gender-determined roles.

> The three structures are rooted in society through numerous abstract, historical, and sociopolitical forces that consistently segregate power and ascribe norms on the basis of gender-determined roles.

The three structures are also evident at a lower level, the ***institutional level***. Social institutions include, but are not limited to, families, relationships, religious institutions, the medical system and the media. The three main institutions that correspond to the three social structures of gender relations are the labor market, the state and the family, are examples of what Connell calls gender regimes. The social structures are maintained within institutions through social mechanisms such as unequal pay for comparable work, the imbalance of control within relationships, and the degrading images of women as portrayed in the media. The presence of these and other social mechanisms constrain women's daily life by producing gender-based inequities in women's economic potential, in their control of resources, and in gender-based expectations. The inequities resulting from social mechanisms which occur within each of these structures are manifested in the public health field as ***exposures*** and in the psychosocial domain as ***risk factors.*** The configuration of the three structures and how they become manifested as exposures and risk factors and then translated into **variables** is described below.

THE SEXUAL DIVISION OF LABOR

A fundamental structure in this theory is the sexual division of labor (Connell, 1987). At the *societal level* the sexual division of labor refers to the allocation of women and men to certain occupations. Often women are assigned different and unequal positions relative to men. Women are often delegated the responsibility of "women's work." This assignment constrains women because the nature and organization of "women's work" limits their economic potential and confines their career paths.

At the *institutional level* the sexual division of labor is most apparent in institutions such as the worksite, the family, and school systems. At the institutional level the sexual division of labor is maintained by social mechanisms such as the segregation of "unpaid nurturing work" for women, namely, child care, caring for the sick and elderly, and housework. Because this work is uncompensated, an economic imbalance occurs in which women often have to rely on men financially. Other social mechanisms occurring within the sexual division of labor include practices that favor male educational attainment, and the segregation of "income-generating work" for men, allowing men control of the family income. While women do participate in the paid labor force, their participation is often less than that of males and remains highly sex-segregated. Further, while "men's work" is often valued either directly through paid remuneration or indirectly through its high status, "women's work" often fails to be recognized as work and is valued at a lower status.

The structure of labor is maintained within institutions through social mechanisms. The presence of these social mechanisms constrains women's daily life by producing gender-based inequities in women's economic potential. The inequities resulting from social mechanisms that occur within the sexual division of labor are manifested in the public health field as *economic exposures* and in the psychosocial domain as socioeconomic risk factors (Figure 14.1).

FIGURE 14.1 *Theory of Gender and Power on Women's Health*

The Societal Level	The Institutional Level	The Social Mechanisms	Exposures	Risk Factors	Biological Factors	Disease
Sexual Division of Labor	Worksite School Family	Manifested as unequal pay produces economic inequities for women.	Economic Exposures	Socio-economic Risk Factors		
Sexual Division of Power	Relationships Medical System	Manifested as imbalances in control power for women.	Physical Exposures	Behavioral Risk Factors	Pregnancy Contraception	HIV
Structure of Cathexis: Social Norms and Affective Attachments	Relationships Family Church	Manifested as constraints in expectations produces disparities in norms for women.	Social Exposures	Personal Risk Factors		

According to the sexual division of labor, as the economic inequity between men and women increases and favors men, women will be more likely to experience adverse health outcomes. Therefore, the theory posits that women having more adverse economic exposures and socioeconomic risk factors will be more burdened by the sexual division of labor, compared to women not having these exposures and risk factors, and subsequently will experience poorer health outcomes. Thus, as the economic inequity between men and women increases and favors men (making women more dependent on men) women will be at greater risk for HIV. Table 14.1 illustrates the economic exposures and socioeconomic risk factors associated with the structure of labor.

THE SEXUAL DIVISION OF POWER

Another fundamental structure in this theory is the sexual division of power (Connell, 1987). At the *societal level* inequalities in power between the sexes form the basis for the sexual division of power. Power has been conceptualized differently by several different disciplines (Wingood and DiClemente, 2000). Gender is negotiated in part through relationships of power. Microlevel power practices contribute to the social transactions of everyday life. These transactions help to sustain and reproduce broader structures of power and inequality. These power relationships are located and constituted in the practice of health behavior. The systematic subordination of women, or patriarchy, is partially made possible through these gendered demonstrations of beliefs and behaviors. It is men's use of their beliefs and behaviors to demonstrate dominant and hegemonic masculine ideals that clearly establish them as men. Hegemonic masculinity is the form of masculinity which is culturally dominant in a given setting (Connell, 1995). This hegemonic masculinity is the expression of the privilege men collectively have over women. It is this socially dominant gender construct that subordinates femininities, that reflects and shapes men's social relationships with women, and that represents power and authority.

The social psychological literature defines power as having the capacity to influence the action of others, conceptualizing power in terms of power over others (Wingood and DiClemente, 2000). This ability resides primarily at the interpersonal level and occasionally at the institutional level. The empowerment literature defines power as having the ability to act or to change in a desired direction (Wingood and DiClemente, 2000). This ability can reside at the, interpersonal, institutional individual, and/or community level. Thus, power can be defined as having the *power to act or change* or having *power over* others. Further, the sources of power can be interpersonal *or* they can be distributed, such that access to power can be shared (Wingood and DiClemente, 2000).

Gender and gender relations associated with the structure of power are often defined and sustained within institutions, such as social and sexual relationships, the medical system and the media. Thus, at the *institutional level* the sexual division of power is maintained by social mechanisms such as the abuse of authority and control in relationships. Women in power-imbalanced relationships tend to depend on their male partner because men usually bring more financial assets (that is, money, status) to the

TABLE 14.1   The Theory of Gender and Power: Exposures and Risk Factors.

The Sexual Division of Labor:	
Economic Exposures	**Socioeconomic Risk Factors**
Women who:	Women who:
• live at the poverty level • have less than a high school education • have no employment or who are underemployed • have a high demand/low control work environment • have limited or no health insurance • have no permanent home (are homeless)	• are ethnic minorities • are younger (under eighteen years of age)

The Sexual Division of Power:	
Physical Exposures	**Behavioral Risk Factors**
Women who have:	Women who have:
• a history of sexual or physical abuse • a partner who disapproves of practicing safer sex • a high-risk steady partner • a greater exposure to sexually explicit media • limited access to HIV prevention (such as drug treatment, female controlled methods, school-based HIV prevention education)	• a history of alcohol and drug abuse • poor assertive communication skills • poor condom use skills • lower self-efficacy to avoid HIV • limited perceived control over condom use

The Structure of Social Norms and Affective Attachments:	
Social Exposures	**Personal Risk Factors**
Women who have:	Women who have:
• a partner who is older • desire to conceive or whose partner desires to conceive • conservative cultural and gender norms • a religious affiliation that forbids the use of contraception • a strong mistrust of the medical system • family influences not supportive of HIV prevention	• limited knowledge of HIV prevention • negative beliefs not supportive of safer sex • perceived invulnerability to HIV/AIDS • a history of depression/psychological distress

relationship. At the institutional level, the sexual division of power is also maintained by social mechanisms such as the disempowering of women by the media, as observable in the sexual degradation of women in the media, to a much greater degree than men. Moreover, at the institutional level the sexual division of power may be maintained by social mechanisms, such as the stigma experienced by women (compared to men).

The structure of power is maintained within institutions through social mechanisms. The presence of these social mechanisms constrains women's daily life by producing gender-based inequities in women's control of resources. The inequities resulting from social mechanisms that occur within the sexual division of power are manifested in the field of public health as *physical exposures* and are manifest in the psychosocial domain as *behavioral risk factors* (Figure 14.1). According to the sexual division of power, as the power inequity between men and women increases and favors men, women will be more likely to experience adverse health outcomes. Therefore, the theory posits that women having more adverse physical exposures and behavioral risk factors will be more burdened by the sexual division of power, compared to women not having these exposures and risk factors, and subsequently will experience poorer health outcomes. Thus, as the power inequity between men and women increases and favors men, women's sexual choices and behavior may be constrained, thereby enhancing their risk for HIV acquisition.

> As the power inequity between men and women increases and favors men, women's sexual choices and behavior may be constrained, thereby enhancing their risk for HIV acquisition.

Table 14.1 illustrates the physical exposures and behavioral risk factors associated with the structure of power.

THE STRUCTURE OF CATHEXIS

The newest structure in this theory is the structure of cathexis (Connell, 1987). To emphasize the affective and stereotypical components of this structure, it is herein referred to as the *structure of affective attachments and social norms*. At the *societal level* this structure dictates appropriate, normative, or stereotypical sexual behavior for women and is characterized by the emotional and sexual attachments that women have with men. This structure constrains the expectations that society has about women with regard to their sexuality and, as a consequence, this structure shapes our perceptions of ourselves and others, and limits our experiences of reality. This structure also describes how women's sexuality is attached to other social concerns, such as those related to impurity and immorality.

Gender stereotypes (for example, having sex prior to marriage is unacceptable for women but acceptable and almost expected for men) are among the meanings used by society in the construction of gender, and are characteristics that are generally believed to be typical either of women or of men. These stereotypes provide collective, organized, and dichotomous meanings of gender and often become widely shared beliefs about innate qualities of men and women. Women and men are encouraged to conform to stereotypical beliefs and behaviors, and commonly do conform to and adopt dominant norms of femininity and masculinity (Bohan, 1993).

At the *institutional level* the structure of affective attachments and social norms is most apparent in institutions such as the social and sexual relationships, the family and faith-based institutions. At the institutional level the structure of social norms and affective attachments is maintained by social mechanisms such as biases people have regarding how women and men should express their sexuality. These biases produce cultural norms, the enforcement of strict gender roles, and stereotypical beliefs such as believing that women should have sex only for procreation, creating taboos regarding female sexuality (that is, being labeled as a "bad girl" for having premarital sex), restraining women's sexuality (that is, being monogamous as opposed to having multiple partners is an accepted norm for men but not women) (Krieger, 1990), and believing that women should refrain from touching their own bodies.

The presence of these and other social mechanisms constrain women's daily life by producing gender-based inequities in gender-based expectations. The inequities resulting from the social mechanisms occurring within the structure of social norms and affective attachments are manifested within the field of public health as *social exposures* and are manifested in the psychosocial domain as *personal risk factors* (Figure 14.1). According to the structure of social norms and affective attachments, women who are more accepting of conventional social norms and beliefs will be more likely to experience adverse health outcomes. Therefore, the theory posits that women who have more social exposures and more personal risk factors will be more burdened by the structure of social norms and affective attachments, compared to women not having these exposures and risk factors, and subsequently will experience poorer health outcomes. Thus, women who are more accepting of conventional social norms and beliefs will be at greater risk of HIV. Table 14.1 illustrates the physical exposures and behavioral risk factors associated with the structure of affective attachments and social norms.

EACH STRUCTURE IS COMPOSED OF EXPOSURES AND RISK FACTORS

The gender-based inequities and disparities in expectations that arise from each of the three structures (sexual division of labor, sexual division of power, structure of affective attachments and social norms) generate different risk factors and exposures that influence women's risk for HIV. Although the term "risk factor" is traditionally used to denote *any influence* that enhances risk for HIV, the theory of gender and power reserves this term specifically to denote intrapersonal variables that emanate from within women and influence their risk for HIV. In the theory of gender and power, exposures are defined as variables that are external to women that may influence their sexual risk behavior. To illustrate the current gender-related risk factors and exposures in the theory of gender and power that are associated with HIV risk taking among women we will describe a national survey known as **SHAWL**.

The gender-based inequities and disparities in expectations that arise from each of the three structures (sexual division of labor, sexual division of power, structure of affective attachments and social norms) generate different risk factors and exposures that influence women's risk for HIV.

The *SHAWL* Study

To facilitate our understanding how gender-related risk factors and exposures associated with the theory of gender and power influence women's risk of HIV, the lead author and her study colleagues conducted a nationally representative random-digit dial telephone household survey of 1,509 women between October 2006 and May 2007. Potential participants who self-reported being female, African American or white, ages 20–45, and unmarried or not currently in any relationship equivalent to marriage were eligible for inclusion. Sampling employed a dual-frame design, incorporating two selection stages without stratification in each frame. The larger frame was designed to provide coverage of the eligible population (both white and African American) on a national basis, defined as all counties with an eligible household incidence of 10 percent or greater; this frame included 1,096 of 3,140 counties. The second frame targeted areas containing a high density of African American women and was restricted to counties with a household incidence of African American women of 7 percent or greater. Because the aim of the study was to assess variables known to increase exposure to HIV risk among women, the primary study outcome was, unprotected sexual intercourse, defined as the number of times they had vaginal sex with a steady partner in the past three months and the number of times they used condoms during vaginal sex with a steady partner in the past three months. A second study outcome, having multiple sexual partners, was defined as the number of different male sexual partners (men other than the women's steady partner) women have had in the past six months. However, in addition to these outcome variables a range of critical risk factor and exposure variables related to the theory of gender and power were assessed.

Moving from Gender-Related Risk Factors and Exposures to Creating Variables

Translating the risk factors and exposures into variables represents a significant and exciting phase in the development of the emergence of the theory of gender and power as it relates to understanding women's risk of HIV. Variables are the measurable or objective forms of risk factors and exposures. Variables indicate how the risk factors and exposures should be measured. As part of the SHAWL study, variables were created to match with the risk factors and exposures articulated within the theory of gender and power. Future phases of the SHAWL study will allow greater ascertainment of which variables and which structures are most predictive of HIV risk behavior in women. The creation of variables is a critical step as HIV interventions, guided by the theory of gender and power, may now administer these measures when attempting to evaluate intervention efforts. Subsequently, in an attempt to design more efficacious HIV interventions tailored to women, HIV interventions using the theory of gender and power can intervene on the variables most predictive of HIV risk.

Within the division of labor variables selected that correspond with the economic exposures are income, employment status, education, health insurance status, and number of dependents. Variables that correspond to the socioeconomic risk factors include the participant and her partner's age and ethnicity as well as a measure of economic hardship. Within the division of power variables selected that correspond with the physical exposures are sexual and physical abuse, community violence, racial and gender discrimination, an assessment of relationship status, and a measure assessing the influence of economic pressure on sexual decision making. Variables that correspond to the behavioral risk factors include drug use, binge drinking, coping with racial and gender discrimination, sexual communication self-efficacy, and perceived ability of the male partner to provide protection from community violence. Within the structure of cathexis variables selected that correspond with the social exposures are sexual stigmas, the age discrepancy between sexual partners and the participant and her partner's desire to conceive. Variables that correspond to the personal risk factors include depression, perceived gender norms, perceived availability of partners, and perceived influence of spirituality on sexual practices. The variables associated with each structure, and an example of an item describing each variable are depicted in Table 14.2. Values for Cronbach's alpha, a measure of inter-item reliability, are presented for variables assessed by scales.

APPLICATION EXAMPLES

To illustrate how the theory of gender and power has been applied to design HIV prevention intervention for women, we present three CDC-defined evidence-based HIV interventions developed for women. These three HIV interventions have been referred to as a "suite" of HIV interventions for women. All three of these interventions were designed to focus on reducing HIV sexual risk behaviors for different subpopulations of African American women. Additionally, all three of these interventions used the theory of gender and power to assist in guiding the intervention content. However, the theory of gender and power was applied differentially for each of the three subgroups of African American women targeted (Wingood and DiClemente, 2006, Table 3).

Moreover, the theoretically derived HIV intervention activities were tailored differentially for each of the three target populations (Table 14.4). We describe each of the three CDC-defined evidence-based HIV interventions below.

THE SISTA INTERVENTION FOR YOUNG ADULT WOMEN

In the 1990's the epidemiology of the HIV epidemic identified young adult African-American women's enhanced vulnerability. In response to these findings, SiSTA (*Sistas' Informing Sistas about Topics on AIDS*), an HIV prevention intervention for young adult African American females, was designed, implemented, evaluated, and was subsequently published in 1995 (DiClemente and Wingood, 1995). The aim of SiSTA was to reduce the risk of HIV among young adult African American women residing in an urban community in California. Relative to a comparison condition, participants randomized to the intervention demonstrated an increase in consistent condom use, greater sexual self-control, greater sexual assertiveness, and reported an increase in partner norms supportive of safer sex over a three-month follow-up period.

TABLE 14.2 Variables Assessed as Part of the SHAWL study.

Variable	Example of a Response	Alpha
I. Division of Labor		
Economic Exposures		
Income (n = 10 responses)	Is your annual household income from all sources . . . (1) Less than $10,000?	
Employment status (n = 9 responses)	Are you currently . . . (1) Employed full-time?	
Education (n = 13 responses)	Is the highest level of education you have completed . . . (1) Grade school (from years 1–4)?	
Health insurance status (n = 3 responses)	Do you have any kind of health care coverage, including health insurance, prepaid plans such as HMOs, or government plans such as Medicare? (1) Yes	
Dependents (n = 3 responses)	Other than yourself, how many people depend on you for financial support? (1) Number of people	
Socioeconomic Risk Factors		
Participant race (n = 8 responses)	Which one or more of the following would you say is your race or ethnicity . . .? (1) Black or African American	
Participant age (n = 3)	In what year were you born?	
Economic hardship[25] (n = 3 responses)	In the past twelve months, was there a time when you didn't meet basic expenses such as food, clothing, or shelter? (1) Yes	
Male sexual partner economic status[3] (n = 7 responses)	Please think about your most recent partner's income at the end of your relationship. How would you say it compared to your income at the end of the relationship? Was it . . . (1) About the same?	
II. Division of Power		
Physical Exposures		
Relationship status[27] (n = 6 responses)	How would you describe your relationship with this person . . .? (1) Dating	

(Continued)

TABLE 14.2 *(Continued)*

History of sexual abuse[28] (n = 7 items)	In any of your relationships with a main partner or someone you were dating, did the person you were involved with ever force you to have sexual activities against your will? (1) Yes
History of physical abuse[28] (n = 22 items)	In any of your relationships with a main partner or someone you were dating, did the person you were involved with ever hit, slap, kick, or otherwise physically hurt you? (1) Yes
Community violence[29] (n = 6 items)	In the past year, in your neighborhood, how many times have you been . . .? (1) A victim of a robbery or mugging?
Gender discrimination (n = 6 items)[25,26]	In your lifetime, how often have you experienced gender discrimination . . .? Please say Never, Once, More Than Once, or Not Applicable. (1) At work
Racial discrimination (n = 9 items)[25,26]	In your lifetime, how often have you experienced racial discrimination . . .? Please say Never, Once, More Than Once, or Not Applicable. (1) From the police or in the courts
Economic pressure and sexual decision making (n=11 items)	I have stayed with a main partner longer than I wanted to because I was worried about . . .? (1) Having a place to live or paying for groceries, utilities, or other bills
High risk sexual partner (n = 6 items)[30]	Do you think your main partner . . .? (1) Has ever spent more than twenty-four hours in jail, prison, or a detention center

Behavioral Risk Factors

Binge drinking[31] (n = 1 item)	Over the past two weeks, on how many occasions have you had Four or more drinks in a row in a two-hour period?
Drug use[32] (n = 2 items)	In the past year, have you used any nonprescription drug that you inject?
Gender discrimination coping (n = 4 items)[25,26]	When you experienced gender discrimination how often did you . . .? Please say Never, Sometimes, Often, or Very Often. (1) Talk to other people about it

TABLE 14.2 *(Continued)*

Racial discrimination coping (n = 4 items)[25,26]	When you experienced racial discrimination how often did you . . .? Please say Never, Sometimes, Often or Very Often (1) Keep it to yourself	
Condom negotiation efficacy (n = 3 items)[33]	I can insist on condom use even if my partner does not want to use one. (1) Strongly Agree	0.67
Perceived ability of male partner to provide protection (n = 3 items)	How important to you is it that your main partner . . .? (1) Makes you feel safe from crime in your neighborhood	0.83

III. Structure of Cathexis

Social Exposures

Sexual stigma[3]	Is it not embarrassing, somewhat embarrassing or very embarrassing to . . .? (1) Ask your partner to use a condom	
Women's desire to conceive	On a scale of 1 to 5 where 1 is not at all and 5 is very much, how much . . .? (1) Do you want to be pregnant at this time?	
Male partner's desire to conceive	On a scale of 1 to 5 where 1 is not at all and 5 is very much how much . . .? (1) Do you think your current partner wants you to be pregnant at this time	
Sex partner age difference	Computed from the respective reported ages	

Personal Risk Factors

Distress[34] (n = 4 items)	How many days in the past week have you . . .? (1) Felt depressed	0.82
Perceived gender norms	Have you relied on your partner to . . .? (1) Teach you about sex	0.62
Perceived male sexual partner availability (n = 3 items)	There are enough suitable potential partners available for me to . . .? (1) Marry	
Perceived influence of spirituality on sex[3] (n = 3 items)	Please answer no effect, or make you more likely or less likely to . . .? (1) Say no to having sex with a partner who doesn't want to use a condom	0.78

TABLE 14.3 Applying the Theory of Gender and Power to Examine Gendered Exposures and Risk Factors for Different Subpopulations of African American Women.

SIHLE	SiSTA	WiLLOW
Division Labor (Women who have:)		
• Economically depended on males	• Older male partners	• Limited practical support
Power (Women who have:)		
• A power-imbalanced relationship • Limited availability of partners	• Violent dating partner(s) • Been stereotyped by the media	• Violent domestic partner(s) • Been stigmatized as an HIV vector
Cathexis (Women who have:)		
• Been discriminated against by society • Long-term relationships • A desire for pregnancy • Limited assertiveness skills	• Been discriminated against as teens • Engaged in serial monogamy • Experienced peer pressure • Limited assertiveness skills	• Been discriminated against because of serostatus • Limited emotional support • Limited appraisal support[1] • Limited assertiveness skills

In the SiSTA HIV intervention, the theory of gender and power was applied to enhance its relevance for young adult African American women (Table 14.3). Applying this gender-relevant theoretical framework was critical in acknowledging and addressing the underlying social factors, prevalent in the lives of African American women such as; being economically dependent on males, being in power-imbalanced relationships, perceiving limited partner availability, perceiving society as having a limited regard for African American women, having long-term relationships, desiring pregnancy, and communicating nonassertively about safer sex (Wingood and DiClemente, 2006, Table 3). Through a systematic process of theory mapping (linking programmatic activities to theoretical constructs), intervention activities were designed to address these social realities prevalent among young African American women (Table 14.4). Additionally, the thematic focus of the intervention, *"SiSTA love is strong, SiSTA love is safe, SiSTA love is surviving,"* was designed to promote a sense of a shared challenges and gender and ethnic pride among participants, and may have inspired them to modify

TABLE 14.4 Application of the Theory of Gender and Power to Design HIV Intervention Content for Women.

	SiSTA (5-session intervention)	SIHLE (4-session intervention)	WiLLOW (4-session intervention)
Session Content			
1	• Praise strengths of AA women • Identify AA female role models	• Praise strengths of AA teens • Identify AA teen role models	• Praise strengths of HIV+ women • Identify women's social networks
2	• Explore HIV vulnerabilities: (long-term relationships, desire to be pregnant, financial situation)	• Enhance coping with emotions that interfere with safer sex	• Define practical, emotional, informational and appraisal support • Identify sources of support
3	• Define and model assertive communication	• Explore HIV vulnerabilities: (serial monogamy, peer pressure, stereotypical media messages) • Define and model assertive communication	• Explore HIV vulnerabilities: (stigmatizing media messages) • Define and model assertive communication • Enhance coping with emotions that interfere with safer sex
4	• Enhance coping with emotions that interfere with safer sex	• Define dating violence and implications for safer sex • Discuss challenges of dating older males • describe and characterize "healthy relationships" • identify community resources for participants in unhealthy relationships	• Define domestic violence and implications for safer sex
5	• Discuss and define power imbalanced relationships • Discuss partner selection	• N/A	• N/A

risk behaviors for altruistic motives; by enhancing their health they were also enhancing the health, destiny, and quality of life for other African American women in their community. The CDC has defined SiSTA as an evidence-based HIV intervention and has cited this publication in their *Compendium of HIV Prevention Interventions with Evidence of Effectiveness* (CDC, 1999).

THE SIHLE INTERVENTION FOR AFRICAN AMERICAN FEMALE ADOLESCENTS

The Sistas, Informing, Healing, Living and Empowering (SIHLE) intervention is an HIV prevention intervention for African American female adolescents with established efficacy (DiClemente, Wingood, and Harrington, 2004). The aim of SIHLE was to reduce the risk of HIV among sexually active African American adolescent females residing in nonurban communities in the South. Relative to a placebo-attention comparison condition, participants in the SIHLE intervention were more likely to use condoms consistently, to use condoms at last sexual intercourse, had better condom application skills, communicated with their sexual partners more frequently, reported a higher percentage of condom-protected sex acts, had higher scores on mediators of safer sex, and were less likely to have a new partner. Positive effects were also observed for reductions in incident chlamydia infections and self-reported pregnancy.

In the SIHLE HIV intervention, the theory of gender and power was applied to enhance its relevance for African American female adolescents (Table 14.3). The application of the theory of gender and power in SIHLE highlights HIV-related social processes prevalent in the lives of African American female adolescents, such as having older male sex partners, having abusive dating partners, being stereotyped by the media, perceiving society as having a limited regard for African American teens, engaging in serial monogamy, experiencing peer pressure to engage in risky sex and communicating nonassertive about safer sex (Wingood and DiClemente, 2006). By using theory mapping, intervention activities associated with constructs articulated in the theory of gender and power were designed to address the social realities that are more prevalent among African American female adolescents (Table 14.4). Additionally, the thematic focus of the intervention, *"Stay Safe for Yourself, Your Family, and Your Community"* was designed to promote a sense of solidarity and ethnic pride among participants, and may have inspired them to modify risk behaviors for altruistic motives; by enhancing their health they were also enhancing the health of their family and the broader African American community. The CDC has defined SIHLE as an evidence-based HIV intervention and has cited this publication in their publication on best-evidence HIV Interventions (Lyles et al. 2007).

THE WILLOW EVIDENCE-BASED HIV INTERVENTION FOR WOMEN LIVING WITH HIV

WiLLOW (*Women Involved in Life Learning from Other Women*) was designed as an HIV transmission risk-reduction program for women living with HIV in urban, nonurban and rural communities in the South (Wingood et al., 2004). The vast majority (85 percent) of the participants in WiLLOW were African American, the remaining women were Caucasian (8 percent), Hispanic (5 percent), Native American (1 percent) and Asian (1 percent). Relative to a placebo-attention comparison condition, participants in the WiLLOW intervention were less likely to have unprotected vaginal sex, were less likely to acquire an incident bacterial infection, reported greater HIV knowledge, reported having more supportive members in their social networks, had fewer partner-related barrier to condom use, and demonstrated greater skill in using condoms.

In the WiLLOW intervention, the theory of gender and power emphasized the limited social networks among women living with HIV, how societal expectations of women's role as caregivers constrains their ability to seek new social network members or ask existing network members for support (Table 14.3) (Wingood and DiClemente, 2006). Furthermore, the intervention addressed how women living with HIV may be less likely to seek support due to the fear of being stigmatized as either promiscuous or as transmitters of HIV. Applying the theory of gender and power in WiLLOW highlighted social conditions prevalent in the lives of women living with HIV, such as having limited practical support (that is, money for food, child care), having violent domestic partners, being stigmatized as an HIV transmitter, receiving limited emotional and appraisal support (provision of information that is useful for self-evaluation, such as positive feedback and affirmations) from family members and non-family members, AIDS social service organizations, and communicating nonassertively about safer sex (Wingood and DiClemente, 2006) (Table 14.3). Thus, the intervention activities associated with the theory of gender and power were designed to address the social conditions prevalent in the lives of HIV positive women (Table 14.4). Additionally, the thematic focus of the intervention, "*Women Involved in Life Learning from Other Women*," was designed to promote a sense of solidarity among women living with HIV, and may have encouraged them to modify risk behaviors by seeking support from nonjudgmental social network members or by expanding their social network to include additional supportive member such as other WiLLOW participants. The CDC has defined WiLLOW as an evidence-based HIV intervention, and has cited this publication in their publication on best-evidence HIV Interventions (Lyles et al., 2007).

While these three HIV prevention interventions briefly describe how the theory of gender and power has been applied to guide the design of HIV prevention interventions nationally. The study author has also applied the theory to guide the design of HIV prevention interventions in the Caribbean, St. Maarten; Armenia; and in Cape Town, South Africa.

FUTURE DIRECTIONS

A refinement that is being made to the theory of gender and power is the inclusion of macrosocial factors. Macrosocial factors may be defined as dimensions of "the social, economic, and political environments that shape and constrain individual, community, and societal health outcomes" (Raphael et al., 2006). These factors have also been referred to as "structural determinants of health" and "contextual factors." In the theory of gender and power, macrosocial factors are conceptualized as a domain of exposures. Consonant with exposures within this theory, macrosocial exposures arise from the sexual division of labor, the sexual division of power, and cathexis. We bring this domain of exposures into focus here because macrosocial factors are widely posited to be potent determinants of racial/ethnic disparities in sexually-transmitted HIV (Aral, Adimora, and Fenton, 2008; Adimora, Schoenbach, and Doherty, 2006; Thomas, 1999).

To date, however, empirical investigations lag behind these propositions.

Plans to elaborate exposures within the theory of gender and power could include intensifying efforts to explore the role of select macrosocial processes, arising from the sexual division of labor, the division of power, and the structure of cathexis in shaping African American girls and women's risk of HIV. Macrosocial factors arising from the division of labor could include: local rates of poverty, wealth, high school graduation, and income inequality.

Macrosocial processes that arise from and capture the sexual division of power, such as, local male-to-female sex ratios among African Americans, and local rates of violence against women (both sexual and domestic), and local rates of racially-motivated hate crimes. Finally, macrosocial factors that arise from and capture social norms and affective attachments, may include local marriage rates and rates of religious congregation membership among African American adults.

Macrosocial factors arising from the division of labor could include: local rates of poverty, wealth, high school graduation, and income inequality.

IMPLICATIONS FOR HEALTH EDUCATION RESEARCH AND ACTION

There are several tasks required for health educators interested in utilizing the theory of gender and power to assess women's HIV-related exposures and risk factors and to design appropriate HIV interventions. Health educators should: (1) specify the goals and objectives of the HIV risk-reduction program (that is, reduce STDs, increase condom use); (2) define the community of at-risk women (that is, teens, Hispanic women, pregnant women); (3) develop an assessment tool, based on the theory of gender and power, to identify women's exposures and risk factors for HIV, using the variables and scales specified in the text (summarized in Table 14.1) and cited in the references; (4) administer the assessment tool using well-trained women; (5) analyze the assessment tool to determine the most prevalent exposures and risk factors for HIV among the community; (6) share the results of the assessment with the community; (7) use the results of the assessment tool and engage the community in a dialogue to determine which structure(s) to target for intervention; (8) delineate the strategies for intervening with the community (examples of interventions are provided in the text); (9) determine the intervention channel(s) (such as schools, media, church); (9) develop linkages with the channel(s); (10) devise a plan to promote dissemination, implementation and maintenance of the program and; (11) reevaluate women using the same assessment tool (as in Step Four) to assess changes in HIV-related exposures and risk factors.

Applying the theory of gender and power to understand the influence of women's health can be challenging. Social structures are often abstract, difficult to operationalize and do not take into account variations across different cultures. Moreover, when applying the theory of gender and power it can be difficult to isolate and tedious to quantify the effect and impact of a particular social structure on women's health. Further, the social structures are so deeply rooted in our culture, and so routinely taken for granted, that they often go unnoticed. In some ways these very situations make it difficult to empirically test this model. This is the primary reason why it is difficult to construct a cogent empirical case that patriarchy is damaging to women's health. However, utilizing the theory of gender and power to understand women's health specifies a range of gender-based exposures and risk factors for examining women's risk of disease. Employing the theory of gender and power marshals new kinds of data, asks new and broader questions regarding women's health, and creates new options for prevention. Focusing on the social construction of health encourages designing, implementing, and evaluating larger social interventions. Women's social risk for disease can be addressed through a variety of public health strategies, from education to policy. Interventions for women are destined to be less than optimally effective if they ignore the social environment. Similarly, strategies that lack practical programs for social change seem equally shortsighted and, in the long run, futile. Social structural theories such as theory of gender and power can help to chart a course between the two extremes (Wingood and DiClemente, 2000).

SUMMARY

In the first edition of *Emerging Theories in Health Promotion Practice and Research*, we described the theory of gender and power. In this second edition, we have six aims: (1) to discuss conceptualizing gender as a social structure; (2) to provide a brief overview of the theory of gender and power; (3) to discuss a research study, known as *SHAWL (the Social Health of African-American Women)* that describes the gender-related risk factors and exposures in the theory of gender and power; (4) to demonstrate how the theory of gender and power has been applied to HIV prevention interventions for African American women; (5) to describe future directions for the theory of gender and power; and (6) to conclude by exploring the implications for health education, action and research.

REFERENCES

Adimora, A. A., Schoenbach, V. J., and Doherty, I. A. (2006). HIV and African Americans in the southern United States: sexual networks and social context. *Sexually Transmitted Diseases, 33*(7 Suppl), S39–45.

Aral, S. O., Adimora, A. A., Fenton, K. A. (2008). Understanding and responding to disparities in HIV and other sexually transmitted infections in African Americans. *Lancet, 372*(9635), 337–40.

Bayne-Smith, M. (1996). *Race, gender and health*. Thousand Oaks, CA: Sage.

Bohan, J. S. (1993). Regarding gender: Essentialism, constructionism and feminist psychology. *Psychology of Women Quarterly, 17*, 5–21.

Centers for Disease Control and Prevention (CDC). (2002). *Behavioral risk factor surveillance system survey questionnaire*. Atlanta, GA: U.S. Department of Health and Human Services, Centers for Disease Control and Prevention.

Centers for Disease Control and Prevention. (2005). *HIV/AIDS surveillance report, 2004*. Atlanta, GA: U.S. Department of Health and Human Services, *Centers for Disease Control and Prevention, 16*, 1–46.

Centers for Disease Control and Prevention. (2006). Twenty-five years of HIV/AIDS—United States, 1981–2006. *Morbidity and Mortality Weekly Report, 55*(21), 585–589.

Connell, R. W. (1985). Theorizing gender. *Sociology, 19*, 262–264.

Connell, R. W. (1987). *Gender and power*. Stanford, CA: Stanford University Press.

Connell, R. W. (1995). *Masculinities*. Berkeley: University of California Press.

Courtenay, W. H. (2000). Constructions of masculinity and their influence on men's well-being: A theory of gender and health. *Social Science and Medicine, 50*, 1385–1401.

Cranford, J. A., McCabe, S. E., and Boyd, C. J. (2006). A new measure of binge drinking: Prevalence and correlates in a probability sample of undergraduates. *Alcoholism: Clinical and Experimental Research, 30*(11), 1896–1905.

Crawford, M. (1995). Talking Difference: *On gender and language*. Thousand Oaks, CA: Sage.

DiClemente, R. J., and Wingood, G. M. (1995). A randomized controlled trial of an HIV sexual risk-reduction intervention for young African-American women. *Journal of the American Medical Association, 274*, 1271–1276.

DiClemente, R. J., Wingood, G. M., and Harrington, K. F. (2004). Efficacy of an HIV prevention intervention for African American adolescent girls: A randomized controlled trial. *Journal of the American Medical Association, 292*, 171–179.

Gerson, J. S., and Peiss, K. (1995). Boundaries, negotiation, consciousness: Reconceputalising gender relations. *Social Problems, 32*(4), 317–331.

HIV/AIDS Prevention Research Synthesis Project. (1999). *Compendium of HIV prevention interventions with evidence of effectiveness*. Revised ed. Atlanta GA: Centers for Disease Control and Prevention.

Jackson, J. S., Torres, M., Caldwell, C. H., Neighbors, H. W., Nesse, R., Taylor, R. J., Trierweiler, S. J., and Williams, D. R. (2004). The National Survey of American Life: A study of racial, ethnic and cultural influences on mental disorders and mental health. *IJMPR, 13*(4), 196–207.

Kimmel, M. S. (1995). *Manhood in America: A Cultural history*. New York: Free press.

Krieger, N. (1990). Racial and gender discrimination: Risk factor for high blood pressure? *Social Science Medicine, 30*(12), 1272–1281.

Lyles, C., Kay, L. S., Crepaz, N., Herbst, J. H., Passin, W. F., Kim, A. S., Rama, S. M., Thadiparthi, S., DeLuca, J. B., and Mullins, M. M. (2007). Best-evidence interventions: Findings from systematic review of HIV behavioral interventions for US populations at high risk, 2000-2004. *American Journal of Public Health, 97*(1), 133–143.

Marin, B. V., Gomez, C. A., Tschann, J. M., and Gregorich, S. E. (1997). Condom use in unmarried Latino men: A test of cultural constructs. *Health Psychology, 15*(5), 458–467.

McFarland, J., Parker, B., Soeken, S., and Bullock, L. (1992). Assessing for abuse during pregnancy: Severity and frequency of injuries and associated entry into prenatal care. *Journal of the American Medical Association, 267*, 3176–3178.

Melchior, L. A., Huba, G. J., Brown, V. B., and Reback, C. J. (1993). A short depression index for women. *Educational and psychological measurement, 53*, 1117–1125.

Rangel, M. C., Gavin, L., Reed, C., Fowler, M. G., and Lee, L. M. (2006). Epidemiology of HIVand AIDS among adolescents and young adults in the United States. *Journal of Adolescent Health, 39*, 156–163.

Raphael, D. (2006). Social determinants of health: Present status, unanswered questions, and future directions. *International Journal of Health Services, 36*(4), 651–677.

Rusbult, C. E, Martz, J. M., and Agnew, C. (1998). The investment model scale: Measuring commitment level, satisfaction level, quality of alternatives, and investment size. *Personal Relationships, 5*, 357–391.

Sikkema, K. J., Kelly, J. A., Winett, R. A., Solomon, L. J., Cargill, V. A., Roffman, R. A., McAuliffe, T. L., et al., (2000). Outcomes of a randomized community-level HIV prevention intervention for women living in 18 low-income housing developments. *American Journal of Public Health, 90*(1), 57–63.

Thomas, J. C., and Thomas, K. K. (1999). Things ain't what they ought to be: Social forces underlying racial disparities in rates of sexually transmitted diseases in a rural Northern Carolina county. *Social Sciences and Medicine, 49*(8), 1075–1084.

Thomson, C. C., Roberts, K., Curran, A., Ryan, L., and Wright, R.J. (2002). Caretaker-child concordance for child's exposure to violence in a preadolescent inner-city population. *Archives of Pediatrics and Adolescent Medicine, 156*, 818–823.

West, C. and Zimmerman, D. H. (1987). Doing gender. *Gender and Society, 1*(2), 125–151.

Wingood, G. M. and DiClemente, R. J. (2000). Applying a theoretical framework of gender and power to understand the exposures and risk factors for HIV among women. *Health Education and Behavior, 27*, 539–565.

Wingood, G. M., and DiClemente, R. J. (2006). Enhancing diffusion of HIV interventions: Development of a suite of effective HIV prevention programs for women. *AIDS Education and Prevention, 18*, 161–170.

Wingood, G. M., DiClemente, R. J., Mikhail, I., Lang, D., Hubbard, McCree, D., Davies, S. L., Hardin, J. W., Hook, E. W., and Saag, M. (2004). A randomized controlled trial to reduce HIV transmission risk behaviors and STDs among women living with HIV: The WiLLOW Program. *Journal of Acquired Immune Deficiency Syndromes, 37*, S58–S67.

THE LOGICAL AND EMPIRICAL BASIS FOR THE BEHAVIORAL ECOLOGICAL MODEL

Mel Hovell
Dennis Wahlgren
Marc Adams

BEHAVIOR AND ITS EFFECT ON HEALTH OUTCOMES

Reduction and prevention of morbidity and mortality in populations is a public health goal that can be achieved *only* by behavior change. Behavior explains more than 50 percent of the variance in infectious diseases and even more for degenerative diseases and injuries (Cuff and Vanselow, 2004; McGinnis and Foege, 1993). The importance of behavior is much broader than lifestyle practices. There is *no* level of medical care or health promotion that does not involve the behavior of at least one person. This is obvious in some instances—to lose weight one must exercise and eat a healthy diet. However, an individual's health is usually a function of the behavior of many people on multiple levels, and a broader systems approach to understanding both the individual's and the populations' behavior is critical to achieving health promotion for all. The eradication of polio was dependent upon behavior of multiple people acting in a system; the behavior of the scientists who developed the vaccine, the behavior of public health and medical practitioners who delivered the vaccine, and the behavior of parents and their children in obtaining vaccinations. All these people and more contributed to the eradication of most polio in western countries. Complex systems of behavior of subgroups within the overall population were and are operating to influence complex behavioral and health outcomes. We cannot ignore the behavior of politicians who enact legislative policies that influence public health research, the behavior from medical care providers and insurers, and the behavior of people involved in commercial industries (for example, pharmaceuticals, the tobacco industry) that may stand to profit from behavior that prevents disease or from behavior that harms the public. The confluence of all of these specialists and more must be considered as a complex ecological system of behavior.

Need for a New Model of Health Behavior

It is not possible for any clinical care delivery system to keep up with the behaviorally- and environmentally based incidence of disease, such as lung cancer from tobacco smoking, or from newly emerging infections such as SARS. Current approaches to understanding and changing behavior have had limited success, in part due to theoretical foundation, and in part due to focus on individuals and not populations. Jeffrey pointed out that thirty years of empirical obesity research using cognitive models of behavior has not resulted in reliable prediction or influence of diet or physical activity (Jeffrey, 2004). Other scientists have argued that rational choice models neglect the complex interactions of associative learning (Adams et al., 2009; West, 2005).

Thus, a new model of health behavior and health behavior change is critical in order to stem the tide of disease. Such prevention efforts will require understanding and effecting change in whole populations. Clinical medicine and psychology, while variously effective in treating individuals, are not equipped to solve some of the most pressing health problems of today and those for which we are at risk in the future (National Cancer Institute, 2007). Population control remains an unrealized goal in developing countries, and the global population, in concert with the lifestyles and practices (especially in developed countries), exhausts resources and adds to environmental damage to the point that may exceed the carrying capacity of the world (Daily et al., 1994; Ehrlich and Ehrlich, 2004). These problems and their associated behaviors contribute to unsafe drinking water, unsustainable agriculture, starvation, inadequate sanitation, global warming, spread of reemerging and new infectious diseases, and the worldwide export of chronic diseases such as diabetes. Indeed, war, political unrest, displacement of populations, and epidemics are likely to increase due to the size of the human population and the way we exploit our physical ecology. Ecologists now suggest that, without radical change in both the size of the population and the way we live, catastrophic damage to life on the planet may be unavoidable (Ehrlich and Ehrlich, 2004).

A focus on small units is appropriate and even essential during the early development of any science. While behavioral science has produced remarkable understanding of individual behavior, it has had less success when applied to large groups or to the maintenance of lifestyle practices in individuals and populations. To change behavior of entire populations of people requires understanding of the behavior of populations, especially when the behavior is relatively consistent across members (that is, cultural practices).

The Behavioral Ecological Model (BEM): A Work in Progress

We present the BEM as a work in progress to which others may contribute. The BEM links behavioral science to basic biological sciences, as foundations for behavior and learning, with an emphasis on ecological principles of selection by environmental consequences at individual and group/cultural levels. From these foundations, the BEM extends selectionistic mechanisms to a hierarchical model of environmental factors that interact to cause behavior in individuals and populations.

The BEM is derived from philosophical tenets of *functional contextualism* (Biglan and Hayes, 1996) and *radical behaviorism* (Skinner, 1953) and general philosophies of science regarding the logic of causal mechanisms. We start with the premise that because living organisms are part of nature, people's behavior is also part of nature and follows "natural laws." Behavior analysis strives to successfully predict and change human behavior, and to do so using procedures following the same rules of empirical science as employed by the natural sciences (Baum, 2005; Biglan, 1995; Sidman, 1960; Hill, 1965). Like all natural science disciplines, the BEM and its roots are based on a contextualistic approach: causes are to be found in the environment external to the phenomenon to be explained. The physicist explains motion of an object as a function of external forces applied to it. The biologist explains the color of a tree's leaves as a function of sunlight and chlorophyll physiology. In neither case is a hypothetical "agent" inside the object invoked as the explanation of behavior—behavior of matter or a tree's physiology. We study the behavior of living organisms as a function of events in the organism's environmental context, both current and past. This approach avoids "mentalism," or hypothetical explanations of behavior (other than physiology) inside the organism. Mentalism is a dualistic (mind-body) approach that results in circular explanations: if your friend orders a salad with a low-fat dressing, you might surmise that she desires to lose weight, and that it is this desire that causes her to order low-calorie food. The desire is inferred from the behavior and then used to explain the behavior—a violation of the rules of logic. Mentalistic explanations are also superfluous; if one has to "make up one's mind" in order to decide which salad to order, the behavioral scientist is now obligated to determine what causes the "mind" to decide and the mechanism by which it controls one's behavior. Contextual accounts are more parsimonious— your friend has been exposed to media that portrays thinness as the ideal, may have been advised by her physician to eat a low-calorie diet to lose weight and avoid diabetes. Examining historical and current contextual events also avoids the logical dilemma of "purposive" or "goal-directed" behavior (that is, future events cannot cause current behavior). These contextual events, while not necessarily complete, are objective, measurable, and manipulable (Baum, 2005). Avoiding mentalism is consistent with all natural sciences and protects behavioral scientists from the inherent bias due to common cultural explanations of behavior. For more complete discussion of the philosophical bases of behavior analysis and the BEM, see Baum (2005), Chiesa (1994), Sidman (1960), Biglan and Hayes (1996), and Skinner (1953, 1974).

The BEM relies on concepts and principles of behavior derived from respondent and operant conditioning and Applied Behavior Analysis (ABA), a scientific field that employs research methods designed to identify factors responsible for human behavior in real life contexts (Baer, Wolf, and Risley, 1968, 1987). We offer the BEM as a means of unifying biological, behavioral, and cultural sciences for explanation of and guidance for modifying human behavior in populations. This requires new research in real life situations.

Figure 15.1 builds upon our previous work (for example, Hovell, Kaplan, and Hovell, 1991; Hovell, Wahlgren, and Gehrman, 2002; Hovell, Wahlgren, and Russos, 1997) and depicts two interacting hierarchical systems that combined help explain both individual and population behavior. The figure is a simple representation of known complex mechanisms of biology and behavior and their interactions. With the vertical axis, we show how behavior bridges biological and learning mechanisms operating both within and outside the body. The horizontal axis shows that behavior flows through time in the context of dynamic stimuli that act as both antecedents and postcedents to behavior.

The two triangles summarize the types of levels of society (upper triangle) and factors within the organism or his/her genetic history (lower triangle) that combine to determine the likelihood of a specific behavior and determine those behaviors that are routinely practiced versus those that are never or rarely practiced. The point of this illustration is to focus attention on the interactions and summary influences of factors at all levels of physiology and society to understand behavior and ultimately influence its routine performance in whole populations. This requires special attention to

FIGURE 15.1 *BEM Diagram of Two Hierarchical Systems that Combined Help Explain Both Individual and Cultural Practices*

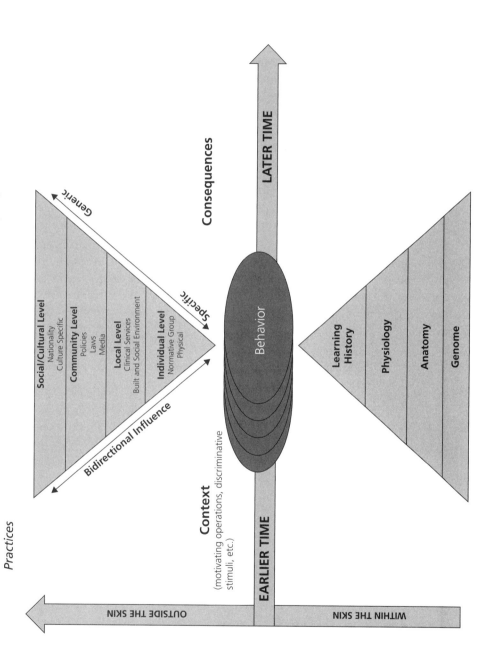

cultures and ultimately how principles of behavior apply to cultures and from which it might be possible to engineer cultures that sustain healthy behavior.

Integrating Behavior and Biology: A Selectionist Model

Similar to biopsychosocial models of behavior, disease, and disparities, the BEM assumes the role of genetics and evolutionary processes as part of the explanation of behavior. A recent version of such a biopsychosocial model was presented by Fernander et al. (2007), making a strong case for physiological factors interacting with both genetic and behavioral factors (for example, other lifestyle practices) as an explanation of tobacco addiction. Recent models of natural selection further extend selectionistic mechanisms to both individual organisms and the social group as a single organism to explain culture advancement (Wilson, Vugt, and O'Gorman, 2008). These examples are complex models with substantial research bases in biology, social psychology, and sociology. However, what they lack and what the BEM provides is a *selectionist foundation across all systems* for classifying environmental conditions and their complex interactions that change or support behavior. *The selectionistic mechanisms are contingencies of reinforcement, their specific features (for example, schedule), and interactions among multiple concurrent contingencies from all levels of biology and society.* The BEM extends the role of contingencies from that of individual behavior to that of whole populations and cultural practices. While the BEM requires substantial additional research for refinements, we believe that the emphasis on contingencies provides a translational foundation that can tie together ecology, physiology, genetics, and behavioral and social sciences.

The BEM is a hierarchical model that relies heavily (not exclusively) upon *variation* and *selection by consequences* that operate at three levels to select for the more adaptive variants within populations of species, and within an individual's repertoire, and within a given culture.

1. Natural Selection Within a population of organisms, the members most adapted to their environment are more likely to reproduce and pass along genes associated with survival traits (phylogeny). The early SubSaharan African population's environment included malaria organisms and the mosquito vectors that transmitted them efficiently. There was also, however, genetic variability among the humans that resulted in some individuals who were relatively resistant to malaria; individuals who were heterozygous for sickle cell anemia were more likely to survive malaria infections than those who were homozygous or did not carry the gene at all. Unfortunately, those individuals who were born without the genes for sickle cell were more likely to die of malaria than those that were heterozygous; those homozygous for sickle cell obtained abnormal sickle-shaped red blood cells, developed anemia, and most died. Environments select for genetic variants within and across species. Selection of genetic variants can define structure, physiology, and *certain aspects of behavior such as reflexes and the general ability to learn (that is, for behavior to be changed by* *one's context within an individual's lifetime).* Thus, the behavior of individuals and groups is dependent on genetic foundations for learning.

2. Operant Selection Within an individual's repertoire ("population of responses"), differential reinforcement selects for certain variants in operant behavior. If a child grows up in an English-speaking community, the community provides differential attention for English sounds and eventually syntax that defines speaking English. If one leaves work at varying times of the day, one may encounter heavy traffic (a punishing consequence) between 4 P.M. and 5 P.M. and light traffic (a reinforcing consequence) before and after those times. Over time, the commuter will leave more often before 4 P.M. or after 5 P.M. Not only may this change in departure behavior reduce the driver's experience of aversive delays in traffic, it may reduce his/her risk of an automobile accident, injury and the possible health effects of anger and frustration reactions of aversive delays in traffic. The important point here is that community-based social reactions or the delays inherent in dense traffic (versus relatively little delays in light traffic) produce differential contingent consequences for learning English or for commuting during times of light traffic. This principle of selection and extinction places incredible importance on understanding selecting environments and should direct research accordingly outside the individual (person or population) for most explanations of complex behavior of individuals and groups.

3. Cultural Selection Broadly speaking, the third level of selection involves variations in cultural practices and the selection for or against those practices by interactions from contingencies derived from multiple cultures within larger cultures (for example, nations) and from interactions between specialized subcultures and changes in the physical environment. While discussion of culture from a behavior analytic standpoint is not new (for example, Skinner 1953, 1981), recently attention has been paid to defining new concepts (for example, Glenn 1988; Houmanfar and Rodrigues, 2006; Malagodi, 1986). To fully appreciate the cumulative and interactive nature of the BEM, it is important to understand both basic and advanced principles of operant behavior of individuals and small groups. This sets the stage for understanding complex concepts defining culture.

BASIC PRINCIPLES OF BEHAVIOR

Some of the basic principles that explain how contextual variables influence behavior are summarized below as a foundation for the BEM. These principles are based on well over a hundred years of cross-species (including human) research. More detailed treatments are available in Fantino and Logan (1979), Catania (1998) and Cooper, Heron, and Heward (2006).

Respondent Conditioning

The physiologist Pavlov showed that reflexive behavior could be brought under the control of novel stimuli. Dogs would naturally salivate when meat powder was placed in their mouths. When a bell was rung just prior to placing the meat powder in the dog's mouth, the dog would begin to salivate in response to a bell alone after a few pairings (Pavlov, 1927). He called this a "conditional reflex" because learned salivation was conditional upon experience with bell/powder pairings. Thus, respondent behavior can be innate (that is, unlearned) or a learned reflex. The proximal determinant ("cause") of each response is the *antecedent* stimulus (meat powder or bell). The distal controlling relation of each response is the historical selecting experience that accounts for the effect of each proximal cause (for meat powder, natural selection in the history of the species; for the bell, the pairings with meat powder in the lifetime of the individual).

The immune system of mice can be similarly conditioned to respond to neutral stimuli, thereby making it possible for mice with autoimmune disease to live about 50 percent longer when treated with lower dosage of medication than untrained mice (Ader, Felten, and Cohen, 1991). Siegel (1975) demonstrated that narcotic tolerance— physiological responses that counteract the effect of the drug—could be elicited by environmental stimuli paired with drug administration. These previously neutral stimuli can elicit physiological responses that compensate for higher and higher doses of narcotic, thereby reducing the risk of death from overdose. This conditioning may account for dependence, as a wide variety of stimuli may come to elicit the compensatory response—experienced as withdrawal symptoms—prompting drug use to abate them. Siegel et al. (1982) showed that heroin-tolerant rats were more likely to die of overdose when the narcotic was given in a novel environment lacking the *inferred* conditioned stimuli that elicited the protective physiological tolerance response.

Drug use and death in novel environments may be explained by failure of conditioned compensatory responses that enable the body to tolerate high doses of narcotic. These studies suggest that physiological responses can be learned in response to different specific external environments. The general principles rely on manipulable environmental variables that may serve as the foundation for designing prevention interventions (Poulos, Hinson, and Siegel, 1981).

These examples of respondent conditioning show the link between innate reflexive behavior and the ability to learn new reflex-like behavior within the life span of the organism. This observation clearly ties biology and behavior together, and their relationship suggests that both biological and behavioral sciences should look for additional links to provide a more complete model of human behavior, diseases and premature mortality.

Operant Conditioning

Skinner (1938) defined operant behavior as a response that operates on or changes the environment. The consequence produced by the behavior may function to make the behavior more likely (referred to as reinforcement) or temporarily less likely (referred to as punishment) in the future. The controlling relation is in the *contingency* (dependency) between the behavior and the *postcedent* consequence it produces—it serves to make the behavior more or less probable in the future. Drawing on

Darwinian logic of selection of species, unique responses from a large or almost infinite array of possible responses are selected (that is, increase in frequency) based on contingent changes in the environment immediately following these unique responses. Responses that do not yield contingent changes in the environment tend to decrease in frequency sometimes to the point of disappearing from the individual's repertoire. This was named extinction to draw on the natural selection analogy. Intermittent reinforcement (reinforcement following multiple responses) tends to take longer to establish high rate behavior, but also tends to establish patterns of behavior more resistant to extinction. Numerous types, or *schedules* of reinforcement have been identified, each producing characteristic patterns of behavior (Ferster and Skinner, 1957; Galbicka, 1994; Lattal and Neef, 1996).

Unlearned and Learned Reinforcers

Contingent consequences that function as reinforcers may be innate (unlearned), selected for in the evolutionary history of the species (for example, food, water, sexual stimuli), or may be acquired (learned) as a function of pairings between neutral stimuli (for example, a parent's smile) and already-established reinforcers for example, food). Once Pavlov's bell had acquired the ability to elicit salivation, it could have served as a reinforcer for training his dogs to sit on command. Such *conditioned reinforcers* can become extremely powerful if paired with multiple established reinforcers. Money is highly reinforcing (that is, a generalized reinforcer) by virtue of its pairing with numerous reinforcers. Again, the link between inherently reinforcing stimuli and learned reinforcers illustrates the bridge between genetic history (phylogeny) and learning history (ontogeny). This linkage provides a more complete model of human behavior than do models that ignore either biological or behavioral principles.

Discriminative Stimuli

Contextual stimuli paired with both the behavior and its reinforcing consequence will acquire the ability to evoke the behavior. These antecedent stimuli occasion (that is, make more likely) the response. The individual learns to *discriminate* whether reinforcement will be available for the behavior. Asking for a bagel at the corner deli is only reinforced (by being given a bagel) when there are bagels in the display case. When the bagel section is empty, asking for such a bagel is extinguished. Asking for a bagel when the display is full might be suppressed if in the presence of a family member urging one to lose weight. The bagels and the presence of a family member are *discriminative stimuli*; in their presence the likelihood of asking for bagels is increased or decreased respectively, relative to the absence of bagels in the window or absence of a family member. The addition of an antecedent to the contingency of reinforcement is called a *three-term contingency*, referring to the Antecedent → Behavior → Consequence model.

   Discriminative stimuli can function both as cues to action and as reinforcing consequences for other actions, in a chain of behavior. A wife's lingerie may be highly discriminative for her husband's sexual advances. That is, wearing lingerie occasions sexual advances, which are more likely to be reinforced with sexual activity in the presence of the lingerie than in their absence. In the future, after the husband takes his wife out for a romantic evening, she may don her lingerie, *the sight of which reinforces the husband's "date" behaviors* from earlier in the evening. Thus, a given stimulus may be a reinforcing consequence for one behavior and discriminative stimulus for another in a complex chain of behavior for one individual or for two or more people's interactions.

Response Classes: Function Versus Topography

Because the aim of science is to discover causal principles, we group behaviors together based on causal functions, not on appearances. Thus, respondent and operant classes of behavior are defined by their respective functional relationships to the environment: respondent behavior is caused by antecedent eliciting stimuli and operant behavior by a history of postcedent consequences. They are not defined by topography (appearance). To group responses by topography would equate behavior under different types of control: an eye-blink elicited by dust is functionally very different from a wink to a friend. The former is respondent and the latter an operant response, yet appear the same. Defining responses by a single topography would also mistakenly treat different behaviors that have common causes as members of separate classes: "physical activity" is an operant response class consisting of walking, stretching, running, bicycling, weight-lifting, and so on. While each member produces unique consequences, such as reduction in muscle strains following stretching, each also produce common environmental consequences, such as the ability to walk, lift, run, and to engage in physical exertion related to escape from danger. An *operant response class* is a set of behaviors that function to produce a common reinforcing consequence. To reiterate, in the operant model, antecedent stimuli may have evoking effects on behavior but are dependent on the response-*consequence* contingency. Respondent behavior, by contrast, is elicited as a function of unlearned or learned eliciting *antecedent* stimuli.

ADVANCED PRINCIPLES OF BEHAVIOR

Operant Behavior in the Apparent Absence of Reinforcement

Much of our behavior appears to occur without producing reinforcement, especially novel and "creative" behavior. To understand the more interesting and challenging aspects of our behavior requires that we make use of combinations of basic principles of behavior and the concurrent addition of advanced principles of behavior.

Schedules of Reinforcement

Most operant behavior is a function of intermittent schedules of reinforcement—not every response is reinforced. This results in behavior that persists even in periods during which there is no explicit reinforcement, such as gambling. Parents who endure increasingly longer periods ignoring their child's tantrums before "giving in" (and reinforcing the tantrums) are unknowingly training their child to tantrum relentlessly and more aggressively. In both cases, high-rate dramatic behavior such as gambling or tantruming may take place in the apparent absence of reinforcement (that is, gambling wins, parent attention) and even in the context of apparent punishment such as loss of money or parent demands to "stop or else." The mystery is explained by an incomplete observation in which the intermittent reinforcement is not visible in short observation periods and in which the parents' threats, while having the syntactic structure of criticism and pending punishment, may actually reinforce tantrum behavior by providing attention the child does not otherwise receive. This is also an instance in which the topography of the consequence (parent threats to punish) is very different from its function (reinforcing tantrums). In such cases, threats function as reinforcers and not as punishers.

Two Important Generalized Response Classes: Imitation and Rule-Governance

Response classes are defined by the function of the behavior to yield similar types of reinforcing consequences (Barnes-Holmes and Barnes-Holmes, 2000). Saying hello, saluting, waving, and nodding all might be members of a generalized response class for "greetings." They all result in similar consequences from the person to whom the wave is directed (for example, wave back). Reinforcement of one member of a response class increases the likelihood of other members, even if they have not been reinforced (Baer, Peterson, and Sherman, 1967; Brigham and Sherman, 1968). This can lead to some behavior appearing in absence of reinforcement.

Two important response classes are imitation and rule following. Imitation of others results in novel behavior that has never been emitted and thus never reinforced. However, very early in life, parents reinforce anything their infant child does that approximates the parent's behavior, such as smiling, laughing, clapping hands, and especially oral/verbal responses (Baer and Deguchi, 1985; Baer, Peterson, and Sherman, 1967; Gewirtz and Stingle, 1968). As the child grows older, imitating the behavior of others also results in natural reinforcers: imitating a sibling who asks for candy is likely to result in obtaining candy as well as attention for imitation. Thus, when we imitate others, it may appear as novel behavior taking place in absence of a reinforcing consequence. However, previous imitative responses have been reinforced by a rich variety of consequences, such as praise for matching or candy when imitating a polite request. These past experiences make more probable future imitations, even in situations in which there may be no discrete reinforcing consequence. Strong generalized imitative response classes are most important for the development of language. Children imitate many behaviors, but very quickly learn to make noises and other verbal responses based on parent and other's models. These rudimentary responses are eventually shaped into language skills by the audience's differential reactions.

The development of language leads to rule-governed behavior. Individuals come under the influence of "rules"—instructions, advice, commands—as complex discriminative stimuli. Rules describe contingencies, either explicitly or implicitly. A parent tells a child "if you finish eating your vegetables, you can have dessert" (discriminative stimulus); the child then follows the instruction by eating vegetables and obtains dessert, praise, and other attention. Not only is the specific response (eating vegetables) reinforced with dessert, and so on, but following instructions in general is reinforced. This situation is then repeated across different behaviors, different people providing instructions, in different contexts, generalizing widely. With experience, individuals acquire a *generalized* rule-governed response class, so named because it is generalized across multiple topographic forms of behavior that result in similar reinforcing consequences, and because it takes place across different people who provide the rules and in different contexts in which the rules are stated, followed, and reinforced (see Hayes, 1989 for more details). Thus, some behavior may take place in response to instructions, but in absence of a discrete reinforcement. This may be due, in part, to previous reinforcement for instruction-following.

Motivating Operations

Context can alter the effects of contingencies. Deprivation and satiation change both the momentary effectiveness of a reinforcer, and can make the behavior associated with the reinforcer more or less likely (Michael, 2000, 2007). Working outdoors on a hot day without water makes water and other beverages more reinforcing, and it also makes more likely many behaviors that have in the past been reinforced with beverages (for example, asking for water). Motivating operations refer to contextual (historical and current) antecedent events that alter the momentary effect of reinforcers and the momentary probability of behaviors that produce them. If a child has asthma, her mother's motivation to avoid social criticism for harming a child with an illness may be substantially greater than for families with healthy children. Asthma, as a context factor, may increase the aversive effect of social criticism, and increase behaviors that avoid both criticism and asthmatic symptoms. Thus, any behavior, such as asking family and friends not to smoke in the home, may be more reinforced by avoiding social criticism for parents of an asthmatic child relative to a family without an asthmatic child. Thus, motivating operations, or contexts, may alter the effects of consequences that otherwise might appear as probable reinforcers or probable punishers. In short, without taking context into consideration, the effects of a given observed consequence may not have the expected magnitude of reinforcing or punitive effects.

Variability, Shaping, Extinction and Resurgence

Every time a person performs a specific behavior, it varies in form, even if slightly. This variability offers the possibility of selecting new and creative forms via differential reinforcement. One possibility is to shape behavior not yet part of the individual's repertoire. For example, parents can shape bicycle riding by holding a child on the bike, praising pedaling, and gradually relaxing the physical assistance, as the child acquires greater balance; training wheels are raised in small steps until the child is a competent bicyclist. This can result in well-established new skills and change in frequency or topography of existing complex practices.

Extinction (ceasing reinforcement) increases the variability of behavior. When opening a locked door with a key is unsuccessful, one usually tries a second time. When that is also unsuccessful (not reinforced with opening the door) he may turn the key multiple times, remove and reinsert the key, jiggle the handle, jiggle the handle while turning the key repeatedly, and finally knock on the door. When one has a headache, he may engage in many different behaviors, such as resting, putting a cold compress on the forehead, taking a hot shower, and taking an aspirin, until something is followed by relief from pain. The exact topography of different responses depends on the individual's learning history for opening doors or relief of headache or other pain. These responses are variations of previously reinforced responses. The responses most highly reinforced in the past are the most likely to occur first, followed by ones less frequently or more distantly reinforced in that context. This *resurgence* of previously reinforced responses, the variations of previously reinforced responses, and their *blending* provide opportunities for reinforcement of novel variants of behavior. Epstein (1999) has described these processes and demonstrated experimentally that "creative" problem-solving behavior is based on previously learned components of the creative behavior and one's history of reinforcement. Thus, formal training efforts can rely on shaping procedures to establish higher precision or more complex skills and routine performance. Similar processes can occur in natural environments, in which slowly changing weather can shape changes in farming, dressing, recreation, and so forth. Some of the same principles of variation and past reinforcement for key complex behavior can recur under extinction conditions from which novel behavior may arise and result in reinforcement, and (by definition) as increase in a new and potentially more functional behavior.

This may explain the performance of apparently novel "creative" behavior, which at first appears seemingly in absence of reinforcing consequences. A history of reinforcement for components of the novel and creative behavior in the presence of extinction conditions might evoke a novel response. For some individuals, a rich history of reinforcement for problem solving, puzzle solutions, and so on may lead to a generalized creative response repertoire or response class. Within specific fields, such as art, dance, or even research, certain individuals may be especially adept at creating a remarkable painting, performing a remarkable dance, or even applying highly creative solutions to answer a research question, and may be able to do so more reliably than others in the same field. These professionals are called masters or senior leaders in the field. However, their skills may be understood as a function of a generalized creativity response class in their area of expertise. Recognizing this explanation of seemingly spontaneous behavior directs attention to learning histories and one's environment as the place to find explanations.

EXTENSION TO THE CULTURAL LEVEL

Advanced principles of behavior help explain complex and unusual behavior. *However, they fall short of explaining population behavior and its evolution.* The BEM offers an extended approach. This approach assumes that important behavior always takes place in the context of a complex culture and that the cultural context makes a difference in the probability of sustained practices. Thus, while the BEM includes principles of individual behavior, the model is extended to larger systems in which more than one person's behavior is explained and in which more than one physical or social agent is responsible for practices in the "real world." Larger systems include analyses at the level of groups and cultural practices.

Group Contingencies

One of the methods by which group behavior can be established and sustained is based on group contingencies, in which a group is provided with reinforcing consequences for the groups' collective behavior. For example, a teacher tells the class that they will obtain extra recess time if all students remain quiet for the remainder of the class period. This type of contingency evokes a cascade of social contingencies in which the students prompt, model, and reinforce quiet behavior, and punish one another's disruptive behavior. Thus, the teacher's policy for recess causes the class culture to focus on policing the group and earn the extra recess time. The teacher does not have to shape all individuals to sustain quiet class time.

Cultural Practices

A definition of culture begins with "cultural practices," or the repetition of learned behavior across individuals, within and across generations (Glenn, 1988; Glenn, 2004; Malagodi and Jackson, 1989). "Generations" may refer to offspring, and may also reflect induction of new people to a cultural practice. Birthday celebrations in the United States constitute a cultural practice in that they are relatively consistent from one occasion to the next, and remain relatively consistent when repeated with different participants each time (Glenn, 1991; Glenn, 2004). Biglan noted that cultural practices can be defined not only by prevalence of a given set of behaviors in a population, but also in terms of the *interlocking patterns of behavior* among the participants (Biglan, 1995; Biglan, 2003). "Interlocking behavior" occurs when behavior of one person, or the consequences of that person's behavior, serves as an antecedent for the other person's behavior, and vice versa in a sequential chain among members (Houmanfar and Rodrigues, 2006).

By these definitions, two or more people might define "a culture," if behavior is consistent over time and if it survives the addition of new members to the group. A group of sports fans or religious adherents can each define small to larger distinct cultures. A given individual also may be a member of multiple cultures concurrently—a powerful concept within the BEM. This concept suggests that the social context present for a given individual is defined by unique social contingencies of reinforcement.

As the individual moves from one social context to another context, his or her behavior will change to match the contingencies present in the new social context. Thus, leaving the relatively conservative context of work (one culture) and going to the sports stadium to meet friends and root for the local baseball team (a second culture) will alter the individual's behavior from intense computer work to cheering, eating hotdogs, and drinking beer. Similarities in behavior that define cultures can result from two potential sources: physical and social environmental contingencies of reinforcement that, separately or combined, produce similar behavior across individuals (Glenn, 2004).

Metacontingencies

Metacontingencies parallel behavioral contingencies, but deal with phenomena at a different level of analysis (Houmanfar and Rodrigues, 2006). As noted previously, the behavioral three-term contingency is defined by antecedent-behavior-consequence relationships. The metacontingency also consists of three terms: the cultural context, an aggregate product produced by a group's interlocked behavior, and selection of the aggregate product by a social environment or audience (Figure 15.2). Variants in the product of the cultural group may be selected by social audiences (other cultural groups) external to the specific cultural group (Glenn, 2004; Glenn and Malagodi, 1991). As a level of analysis different from that of individual behavior, the metacontingency can be studied without reference to the behavior of the individual participants. This is analogous to studying the antecedent-behavior-consequence contingency for individual behavior, which need not include analysis of the individual's physiology (for example, neural function) for a functional account of behavior. Rather, the behavior of the group is the central focus for defining functional contingencies that increase or decrease the groups' behavior, even if some members' behavior within the group does not correspond precisely. The BEM acknowledges that all levels—physiological, behavioral, cultural—are functioning at any given time, but one may focus on a given level for an account *at that level of analysis*. Understanding all levels and their interactions may be required to fully understand or engineer sustained health-related practices in populations.

Firefighting may be sustained by societal control at individual and metacontingency levels. When firefighters coordinate their efforts, the coordinated behavior of the group is reinforced and will be more probable in the future as a function of extinguishing the fire more quickly, more completely or with less effort than true in an uncoordinated effort. Simultaneously, but more delayed, successfully extinguishing a community fire results in the appreciation from home owners whose lives and property may have been saved. These audiences are likely to provide reinforcing attention and promote policies that support firefighters more liberally with needed equipment or payment. Even if some individual firefighters were not cooperating efficiently, as long as the groups' performance results in saving homes, the success in putting out fires and the community's collective response by praising firefighters and increasing resources for them may serve as a metacontingency that increases the likelihood of the firefighters' coordinated efforts to put out fires in the future.

FIGURE 15.2 *BEM Diagram of Interlocked Behaviors and Cultural-Level Selection*

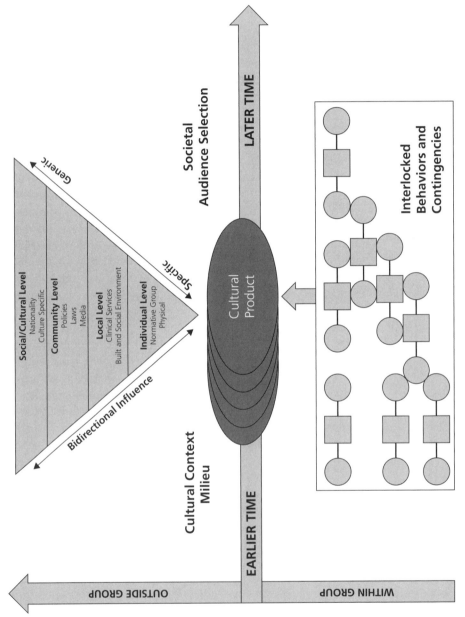

In Fig. 15.2, the metacontingency consists of three terms: the cultural milieu, a cultural product produced by a group's interlocked behavior, and selection of the aggregate product by a social environment. Within a group or culture, the behavior of one individual, or consequences of their behavior, serves as an antecedent for the other person's behavior, and vice versa in a sequential chain among members. Antecedent-behavior-consequence relationships are represented by the circle-square-circles.

Macrocontingencies

Multiple people may engage in similar behavior essentially independently of one another, as a result of similar contingencies independently acting upon each individual. Eating high-fat, high-salt and high-sugar foods is inherently reinforcing for most people in most contexts. Thus, when food is produced easily by a food industry that enables almost all individuals in Western society to avoid the intensive physical labor required to grow, transport and prepare food for consumption, most people buy and eat it, even if it contributes to obesity and consequential diseases. When the behavior of multiple people acting independently produces a cumulative, aggregate outcome, it is termed a *macrocontingency* (Glenn, 2004). Unlike the common product from firefighters' coordinated effort to extinguish a fire, the outcome or product of a large group of people's independent behavior does not function as a reinforcing or punishing consequence for any individual's behavior, nor does any one individual's behavior appreciably affect the outcome. The high prevalence of obesity does not function to make overeating less likely, nor does any one's change in diet markedly change the population prevalence.

A macrocontingency relation is distinguished from a metacontingency in two ways. First, the behavior of the individuals is not necessarily *interlocked* or coordinated in some fashion. Second, the outcome (for example, obesity) does not function to select for or against the recurrence of the highly prevalent behaviors that produce it. Thus, the macrocontingency is a function of common reinforcing consequences that yield high prevalence of similar behavior. In this example, the reinforcing consequences are inherent in consumption of fast food and avoidance of moderate to intensive physical activity. The longer-term outcomes such as obesity and disease rates in the population are side effects of these contingencies. However, delayed weight gain has little consequential influence on eating or activity patterns, even when most individuals are well aware of the relationships between overeating, underexercising, and obesity and disease.

While the macrocontingency concept may appear at first to be of limited use, it can lead to conceptualizing problems and potential solutions differently. Houmanfar and Rodrigues (2006) suggest that promoting attendance to weight-loss groups will require interactions among members of the group and will involve interlocking contingencies as members prompt and differentially reinforce changes in diet and activity of one another. This type of metacontingency might contribute to obesity control. Or, following a macrocontingency logic, a nationwide health promotion media campaign directed to the whole population might prompt diet and activity changes in many of the audience. This would approximate a macrocontingency, where changes in diet and activity might be reinforced (by incidental social reactions of friends and others) for many of individuals so prompted, but their behavior and unique reinforcing contingencies would not be interlocked across the population. While the use of such media might help, it probably would not be sufficient (and has not been to date) for controlling the obesity epidemic in the United States, even if it changes some important proportion of the population's behavior. A more profound macrocontingency dictated by principles of behavior could be a nationwide tax on all fast food and all automobiles. By using a tax, all individuals who buy fast food or use private automobiles for transportation would be discouraged from doing so, and this could lower the rates for both behaviors for the whole population. Thus, laws and other policy mechanisms might serve as powerful contingencies for most if not all individuals in the society. If engineered based on empirically validated principles of behavior, such policies might make marked differences in population practices and their consequential health. The current increase in gasoline prices may eventually have impact on automobile use, price of food, and ultimately both eating and physical activity practices. If so, this macrocontingency might have beneficial health effects.

The BEM includes expected influences of the masses of people who might change their behavior as a function of the density of people responding to a given macrocontingency. In our previous work (Adams, et al., 2006), we speculated that the density of people who use stairs rather than escalators would provide both models to be imitated by others and possible advice (for example, mediated by rule-governed conditioned reinforcers) and social reinforcement for adopting similar practices by friends and acquaintances. Macrocontingencies could promote coordinated interactions that meet the standard of a new culture (for example, healthy eating and activity practice culture) based on the interlocked behavior and interlocking social contingencies prompted by the density of new models generated by a single tax contingency. Thus, macrocontingencies might be engineered to establish a cascade of social metacontingencies that might magnify the effects of the tax in a synergistic fashion and contribute to effects for individuals (for example, the wealthy) not influenced by the tax or to cultures (for example, other cities, states, or nations) where such taxes are not in place. Taxing tobacco sales may have had this effect in many states in the United States and in increasing numbers of whole nations (Martinez-Donate et al., 2008).

Complexity and Selection of Cultures

The BEM emphasizes metacontingencies that define cultures and subcultures within them as an important unit of function and unit of analysis for protecting the health of whole populations. Subcultures are ever evolving. Many will evolve as a function of the immediate reinforcing outcomes derived from interlocked behavior of the group. Our firefighter example earlier illustrates this process.

However, some are created or suppressed by other subcultures. These include institutions whose cultural rules are to protect the population. Armies do this for defense against other national cultures. Public health professionals do this for prevention of ills in whole populations. In a modern society, there are hundreds of specialized subcultures or institutions whose overriding internal metacontingencies define protection or service to the population as the outcome or product for which the group's behavior is reinforced. Federal agencies such as the Centers for Disease Control and Prevention (CDC), Environmental Protection Agency (EPA), National Institute of Occupational Safety and Health (NIOSH), and similar state and local agencies serve as special subcultures for whom contingencies are in place for specialists to look for risks of disease, toxic exposures, and traumatic injury, and then take action that will reduce the risks of morbidity and mortality to high-risk populations. The presence of these agencies is a measure of the complexity of our national culture. These agencies serve as checks and balances on other agencies (for example, commercial businesses) and systems (evolution of new pathogens, such as SARS) that might create risks for the population at large. Relative to other nations, the United States might be viewed as more complex a culture and one that is more likely to detect early warning signs and take corrective action to protect the U.S. population than might be true for other nations. However, this remains to be determined.

Jared Diamond illustrates dramatically what can happen to cultures in the absence of early warning systems for cultural practices gone awry. If delayed effects are potentially disastrous to the population and if a society is blind to the effect of the culture's dangerous practices (or dangerous practices from a subculture), the effect on survival might not be discriminated in time to refine cultural practices and save the members of the culture from extinction (that is, death of a population). Primitive inhabitants of Easter Island built stone totems, and in doing so depleted the natural resources of the island, causing starvation and death of almost all members of the population (Diamond, 2005). Thus, a cultural practice led to the extinction of the island people, and their totem-construction practices with them. The BEM explains this outcome as a function of metacontingencies for totem construction without subcultures that could predict the delayed effects of such construction on resources necessary for survival.

In spite of our illustrations above that suggest that the United States has necessary subcultures such as CDC to protect us, it is no longer clear that such agencies are sufficient. Diamond's theme is that catastrophic damage to the entire globe may well be under way as a consequence of our culture, and most cultures across all nations, and with insufficient attention to the degree of damage taking place and insufficient ability to respond before it is too late to save life on our planet (Diamond, 2005). The BEM offers another means of understanding Diamond's thesis, and a possible means of preventing the catastrophe he foretells. The BEM offers metacontingencies as one of the important units of function that defines cultures, and understanding these contingencies may provide the guide necessary to forestall disasters due to our current culture. However, this requires a more vigorous science of culture, including engineering change in cultures to enhance health. Among the most important directions for such science is increased understanding of how subcultures such as the EPA or CDC evolve to protect us from our own practices. Agencies such as CDC may identify the early outbreak of an infectious disease due to lifestyle practices such as sharing water pipes for smoking perfumed tobacco in commercial hookah bars. In such a plausible scenario, the CDC professionals would send out alarms concerning a new infectious disease epidemic, might suggest patrons avoid hookah bars and might even suggest that such bars be banned. In all likelihood, they would recommend physician visits to obtain treatment for possible bacterial infections.

However, most government agencies could not now provide clear warnings about the complex metacontingencies that define hookah bars, their popularity and the financial contingencies that result in many city governments allowing such commercial tobacco smoking agencies to operate legally or to operate in absence of enforcement of existing laws that prevent smoking in public (World Health Organization, 2005). Cultural specialists at organizations like CDC should be promoted in order to establish expertise in cultural contingencies and from which early warning measures of developing metacontingencies in businesses, such as hookah bars, could be developed. Such expertise also could provide an early warning system to local governments and provide the expertise to suggest countercontingencies necessary to suppress such businesses or to redirect them to business practices that do not increase risk of disease. As such CDC could serve as a more profound specialized subculture that could *select* for businesses that promote healthy recreational practices versus those that promote dangerous and morbidity-producing practices.

To our knowledge, when government or other agencies establish new policies to protect the health of populations, they do so with little or no guidance from the principles of behavior described in this chapter. Thus, there is as yet no subculture of experts that promotes use of the BEM to inform new policies and effective contingencies that might select for health-promoting subcultures and extinguish subcultures that promote risk. In this context, "risk" is defined broadly, such that a home developer who promotes suburban housing contributes to both global warming and sedentary behavior, from which destruction of life as we know it might take place and in the meantime most of the U.S. population will suffer from obesity and consequential diseases. Thus, policies should be developed based on our knowledge of principles of behavior to alter the typical home builder's promotion of suburban and inefficient housing to that of efficient and urban living. This will require aggressive new science and professional advisors to policy makers to determine the most effective policies that do not also have unintended iatrogenic effects on society. Ultimately, the BEM implies the need for a defined subculture institution (for example, the EPA) that could inform the design of policies (that is, macrocontingencies and metacontingencies) directed to changing population behavior most effectively, based on a public health ethical standard that ranks protection of the public from delayed harm or death above short-term gains from risky practices; that takes into account the redirection of existing industries to services that will contribute to health instead of illness or injury; and that does so based on empirically validated principles of behavior of both individual and groups.

Summary of the Model

The BEM defines separate but integrated levels of analysis, in which the physical environment selects for genetic variants suitable to the current world; in which individual contingencies select the repertoire of an individual and some cultural practices; and in which aggregate products of group practices are involved in selecting for the complex and coordinated behavior of cultural groups. Behavioral phenomena are built on physiology, but cannot be explained well by physiological principles alone. Similarly, culture is based on operant principles but cannot be explained completely by reduction to an individual's contingencies (Glenn and Malagodi, 1991). The BEM emphasizes the interaction among individual contingencies, metacontingencies, and macrocontingencies. Systems in which consequence-based contingencies at each level of consideration may be immediate or delayed, continuous or intermittent, and true for few people in the population or nearly universal, interact to influence individual and group behavior. Understanding these principles and advancing the science of culture following the BEM may enable integration of biology, behavioral, and social sciences to effect health-promoting cultures and maximize the survival of the species.

EMPIRICAL EVIDENCE FOR THE BEM

Table 15.1 highlights studies that were based on the BEM or were sufficiently close to its axioms to provide empirical evidence for the model. The complexity of these mechanisms makes it impossible for one study to address all aspects. Several scientists have demonstrated key aspects of the BEM by directly or indirectly following its logic. Genetics, evolutionary biology, ecology, and basic operant and respondent psychology and decades of Applied Behavior Analysis have contributed to the foundation of the BEM, offering an important degree of construct validity to the logic of the model. What we have described here focuses on the cultural, ecological, and dynamic interactive aspects of hierarchical interactions within and across all societies as critical to understanding and effecting population-wide changes in health behavior. We have selected examples from four classes of studies to illustrate tests and empirical evidence supporting components of the BEM. This brief review of empirical evidence is a highly selected sample of studies that suggest features of the BEM may be valid and generalizable. However, it is not complete and it does not represent a search of literature that might refute or demonstrate inaccuracies in the current level of development of the model. As a work in progress, we welcome peers to join us in identifying existing empirical evidence and contributing to new science that will refine the model.

Legal Contingencies, Public Policies, and Enforcement

Laws and public policies are behavioral contingencies specified through rules. Politicians, at various levels of government and through various interactions with

TABLE 15.1 Selected Studies Supporting the BEM.

Behavior/ Outcome	Authors	Sample	Design
Acculturation, cultural contingencies, and health behavior			
Physical Activity	Hofstetter et al., 2008	Korean adults in California	CS
Tobacco use/Alcohol use/ Diet	Landrine and Klonoff, 2004	Mexico, Japan, US	Review article
Tobacco control	Hovell et al., 2004	Medical providers	Theory article
Tobacco use	Hofstetter et al., 2004	Korean adults in California	CS
Tobacco use/ Diet	Song et al., 2004	Korean adults in California and Korea	CS
Tobacco use/cessation	Martinez-Donate et al., 2007	Mexican-descent adults in CA	CS
Tobacco use/cessation	Martinez-Donate et al. 2008	Mexicans in CA and Mexico	QED
Laws, policies, and enforcement			
Child safety seat use	Lavelle, Hovell, West, and Wahlgren, 1992	Police officers	2 group ABA
Political lobbying	Schroeder, Hovell, Kolody, and Elder, 2004	Beach business managers	RCT

Reengineering health service contingencies			
Alcohol use	Myers, Hovell, Elder, and Hall, 1991	College students	RCT
Alcohol use/illicit drug use	Bousman et al., 2005	Homeless adolescents	CS
Clinician leadership/ tobacco use	Hovell et al., 1995	Orthodontists	Group RCT
Condom acquisition	Zellner et al., 2006	High school students	Two-group repeated measures
ETS avoidance/ Smoking cessation	Zakarian et al., 2004	Mothers w/ETS exposed child	RCT
ETS exposure/asthma symptoms	Wahlgren, Hovell, Meltzer, Hofstetter, and Zakarian, 1997	Parents w/asthmatic children	RCT
Junior high school education	Schumaker, Hovell, and Sherman, 1977	Junior high school students	MBL
Medical referral services	Johns, Hovell, Drastal, Lamke, and Patrick, 1992	Medical providers	Hybrid MBL and ABA
Smoking incidence	Wahlgren et al., 1997	Adolescent patients	One-group prospective
Tobacco use prevention	Elder et al., 1993	Junior high school students	Group RCT

(Continued)

TABLE 15.1 (Continued)

Behavior/Outcome	Authors	Sample	Design
Tobacco use prevention/cessation	Russos et al., 1999	Orthodontists and youth	Group RCT
Vaginal and anal sex/condom use	Martinez-Donate et al., 2004b; Martinez-Donate et al., 2004a	Mexican high school students	Group RCT
WIC participation	DeBate and Pyle, 2004	WIC mothers	CS
Media contingencies			
Marketing and childhood overweight	Dresler-Hawke and Veer, 2006	None	Theory article
Behavioral modeling and transmission of behavior			
Physical activity/sedentary behavior	Sallis et al., 1990	Adults	CS
Physical activity/stair use	Adams et al., 2006	Airport patrons	Alternating treatment

RCT = Randomized Controlled Trial; QED = Quasi-Experimental Design; ABA = Withdrawal Design ; MBL = Multiple Baseline Design; CS = Cross-sectional Design other politicians, create these rules, often without clear evidence of their effect on behavior. The passage of certain legislation is the aggregate product of politicians' interlocked behavior. A passage of legislation can be influenced by various industry lobbyists, usually through campaign contributions and other social consequences, by individual constituents—who usually are neither organized nor resource rich—or by organized groups of constituents (for example, labor unions) who share a common issue. The politicians' social environment selects for or against certain types of legislation over time. Therefore, to change politicians' behavior, one could change the politicians' social environment. Schroeder and colleagues (2004) tested whether a newsletter intervention could increase coastal business managers' political lobbying actions by associating water quality with potential store sales. Environmental damage resulting from human actions can have serious economic and health consequences for a community and repercussions for its tourist industry. Business managers received two one-page newsletters each week for six weeks that emphasized economic, tourism, health, and other consequences of coastal water quality. The newsletters linked good water quality with higher tourist income and poor quality with lower income. The newsletters also provided managers with telephone numbers to contact politicians and environmental organizations. At the end of six weeks, the intervention group reported greater political contact than a control group of business managers (46 percent versus 15 percent). Delivery of prompts that highlight the existing economic contingencies associated with water quality to business managers can foster managers' political action directed to improve water quality and the physical ecology in general, sometimes because protecting the ecology was reinforcing to some managers and in other instances only because it might enhance their business income. This suggests that use of media to prompt behavior that is likely to take place in the context of existing financial contingencies may be a means of changing a large proportion of a given subculture's (for example, tourist beach businesses) political lobbying practices, which could in turn affect the larger culture should it translate to new public policy. This study illustrated the use of a macrocotingency or prompt to a large number of independent business owners who, in turn, created a cumulative political prompt to selected local politicians.

Legal contingencies are not always designed well or upheld. Thus, laws can have their effects attenuated when principles of behavior are not considered. Lavelle and colleagues (1992) tested an intervention to increase police officers' enforcement of child safety seat use laws between two geographically separated cities with similar incidence of vehicle crashes with injuries. In the intervention town, the study aimed to increase safety seat use by reengineering the existing contingencies for both officers and noncompliant motorists. Police officers suggested that issuing the standard $50 ticket to otherwise law-abiding citizens was an (immediately) aversive practice for the officers, even though they understood tickets could reduce children's injury or death. In collaboration with the officers, the intervention staff designed an alternative to the traditional citation process. Noncompliant motorists ticketed by the police were given a $50 ticket accompanied by a referral coupon. The coupon entitled the cited motorists to have the fine waived for attending a forty-five-minute educational class from the health department and for acquiring a safety seat at no charge. Using a two-group withdrawal design with repeated measures over four years, both the intervention and control cities had similar rates of ticketing for non-use of safety seats (<1 percent of all traffic-related tickets) for the two years prior to the intervention. During the intervention, officers' rate of citations for noncompliance increased to 4.8 percent and remained higher than baseline (1.32 percent) after the intervention was withdrawn. The control city remained at a near-zero rate throughout the intervention and follow-up. Trends in all other citations were unchanged over time. This study showed that officers' enforcement of child safety-seat laws increased once a contingency was designed that allowed noncompliant motorists to escape the aversive economic consequences of an officer's ticket and allowed officers to maintain or increase their positive standing. This new contingency decreased the aversive consequences previously true for both the officers' and motorists' ticketing and child car seat practices. Had this program been promoted outside the specific law enforcement agencies and research team involved, it might have reduced children's injuries by engineering a metacontingency among the officers, the court system, the health department, and drivers, in which the community selected for the aggregate product (reduced child injury) by providing financial, legislative, and other support for the new infraction penalty structure.

Acculturation, Cultural Contingencies, and Health Behavior

It has been observed that the experience of acculturating to another society—that is, changing one's behavior to be more similar to that most prevalent in the new culture—can affect health behavior differently for different ethnic groups, and for men and women within the same ethnic group. Landrine and Klonoff's recent review (2004) showed that the existing acculturation literature, which finds that recent immigrants to the United States have differential rates of tobacco use, fruit and vegetable consumption, and alcohol use when compared with their native cultures, could be reinterpreted and expanded by using operant and cultural selection concepts. After outlining the limitations of current bidirectional and multidirectional acculturation models, the authors reviewed the recent sex-specific findings of acculturation on these health behaviors for Latino, black, and Asian racial/ethnic groups in the United States.

If cultures differ in their prevalence and use of social and cultural contingencies, then studying the same population within cultural settings *known to differ in certain contingencies* should show differential rates of behavior. Obviously, randomizing individuals to different cultures is impossible. One alternative may be to study recent arrivals and longer-term members from one ethnic group to a society and their counterparts living in their native culture. In a study of Korean-descent adults living in California and Seoul, Korea, we demonstrated that acculturated women currently smoke at a higher rate in the United States than do women in Korea (17 percent versus 7 percent), but acculturated males smoke at a drastically lower rate than do men in Korea (36.2 percent versus 62.1 percent) (Song et al., 2004). Differences in smoking rates between the indigenous and current cultures may be a function of different macrocontingencies, or the relative density of community-wide social modeling, reinforcement, and punitive contingencies that occur interpersonally in neighborhood and community settings, and the media. For Korean women in the United States, there may be lower density of punitive contingencies and higher density of reinforcing contingences for smoking relative to Korea, and for Korean men in the United States, a higher density of punitive and lower density of reinforcement contingencies for smoking relative to Korea. These results suggest that the relative difference in the prevalence of reinforcing contingencies for each culture by gender, and potentially by other variables such as ethnic group or rural versus urban areas, may produce both protective and deleterious effects for health behavior.

Stronger evidence of the effects of community-wide contingencies would be a quasi-experimental test in which contingencies are redesigned to target a specific behavior, and that behavior could be monitored on a population level by differing exposures to these contingencies. The California Tobacco Control Program (CTCP) is an exemplar of some of the components of the BEM for tobacco-related behaviors (Hovell, Wahlgren, and Gehrman, 2002). The CTCP includes smoke-free laws, tobacco taxation, restrictions in tobacco advertising and promotion, community involvement, media campaigns, and cessation services. These antismoking components attempt to reengineer community-wide contingencies that were developed and continue to be developed by the tobacco industry to promote smoking. To test the influence and strength of the reengineered antitobacco contingencies, Martinez-Donate et al. (2008) conducted three concurrent population surveys among Mexican-descent adults residing in three cities that represent implicit full, partial, and no exposure to the CTCP: San Diego (California, United States), Tijuana (Baja California, Mexico), and Guadalajara (Jalisco, Mexico). The study found significantly different rates of smoking, exposure to secondhand smoke (SHS), prevalence of home smoking bans and tobacco-related diseases, all in the hypothesized directions among residents of San Diego, Tijuana, and Guadalajara. San Diego had the lowest rates of current smoking, exposure to secondhand smoke and tobacco-related diseases, and highest rates of smoking bans. Guadalajara had the highest rates of smoking, exposure to SHS and tobacco-related diseases, and the lowest rates of bans. Tijuana's rates were significantly different from Guadalajara for SHS exposure, smoking bans, and tobacco-related diseases. These findings suggest a dose-response relationship between exposure to the CTCP and the prevalence of tobacco-related behaviors that parallels the different levels of antitobacco contingencies generated by the CTCP. This study provided evidence of construct validity by evaluating the degree of modeling, social criticism or praise for tobacco use, SHS exposure and home bans. Most of these variables followed the same city pattern with more criticism for tobacco use in San Diego and the least in Guadalajara. This suggests that the California culture with respect to tobacco control has influenced the culture of Tijuana, as compared to that of Guadalajara. If these results are valid, it suggests that cultural contingencies may be transmitted through social interaction with populations of other nations even in absence of similar tobacco control taxation and restriction policies in those other nations. We believe California's CTCP has served as a model for the rapid increase in the number of countries that have banned smoking in public buildings. If our assumption is correct, it provides an example of cascading contingencies as predicted by the BEM.

Sexual Behavior

Sexual behavior is a culturally sensitive topic and yet one that must be addressed in order to provide a complete accounting of human health-related behavior and in order to control sexually transmitted diseases. In this context, Cohen and colleagues followed an early ecological model and distributed free condoms in New Orleans and showed that African American women obtained and reported using condoms at a higher rate than was true prior to the free distribution (Cohen, 1999). However, Anglo women and males did not report these changes in response to free distribution. This led to consideration of how condom retrieval and use might well be context-driven. Martinez-Donate and colleagues conducted a quasi-experimental study of sex education and condom distribution for Mexican adolescents in order to test hypothesis about possible motivating operations (moderating context variables) that might alter the use of a free condom kiosk on school grounds (Martinez-Donate, Hovell, et al., 2004; Zellner et al., 2006). This study was based on the BEM and showed that workshop education changed youth attitudes about condoms and sexual initiation. When a condom distribution kiosk was added to schools with and without previous workshop educational programs, results showed that youth who had access to the workshop and a condom kiosk distribution service obtained more condoms and decreased reported sexual initiation compared to kiosk or workshop-only conditions. While these associations do not fully test motivating operations, they are congruent with the BEM, where the workshop education enhanced the use of a condom distribution kiosk on campus. This pilot study relied on self-reported practices and, as such, remains to be replicated with more objective outcome measures.

Literature concerning professional sex workers suggests that higher rates of condom use and lower rates of infection are observed for those who work in brothels where condom use is required and where medical examinations, including HIV testing, are routine, where condoms are provided and where supervision requires adherence to condom use. The 100 percent condom use program in Thailand provides a remarkable quasi-experimental test of such contingencies. In this program condoms were provided in brothels, a policy of 100 percent use of condoms was initiated nationwide, and brothel staff supervised the use of condoms, medical examinations were provided periodically, and media programs promoted the program. Over ten years, the rates of sexually transmitted infections decreased dramatically and the rates of condom use increased equally dramatically (Rojanapitahayakorn, 2006).

This type of program required a cultural foundation in Thailand that enabled a profoundly different approach from that normally employed in the United States.

The approach was coordinated nationally, funded nationally, and involved means of preventing disease instead of means of preventing or suppressing sexual practices. This difference almost certainly made a major difference in the success of the program. Understanding which cultures might approach HIV or other sexually transmitted infections in this manner might enable this program to be replicated more efficiently. Understanding how to engineer cultures might enable the promotion of cultural contingencies that would avoid most sexually transmitted diseases without requiring abstinence.

These few examples concerning sexual behavior and control or prevention of HIV infections suggest that complex motivating operations and race/ethnicity-specific cultures can alter the effects of traditional sex education on the use of a free condom distribution service. The larger literature also suggests that relatively powerful social penalties can alter condom use among professional sex workers supervised in brothels. While these examples do not point to means of completely preventing HIV and AIDS, they do suggest that powerful contingencies may alter the behavior that is normally a function of very powerful natural contingencies supporting sexual behavior in absence of condoms.

Physical Activity, the Physical Environment, and Cultural Practices

Sallis and colleagues (1990) showed that persons who lived near fee-for-service exercise facilities, such as fitness centers, were more likely to engage in vigorous physical activity. We hypothesized that these facilities served as cues—that people entering, leaving, and exercising in and around fitness centers serve as behavioral models for exercising and that the incidental interaction with individuals who exercise in the fitness center or nearby might provide social reinforcement for physical activity. Thus, the density of models and social contingencies may account for the relationship between activity and exercise centers.

These types of associations raise questions about direction of causation. It is difficult to know whether fitness centers cause people to be more active or whether already-active people are more likely to live where fitness centers are located. Both are likely. Experiments can disentangle these relationships by studying sedentary immigrants to a neighborhood with fitness centers, or vice versa. The BEM calls for these types of interventions.

To test the effects of behavioral modeling in a natural setting, our recent study based on the BEM employed individuals to ascend and descend a public staircase adjacent to an escalator, thereby producing behavioral models for stair use (Adams et al., 2006). Using direct observation, we found that participants' stair use increased by two to three times in the presence of models compared to no model conditions, after controlling for participants personal characteristics, clothing, social interactions, and baggage.

Our behavioral modeling study may have cultural implications. Three prior stair-use studies, not based on the BEM, observed the effect of sign prompts on stair use (Blamey, Mutrie, and Aitchison, 1995; Brownell, Stunkard, and Albaum 1980; Kerr,

Eves, and Carroll, 2001) at a number of commuter stations and shopping malls. These long-term studies concluded that their effects persisted up to sixteen weeks after sign prompts were removed. While those initially exposed to the signs may continue to use the stairs, these studies did not explain how stair use could persist even among people who never previously saw the signs. Our theory postulates, and our modeling study suggests, that the sign prompts establish a base rate of models engaging in stair use, and that the greater number of people using the stairs can act as interlocked behavioral models that prompt others to use the stairs. Second-generation converts (people not exposed to the sign, but prompted by people who were exposed to the sign) may become models for even more people. This cascading transmission of behavior could explain sustained stair use without repeated exposure to the sign intervention. This may set the stage for development of a stair climbing "culture," especially if individuals who have been exposed to it in commuter stations or shopping malls begin to use stairs more frequently in other settings. Behavioral models can "recruit" new individuals to stair use and as such can be viewed as recruiting new members to the culture of stair use in a given setting. While the threshold density of models and/or reinforcement contingencies required to tip the current culture to an alternative healthy behavior is currently unknown, this type of behavioral evolution is predicted by the BEM, might be engineered, and should be studied using both observational and experimental procedures.

SUMMARY

The BEM offers a logical means of integrating natural sciences, especially biology, physiology and ecology, with behavioral and social sciences. This potential integration is based on adoption of principles of evolution of species, specifically the assumption of variability and selecting environments that define the species on the globe today. This selectionist model is extended to the selection of responses in the repertoire of an individual based on reinforcement contingencies from the physical and social environment of the individual. However, this alone does not integrate the social sciences. Borrowing again on the selectionist concepts, metacontingencies involve interlocking behavior and interlocking contingencies among members of a defined group of people and their larger cultural society. Their collective behavior yields one or more common product not possible by individual behavior alone (for example, firefighters who can put out home fires efficiently) and who garner the social reinforcement from community members and agencies (for example, city councils) based on the common product (for example, successful firefighting results). The BEM also asserts that metacontingencies contribute to the establishment and maintenance of cultures and subcultures, and that specific subcultures may select for other subcultures. However, we freely admit that the science that follows the BEM for study of cultures is rare and that leaves us with little to no library of predictable effects from observation of one cultural metacontingency to another. The infinite number of complex relationships among biological, intrapersonal and social systems is overwhelming, similar to the task of understanding the human genome and the infinite interactions possible among genes, among epigenetic factors, let alone their interactions with varying environments. Applied Behavior Analysis offers a model science for the study of behavior in the real world. This is important for testing and refining the BEM, because the very features of the BEM that warrant study are hierarchical and interacting factors from the larger society all the way "down" to the biology of individuals. The factors present in a given national culture, for instance, cannot be easily duplicated in an analogue laboratory context. The BEM requires extensive study of existing systems, using observational, quasi-experimental or natural experimental designs to confirm hypotheses, refine others and add to the depth of mechanisms implied by the current model. No doubt the empirical foundation for this model, as we have conceptualized it, is stronger than what we have presented in this brief chapter. Indeed it is founded in part on the already-established sciences of evolutionary biology and behavior analysis, among others. Similarly, new science will no doubt require modification in some of the concepts or in our interpretation of probable effects of complex interacting factors across biological through international social systems. This chapter might prompt others to help with the spadework necessary to test the model and add to the details of mechanisms by which health behavior of populations evolves and how we might use these principles to engineer cultures that insure health practices of all members of society.

Finally, because the BEM is focused on human behavior at the population level, it offers the possibility of making huge differences in whole cultures and doing so

relatively fast. This is likely to be derived from careful and experimental study of policy and laws, as special cases of contingencies that might impact whole cultures and subcultures and even most individuals simultaneously. The World Health Organization is a relatively new invention by humankind. It has limited support from member countries but even with this limitation it has evolved in its ability to influence health policies worldwide. This is evident in the first international health treaty signed by most of the member nations (168 to date, excluding the United States) for tobacco control ("Framework Convention Alliance," n.d.; "WHO Framework Convention on Tobacco Control," n.d.). Even without financial reinforcers or penalties or other policing powers, this policy has had major impact on governments' compliance with tobacco control guidelines. This illustrates the potential for international policies to have impact on health behavior nationally and internationally. Making entry into the European Union contingent on the WHO standards has undoubtedly helped move compliance with the tobacco treaty for countries in Central Europe, where such membership offers substantial financial benefit. Imagine how powerful such a treaty might be if large financial assistance were contingent on the decreasing national prevalence of smoking and tobacco sales, and on increasing the number of places in which smoking is banned (such as workplaces, public places). We humbly submit that the BEM offers the possibility of science that will make such policies more effective and more efficient; that will teach us how to eliminate the health risk behavior of specific subcultures, while selecting for subcultures (other group practices) that insure health.

ACKNOWLEDGMENTS

This report was supported, in part, by grants (*National Children's Study* NIH, # NIH-NICHD-NCS-07–11W (HHSN267200700021C); *Sirocco* NIH, NHLBI, #1RO1 HL066307; *Mechanisms of Physical Activity* NIH, NCI, #RO1 CA113828) and from intramural funds from the Center for Behavioral Epidemiology and Community Health (CBEACH), San Diego State University. We acknowledge many colleagues and students who have helped shape the concepts presented in this chapter.

REFERENCES

Adams, M. A., Hovell, M. F., Irvin, V., Sallis, J. F., Coleman, K. J., and Liles, S. (2006). Promoting stair use by modeling: An experimental application of the behavioral ecological model. *American Journal of Health Promotion*, *21*, 101–109.

Adams, M. A., Norman G. J., Hovell M. F., Sallis J. F., and Patrick, K. (2009). Reconceptualizing decisional balance in an adolescent sun protection intervention: mediating effects and theoretical interpretations. *Health Psychology*, *28*, 217–225.

Ader, R., Felten, D. L., and Cohen, N. (Eds.) (1991). *Psychoneuroimmunology*. San Diego, CA: Academic Press.

Baer, D. M., and Deguchi, H. (1985). Generalized imitation from a radical-behavioral viewpoint. In S. Reiss and R. R. Bootzin (eds.), *Theoretical issues in behavior therapy*, (pp. 176–217). Orlando, FL: Academic Press.

Baer, D. M., Peterson, R. F., and Sherman, J. A. (1967). The development of imitation by reinforcing behavioral similarity to a model. *Journal of the Experimental Analysis of Behavior*, *10*, 405–16.

Baer, D. M, Wolf M. M., and Risley T. R. (1968). Some current dimensions of applied behavior analysis. *Journal of Applied Behavior Analysis*, *1*, 91–97.

Baer, D. M, Wolf M. M., and Risley T. R. (1987). Some still-current dimensions of applied behavior analysis. *Journal of Applied Behavior Analysis*, *20*, 313–327.

Barnes-Holmes, D., and Barnes-Holmes, Y. (2000). Explaining complex behavior: Two perspectives on the concept of generalized operant classes. *The Psychological Record*, *50*, 251–265.

Baum, W. M. (2005). *Understanding behaviorism: Behavior, culture, and evolution*. Malden, MA: Blackwell Publishing.

Biglan, A. (1995). *Changing cultural practices: A contextualist framework for intervention research*. Reno, NV: Context Press.

Biglan, A. (2003). Selection by consequences: One unifying principle for a transdisciplinary science of prevention. *Prevention Science*, *4*, 213–232.

Biglan, A., and Hayes, S. C. (1996). Should the behavioral sciences become more pragmatic? The case for functional contextualism in research on human behavior. *Applied and Preventive Psychology. Current Scientific Perspectives*, *5*, 47–57.

Blamey, A., Mutrie, N., and Aitchison, T. (1995). Health promotion by encouraged use of stairs. *British Medical Journal*, *311*, 289–290.

Bousman, C. A., Blumberg, E. J., Shillington, A. M., Hovell, M. F., Ji, M., Lehman, S., et al. (2005). Predictors of substance use among homeless youth in San Diego. *Addictive Behavior*, *30*, 1100–1110.

Brownell, K. D., Stunkard, A. J., and Albaum, J. M. (1980). Evaluation and modification of exercise patterns in the natural environment. *American Journal of Psychiatry*, *137*, 1540–1545.

Brigham, T. A., and Sherman, J. A. (1968). An experimental analysis of verbal imitation in preschool children. *Journal of Applied Behavior Analysis*, *1*, 151–158.

Catania, A. C. *Learning* (4th ed.). Upper Saddle River, NJ: Prentice Hall. 1998.

Chiesa, M. *Radical behaviorism: the philosophy and the science*. Boston: Authors Cooperative. 1994.

Cohen, D. A. (1999). Condom availability for HIV/STD prevention. *AIDS Patient Care and STDs, 13*, 731–737.

Cooper, J. O., Heron, T. E., and Heward, W. L. (2006). *Applied behavior analysis*. Columbus, OH: Prentice Hall.

Cuff, P. A., and Vanselow, N. (2004). *Improving medical education: Enhancing the behavioral and social science content of medical school curricula*. Washington DC: National Academy Press.

DeBate, R. D., and Pyle, G. F. (2004). The behavioral ecological model: A framework for early WIC participation. *American Journal of Health Studies, 19*, 138–147.

Diamond, J. (2005). *Collapse: How societies choose to fail or succeed*. New York: Viking.

Daily, G. C., Ehrlich, A. H., and Ehrlich, P. R. (1994). Optimum human population size. *Population and Environment, 15*, 469–475.

Dresler-Hawke, E., and Veer, E. (2006). Making healthy eating messages more effective: Combining integrated marketing communication with the behaviour ecological model. *International Journal of Consumer Studies, 30*, 318–326.

Ehrlich, P. R., and Ehrlich, A. H. (2004). *One with Nineveh: Politics, consumption, and the human future*. Washington, DC: Island Press.

Elder, J. P., Wildey, M., de Moor, C., Sallis, J. F., Eckhardt, L., Edwards, C., et al. (1993) The long-term prevention of tobacco use among junior high school students: Classroom and telephone interventions. *American Journal of Public Health, 83*, 1239–44.

Epstein, R. (1999). Generativity theory. In M. Runco and S. Pritzker (eds.) *Encyclopedia of creativity, Vol 1*. San Diego CA: Academic Press.

Fantino, E., and Logan, C. A. (1979). *The experimental analysis of behavior: A biological perspective*. New York: Freeman.

Fernander, A. F., Shavers, V. L., Hammons, G. J. (2007) A biopsychosocial approach to examining tobacco-related health disparities among racially classified social groups. *Addiction, 102* (suppl.2) 43–57.

Ferster, C. B., and Skinner, B. F. (1957). *Schedules of reinforcement*. New York: Appleton-Century-Crofts.

Framework Convention Alliance. (n.d.). Retrieved January 11, 2008, from http://www.fctc.org.

Galbicka, G. (1994). Shaping in the 21st century: Moving percentile schedules into applied settings. *Journal of Applied Behavior Analysis, 27*, 739–760.

Gewirtz, J. L., and Stingle, K. G. (1968). Learning of generalized imitation as the basis for identification. *Psychological Review, 75*, 374–397.

Glenn, S. (1988). Contingencies and metacontingencies: Toward a synthesis of behavior analysis and cultural materialism. *The Behavior Analyst, 11*, 161–179.

Glenn, S. (1991). Contingencies and metacontingencies: Relations among behavioral, cultural, and biological evolution. In P. A. Lamal, (ed.), *Behavior analysis of societies and cultural practices* (pp. 39–73). Washington, DC: Hemisphere Publishing.

Glenn, (2004). Individual behavior, culture and social change. *The Behavior Analyst. 27*, 133–151.

Glenn, S. and Malagodi, E. F. (1991). Process and content in behavioral and cultural phenomena. *Behavior and Social Issues, 1*, 1–14.

Hayes, S. C. (1989). *Rule-governed behavior: Cognition, contingencies, and instructional control*. New York: Plenum Press.

Hill, A. (1965). Environment and disease—association or causation. *Proceedings of the Royal Society of Medicine—London. 58*:295–300.

Hofstetter, C. R., Hovell, M. F., Lee, J., Zakarian, J., Park, H., Paik, H. Y., et al. (2004). Tobacco use and acculturation among Californians of Korean descent: A behavioral epidemiological analysis. *Nicotine and Tobacco Research, 6*, 481–489.

Hofstetter, C. R., Irvin, V., Schmitz, K., Hovell, M. F., Nichols, J., Kim, H. R., et al. (2008). Demography of exercise among Californians of Korean descent: A cross-sectional telephone survey. *Journal of Immigrant and Minority Health, 10*, 53–65.

Houmanfar, R., and Rodrigues, N. J. (2006). The metacontingency and the behavioral contingency: Points of contact and departure. *Behavior and Social Issues, 15*, 13–30.

Hovell, M. F., Kaplan R., and Hovell F. (1991). Analysis of preventive medical services in the U.S. In P. A. Lamal, (ed.), *Behavior analysis of societies and cultural practices* (pp. 181–200). Washington, DC: Hemisphere Publishing.

Hovell, M., Russos, S., Hill, L., Johnson, N. W., Squier, C., and Gyenes, M. (2004). Engineering clinician leadership and success in tobacco control: Recommendations for policy and practice in Hungary and Central Europe. *European Journal of Dental Education*, *8*, 51–60.

Hovell, M. F., Russos, S., Beckhelm, M. K., Jones, J. A., Burkham-Kreitner, S. M., Slymen, D. J., et al. (1995). Compliance with primary prevention in private practice: Creating a tobacco-free environment. *American Journal of Preventive Medicine*, *11*, 288–293.

Hovell, M. F., Wahlgren, D. R., and Gehrman, C. A. (2002). The behavioral ecological model: Integrating public health and behavioral science. In R. J. DiClemente (Ed.), *Emerging theories in health promotion practice and research: Strategies for improving public health, first edition* (pp. 347–385). San Francisco: Jossey-Bass.

Hovell, M. F., Wahlgren D. R., and Russos S. (1997). Preventive medicine and cultural contingencies: The great natural experiment. In P.A. Lamal, (ed.), *Cultural contingencies: Behavior analytic perspectives on cultural practices* (pp. 1–29). Westport, Connecticut: Praeger Publications.

Jeffery, R. W. (2004). How can Health Behavior Theory be made more useful for intervention research? *International Journal of Behavioral Nutrition and Physical Activity*, *1*, 10.

Johns, M. B., Hovell, M. F., Drastal, C. A., Lamke, C., and Patrick, K. (1992). Promoting prevention services in primary care: A controlled trial. *American Journal of Preventive Medicine*, *8*, 135–140.

Kerr, K. Eves, F., and Carroll, D. (2001). Six-month observational study of prompted stair climbing. *Preventive Medicine*, *33*, 422–427.

Landrine, H., and Klonoff, E. A. (2004). Culture change and ethnic-minority health behavior: An operant theory of acculturation. *Journal of Behavioral Medicine*, *27*, 527–555.

Lattal, K. A., and Neef, N. A. (1996). Recent reinforcement-schedule research and applied behavior analysis. *Journal of Applied Behavior Analysis*, *29*, 213–230.

Lavelle, J. M., Hovell, M. F., West, M. P., and Wahlgren, D. R. (1992). Promoting law enforcement for child protection: a community analysis. *Journal of Applied Behavior Analysis*, *25*, 885–892.

Malagodi, E. F. (1986). On radicalizing behaviorism. A call for cultural analysis. *The Behavior Analyst*, *9*, 1–17.

Malagodi, E. F., and Jackson, K. (1989). Behavior analysts and cultural analysis: Troubles and issues. *The Behavior Analyst*, *12*, 17–33.

Martinez-Donate, A. P., Blumberg, E. J., Hovell, M. F., Sipan, C. L., Zellner, J. A., and Hughes, S. (2004). Risk for HIV infection among adolescents in the border city of Tijuana, Mexico. *Hispanic Journal of Behavioral Sciences*, *26*, 407–425.

Martinez-Donate, A. P., Hovell, M. F., Hofstetter, C. R., Gonzalez-Perez, G. J., Kotay, A., and Adams, M.A. (2008). Crossing borders: Impact of the California Tobacco Control Program on both sides of the U.S.-Mexico border. *American Journal of Public Health*. *98*(2), 258–267.

Martinez-Donate, A. P., Hovell, M. F., Hofstetter, C. R., Gonzalez-Perez, G. J., Adams, M. A., and Kotay, A. (2007) Correlates of home smoking bans among Mexican-Americans. *American Journal of Health Promotion*, *21*, 229–236.

Martinez-Donate, A. P., Hovell, M. F., Zellner, J., Sipan, C. L., Blumberg, E. J., and Carrizosa, C. (2004). Evaluation of two school-based HIV prevention interventions in the border city of Tijuana, Mexico. *Journal of Sex Research*, *41*, 267–278.

McGinnis, J. M., and Foege, W. H. (1993). Actual causes of death in the United States. *Journal of the American Medical Association*, *270*, 2207–2212.

Michael, J. (2000). Implications and refinements of the establishing operation concept. *Journal of Applied Behavior Analysis*, *33*, 401–410.

Michael, J. (2007). Motivating operations. In J. O. Cooper, T. E. Heron and W. L. Heward, *Applied behavior analysis* (2nd ed.) Upper Saddle River, NJ: Prentice Hall/Merrill.

Myers, C. A., Hovell, M. F., Elder, J. P., and Hall, J. A. (1991). Paradoxical effects of blood alcohol concentration charts. *Preventive Medicine*, *20*, 431–435.

National Cancer Institute. Greater than the sum: Systems thinking in tobacco control. *Tobacco control monograph No. 18*. Bethesda, MD: U.S. Department of Health and Human Services, National Institutes of Health, National Cancer Institute. NIH Pub. No. 06–6085, April 2007.

Pavlov, I. P. (1927). *Conditioned reflexes*. (Tr. by G. V. Anrep) London: Oxford University Press.

Poulos, C. X., Hinson, R. E., and Siegel, S. (1981). The role of Pavlovian processes in drug tolerance and dependence: implications for treatment. *Addictive Behaviors*, *6*, 205–211.

Rojanapithayakorn, W. (2006). The 100 percent condom use programme in Asia. *Reproductive Health Matters 14*, 41–52.

Russos, S., Keating, K., Hovell, M. F., Jones, J. A., Slymen, D. J., Hofstetter, C. R., et al. (1999). Counseling youth in tobacco-use prevention: determinants of clinician compliance. *Preventive Medicine*, *29*, 13–21.

Sallis, J. F., Hovell, M. F., Hofstetter, C. R., Elder, J. P., Hackley, M., Caspersen, C. J., et al. (1990). Distance between homes and exercise facilities related to frequency of exercise among San Diego residents. *Public Health Reports*, *105*, 179–185.

Schroeder, S. T., Hovell, M. F., Kolody, B., and Elder, J. P. (2004). Use of newsletters to promote environmental political action: An experimental analysis. *Journal of Applied Behavior Analysis*, *37*, 427–429.

Schumaker, J. B., Hovell, M. F., and Sherman, J. A. (1977). An analysis of daily report cards and parent managed privileges in the improvement of adolescents' classroom performance. *Journal of Applied Behavior Analysis*, *10*, 449–464.

Sidman, M. (1960). *Tactics of scientific research: evaluating experimental data in psychology*. Boston: Authors Cooperative.

Siegel, S. (1975) Evidence from rats that morphine tolerance is a learned response. *Journal of Comparative and Physiological Psychology*, *89*, 498–506.

Siegel, S. (1982). Heroin "overdose" death: contribution of drug-associated environmental cues. *Science*, *216*, 436–437.

Skinner, B. F. (1938). *The behavior of organisms*. New York: Appleton-Century-Crofts.

Skinner, B. F. (1974). *About behaviorism*. New York: Vintage Books.

Skinner, B. F. (1953). *Science and human behavior*. New York: Macmillan.

Skinner, B. F. (1981). Selection by consequences. *Science*, *213*, 501–504.

Song, Y. J., Hofstetter, C. R., Hovell, M. F., Paik, H. Y., Park, H. R., Lee, J., et al. (2004). Acculturation and health risk behaviors among Californians of Korean descent. *Preventive Medicine*, *39*, 147–156.

Wahlgren, D. R., Hovell, M. F., Meltzer, S. B., Hofstetter, C. R., and Zakarian, J. M. (1997). Reduction of environmental tobacco smoke exposure in asthmatic children. A two-year follow-up. *Chest*, *111*, 81–88.

Wahlgren, D. R., Hovell, M. F., Slymen, D. J., Conway, T. L., Hofstetter, C. R., and Jones, J. A. (1997). Predictors of tobacco use initiation in adolescents: A two-year prospective study and theoretical discussion. *Tobacco Control*, *6*, 95–103.

West, R. (2005) Time for a change: putting the Transtheoretical Model to rest. *Addiction*, *100*, 1036–1039.

WHO Framework Convention on Tobacco Control. (n.d.). Retrieved January 11, 2008, from http://www.who .int/tobacco/framework/en/.

WHO study group on tobacco product regulation, advisory note: waterpipe tobacco smoking: Health effects, research needs and recommended actions by regulators. (2005). Geneva, Switzerland: World Health Organization. Available at: http://www.who.int/tobacco/global_interaction/tobreg/waterpipe/en/index.html.

Wilson, D.S., Van Vugt, M., O'Gorman, R. (2008) Multilevel Selection Theory and major evolutionary transitions: implications for psychological science. *Current Directions in Psychological Science*, *17*, 6–9.

Zakarian, J. M., Hovell, M. F., Sandweiss, R. D., Hofstetter, C. R., Matt, G. E., Bernert, J. T., et al. (2004). Behavioral counseling for reducing children's ETS exposure: implementation in community clinics. *Nicotine and Tobacco Research*, *6*, 1061–1074.

Zellner, J. A., Martinez-Donate, A. P., Hovell, M. F., Sipan, C. L., Blumberg, E. J., Carrizosa, C. M. et al. (2006). Feasibility and use of school-based condom availability programs in Tijuana, Mexico. *AIDS and Behavior*, *10*, 649–657.

CHAPTER

16

THE THEORY OF TRIADIC INFLUENCE

Brian R. Flay
Frank J. Snyder
John Petraitis

INFLUENCING HEALTH-ENHANCING BEHAVIOR

Anyone in the business of health promotion (HP) must know two things: what causes health-related behaviors (HRBs), and how to effectively promote health-enhancing behaviors (like wearing seatbelts) or deter health-compromising behaviors (like smoking cigarettes). This knowledge, however, has been evasive because (1) the causes of behavior are many and varied, each cause being just one piece in a complex puzzle of causes (Petraitis, Flay, and Miller, 1995); (2) different theories of behavior have focused on different aspects of the puzzle; (3) theories are difficult to confirm, clouding our understanding with uncertainty; and (4) the translation of any theory into HP programs is limited by the scope of the theory, such that narrowly focused theories lead to narrowly focused interventions. For example, some theories of health behavior (HB) focus on proximal affective/cognitive predictors of behavior like self-efficacy, social normative beliefs, attitudes and intentions (for example, Ajzen, 1991; Fishbein and Ajzen, 1975), while others focus on ultimate or underlying causes in the broad sociocultural environment (Biglan, 2004), social situations (Magnusson, 1981), or biology (for example, Frankenhaeuser, 1991; Sher, 1991) and personality (Digman, 1990; Zuckerman, Ball, and Black, 1990). Yet other theories focus on interpersonal situations, social support, and bonding processes (for example, Elliott, Huizinga, and Ageton, 1985; Hawkins and Weis, 1985; Oetting and Beauvais, 1986), or social learning processes (for example, Akers, Krohn, Lanza-Kaduce, and Radosevich, 1979; Bandura, 1977). Very few extant theories of HB incorporate several of these viewpoints (for example, Bandura, 1986; Jessor and Jessor, 1977; Jessor et al., 2003), and those that do are limited in various ways.

We believe that some new ideas about HRBs and HP can be found in our integrative theory, the theory of triadic influence (TTI) (Flay and Petraitis, 1994). The TTI provides a meta-theoretical orientation that suggests higher-order descriptions and explanations of HRB, offers a detailed ecological approach to HB change, and suggests that an increased focus on distal and ultimate levels of influence will produce greater and more sustainable HP effects than the traditional (at least in the United States) focus on affective/cognitive approaches. This chapter provides a brief explanation of why a comprehensive theory of HB is needed, a general overview of the TTI, examples of how it explains a variety of HRBs, empirical evidence for its propositions, a description, some examples of how it can be applied in HP, and some conclusions and comments about future developments.

GENESIS OF THE THEORY OF TRIADIC INFLUENCE

Before introducing the TTI, we explain the need for an integrative theory of HRBs. Scholars have proposed dozens of different theories of various HRBs. For example, Lettieri, Sayers, and Pearson (1980) identified forty-three different theories that attempted to explain the development of substance use. These theories spanned a broad range of disciplines (from neuroscience to political science) and an even broader range of variables (from disorganized social institutions to the spur-of-the moment decision to use substances). Most of these forty-three theories were rather narrow in scope, simply because earlier attempts to develop health behavior theories had to focus on smaller, manageable, and measurable components that contribute to a specific HB. In the decades since the review by Lettieri et al. the number of theories and variables that contribute to HB has grown, leaving planners of HP programs with a puzzle that had scores of pieces (variables), different ways of putting the pieces together (theories) and different sections of the puzzle complete or incomplete. Unfortunately, this predicament leads to considerable confusion and little agreement about how to design HP programs.

After carefully reviewing theories of HB (Petraitis et al., 1995), we recognized that theories and variables could be organized along two dimensions (Table 16.1), levels of causation and streams of influence, and we proposed the TTI (Flay and Petraitis, 1994) to reduce confusion and to integrate the scores of potentially relevant variables and theories in a conceptually meaningful way. Our focus was on developing a more comprehensive theory that would provide a set of testable and practical guidelines for both understanding the causes of HRBs and developing effective HP programs. Thus, in the terms of Glanz, Rimer, and Lewis (2002, pp. 25–26), the TTI represents both (1) a theory of the problem, in which the focus is on explanation and prediction of HB, and (2) a change theory, or theory of action, in which the emphasis is on guiding the development of HP interventions.

The TTI proposes that theories and variables can be arranged by different *levels (or tiers) of causation* (see Table 16.1). Some variables (like intentions) have direct effects on behavior and are *causally proximal or immediate*; some variables (like motivation to comply with or please others) have effects that are mediated through other variables (like social normative beliefs) and are more *causally distal or predisposing*; other variables (like the style of parenting one experienced during childhood or taxes on cigarettes) are mediated by even more variables and are even more *causally distal*; and yet other variables (like ethnic culture, neighborhood poverty, or personality) represent the *underlying or ultimate causes* of behavior.

The TTI also proposes that theories and variables can be arranged into three relatively distinct types or *streams of influence* (see Table 16.1), corresponding to the Person, Situation, and Environment of other theorists (Bandura, 1986; Frankenhaeuser, 1991; Lewin, 1951; Magnusson, 1981; Sadava, 1987), each of which acts through the levels of causation:

1. Intra-PERSONAL Influences are intrapersonal characteristics that contribute to one's self-efficacy regarding specific behaviors;
2. Interpersonal SOCIAL Influences are the social situation/context or micro-environment that contribute to social normative beliefs about specific behaviors; and
3. Cultural-ENVIRONMENTAL Influences are multiple sociocultural macro-environmental factors that contribute to attitudes toward specific behaviors.

TABLE 16.1   **A Matrix of Selected Theories of Social and Health Behavior: Streams of Influence and Levels of Causation.**

	Streams of Influence		
Levels of Causation	Intrapersonal (Biological and **P**ersonality) →Self-efficacy	Interpersonal or **S**ocial Situation/Context →Normative Beliefs	Sociocultural **E**nvironment →Attitudinal
Ultimate causes	Biological Psychoanalytic Personality Resilience Self-control	Social control (Elliott) Family systems (Brook) Parenting styles Peer clustering (Oetting)	Class conflict Low SES Anomie Social Disorganization Strain (Merton) Radical theories
Distal influences	Personal competence Self-esteem Self-derogation (Kaplan) Personal control	Social attachment/ bonding Social development (Hawkins) Differential association Social learning	General knowledge Cultural identity Values theories Motivation theories
Proximal predictors	Social skills Self-regulation Self-efficacy	Conformity Social normative beliefs	Expectancy Subjective utility Attitude
	Theories of decision making and problem solving, Theory of Reasoned Action (Fishbein and Ajzen), Theory of Planned Behavior (Ajzen)		
Integrative	Social Cognitive Theory (Bandura), Problem Behavior Theory (Jessor), Feedback systems theories		

See text and reference list for references

The TTI then proposes that the effects of ultimate and distal causes of behavior flow predominantly within each stream (that is, *personal, social,* and *environmental* factors) and act through a small set of proximal predictors of behavior (self-efficacy, social normative beliefs, attitudes, and intentions), with multiple mediating factors between (Figure 16.1).

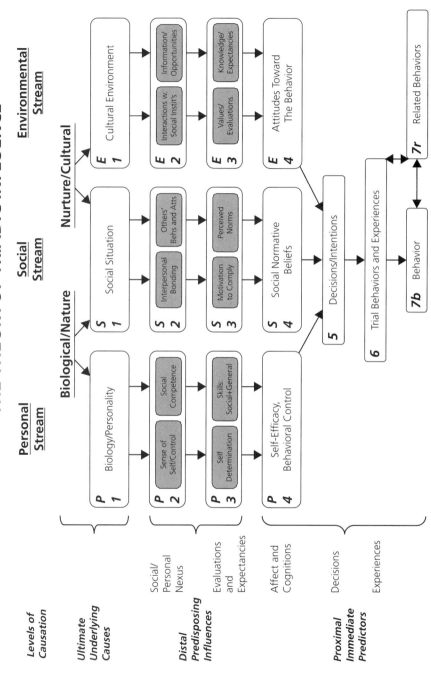

THE THEORY OF TRIADIC INFLUENCE

Note: In this chapter, we consider the three streams and six substreams in the reverse order, or mirror image, compared to our previous presentations. This is in response to suggestions from others that it is a little easier for many people to think from persons outward to the environment and illustratively from left to right.

The TTI is one of the most comprehensive and integrative theories of HB to date and is actually relevant for all types of behavior (for example, saving money for retirement). As can be seen in Figure 16.1, the TTI begins with the simple but important assumption that the trial of a behavior is most immediately determined by one's decisions (Gerrard, Gibbons, Houlihan, Stock, and Pomery, 2008; Reyna and Rivers, 2008; Steinberg, 2008) or intentions (Fishbein and Ajzen, 1975). For example, a person's decisions precede the use of cigarettes, seat belts, or condoms. Consequently, the challenge for health promoters is to influence health decisions. Decisions are sometimes habitual (Wood, Quinn, and Kashy, 2002) and sometimes made in the heat of the moment (compare with hot cognition or emotionally influenced decision-making—Dahl, 2001, 2004); indeed, emotion is integral to both intuition and decision making (Gerrard et al., 2008; Mills, Reyna, and Estrada, 2008; Reyna and Farley, 2006a; Reyna and Rivers, 2008; Rivers, Reyna, and Mills, 2008; Steinberg, 2008; Sunstein, 2008). The TTI then asserts that three relatively independent paths—each ranging from ultimate, through distal, to proximal tiers of influences or causation—converge on health-related decisions/intentions that, in turn, lead to trial behaviors and then, depending on the experience, repeated or alternative behaviors.

The three major streams of influence each include *two sub-streams*. One sub-stream is more *cognitive and rational* in nature, based for example on an objective weighing of the perceived pros (for example, losing ten pounds) and cons (for example, giving up favorite foods) concerning a given behavior (for example, starting a diet). The other sub-stream that influences behavior is more *affective* or emotional and less rational (for example, wanting to look good for a high-school reunion, or no longer caring how one looks). Thus, decisions are not always entirely rational; they may include an affective or emotional component (compare with *hot cognition*) as well as a cognitive or rational component.

The theory also recognizes that influences in one path are often mediated by or moderate (or interact with) influences in another path. The TTI also recognizes that engaging in a behavior may have effects that feed back and alter the original causes of the behavior. Finally, the theory leads to implications for both understanding the causes of behavior and the development of effective forms of HP.

In summary, the TTI consists of multiple tiers/levels of causation, three major streams each with two sub-streams of influence, dozens of predictions about direct and indirect (mediated) pathways and interactions (moderation) between variables, and feedback loops. In the next section, we provide an in-depth overview of the TTI.

AN IN-DEPTH OVERVIEW OF THE THEORY OF TRIADIC INFLUENCE

Levels of Causation, Influence, and Prediction

As noted above, the TTI arranges the myriad causes of behavior into a set of tiers or levels that represent their causal distance from behavior. We use the term "cause" in the probabilistic sense (Eells, 1991; Suppes, 1970), not in the deterministic sense of Galileo or Hume. Epidemiologists and some behavioral scientists use the terms "risk factors," "protective factors," or "risk regulators" (Glass and McAtee, 2006; Hawkins, Catalano, and Miller, 1992; Jessor et al., 2003; Jessor, Van Den Bos, Vabderryn, Costa, and Turbin, 1995; Rutter and Garmezy, 1983; Werner and Smith, 1992) instead of "causes" because they are not deterministic. However, we think it is appropriate to think in terms of *probabilistic causation*, whereby a cause increases the probability of a consequence. See Glass and McAtee (2006) for an extensive discussion of this issue. In addition, as we will describe below, these probabilistic causes occur at different levels of causation with regard to (1) the strength of the causal link, and (2) the distance between the cause and the behavior in terms of the number of mediating links that may exist between a particular cause and behavior. Thus, the causes of behavior within each stream are arranged from those causally most distant (ultimate or underlying causes), to those that are causally distal (predisposing influences), to those that are causally closest (proximal or immediate predictors).

Ultimate or underlying causes are the furthest removed from behavior (for example, biological susceptibility, rigid parenting style, poverty rates). They are largely beyond the easy control of any individual and are relatively stable (for example, cultural characteristics of a country or basic personality traits that do not change much). Their effects, however, are the most pervasive (having effects on multiple behaviors), the most mediated, and often the most difficult for any one person or program to change, but, if changed, are likely to have the greatest and longest-lasting influence on a broad array of behaviors. The well-known debate over the relative effects of nature and nurture on behavior usually focuses on ultimate causes (Institute of Medicine, 2006); thus, we place nature and nurture above the three streams of the TTI (Figure 16.1).

Distal influences are one step closer to behavior. The first level of distal causes is at the *social-personal nexus* (for example, rebelliousness, bonding to parents or deviant role models, religious participation), variables that reflect the quality and quantity of contact between individuals and their sociocultural environments, social situations or personality.

Second-order distal influences, another step closer to behavior, are a set of affective/cognitive influences, called *evaluations and expectancies*. They are general values and behavior-specific evaluations as well as general knowledge and specific beliefs that arise out of the contact between individuals and their surroundings. Compared to ultimate-level causes, distal-level influences are less removed from behavior, have effects on behavior that are less mediated, and usually more changeable. At the same time, however, when compared to ultimate-level influences, some distal-level influences are somewhat narrower and more behavior-specific. For instance, as an ultimate-level variable, the quality of healthcare options in a community might have diffuse and indirect effects on cancer screening; by contrast, as a distal-level variable, an individual's health locus of control (which might be influenced by community health care options) probably has more targeted and less mediated effects on her attitudes towards cancer screening.

Proximal predictors of behavior are even closer to behavior and closer to the bottom of Figure 16.1. Self-efficacy, social normative beliefs, and attitudes are (1) less general than evaluations and expectancies on the previous tier, (2) are always specific to a targeted behavior, and (3) have direct effects on decisions/intentions to engage in that behavior.

The more proximal the predictor to a behavior, the more likely it is to be specific to that behavior. For example, attitudes toward cancer screening will be more predictive of cancer screening, but less predictive of hypertension screening or attempts at smoking cessation. Proximal predictors of behavior are also less stable, more likely to change (people's attitudes change, after all, more quickly than their personalities); they might be the easier targets of health programs in the short run, but might have the smallest or shortest-lasting influence and the least generalization to other behaviors.

Within any one level, the variables are usually correlated to some degree (not shown in Figure 16.1). For example, at the ultimate level, a child's personal development is correlated with family structure, which, in turn, is correlated with socioeconomic status (Krieger, 2007). Indeed, modern concepts from developmental psychology were derived from the fusion of biological and contextual levels of organization (Lerner, 1978; Overton, 1973). Similarly, at the proximal level, self-efficacy, social normative beliefs and attitudes regarding a specific behavior are usually correlated (Ajzen, 1988).

We distinguish between the three levels of influence not only by the ultimate, distal and proximal labels, but also by labels of differing degrees of causation—namely underlying causes (that are ultimate), predisposing influences (that are distal) and immediate predictors (that are proximal). Proximal or immediate predictors are usually the strongest predictors of particular behaviors because they are (1) causally closest (most proximal) to the behavior; (2) behavior specific; and (3) because they are behavior-specific, they usually correlate with the behavior being predicted more highly than the more distal influences or ultimate causes. Although ultimate causes often have lower correlations with any particular behavior, they have a causal relationship to many behaviors. In contrast, proximal predictors usually have higher correlations with a particular behavior and not with others. That is, proximal predictors are very specific to a behavior, while ultimate causes have more widespread effects. For example, attitudes toward smoking cigarettes will be highly predictive of cigarette smoking, but probably not of delinquency, whereas social disadvantage might be very predictive of both smoking and delinquency (see Figure 7 in Flay and Petraitis [1994] for one way of depicting this).

Streams of Influence

Figure 16.1 shows that causal effects flow primarily within three streams of influence, converging on behavioral intentions and behaviors. The TTI's intra-PERSONAL stream begins at the ultimate level with relatively stable biological predispositions (for example, testosterone levels) and personality characteristics (for example, the

Big Five: openness to experience, consciousness, extraversion, agreeableness, and neuroticism). The TTI predicts that these ultimate-level intrapersonal influences (labeled as P1 variables in Figure 16.1) have direct effects on social/personal nexus variables in the intrapersonal stream (labeled as P2 variables), including views of one's self (for example, self-esteem), and one's general competencies (for example, locus of control). These P2 variables then have, according to the TTI, direct effects on P3 variables. The P3 variables are more targeted to a specific behavior (for example, attempting to quit smoking), and include one's will or determination to engage in the behavior and one's perceived skills to succeed in the behavior. Rick Snyder (2002; Snyder, Feldman, Taylor, Schroeder, and Adams, 2000) calls this "hope"—the perceived capability (skill) to derive pathways to desired goals, and motivate oneself (will) via agency thinking to use those pathways. Finally, the TTI predicts that P3 variables converge on one's sense of self-efficacy regarding a particular behavior.

A similar flow exists within the TTI's SOCIAL stream. The social stream begins with S1 variables (ultimate-level characteristics of one's immediate social surroundings) that are largely outside the control of individuals (for example, parenting practices during their childhoods, or negative evaluations from family members). It continues through S2 variables (social/personal nexus variables in one's immediate social surroundings), including the strength of the interpersonal bonds with immediate role models, and the relevant behaviors of those role models (for example, whether older family members practice cancer screening). The flow then continues through S3 variables, including one's motivation to comply with various role models (for example, whether to comply more with family members or peers), and perceptions of what behaviors those role models are encouraging. Finally, social influences converge on one's social normative beliefs regarding the specific behavior, that is, the perceptions of social pressures to engage in that particular behavior.

The TTI's third stream, the cultural-ENVIRONMENT stream, follows the same pattern as the previous two streams. It begins with E1 variables—characteristics of one's broader culture that are largely beyond one's personal control, including political, economic, religious, legal, mass media, and policies environments (Minkler, Wallace, and McDonald, 1995). The third stream flows into E2 variables, including the nature of the interactions people have with social institutions (for example, the nature of their relationship with political, legal, religious, and governing systems) and the information they glean from their culture (for example, what they learn from exposure to mass media). The stream then flows through E3 variables, the consequences one expects from a behavior (for example, whether cancer screening is accurate, how much it will cost, and so on) and how one evaluates, favorably or unfavorably, the various consequences of a behavior. Finally, environmental influences converge on one's attitudes toward the specific behavior.

Affective and Cognitive Sub-Streams of Influence

Figure 16.1 shows obvious parallels in how each of the three major streams flow from ultimate-level influences, through distal-level influences and into proximal influences that then converge on intentions. In addition, there are two sub-streams within each of the three major streams. Separately, these sub-streams represent affective and cognitive flows within the major streams. For example, the cultural-ENVIRONMENTAL stream consists of (1) the control/affective domain of the *values environment* (culture, religion, and so on) that informs values and evaluations of consequences, and (2) the cognitive domain of the *informational environment* (media, laws, politics, and so on) that informs knowledge and expectations of the consequences (or expectancies) of a behavior. Classic sociological theorists label the affective sub-stream as *control* (rather than affective), emphasizing how values-forming institutions (religions, laws, and so on), social bonding, and sense of self (and self-control) act as control mechanisms on, or reinforcers of, behavior. Both basic learning theories (Mowrer, 1960) and social learning theories (Akers, 1977; Bandura, 1977) also emphasize how behaviors are reinforced, shaped or controlled (Biglan, 1995; Glenn, 1988).

The affective and cognitive sub-streams both include ultimate causes that are common in multiple political-economy theories of subjective expected utilities (Bauman, 1980; Bauman and Fisher, 1985; Edwards, 1954, 1961) and the related distal and proximal influences common in expectancy-value theories (Atkinson, 1957; Eccles et al., 1983; Feather, 1982). The existence of so many related theories (subjective utility and expectancy-value) underlies the obvious importance of information/knowledge/expectancies and values/evaluations to our behaviors. However, the failure of so many educational campaigns designed to increase awareness of the dangers of health-compromising behaviors also points to the limitations of relying on just these theories or just the proximal levels of this one stream of the TTI for designing effective interventions.

For some readers, the proximal levels of all streams (self-efficacy, social normative beliefs and attitudes) may seem like they are intrapersonal factors. However, we distinguish these affective/cognitive factors that originate from social/interpersonal (social situation → social normative beliefs) or sociocultural (sociocultural environment → attitudes) factors from those that originate in the person (intrapersonal → self-efficacy). Within the TTI, each and every stream ends in affective/cognitive factors (self-efficacy, social normative beliefs and attitudes) that, in turn, influence the most proximal affective/cognitive predictor of behavior, intentions.

Both of the other streams of the TTI also include affective and cognitive sub-streams. For example, the SOCIAL stream includes social attachment or bonding and the desire to please others (or motivation to comply with others) as the affective sub-stream, and observations of others' behaviors (role models) and perceived norms as the cognitive sub-stream. Similarly, the PERSONAL stream includes the sense of self/control (Diamond, Barnett, Thomas, and Munro, 2007; Diamond and Kirkham, 2005) or self regulation (Csikszentmihalyi and Nakamura, 1999) and will or self-determination (Ryan and Deci, 2000) to behave in a certain way as the affective sub-stream, and general and social competence and skills as the cognitive sub-stream. Both the affective and cognitive sub-streams of all three streams of influence affect HBs.

Flows and Interactions between Streams of Influence

So far, much of our in-depth description of the TTI has focused on within-stream paths. Another very important assumption of the TTI concerns the causal connections between the three streams of influence. Although we believe that the three streams represent the major influences on behavior, we also recognize that factors in one stream can influence factors in another stream, and that Figure 16.1 oversimplifies matters in this respect. The TTI recognizes that many intra-PERSONAL factors contribute to more than just self-efficacy, many SOCIAL situational factors have influences that go beyond social normative beliefs, and many cultural-ENVIRONMENTAL factors affect more than just attitudes. These interactions between streams of influence are shown as paths *a–w* in Figure 16.2, a more complete representation of the TTI. The cross-stream interactions "explain" or account for the correlations between variables at the same level of causation mentioned above.

The interactions between streams at the upper levels (paths *a–f*) demonstrate the overpowering importance of characteristics of each of (1) a person's biological and personality dispositions, (2) the social situation/context in which the behaviors occur, and (3) the broader sociocultural environment in which an adolescent is raised and matures, in determining social and HRBs. The HP programs or policies that can address these ultimate causes will obviously have the greatest impact over the long term. Unfortunately, this is often easier said than done.

Many of the most important interactions for intervention purposes occur between the second and third levels of causation, between the social-personal nexus and expectancy-value levels (shown as paths *g–r* in Figure 16.2). For example, the TTI recognizes that adolescents who are impulsive, hyperactive or incapable of controlling their behaviors (all hypothesized sources of low self-efficacy) might place little value on their health (an attitudinal factor—see path *o* in Figure 16.2, from sense of self/control to values/evaluations) and might be motivated to please deviant peers who encourage risky behaviors (a social normative factor—see path *k* in Figure 16.2, sense of self/control to motivation to comply).

The TTI explicitly does not posit paths between an affective variable at one level and a cognitive variable at another level or vice versa. Accordingly, among paths *g–r*, those that are solid are between affective/control variables and those that are dotted are between cognitive variables.

For the analytically sophisticated, note that interactions between streams can be represented statistically as mediation or moderation (or, indeed, as mediated moderation), depending on the level at which it occurs (Baron and Kenny, 1986; MacKinnon and Lockwood, 2003; MacKinnon, Taborga, and Morgan-Lopez, 2002). Figure 16.2 also provides an answer to Nancy Krieger's (1994) question about the "web of causation," namely, "has anyone seen the spider?" Figure 16.2 shows that the causes of HB are, just like spider webs, remarkably complex and interwoven, yet ordered, systematic, and coherent, but that there is not a single causal agent or pathway.

FIGURE 16.2 Formal View of the Theory of Triadic Influence Showing Cross-Stream and Feedback Influences

THE THEORY OF TRIADIC INFLUENCE

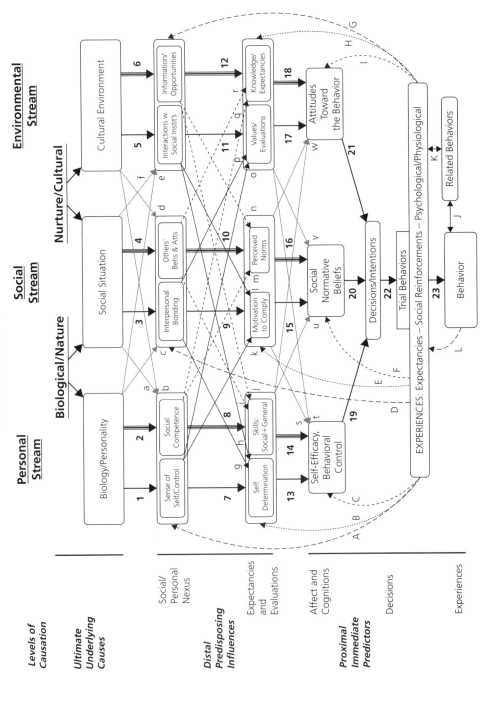

Levels of
Causation

Ultimate
Underlying
Causes

Social/
Personal
Nexus

Distal
Predisposing
Influences

Expectancies
and
Evaluations

Affect and
Cognitions

Proximal
Immediate
Predictors

Decisions

Experiences

THE ROLE OF BEHAVIORAL EXPERIENCE AND FEEDBACK

Once someone tries a behavior, her experience with it influences her future behavior. For example, an adolescent is more likely to repeat a behavior (like smoking) if she feels more accepted by her peers for trying it. The social reinforcement one receives will depend on the strength of social bonding one has with the person giving it. In turn, this reinforcement strengthens the bond with the person giving the reinforcement, and this increases the likelihood of pleasing that person again in the future by repeating the behavior. This is a feedback loop within the SOCIAL stream (path *D* in Figure 16.2). This feedback effect might occur all the way up to the ultimate level, as just described, or it might occur just to the expectancies/evaluation level (path *E*) or the affect/cognitions level (path *F*), depending on the specific context of the experience. For example, if an adolescent perceives that substantially more or substantially fewer of her peers smoke than she earlier believed, then the immediate feedback might be to the proximal (interpersonal bonding—path *F*) or distal (motivation to comply or desire to please—path *E*) levels.

There are also feedback loops in the cultural-ENVIRONMENTAL and intra-PERSONAL streams. The experience of many behaviors is accompanied by emotional or psychological consequences. The emotional or psychological feelings adolescents have from a behavior depend, to some extent, on their current sense of self (DuBois and Flay, 2004; DuBois, Flay, and Fagen, this volume). In turn, these feelings may feed back to alter how they feel about themselves (that is, their self-esteem). In addition, how one performs a new behavior is determined by one's skill; in turn, a good experience with the behavior will improve one's skill. These are the feedback loops in the intra-PERSONAL stream (paths *A, B* and *C*). The many theories of self-control, self-regulation, and self-monitoring rely on feedback loops to influence behavior change (Bandura, 2000, 2005; DiClemente, Marinilli, Singh, and Bellino, 2001; Gross, 2002; Karoly, 1993; Zimmerman, 2001).

How people experience a behavior depends, to some extent, on their expectations regarding it. In turn, performance of a behavior gives people immediate feedback of some of the consequences, both good and bad. Whether these experiences are the same as or different from those expected, the experience adds to firsthand knowledge about that behavior. This modified or reinforced knowledge then influences their future behavior. These are the feedback loops within the cultural-ENVIRONMENTAL stream (paths *G, H* and *I*).

Habitual Behaviors

Habitual behaviors are those for which the experiences of the behavior take on ever-increasing importance over time. Once they have been experienced a few times, habitual behaviors may be driven by social reinforcement (for example, sunbathing because all of one's friends are doing it and because having a tan increases acceptance by one's peers), psychological dependencies (the way it makes one feel), or physiological addictions (biochemical reactions within the body that are beyond one's control).

As a behavior becomes habitual, the relative strength of other factors weakens over time, and future behavior may be best predicted by past behavior (see path *L* in Figure 16.2) or affective-motivational processes. Most everyday behavior consists of routine activities (Hanson and Hanson, 1993) or is habitual, and does not involve active or conscious decision making or intentions—it essentially follows a very tight and well-worn feedback loop (defined by paths *L* and *23* in Figure 16.2) (Aarts and Dijksterhuis, 2000; Neal, Wood, and Quinn, 2006; Ouellette and Wood, 1998; Wood et al., 2002). It is important to remember, however, that habitual behaviors are intentional in the sense that they are goal-oriented (Aarts, 2007; Verplanken and Aarts, 1999).

Habitual behaviors (and dependencies and addictions) are the most difficult for health professionals to change, because one has to first "slow down the action," so as to make other determinants of behavior salient once again. One has to first motivate the person to want to change, then provide adequate positive social and personal skills (and reinforcement for using those skills) and engage the person in the changed behavior to overcome the strength of the habit.

The Role of Related Behaviors

Related behaviors influence or relate to each other in at least two ways. First, they have many of the same ultimate and distal causes. For example, youth who have high levels of sensation seeking or risk taking, or youth who are raised in disadvantaged communities or by unconventional parents, are more likely to engage in multiple problem behaviors (Biglan, Brennan, Foster, and Holder, 2004). Second, engaging in one problem behavior alters, through the feedback mechanisms described above (and through paths J, K and 23 in Figure 16.2), the causes of that behavior and closely related behaviors. For example, engaging in smoking cigarettes may change one's attitudes toward trying other substances (Kandel, Wu, and Davies, 1994).

The Role of Human Development

Adolescence provides its own unique developmental challenges. Besides integrating prominent theories of HB, another feature of the TTI is that its three streams of influence should remind health promoters and researchers that there are also three developmental features of adolescence that threaten adolescent health. It is clear that the *plasticity* of biological and social development plays an important role in determining behavior (Lerner, 2006; Lerner et al., in press; Merzenich, 2001). The multiple causes of behavior compose a *dynamic system* that changes as people develop and have new experiences with particular behaviors (Lerner, 1978, 2006).

The relative importance of self-efficacy, social normative beliefs, and attitudinal variables changes as children develop. Attitudinal influences are most important for younger children, social and normative processes become more important during adolescence, and self-efficacy becomes more important as youth gain more experience. First, adolescents begin to exert their independence from their parents, often by bonding more closely with their peers. Usually beginning at puberty, positive interactions between adolescents and parents diminish (Steinberg, 1991) and adolescents begin seeking independence from their parents (Montemayor and Flannery, 1991). Their independence from parents is replaced by greater dependence on peers, and relations with peers "become more pervasive, more intense, and carry greater psychological importance" (Foster-Clark and Blyth, 1991, p. 786). Not too surprisingly, adolescents are more susceptible to and compliant with social pressures than are children or adults (Berndt, 1979; Landsbaum and Willis, 1971). This is especially true of pressures to engage in deviant acts like substance use (Brown, Clasen, and Eicher, 1986; Flay et al., 1994).

Second, during early adolescence, the delicate search for self-identity begins and adolescents start "trying out" different adult behaviors and roles. The search is not easy, and during it adolescents are psychologically vulnerable (Konopka, 1991), self-conscious, concerned about social appearances (Elkind and Bowen, 1979), and highly self-critical (Lowenthal, Thurner, and Chiriboga, 1975; Rosenberg, 1985), possibly because, for the first time, they can envision discrepancies between who they are and who they want to be or ought to be (Damon, 1991; Higgins, 1987). However, the finding about adolescents being highly self-critical might be a cohort effect. Compared to earlier generations, people born after the early 1970s (dubbed "Generation Me") seem less inclined toward self-criticism and higher in self-esteem; however, they often face a crisis in early adulthood when their high, but rarely tested/confirmed, self-esteem hits reality. As a result, self-esteem is at an all-time high, but so is anxiety (Twenge, 2006). Risky behaviors, such as substance use, might serve as a coping mechanism as adolescents search for an identity and feel vulnerable and self-conscious during this stage of intrapersonal flux (DuBois et al., this volume; Flammer, 1991).

Third, prior to adulthood, cognitive and affective skills are not fully developed and, to varying degrees, children and adolescents have difficulty understanding abstract information, appreciating events which might occur in the distant future (Orr and Ingersoll, 1991), or reacting calmly to emotional situations (Dahl, 2001, 2004; Reyna and Farley, 2006b; Steinberg et al., 2004). These, paired with generally good health (Brindis and Lee, 1991), might contribute to an adolescent's cavalier attitudes about health (Levenson, Marrow, and Pfefferbaum, 1984) and tendency to underestimate personal risks from health-compromising behaviors (Millstein, 1991), such as substance use.

The absence of fully developed cognitive skills, the immature state of affective control, the desire to be "grown up," and deepening attachment to peers makes adolescence a period when adolescents are particularly susceptible to health risks. They may, for example, begin smoking cigarettes because they (1) feel anxious or insecure and want to look "mature"; (2) feel pressure to smoke from peers who smoke and want to feel like they "belong"; or (3) cannot fully appreciate the long-term dangers of smoking. Each of these developmental features of adolescence—personality, social and cognitive development—poses special challenges for health promoters.

An Ecological View of the Theory of Triadic Influence

The three streams of influence in the TTI and the notion of inter-related influences are similar to the rings of influence in Bronfrenbrenner's (1979, 1986, 2005) ecology systems theory or social ecology model. However, most conceptions of the social ecology model, including those used in HP (Glass and McAtee, 2006; Hovell, Wahlgren, and Gehrman, 2002; King, Stokols, Talen, Brassington, and Killingsworth, 2002; McLeroy, Bibeau, and Glanz, 1988; Stokols, 1992), do not consider the levels/tiers of causation within its rings. In the TTI, intrapersonal factors can be seen to be nested within social factors that, in turn, are nested within broader sociocultural environmental factors, just as in the basic ecological models. However, within the TTI, all three rings/streams also have causal influences at multiple levels; ultimate/underlying, distal/predisposing, and proximal/immediate. See Figure 16.3 for a depiction of the TTI that emphasizes both the ecological rings and the levels of causation.

FIGURE 16.3   *The TTI Ecological System, showing how the intrapersonal factors lie inside the situation (contextual or interpersonal) factors that, in turn, lie inside the broad sociocultural environmental factors. Unlike most ecological systems, however, the TTI includes levels/tiers of causation within each circle.*

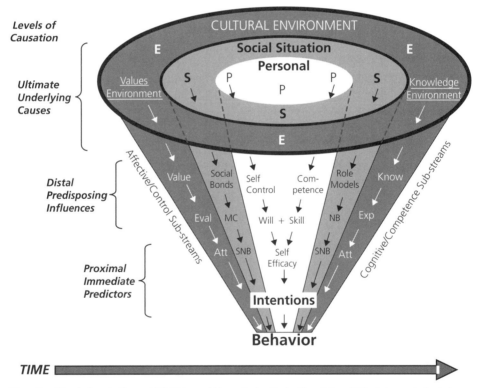

Note: For abbreviations in Figure 16.3: Value = Values, Eval = Evaluation, Att = Attitude towards the behavior, MC = Motivation to comply, SNB = Social Normative Beliefs, Know = Knowledge, Exp = Expectancies.

By incorporating both (1) levels of ecology and (2) levels of causation as independent dimensions, the TTI overcomes many of the problems of terminology and understanding about levels of causation outlined recently by Nancy Krieger (2008). We make it clear that levels of causation exist within every ecological domain; this is in contrast to some usages, that suggest that person-centered causes are proximal, social causes are distal and societal causes are ultimate or fundamental (Kuh and Yoav, 2004; McKinlay and Marceau, 2000). Note also that "level" is not a spatial or temporal dimension; rather, it is a "relational construct that organizes and distinguishes (conceptually or structurally) different orders of hierarchically linked systems and processes (including both nested and non-nested hierarchies)" (Krieger, 2008, page 226). Causal "distance" does not involve spatiotemporal separation; actually all levels co-occur simultaneously. However, space and time do matter for levels in the case of nested hierarchies, whereby processes at lower levels typically are smaller and involve faster processes than processes at higher levels. Whereas some usage of the proximal-distal terms "inherently cleaves levels rather than connects them, thereby obscuring the intermingling of ecosystems, economics, politics, history, and specific exposures and processes at *every* level, macro to micro, from societal to inside the body" (Krieger, 2008, page 227), the structure of the TTI separates levels of causation from ecological domains. As Krieger suggests, we need levels of causation as well as pathways that link them within and across ecological levels. This is achieved by the TTI.

Linking Ecologies, Development and Feedback
—A Life-Course Perspective

Development, of course, does not end at adolescence; nor do the influences on and theories about health. An important third dimension of the TTI is time (shown with the large arrow from left to right in Figure 16.3) or development (Giddens, 1987; Glass and McAtee, 2006). Rather than solely focusing on the building blocks of social ecologies, Bronfrenbrenner's ecological model describes "the way in which these entities are related to each other and to the course of development" (1979, page 8). However, the developmental emphasis in Bronfenbrenner's model (and most other ecological models used) is missing from its application in HP (Li, 2008). A temporal (life-span and life-course) perspective can inform the timing of interventions regarding the needs, risks, and opportunities to change at a particular time in the life course, and the development of strategies at the individual, social, and socio-cultural environmental levels that match the timing of interventions (Settersten, 2005). The meanings associated with life transitions are often socially constructed. Furthermore, life transitions typically encompass changes in social roles and responsibilities that may have transformational experiences that lead to major changes in an individual's life (Resnicow and Vaughan, 2006).

Extended from the ecological models that link an individual's life to the physical and social context, the life-course perspective connects the past to the present and examines the social pathways in their historical context (George, 2004). Cumulative positive experiences with a behavior, with their feedback experiences, can lead into developmental trajectories and, eventually, to habituation. On the other hand, cumulative negative experiences with a behavior, new experiences or ecological transitions (Bronfrenbrenner, 1979), can lead to dropping a behavior, transitions in behavior (for example, post-marriage weight gain), teachable moments (McBride et al., 2008) or turning points (Baxter and Bullis, 1986; Graber and Brooks-Gunn, 1996; Kearney and O'Sullivan, 2003; Laub and Sampson, 1993; Wheaton and Gotlib, 1997).

EMPIRICAL SUPPORT FOR THE THEORY OF TRIADIC INFLUENCE

There are many components of the TTI for which we could review the empirical support. For this chapter, we chose to examine one of the most important of these, the mediated pathways included in the TTI. Mediated pathways are where the effects of an ultimate or underlying cause (for example, repeated exposure to a religious affiliation) or a distal or predisposing influence (for example, acceptance of Christian values) are mediated through some intervening variable (for example, attitudes toward substance use) on their way to influencing behavior (for example, substance use). The following is a review of the extant literature that (1) explicitly used the TTI and (2) empirically tested for mediation. Multivariate statistical analyses provide considerable support for the streams of influence and mediated pathways included in the TTI.

We reviewed findings from ten studies of various behavioral domains (that is, substance use, risk behavior, dietary behavior and physical activity, breast self-examination, and breast cancer screening) and, for the ease of discussion, we categorized each study in a particular stream based on the study's most distal variable (X). We classified studies that included variables that could be categorized in multiple streams (for example, ethnic group) or combined variables from several streams (for example, perceived behavioral control, social normative beliefs, and attitudes) as a single composite variable in the stream with the most outer ecological ring in the TTI Ecological System (see Figure 16.3). We created a separate category for studies that included feedback or past behavior as the most distal variable separately.

We coded mediation pathway findings from the ten studies using the construct labels (for example, P1) presented in the basic version of the TTI (Figure 16.1) and summarize them in Table 16.2. We classified mediation as complete, partial or non-significant as follows:

1. Complete mediation when the pathway from the more distal predictor (X) to the behavioral outcome (Z) was significantly mediated by a variable (Y), with no significant direct effect from the predictor (X) to the behavioral outcome (Z) remaining;
2. Partial mediation when the pathway from the most distal predictor (X) to the behavioral outcome (Z) was significantly mediated by an endogenous variable

TABLE 16.2   The TTI Mediation Literature.

Study	Behavioral Domain	Population	Design	X Variable Label[A]	X Variable Name	Mediator 1: Label	Mediator 1: Name	Y Mediator 2: Label	Mediator 2: Name	Z Dependent Variable	Mediation[B]
Personal Kear, 2002	Substance Use: Tobacco	224 U.S. college students	Cross-sectional	p3/s3/e3	Risk-taking tendency	s4	Social normative beliefs	p4	Resistance self-efficacy	Smoking	c
				p2	Depression	p4	Resistance self-efficacy			Smoking	c
				p2	Depression	s4	Social normative beliefs	p4	Resistance self-efficacy	Smoking	c
Social Schofield et al., 2003	Substance Use: Tobacco	Over 1300 Australian Adolescents	Longitudinal	6	Experiences with smoking	e4	Attitudes	5	Intention	Smoking	p
				6	Experiences	5	Intention			Smoking	p
				6	Experiences	s4	Subjective norm	5	Intention	Smoking	p
				6	Experiences	p4	Self-efficacy	5	Intention	Smoking	p
				s4	Experiences	e4	Attitudes	5	Intention	Smoking	p
				s4	Peer-group norm	e4	Subjective norm	5	Intention	Smoking	p
				s4	Peer-group norm	5	Intention			Smoking	p
				s4	Peer-group norm	p4	Self-efficacy	5	Intention	Smoking	p

(Continued)

TABLE 16.2 (Continued)

Study	Behavioral Domain	Population	Design		X		Y			Z	Mediation[B]
Sieving et al., 2000a	Substance Use: Alcohol Use	413 U.S. adolescent-parent dyads	Longitudinal	s1	Parent norms: Time 1	p4/e4/5	Alcohol-related cognitions: Time 1	p4/e4/5	Alcohol-related cognitions: Time 2	Alcohol use: Time 3	c
Environmental Carvajal et al., 2004	Substance Use: Tobacco	2,004 U.S. middle school students	Cross-sectional	p1/s1/e1	Age	p3	Grade point average	p4/s4/e4/5	Self-efficacy, norms, attitudes, impediments, intention	Smoking	p
				p1/s1/e1	Age	p2/s2	Depression, parental relatedness, maladaptive coping, academic aspirations			Smoking susceptibility among nonsmoker	p
Carvajal and Granillo, 2006	Substance Use: Tobacco	1137 U.S. Adolescents	Prospective cohort study	p1/s1/e1	Age, gender, ethnicity, SES	p3/s2/s3/e3	Depression, school connectedness, parent relatedness, global expectancies, coping, academic aspirations, GPA	p4/s4/e4/5	Intentions, perceived risk, attitudes, impediments, norms, self-efficacy	Smoking: Time 2	p

De Bruijn et al., 2005	Physical Activity and Diet	3,895 Dutch adolescents	Cross-sectional	p1/s1/e1 p2/p3/s2	Home situation, urbanization, school type, gender, self-esteem, relation with parents	p4/s4/e4	Perceived behavioral control, subjective norm (marginally significant), attitude	5	Intention	Snacking	p
				p1/s1/e1	Ethnicity, school type, degree of urbanization	p4/s4/e4	Perceived behavioral control, subjective norm (marginally significant), attitude	5	Intention	Bicycle use	p

(Continued)

TABLE 16.2 (Continued)

	Study	Domain	Population	Design	X		Y		Z	Mediation[B]
Feedback & Past Behavior	Carvajal et al., 2002	Substance Use	525 Adolescents	Prospective cohort study	f	Substance use: Time 1	e3	Global positive expectancies	p4→5 (i.e., 5 is mediator 3) Self-efficacy→Intentions to avoid substance use	Substance use: Time 2	c
					f	Substance use: Time 1	p4	Self-efficacy	5 Intentions to avoid substance use	Substance use: Time 2	c
					f	Substance use: Time 1	e3	Global positive expectancies	e4→5 (i.e., 5 is mediator 3) Attitudes→Intentions to avoid substance use	Substance use: Time 2	c
					f	Substance use: Time 1	e4	Attitudes	5 Intentions to avoid substance use	Substance use: Time 2	c
					f	Substance use: Time 1	5	Intentions to avoid Substance use		Substance use: Time 2	c

Study	Behavior	Sample	Design	f	Predictor (code)	Mediator 1 (code)	Mediator 2 (code)	Outcome	Mediation
				f	Substance use: Time 1 (p2)	Self-esteem (p4, s4, e4)	Self-efficacy, Social norms, Attitudes		ns
				f	Substance use: Time 1 (e3)	Global positive expectancies (s4 → 5)	Social norms → Intentions to avoid substance use (i.e., 5 is mediator 3)		ns
Lechner et al., 1997	Breast cancer screening	395 Dutch women	Longitudinal	f	Past behavior (e4/p4)	Perceived consequences, anticipated regret, modeling (5)	Intention	Participation in second screening	c
Lechner et al., 2004	Breast-self examination	364 Dutch women	Longitudinal	f	Past behavior: Time 1 (p4/s4/e4)	Self-efficacy, social influence, attitude, intention (5)	Intention: Time 2	Breast self-examination	p
				f	Past behavior: Time 1 (p4/s4/e4)	Self-efficacy, social influence, attitude, intention (5)	Intention	Intention	p

[A] Variables are coded using the construct labels presented in Figure 1. f: feedback or past behavior.

[B] Mediation: c:complete, p: partial, ns: final pathway non-significant.

(Y), with a significant, but reduced, direct effect remaining from the predictor (X) to the outcome (Z); and

3. Nonsignificant when mediation was tested for and found to be nonsignificant.

See Baron and Kenny (1986) and MacKinnon and colleagues (2002) for more detailed discussions of mediation.

PERSONAL Stream: Intrapersonal Characteristics → Self-Efficacy

Only one study examined a model with the most distal variables from the TTI's PERSONAL stream. Kear (2002) explored psychosocial predictors of smoking among a cross-sectional sample of 224 college students. A Web-based survey assessed depression, risk-taking tendency, self-efficacy to resist smoking, and social normative beliefs. Depression and risk-taking tendency were the most distal variables examined. Results indicated that all four predictors of smoking behavior were significant, with self-efficacy to resist smoking being the strongest predictor. Self-efficacy (a proximal variable in the TTI) had the only direct effect on smoking behavior and completely mediated the effects of depression, risk-taking tendency (both more distal variables in the TTI), and social normative beliefs (a proximal variable in the TTI). Further, the study's model provided an example of cross-stream effects displayed in the TTI—social normative beliefs mediated the effects of depression on smoking behavior.

SOCIAL Stream: Interpersonal Situations/Contexts →
Social Normative Beliefs

Two studies tested models with the most distal variables from the TTI's SOCIAL stream. In a longitudinal study of more than one thousand Australian adolescents, Schofield and colleagues (2003) investigated predictors of future smoking. They found that intentions (on a lower tier in the TTI) were predicted from attitudes and self-efficacy, and these, in turn, were predicted by peer-group norms (on the expectancies/evaluation tier of the TTI) and experiences with smoking (consistent with the TTI's feedback loops). Although the authors concluded that the addition of peer-group norms to the TTI model enhanced the model's performance, we note that peer group norms are already included in the TTI as part of subjective norms. Despite the study's limitations, support was provided for the mediated pathways included in the TTI from proximal predictors (for example, self-efficacy, social normative beliefs, and attitudes) through intentions to behavior. Additionally, the study provided an example of how past behavior (that is, personal experiences with smoking) can have a strong feedback effect.

A second study in the SOCIAL stream was conducted by Sieving and colleagues (2000a) to examine parental influences on adolescent alcohol use. Participants were 413 adolescent-parent dyads who were participants in Project Northland, a multi-component intervention designed to reduce adolescent alcohol use. A structural equation modeling approach was used to examine mediated pathways to adolescent alcohol use. Consistent with the TTI, parent norms (on the expectancies/evaluation tier) had significant indirect relationships with alcohol use at one- and two-year follow-up. The relationships, in turn, were mediated by adolescents' alcohol-related cognitions (proximal predictors). Overall, the study emphasized the importance of adolescents' social situation and underscored the key role of parental influence on initial alcohol use.

ENVIRONMENTAL Stream: Sociocultural Environments → Attitudes

Several studies tested models with distal variables among the TTI's cultural-ENVIRONMENTAL stream. Using a cross-sectional sample of over two thousand middle-school students, Carvajal and colleagues (2004) found that ultimate causes, distal influences, and proximal predictors explained approximately 55 percent of the variance in smoking, with variables from each level significantly predicting current smoking. The researchers concluded that their model supported the TTI's structure of tiers and found adolescents were more likely to be current smokers if they had fewer impediments to smoking, greater positive attitudes toward smoking, lower self-efficacy, and a greater intention to smoke.

More recently, Carvajal and Granillo (2006) tested numerous predictors of smoking initiation among a sample of more than eleven hundred early adolescents (aged eleven to fourteen). The prospective cohort study examined an assortment of ultimate causes, such as ethnicity, as well as distal influences and proximal predictors. Within the ten-month follow-up period, in contrast to the previous cross-sectional analyses, more distal causes were more predictive of smoking than proximal predictors. However, consistent with TTI, relationships between ultimate causes and smoking initiation were mediated by distal influences and/or proximal predictors. The researchers, supporting the TTI's inclusion of multiple tiers of influence, highlight the importance of interventions not only targeting proximal predictors, but also targeting more ultimate causes and distal influences of behavior.

Similar analyses have been conducted by researchers in the Netherlands to investigate predictors of dietary behavior and physical activity (de Bruijn, Kremers, Schaalma, van Mechelen, and Brug, 2005). Using a cross-sectional sample of almost four thousand Dutch adolescents, the researchers examined predictors of bicycle use and snacking behavior. Paths from ultimate causes, such as degree of urbanization and type of school, along with paths from distal influences and proximal predictors were examined. Results indicated that more distal variables had associations with both bicycle use and snacking behavior that were partially mediated. The researchers concluded that there is a need to include more distal factors to fully understand dietary behaviors and physical activity.

Feedback and Past Behavior

Several studies included feedback or past behavior as the most distal variable. Carvajal and colleagues (2002) conducted a prospective cohort study of 525 adolescents in March (Time 1) and October (Time 2), 1995. Using substance use at Time 1 as the more distal variable, they investigated a model that included self-esteem, self-efficacy, social norms, attitudes, global positive expectancies (general positive expectancies toward oneself and future outcomes), and intentions to avoid substance use. Results demonstrated that Time 1 substance use predicted all other endogenous variables in the model, with the exception of Time 2 substance use. That is, consistent with the TTI's feedback loops, the pathway from Time 1 to Time 2 substance use was completely mediated by variables on the TTI's several tiers. In addition, the relationship between global positive expectancies and substance use at Time 2 was mediated by self-efficacy, subjective normative beliefs, attitudes, and intentions.

Past breast cancer screening behavior (classified as the most distal variable) was examined by Lechner and colleagues (1997) in a study of participation in the Dutch national breast cancer screening program. The longitudinal study (at three time points over two years) of 395 women investigated the relationship between (1) past behavior, perceived consequences, anticipated regret (that is, not participating would cause feelings of regret), modeling (that is, female acquaintances received invitations to the screening or participated), and intention; and (2) breast cancer screening participation at a second screening. Results (Table 16.3) indicated intention and past behavior (that is, a feedback loop) were significant predictors of future screening participation. Further, using another model, the researchers concluded that self-efficacy, attitudes, and previous screening experiences significantly predicted intention to participate in future screening.

Subsequently, Lechner and colleagues (2004) conducted a longitudinal study (three time points over six months) to investigate the relationship between past breast self-examination, self-efficacy, social influence, attitude- and intention, on future breast self-exam behavior among 364 Dutch women. Consistent with the TTI's structure, they found that psychosocial determinants and past behavior directly predicted breast self-examination.

All three of these studies provided considerable support for the feedback loops of the TTI.

The Complete TTI Framework

Teena Willoughby and colleagues at Brock University in Ontario, Canada have provided the only attempt to date to test the complete TTI in one study (Busseri, Willoughby, Chalmers, and YLC-CURA, 2005, April; Willoughby et al., 2008). Using a longitudinal sample of almost sixteen hundred students from eight high schools, they used a twenty-eight-page questionnaire to assess: (1) six ultimate causes (neighborhood quality, school climate, parental education, difficult temperament, age, and gender); (2) ten distal influences (religiosity, parental relationships, curfew, friendship quality, peer victimization, sibling behavior, academic orientation, structured activities, unstructured activities, well-being); (3) six proximal predictors related to attitudes (tolerance of deviance), beliefs (how risky the behaviors were for oneself and for peers), expectations (how upset friends would be, how upset parents would be), and thoughts (how often youth think about risk behaviors concerning risk behavior involvement); to predict (4) a wide range of risk behaviors, including substance use, direct and indirect aggressive behaviors, and a variety of minor and major delinquent behaviors. All measures were collected on two occasions approximately eighteen months apart. Though this list of variables does not cover all possible variables included in the TTI, it covers many of them and certainly more than any other single study. In both cross-sectional and longitudinal models of predictors of a composite of the risky behaviors, they found that: (1) most of the relationships between ultimate causes and a composite of proximal predictors were mediated by distal influences; (2) most of the relationships between ultimate causes and behavior were mediated by distal influences and/or proximal predictors; and (3) most of the relationships between distal influences and behavior were mediated by proximal predictors. This study presents a demonstration of the flow of causation from multiple ultimate causes through multiple distal influences and a composite of multiple proximal predictors to a composite of multiple behaviors.

The evidence from studies of pathways in the TTI consistently shows that more ultimate or distal variables are mediated by distal or proximal variables in the prediction of a range of HRBs across a range of populations (adult and adolescent) in several countries. Many other studies of the etiology of HBs that did not cite the TTI also support this pattern of findings.

APPLICATIONS OF THE THEORY OF TRIADIC INFLUENCE

By integrating and organizing so many risk and protective factors, hierarchical tiers, streams, sub-streams, mediated and moderated paths, and feedback loops, the TTI has utility for researchers who are studying the etiology of a HRB (like substance use or seat belt use) and for program planners who are designing and evaluating HP interventions. Etiology researchers and program planners might do well to study the TTI when designing their questionnaires, analyzing their data, and planning their interventions. With so many variables implicated in HRBs, the TTI can bring some order to the chaos that etiology researchers and program planners face.

Applications in Etiology Research

For etiology researchers, the TTI is designed to give insight into the multitude of causes of HRBs and how they relate to each other and to behavior. When compared to other theories of HB, the TTI's functionality for etiological research is apparent. With multiple hierarchical tiers, three thematic streams, and two sub-streams (affective and cognitive), the TTI has an explicit ability to organize coherently the factors influencing behavior. The TTI also offers a structured outline of multivariate hypotheses about how numerous predictor variables within a stream are linked to each other (through mediation) and to a behavioral outcome, as well as how numerous predictors between streams are linked to each other (through moderation) and to a behavioral outcome.

Since the introduction of the TTI (Flay and Petraitis, 1994; Petraitis et al., 1995), much of the etiological research regarding the TTI's tiers, streams, and sub-streams has focused on the etiology of substance use. However, in recent years, researchers from various disciplines have utilized the TTI in examining an assortment of behavioral domains including: dietary behaviors and physical activity; mental health; problem behaviors, such as violence and delinquency; positive youth development; and sexual behaviors (see Table 16.3, second column, for references).

TABLE 16.3   Literature Referring to the TTI by Behavioral Domain and Type of Study.

Behavioral Domain	Etiology	Intervention
Dietary Behaviors	Brug et al., 2006; Kamphuis et al., 2006	Brug et al., 2003; Klepp et al., 2005; McCall et al., 2005; Sandvik et al., 2005; Schols and Brug, 2003; te Velde et al., 2006; Wind, 2006; Wind et al., 2006
Dietary Behaviors and Physical Activity	Brug et al., 2006; de Bruijn et al., 2005; de Bruijn et al., 2005; Kremers et al., 2005	Wang et al., 2006
Health-Related Behaviors	Flay and Petraitis, 1994; Freudenberg et al., 1995; Perry, 2004	Brug et al., 2005
Mental Health	Fuemmeler, 2004; Mann et al., 2004	Bell and McKay, 2004; Breland-Noble et al., 2006
Multiple Risk Behaviors/Problem Behaviors	Busseri et al., 2007; Hirschberger et al., 2002; Willoughby et al., 2008	Browne et al., 2001; Flay and Collins, 2005; Flay et al., 2004
Physical Activity	Baranowski et al., 1998; Ferreira et al., 2007	
Positive Youth Development / Character Development	Flay, 2002	Flay and Allred, 2003; Flay et al., 2001; Ji et al., 2005
Sexual Behaviors	Bearinger and Resnick, 2003; Hellerstedt et al., 2006; Kocken et al., 2006; Sieving et al., 2006; Sieving et al., 2000b	Bell et al., 2007; Kugler et al., 2007; Tortolero et al., 2005; Weeks et al., 1995

Substance Use	Abrams, 1999; Anderson, 1998; Carvajal and Granillo, 2006; Carvajal et al., 2002; Carvajal et al., 2004; DiRocco et al., 2007; Drobes, 2002; Ertas, 2007; Flay, 1993; Flay, 1999; Flay, 2000; Flay and Petraitis, 1991; Flay and Petraitis, 2003; Flay et al., 1994; Flay et al., 1995; Flay et al., 1999; Foshee et al., 2007; Haug, 2001; Holder et al., 1999; Hover et al., 2000; Karlsson, 2006; Kear, 2002; Kobus, 2003; Komro and Toomey, 2002; Kumar et al., 2002; Leatherdale and Manske, 2005; Leatherdale and Strath, 2007; Mohatt et al., 2004; Murnaghan, 2007; Nierkens et al., 2006; Petersen et al., 2005; Petraitis et al., 1995; Petraitis et al., 1998; Schofield et al., 2003; Schulenberg et al., 2001; Shadel et al., 2004a; Shadel et al., 2004b; Sieving et al., 2000a; Sussman et al., 2000; Thorner et al., 2007; Turner et al., 2004; Victoir et al., 2007; Wiefferink et al., 2006; Wiefferink et al., 2008	Fogg and Borody, 2001; Komro et al., 2004a; Midford et al., 2005; Perry et al., 2008; Perry et al., 2002; Scheier, 2001; Stigler et al., 2006
Violence	Botvin et al., 2006	Jagers et al., 2007a; Komro et al., 2004a
Other: (for example, gambling, skin cancer protection, colorectal cancer screening)	Biglan, 2003; Biglan, 2004; Commers et al., 2007; Chalmers and Willoughby 2006; de Vries and Lechner, 2000; DuBois and Flay, 2004; Kremers et al., 2000; Lechner et al., 2004; Lechner et al., 1997; Stanton et al., 2005; Wolf, 2002	Freudenberg et al., 2000

Applications in Health Promotion

The utility of the TTI might be even stronger for those who are developing HP programs. HB theory should provide a guide for the treatment or prevention of health-compromising or other risky behaviors, and the promotion of health-enhancing behaviors. The TTI has been referenced as helping guide the development of multiple HP programs designed to influence a variety of behavioral outcomes, such as: reducing substance use, reducing risky behaviors among adolescents, improving mental health, increasing healthy dietary behaviors and physical activity, and improving youths' academic achievement and behavior (see third column of Table 16.3). Presumably, the TTI has been useful to program planners because it is more comprehensive than other theories, addressing the myriad causes of a particular behavior or class of behaviors (see Table 16.1), providing coherent suggestions of how causal processes operate (mediating and moderating processes [Figure 16.2]), and providing program developers some guidelines when planning a program.

The TTI is useful for health promoters applying planning and evaluation models such as the PRECEDE-PROCEED model (Green, 1992; Green and Kreuter, 2005), Intervention Mapping (Bartholomew, Parcel, Kok, and Gottlieb, 2006) and the culturally appropriate PEN-3 planning approach (Airhihenbuwa, 1995). Specifically, the TTI is helpful in (1) identifying predisposing, enabling and reinforcing factors that influence behavior; (2) selecting, or including, strategies in an intervention; and (3) predicting and understanding a program's impact. We now review some of the ways the TTI can help in the development of interventions.

First, the TTI reminds program planners that they have options. Programs generally try to change a behavior by trying to alter variables that cause the behavior. By reminding program planners that any given HRB has multiple causes, the TTI reminds program planners that there are many different causes that they can alter. Beyond that, however, the TTI can help in the identification of modifiable risk and protective factors and help program planners decide what to provide. This is the first function of theory: to guide the development of interventions by helping identify protective factors (like knowledge about the dangers of substance use) and risk factors (like lack of adult supervision after school). It is no coincidence that substance use prevention programs only started teaching refusal skills after Bandura (1977) presented his theoretical work on self-efficacy. In this and countless other cases, theories have suggested the basic content that has gone into developing new and more effective approaches to prevention. By including so many risk and protective factors in one model, the TTI reminds program planners of more and more ways to affect HRB.

Table 16.4 provides another view of the TTI matrix, illustrating what we call the Big Three (the three streams) and the six (the six sub-streams) causes of behavior, and the parallel Big Three and six reasons for changing behavior. The table also shows the six parallel strategies for contextual change (that would lead to behavior change) and the six parallel strategies for individual-level behavior change, as well as the modes or channels that can be used to effect change. We elaborate on these ideas below.

TABLE 16.4   Causes of Behavior, Reasons for Behavior Change, and Strategies for Contextual and Behavior Change.

The Big three Causes of Behavior	IntraPersonal Genetic/Biological, Personality		Social Situation/Context Family, School, Friends		Sociocultural Environment Culture/Ethnicity, SES, Media Exposure, Social (Dis)organization	
The six Causes of Behavior	*Sense of self, self determination, self control*	General competence, *social skills*	*Social attachment to (bonding with) family, friends, school*	Observed (modeled) *behaviors and attitudes of others*	*Value of expected* consequences	*Knowledge of expected* consequences
Big three Reasons for Behavior Change	*Self-Efficacy:* "I have the behavioral skills and self-determination (Skill + Will)"		*Social Normative Behaviors* "Important others would like me to"		*Attitudes toward the behavior:* "It will be good for me"	
Six Reasons for Behavior Change	I really want to OR I can't help myself	I find it easier to do than not to	To please others—social acceptance	Because "everyone else is doing it"	To improve myself (or my health) in ways I value	To avoid negative consequences or gain positive ones
Six Classes of Strategies For Contextual Change*	**Improve group empowerment**	**Improve general/social competencies**	**Change sources and levels of social support**	**Change normative environment, role models**	**Change the socio-cultural values environment**	**Change the informational environment**
Six Classes of Strategies For Behavioral Change	Improve self control/image; *Provide cues and reminders*	Teach, learn, practice improved *(social) skills*	Increase social attachments; *Provide/find sources of social support*	*Model* desired behavior; Correct or alter normative expectations	Teach cultural values, clarify or (re)develop *values/evaluations* Teach problem solving and decision making	*Provide information,* change expectations
Modes or Channels of Change	Individual counseling, small groups, schools; media for modeling and cues		Modeling and increasing opportunities, in communities, schools, families and small groups, parent training, support groups,		Societal opportunities, legislation, policies, taxes, media (messages, counter advertising), communities, schools, health care systems	

* *Note:* The bolded row indicates our belief that future health promotion interventions need to focus on the distal and ultimate causes of health behavior, where they can influence multiple behaviors more efficiently and in a more sustained way than most of our current affectively/cognitively-focused interventions.

Each stream of the TTI suggests multiple approaches to HB change. For example, the TTI's PERSONAL stream suggests that there are two means by which health promoters can improve health-related self-efficacy (Figure 16.1 and Table 16.4). First, health promoters can teach self-regulation and self-management skills to adolescents and adults with weak self-concept or self-control, because they are otherwise at elevated risk for health-compromising behaviors (Bandura, 2005). Second, health promoters can improve people's skills and confidence so that they know how to handle situations where their health is at risk. For example, educators can help adolescents with their abilities to resist social pressures to use substances and engage in unsafe sexual activities.

The SOCIAL stream of the TTI suggests that health promoters can provide people with prominent role models who practice healthy lifestyles (Bandura, 1986; Jessor et al., 2003). Health promoters also can try to change the behaviors of peer and family members (and themselves) who serve as role models of health-compromising behavior (Flay, 2000). For example, by directly encouraging one employee or parent to quit smoking, educators can indirectly affect other coworkers' or children's perceptions that smoking is not normative. Health promoters can also help alleviate social pressure by correcting people's (1) distorted perceptions (knowledge or cognitions) about how people engage in health-compromising behaviors, and (2) their bonds and motivation to comply with or please people (an affective component) who engage in health-compromising behaviors. Finally, once an HRB has been changed, it can be maintained better if social support is available from important others (Duncan and McAuley, 1993; Gallant, 2003; Hurdle, 2001; Jessor et al., 2003; Verheijden, Bakx, Weel, Koelen, and Staveren, 2005).

The cultural-ENVIRONMENTAL stream of the TTI suggests several ways that health promoters can improve people's health. The most obvious way is to provide people with information and knowledge about the consequences of HRBs. Attempts at HP have often assumed that knowledge is power, and that the key to changing HRBs is to provide people with new information about health. It is widely assumed, for example, that if adolescents truly appreciate the dangers of cigarettes and unsafe sex, they would rationally decide to avoid smoking and use condoms. Similarly, it is assumed that if adults knew about the benefits of low-sodium diets they would reduce their salt consumption. The assumption that knowledge is power has shaped the foundation of many HP efforts (historically, the first approach to be used—Dusenbury and Botvin, 1990) and many well-known models of HB, such as the Health Belief Model (Janz and Becker, 1984; Rosenstock, 1974).

Knowledge, attitudes, decisions, and behaviors do not always fall into line with each other, and providing accurate information and expecting people to act in their best interests often fails to change them. However, as the TTI and expectancy-value theories (Feather, 1982) make clear, new knowledge is often worthless without new values. For example, teaching adolescents that smoking might cause cancer in decades to come will not deter them if they discount the value of their long-term health or if they place a higher value on getting along with peers now. Similarly, adults might not heed warnings about high-sodium diets if they believe that low-sodium diets are bland and greatly reduce the quality of their lives. Consequently, the second means (and the second to be used historically in HP research—Dusenbury and Botvin, 1990) of boosting health-encouraging attitudes among people is to change their general health and social values. Historically, the third approach to prevention to heath promotion was to teach decision-making and problem-solving skills (Dusenbury and Botvin, 1990), which teaches people how to combine their values with their knowledge to reach informed decisions.

A second way that the TTI can help in the development of interventions is by encouraging developers to take advantage of multiple options. Looking at Figures 16.1 or 16.2 should make it clear to program developers that a program's effectiveness might be determined by its ability to affect more—rather than fewer—risk and protective factors. Therefore, the TTI reminds us that the most effective interventions are probably those that target a wide range of such factors.

For example, the TTI makes it clear that teaching about information, values and decision making may not be enough to change behavior, especially if people are exposed to multiple conflicting messages and the ultimate causes remain unchanged. Health promoters might do better by contributing to the sociocultural environment in which people mature and live day to day. As examples, health promoters might aim at (1) influencing health-related legislation, taxation, and public policy; (2) guiding selection of school curricula, food choices, and opportunities for physical activity; and (3) employing the mass media and popular public figures, as means of shaping the health-related values upon which people build their health-related attitudes, limiting or providing opportunities for behavioral choices (compare with Jessor et al., 2003), and reinforcing desired behaviors. One glance at Figure 16.1 reminds prevention planners that behaviors have their roots in all three streams, and reminds planners that simple interventions that target few risk or protective factors, or focus within only one stream, are likely to have modest effects. Moreover, Figure 16.1 reminds planners that among the three streams of influence, only a few factors probably affect a behavior fairly directly (such as attitudes toward the behavior) and that most factors probably have indirect effects (for example, religious involvement).

With such advice in mind, Bell and colleagues (Bell, Bhana, McKay, and Petersen, 2007; Bell et al., 2008) applied the TTI to guide the design of the Collaborative HIV Prevention and Adolescent Mental Health Project-South Africa (CHAMPSA). CHAMPSA is a South African version of the Collaborative HIV Prevention and Adolescent Project (CHAMP): a family-based HIV prevention research project originally conducted in Chicago (Bell and McKay, 2004). The TTI was used by these program developers to derive seven principles for interventions that CHAMPSA incorporated: individual, peer and family group, and community-based interventions, reflecting the TTI's PERSONAL, SOCIAL and cultural-ENVIRONMENTAL streams, respectively. Thus, CHAMPSA had a greater likelihood of success and could expect greater results by addressing more rather than fewer risk and protective factors.

Logically following the above two points, a third advantage of using the TTI in program planning is that it can help planners anticipate the size of their program's impact. Programs with modest resources that can only target one or two of the proximal causes of a behavior (like simply teaching kids about the dangers of drugs) should anticipate modest effects. At the same time, programs with many more resources and plans to target multiple causes, especially more distal and ultimate causes, should run long enough to produce larger and more lasting effects before being considered (un)successful. Therefore, program planners and funding agencies might do well to study Figure 16.1 before designing a program or approving of its funding to arrive at a more realistic estimate of their program's potential impact.

Fourth, not only can the TTI provide a preliminary estimate of the magnitude of a program's impact, the TTI's mediated pathways also point toward the location of a program's impact. Programs are designed to have an immediate effect on some variables that are expected to have subsequent effects on the targeted behavior. For instance, substance use prevention programs might try to correct perceptions about the extent of a behavior among peers in the hope that corrected social normative beliefs will change intentions toward substance use and, eventually, reduce substance use. By spelling out the intervening (mediating) variables, the TTI allows us to measure the appropriate variables and helps us locate the immediate, intermediate, and long-term effects of a program.

Fifth, whereas the TTI's within-stream mediated paths point toward the location of likely effects, the TTI's between-streams moderator paths should remind program planners about interactions and encourage careful thought about identifying appropriate target audiences for interventions. Not all people have the same level of risk or the same reaction to a program. For instance, a program that emphasizes the dangers of drug use might reduce the drug use of low risk takers but might promote drug use among high risk takers. Thus, the TTI, because it articulates moderating or interaction effects, encourages program planners to think about the populations for whom programs are more appropriate, and whether prevention efforts should be universal, selective, or indicated (Airhihenbuwa, 1995; Gordon, 1983, 1987).

Sixth, the TTI suggests to program developers that it is better, in the long term, to address ultimate or more distal factors rather than less distal or proximal factors. If a program focuses on proximal predictors rather than ultimate and more distal determinants of a behavior, the behavior might change temporarily but soon revert back to prior levels as underlying influences in the individuals' homes, schools, and broader sociocultural environments remain unaltered. For instance, a one-shot program that encourages adolescents to "just say 'no'" to offers of substances, although important, targets only proximal-level predictors, leaves unaltered more distal influences, and, therefore, is unlikely to have much long-term success. If program developers understand the short-term causal processes, the long-term causal processes, and intervening variables, they are in a better position to develop an effective program.

Theories, in conjunction with empirical support, explicitly articulate the intervening causal processes that link unmodifiable variables with behavior. Consequently, the TTI gives program developers more than a list of risk and protective factors: it also gives developers a comprehensive list of those factors that can be modified by the program. Thus, to be long lasting, HP programs must not only be sustained, but they must also change the social ecologies in which people live. The influences in peoples' sociocultural environments to engage in health-compromising behavior do not go away, so programs must continue to influence or counteract them.

It is obvious by now that the many determinants of behavior need to be considered when planning a preventive or HP intervention. One cannot assume that information alone will do much to alter behavior. In many cases it has not, and in some cases has actually made things worse (Goodstadt, 1978, 1980). In part, information is usually not enough to change behavior because there are so many other determinants of the targeted behavior. Educational programs that address social skills (and self-efficacy) and norms, as well as information (and attitudes) are an improvement. However, given that the underlying/ultimate causes of behavior are at the level of families and neighborhoods (within the SOCIAL stream) and at the level of one's sociocultural heritage and macro-environment (within the cultural-ENVIRONMENTAL stream), one may need to consider educating parents as well as children, or using sociocultural environmental or legal interventions instead of, or in addition to, educational programs or campaigns. For behaviors for which the primary underlying causes are the physiological makeup or psychological adjustment of the person, clinical treatment programs will probably be more appropriate (Bierman et al., 2004; Greenberg, 2004).

A seventh and final way in which the TTI can help in the development of effective HP interventions is by providing a common framework with which to analyze the common elements of effective or evidence-based programs. In one example, Mary Jane Rotheram-Borus' laboratory (for example, Ingram, Flannery, Elkavich, and Rotheram-Borus, 2008) has analyzed the common components of AIDS prevention programs and found that they included structural features (agenda or goal setting), group management strategies (for example, active engagement), and content (for example, cognitive changes, skills/competence development and practice). Surprisingly, to them and us, they found little consistency in the application of positive reinforcement. A Behavior Change Consortium (Ory, Jordan, and Bazzarre, 2002) found the following common factors in interventions: decisional balance (pros and cons), goal setting, outcome expectations, self-determination/ autonomy, (self-) efficacy, social support, and stress management. In another consensus exercise, Michie and colleagues (2005) identified twelve theoretical constructs for use in (1) studying the implementation of evidence-based practice; and (2) developing strategies for effective implementation, and to communicate these constructs to an interdisciplinary audience. The twelve constructs were: (1) knowledge; (2) skills; (3) social/professional role and identity; (4) beliefs about capabilities; (5) beliefs about consequences; (6) motivation and goals; (7) memory, attention and decision processes; (8) environmental context and resources; (9) social influences; (10) emotion regulation; (11) behavioral regulation; and (12) nature of the behavior.

Distinguishing core elements from optional elements of effective interventions could help program implementers to not undermine the program's effectiveness when they modify programs to meet the needs of their target population. The search for core elements in prevention interventions is parallel to the identification of "common factors" in a large body of psychotherapy research (Lambert and Oglesk, 2004) and other mental health interventions (for example, Arnold, Rice, Flannery, and Rotheram-Borus, 2008), as well as consistent with the study of levels of change by a National Institute of Mental Health task force (Bellack et al., 2001). A focus on the common elements in successful interventions, rather than on their theoretical explanations or idiosyncratic packaging, will make an empirically validated knowledge base more accessible to community interventionists (Ingram et al., 2008).

ABAN AYA: AN EXAMPLE OF THE APPLICATION OF THE THEORY OF TRIADIC INFLUENCE

It is clear from the TTI that interventions that (1) target multiple variables, (2) include the social context, and (3) address ultimate-level causes should have more and longer-lasting effects on more behaviors than interventions that target only a few variables, give less emphasis to social context, and/or do not address ultimate-level causes. In this section we describe how the TTI was used to design, implement, and evaluate the Aban Aya Youth Project. Aban Aya was an intervention designed to target the risk behaviors of violence, provoking behavior, substance use, school delinquency, and sexual practices (engaging in sexual intercourse and using condoms) among urban African American youth (Flay, Graumlich, Segawa, Burns, and Holliday, 2004). The culturally grounded project derived its name from two Ghanian symbols, Aban, a fence signifying double (social) protection, and Aya, an unfurling fern signifying standing up to the world, or self-determination.

Violence, substance use, delinquency, and risky sexual practices are major public health concerns confronting urban African American youth (Dahlberg, 1998; Herrenkohl et al., 2000). The Aban Aya Youth Project was a longitudinal randomized control trial of three interventions (two experimental interventions and one "attention-placebo" control) that were implemented in grades five through eight in twelve metropolitan Chicago schools between 1994 and 1998. More in-depth descriptions of research and intervention design, activities, implementation, and evaluation can be found elsewhere (Flay et al., 2004; Jagers, Morgan-Lopez, H. Browne, and Flay, 2007; Jagers, Sydnor, Mouttapa, and Flay, 2007; Ngwe, Liu, Flay, Segawa, and Aban Aya Co-Investigators, 2004; Segawa, Ngwe, Li, and Flay, 2005).

One of the Aban Aya experimental conditions was the social development curriculum (SDC), a four-year, classroom-based intervention consisting of sixteen to twenty-one lessons a year designed to: teach cognitive-behavioral skills to build self-esteem and empathy; manage stress and anxiety; develop interpersonal relationships; resist peer pressure; and develop decision-making, problem-solving, conflict-resolution and goal-setting skills. The SDC was structured to teach application of these skills to avoiding violence, drug use and, unsafe sex. The control condition was a health enhancement curriculum (HEC) that addressed physical HBs (for example, physical activity, nutrition, and sleep) rather than problem behaviors.

The second experimental condition was the school and community intervention (SCI). The SCI echoed the SDC's focus on community-specific issues (that is, violence, provocation, delinquency, drugs, and unsafe sex) but added parental support plus school climate and community components. The parent-support component reinforced the program's classroom lessons and promoted child/parent communication. The school staff and schoolwide youth-support component integrated programmatic skills into the school environment and provide reinforcement of appropriate behaviors. The community component forged linkages among parents, schools, and local businesses. Each SCI school formed a local school task force consisting of school personnel, students, parents, community advocates, and project staff to implement the program components (Comer, 1988), propose changes in school policy, develop other school/community liaisons supportive of school-based efforts, and solicit community organizations to conduct activities to support the SCI efforts. A goal of these linkages was to "rebuild the village" and create a "sense of ownership" by all stakeholders to promote sustainability of these efforts on completion of the project (Bell and Fink, 2000; Bell, Gamm, Vallas, and Jackson, 2001).

With the TTI as its conceptual foundation, Aban Aya included constructs from the PERSONAL, SOCIAL, and cultural-ENVIRONMENTAL streams (see Figure 16.4). For example, both the SDI and SCI incorporated skill building (for example, resistance, assertiveness, conflict resolution, and negotiation) from the PERSONAL stream, norms awareness and clarification from the SOCIAL stream, and values education from the cultural-ENVIRONMENTAL stream. Furthermore, the project included ultimate, distal, and proximal levels of causation. For example, the SCI incorporated more ultimate levels of causation and represented an ecological approach by including (1) a parental component, (2) a school climate component, and (3) a community component (see Figure 16.4). Thus, by addressing ultimate levels of causation, distal influences, and proximal predictors, we expected that the SCI would result in a greater reduction in the growth of negative behaviors than the SDC alone (Flay et al., 2004).

By including contextual components, the TTI would predict that both experimental conditions would improve behavior and that the SCI would have stronger effects than the SDC. Results supported this prediction. For boys in the SDC and SCI conditions, there were significant reductions in the rate of increase in negative behaviors from fifth to eighth grade compared to boys in the HEC condition: violence by 35 percent and 47 percent, from the SDC and SCI conditions, respectively; provoking behavior, 41 percent and 59 percent; school delinquency, 31 percent and 66 percent; drug use, 32 percent and 34 percent; and recent sexual intercourse, 44 percent and 65 percent. Among those who were sexually active, the relative improvements in condom use were 95 percent and 165 percent, respectively. A recent review of violence-prevention interventions (Limbos et al., 2007) indicated that Aban Aya was one of

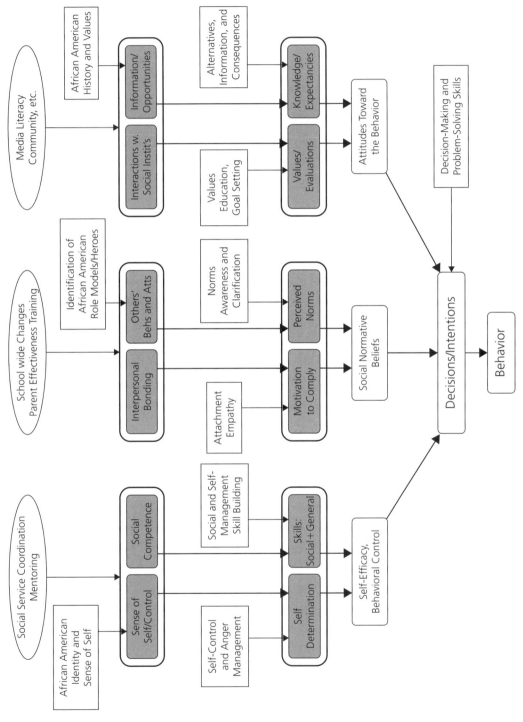

FIGURE 16.4 *The Aban Aya Program Content Mapped onto the TTI*

only two primary-level interventions (that is, implemented universally to prevent inception of violence) that were evaluated with a randomized trial and that demonstrated a significant reduction in violence outcomes.

In addition to providing a framework for the Aban Aya interventions, the TTI also offered a framework to evaluate the interventions and test potential mediators. For example, Ngwe and colleagues (Ngwe et al., 2004) found that, as the TTI would predict, behavioral intentions, attitudes toward violence, estimates of peers' behaviors, and estimates of best friends' behaviors were complete mediators between the intervention and its preventive effects. Likewise, Jagers and colleagues (2007a) investigated if Aban Aya produced differences in changes over time in communal value orientation, empathy, and violence avoidance self-efficacy beliefs. They found that both the SDC and SCI had significant effects on empathy; thereby reducing the likelihood of violent behavior over time. Moreover, they indicated that changes over time in violence avoidance self-efficacy were related to less violent behavior over time.

The TTI provided a ready source of mediation hypotheses for Ngwe et al. (2004) and Jagers et al. (2007a). Consequently, other researchers can select the various constructs incorporated in the TTI to gain a greater understanding of the effects of a particular intervention. Additionally, the TTI provides researchers with a testable model and allows them to study many variables to understand their influence on a particular behavior, allowing researchers to better understand the etiology of behaviors and how to alter them.

STRENGTHS AND LIMITATIONS OF THE THEORY OF TRIADIC INFLUENCE

The TTI provides a single, unifying framework that organizes the constructs from many other theories. Indeed, the TTI is pan-theoretical in orientation and provides a "rapprochement" of competing theories (Flay, 2002) by bringing together constructs and processes from various multivariate theories of behavior, including, but not limited to the following:

■ Theories of ultimate influences like social control theory (Hirschi, 1969) and its extensions (Elliott, Huizinga, and Menard, 1989), social development theory (Hawkins and Weis, 1985), biological vulnerability (Sher, 1991);

■ Theories of distal influences like family attachment (Baumrind, 1985; Brook, Brook, Gordon, and Whiteman, 1990), peer clustering (Oetting and Beauvais, 1986), personality (Digman, 1990; Zuckerman, 1971; Zuckerman et al., 1990);

■ Theories of proximal cognitive-affective predictors of behavior, such as the Health Beliefs Model (Becker, 1974; Janz and Becker, 1984), the theory of reasoned action (Fishbein and Ajzen, 1975), the theory of planned behavior (Ajzen, 1985, 1988, 1991), self-regulation, self-determination, and self-control theories (Aarts, 2007; Deci and Ryan, 1985; Hall and Fong, 2007), numerous expectancy-value theories (Atkinson, 1957; Feather, 1982), and self-efficacy theory (Bandura, 1977);

- Theories that cross levels and streams of influence like social learning (Akers, 1977; Akers et al., 1979), social cognitive theory (Bandura, 1986), social ecological systems (Bronfrenbrenner, 1979, 1986); and

- Other integrative theories (Huba and Bentler, 1982; Jessor and Jessor, 1977; Sadava, 1987).

See Petraitis, Flay, and Miller (1995) for a review of many of these theories.

One major strength of the TTI is that it provides dozens of testable hypotheses about causal processes, including mediation, moderation, and reciprocal effects. The TTI is useful not only for explaining behavior, but also for designing interventions for the treatment or prevention of health-compromising or other risky behaviors, the promotion of health-enhancing and other positive behaviors, and positive youth development (Catalano, Berglund, Ryan, Lonczak, and Hawkins, 2004; Flay, 2002; Lerner, 2006; Lerner et al., in press).

The TTI has major implications for understanding behavior and its change. The most obvious implication is that the determinants of any one behavior are many and varied. They range from proximal (decision/intentions and affective/cognitive predictors) to ultimate causes (those characteristics one brings into the world and the cultural and social environments within which one is raised and matures). These all act through three major streams and multiple levels of causation: (1) intra-PERSONAL characteristics, which are the major determinants of an adolescent's sense of self and competence (social and general) that, in turn, influence their self-esteem and self-efficacy; (2) the SOCIAL situations/contexts or micro-environments, which provide role models and are the major determinants of social bonding that, in turn, influence social normative beliefs; and (3) the cultural-ENVIRONMENTS, which are the major determinants of knowledge and values that, in turn, influence attitudes. There are important interactions between streams of influence, so that features within each stream affect features within others. Finally, feedback loops to and from behavioral experiences and both proximal predictors and the social-personal nexus influence both (1) how a behavior is experienced, and (2) the likelihood of future repetitions of the behavior. We have formalized all of these properties into ten postulates of the TTI as shown in Table 16.5.

IMPLICATIONS FOR BEHAVIOR CHANGE (PREVENTION OR PROMOTION)

The comprehensiveness of the TTI clarifies why informational or didactic educational approaches to prevention have usually failed. They focused toward the bottom of only the cultural-ENVIRONMENTAL stream of influence. Affective approaches have also failed because they also focused near the middle (values clarification) or the bottom (decision making) of only the cultural-ENVIRONMENTAL stream. Only more recent programs have added a focus on the intra-PERSONAL stream by addressing the need for social skills and self-efficacy; however, though some of these

TABLE 16.5 Postulates of the Theory of Triadic Influence.

1. The TTI provides a comprehensive, meta-theoretical view of behavior in which a symmetrical, higher-order system of description and explanation integrates multiple levels of organization. Certainly, no one variable can provide an adequate explanation of behavior—and there is no silver bullet for changing a behavior. In addition, no one existing theory can provide a satisfactory description of behavior. It requires the integration of numerous theories from many disciplines and subdisciplines to provide a full understanding of behavior. The TTI satisfies the requirements of a systems theory in that it is comprehensive, systematic, involves multiple levels and ecologies, includes feedback loops, and is symmetrical (Stewart and Cohen, 1997).

2. All behavioral choices are influenced by the interaction of genetic/nature and environmental/nurture factors.

3. Each behavioral choice is influenced by a complex system of PERSONAL (intrapersonal → self-efficacy), SOCIAL (interpersonal → social normative beliefs) and ENVIRONMENTAL (sociocultural → attitudes) factors.

4. All three (triadic) streams of influence each have two substreams: three control/values/affective/feelings sub-streams, and three information/cognitive substreams.

5. All (sub) streams of influence flow from causes most distant (ultimate) through distal influences to predictors closest (proximal) to the behavior of interest—a cascade of multiple and interacting influences. Proximal influences predict behavior while distal influences and ultimate causes help explain it.

6. Most influences, including all informative/cognitive influences, can have positive or negative values. The more positive influences there are, the more likely are positive behaviors. The more negative influences there are, the more likely are negative behaviors.

7. The most proximal control/affect predictors have values that range from zero to one (probabilities). The higher these probabilities, the more influence the corresponding information/cognitions will have on behavioral choices.

8. Interactions across streams can increase or reduce risks/protection; for example, positive sense of self can reduce risk in disorganized communities, negative sense of self can increase risk in protective families, positive community/family forces can protect against poor sense of self.

9. Once a behavior occurs, the resulting reactions and/or experiences (thoughts and feelings) feed back to change the original causes. For example, engaging in a behavior changes one's self-efficacy, relationships with parents and peers, and attitudes. Feedback changes the likelihood of engaging in the same or a similar behavior in the future. Thus, causes and effects are in a continuous cycle: with each action changing the causes, and the changed causes leading to the same, similar or different behavior over time, involving many mutually influential individual contextual relations and developmental regulation.

10. The reactions to certain behaviors feed back to influence the causes of related behaviors (for example, smoking and other drug use); that is, related behaviors have similar causes, with the more distal causes being the most similar. Less related behaviors (for example, smoking and skiing) have fewer causes in common. Even related behaviors may have some differences in proximal causes.

programs have demonstrated improvements in skills and self-efficacy, only weak linkages have been found between improved skills and subsequent behavior (MacKinnon et al., 1991). We suspect several reasons for this. First, many such programs minimized the informational and values components, so reducing the components that should motivate youth to *want* to behave differently. Second, the SOCIAL stream was still not addressed adequately. Though these programs included components to increase awareness of social influences, few of them deliberately altered social normative beliefs (or actual norms in the surrounding society). Recent studies demonstrate the importance of such components (Hansen and Graham, 1991; Kirby, Barth, Leland, and Fetro, 1991; MacKinnon et al., 1991). Few programs of any type addressed the upper levels of any of the streams of influence. Evidence from multiple studies suggests the power of altering influences on the upper levels of the SOCIAL and cultural-ENVIRONMENTAL streams (for example, school policies, increasing taxes, driving under the influence legislation, speed limits, legislating the wearing of seat belts, activism against billboards).

New interventions need to be broader, longer, and deeper; but we should not throw out all of the content of traditional approaches. We need to include family participation and parenting/communication skills, teach multiple relevant skills, consider special interventions for children in high-risk families, and consider how to impact broad sociocultural influences. Regarding the latter, perhaps we can train students to be advocates, reduce sales/access to minors (alcohol and tobacco), eliminate advertising of alcohol and tobacco on billboards and TV, increase taxes on tobacco and alcohol, change school lunches, reduce exposure to violence on TV and in movies, and so on. In short, the best interventions will use contextual and behavioral change strategies from all six sub-streams and from multiple causal levels (see Table 16.1).

Limitations

Comprehensiveness also leads to complexity—and complexity poses, perhaps, the biggest challenge to the TTI. Simply put, it is difficult to test the predictive power of the entire theory in one study (though Willoughby et al. [2008] made a good attempt) because that study would have to measure—and measure adequately—twenty-two different sets of variables (see Figure 16.1), the more proximal ones separately for each behavior of interest. Some sets of variables might be relatively easy to define and measure, especially TTI's proximal predictors; however, other sets of variables are considerably harder to define and measure. For instance, "cultural environment variables"—the ultimate causes in the cultural-ENVIRONMENTAL stream—need to be measured, but the TTI does not yet offer detailed guidance on which cultural environment variables need to be measured. Similarly, researchers should measure ultimate personality variables, but TTI does not yet say exactly which personality variables to measure. Starting with "the Big Five" (openness to experience, conscientiousness, extraversion, agreeableness, and neuroticism) personality variables would be a good start, but the list could be much longer. As research advances in these twenty-two sets of variables, future versions of the TTI can provide a more complete list of variables to measure. For now, however, the complexity of the TTI leads to piecemeal evidence: one study showing support for one set of paths, another study showing support for another set of paths.

It also may be difficult to incorporate all influences in one intervention. The Aban Aya program (Flay et al., 2004) and other programs such as the Positive Action program (Flay and Allred, 2003; Flay, Allred, and Ordway, 2001; Beets, et al., 2009) demonstrate how it might be done. Future HP needs to focus less on the micro levels of causation and more on the distal and ultimate levels. A focus on distal and ultimate levels will lead to programs that are more efficient because they change multiple behaviors at once, and will lead to programs that are more sustainable because they change the cultural context. David Olds's home nursing program (1997) is an example of an intervention that has long-term effects on multiple youth behaviors. We need to focus more on the big picture, so that HP programs can socially infiltrate society, like fast food and TV have done!

Note that a focus on distal and ultimate levels is NOT the same as a focus on only the environment—it still includes interpersonal-social situations and the person. Some advocates of the focus on the environment leave out the ultimate or distal influences in the interpersonal and intrapersonal domains. We believe that there are distal and ultimate aspects of all three streams that should be focused on, not just of the environmental stream.

FUTURE DIRECTIONS

The TTI will be about fifteen years old when this book is published. The behavioral and health sciences have changed greatly during those years. One change has been the rapid growth in new technologies that can investigate the biological contributions to thoughts, feelings, and behaviors. Results from the Human Genome Project were published in 2001, providing a basis for researchers to look at the relationships between different genotypes and phenotypes. As a result, scientists are learning more about the biology of behavior, and advancing more detailed theory about such influences (Dodge and Pettit, 2003; Reiss and Leve, 2007). For instance, deBry and Tiffany (2008) recently proposed that early initiation of tobacco use has neurotoxic effects that alter the normal progress of neurodevelopment, particularly in the areas of executive functioning and control of inhibitions. In another example, a mediational study highlighted the importance of studying how program-influence variables at the distal level in the PERSONAL stream, namely, students' brain development and functional capabilities (Riggs, Greenberg, Kusché, and Pentz, 2006). In this study, improved neuropsychological functioning, in terms of increased inhibitory control and verbal fluency, partially mediated improvement in behavioral problems. Furthermore, neuroimaging research indicates that learning-oriented interventions can result in positive brain changes (Roffman, Marci, Glick, Dougherty, and Rauch, 2005).

Other research highlights the importance of other biological factors. For example, substance use tends to run in families (Sher, 1991) and is also linked to a variety of biological factors (Cloninger, 1987; Phil, Peterson, and Finn, 1990; Tarter, Alterman, and Edwards, 1985). Along these lines, studies have shown that cigarette use among girls (but not boys) is positively related to testosterone levels (Bauman, Foshee, and Haley, 1992); the early onset of puberty predicts the onset of cigarette use (D. M. Wilson et al., 1994); and levels of serotonin and dopamine influence cocaine consumption among rats (White, 1997). In its original form, the TTI had little to say about such influences. The TTI does, however, have a structure and a location to place biological influences—among the ultimate-level intrapersonal influences. We hope that the future of the TTI will do more than have a place for biological influences; we hope that it spells out the biological mechanisms in more detail.

Another important change in the sciences since the TTI's inception is the rise in systematic research on evolutionary influences on human behavior and the recognition that many behaviors people do today might have genetic roots in behaviors that benefited ancestral humans 200,000 years ago. Evolutionary psychology might, for example, help explain unsafe sex practices, poor diets, and lack of exercise in today's modern world (Cosmides and Tooby, 2003). With hunter-gatherer humans facing a short and strenuous existence with frequent infant mortality and scarce food (especially calorie- and protein-rich foods), cautious sex, dieting, and forgoing opportunities for rest were costly behaviors of ancestral humans. Having inherited our genes from hunter-gatherer humans, modern humans might have inherited genetic inclinations towards unprotected sex; food cravings for fat, protein, and carbohydrates rather than vegetables; and a preference to be sedentary whenever possible. Originally, the TTI had little to say about these and other evolutionary influences (Petraitis, Lampman, and Falconer, 2008). Whereas the biological influences discussed in the previous paragraph might fit neatly into the TTI's PERSONAL influences stream, evolutionary influences also contribute to the SOCIAL and cultural-ENVIRONMENTAL streams (Richerson and Boyd, 2005; Sober and Wilson, 1998; D. S. Wilson, 2007; D. S Wilson and Csikszentmihalyi, 2008). We hope we can spell out the role of evolution in HRBs in more detail in future versions of the TTI.

We also hope that the future of the TTI spells out more specifically the roles of some key demographic factors such as gender, age, ethnic heritage, and socioeconomic status in greater detail. Each of these demographic factors probably affects variables in each of the TTI's streams. For example, being a female might affect one's rebelliousness and sense of self (variables in the PERSONAL stream), how one evaluates the various consequences of a behavior (a variable in the cultural-ENVIRONMENTAL stream) and the quantity and nature of one's social bonds (a variable in the SOCIAL stream). Future versions of the TTI should address the likely cross-stream influence of these key demographic variables.

Finally, we remind readers that the TTI is just as relevant to positive behaviors as to the negative ones on which HB researchers tend to focus. All of the same variables and pathways are involved in the prediction of positive behaviors. One of us has written elsewhere about the role of TTI in positive youth development (Flay, 2002). In the long term, however, the HP field needs to focus less on the micro levels, and more on the common distal and ultimate levels. We need to focus more on the big picture so that our HP programs socially infiltrate society. It is for this reason that we bold one row of Table 16.4.

SUMMARY

The TTI is an ambitious theory: compared to other models of HRBs, the TTI aims to provide a more coherent structure for a more comprehensive set of variables. It should not be viewed, however, as finished. It is a work in progress and as scientists discover more pieces in the puzzle of HRB, we hope that the TTI will expand and will help show how the pieces fit together.

Everything in our biological/personal, social, and sociocultural (including physical) environments—from cells to society, from neurons to neighborhoods (Shonkoff and Phillips, 2000), from global warming to environmental contaminants, from national welfare policies to neighborhood poverty, from politics to religion, from international trade policies to the availability of healthy food and affordable energy—affects our health status both directly, and indirectly through affecting our behavior (Glass and McAtee, 2006). The TTI helps us understand the multiple determinants of our behavior and the complex webs of interacting and cascading linkages between the causes as they flow from ultimate to distal, and from distal to proximal, to ultimately influence multiple behaviors.

It is important to realize that each ultimate cause influences multiple behaviors. Indeed, they also influence many other aspects of human life besides the HRBs of interest in this text. They influence behavior in every realm of life as well as multiple health outcomes (Link and Phelan, 1995; Rose, 1985). For example, socioeconomic status (or education) predicts the risk of engaging in health-compromising behavior as well as morbidity and mortality. Further, socioeconomic status (SES) predicts health status in ways independent of its path through HRBs (Coburn, 2000, 2004); for example, by leading to chronic stress, which, in turn, leads to increased levels of cortisol and adrenalin in the body, leading to increased disease of diabetes, cardiovascular disease, and other morbidities (Adler and Newman, 2002; Coburn, 2000; House, 2002; Kawachi and Subramanian, 2007; Krieger, 2007; Marmot, 2001; Marmot and Wilkinson, 2006).

Ethnicity and culture also play important roles in both behavior and health status. Although the SES-health gradient exists for both whites and African Americans in the U.S. population, the overall level of health is lower for African Americans than it is for whites at every level of SES. This is, in part at least, because of the higher frequency of stressful experiences brought on by racism in the United States, leading to increases in cortisol and adrenalin flowing through the body more frequently for African Americans than whites (Morenoff et al., 2007; Williams and Earl, 2007). Another example concerns brain and language development—both are influenced by SES because of differing exposures to stimuli (Hart and Risley, 1995; Merzenich, 2001).

The point of the above two paragraphs is that the ultimate causes of HRB (biological/PERSONAL, SOCIAL situational or cultural-ENVIRONMENTAL) are also the ultimate or underling causes of many forms of morbidity and many other human developmental experiences. The TTI also makes it clear, however, that there are many pathways through which the effects of these underlying causal influences can be redirected so as to *not* have the influences addressed in these paragraphs! This is the critical work of HP. For example, any particular risk factor need not be predictive of bad outcomes because protective factors in youth's lives may counteract them. Using interventions derived from the TTI could place those protective factors in the lives of children in risky contexts in a strategic and intentional manner that actualizes the goals of HB change so essential to public health (Dodge and Pettit, 2003).

It is also important to understand that each behavior has multiple determinants (in addition to each ultimate cause influencing multiple behaviors). The complex relationships between causes and outcomes can be characterized as a "complex adaptive system" (Gell-Mann, 2003; Trochim, Cabrera, Milstein, Gallagher, and Leischow, 2006; Waldrop, 1992). One can view multiple pathways of influence coming into each behavior, the outcome-oriented view (Elder and Pellerin, 1998), or multiple pathways of influence emanating from each ultimate causal factor, the event-oriented view (Elder and Pellerin, 1998). The outcome-oriented model links multiple events, from proximal to distal, to the outcome of interest. Conversely, the event-oriented model links the events of interest to multiple proximal and distal outcomes. Both the outcome-oriented and event-oriented approaches can be applied to studies of HP. Somewhere in the middle is the complexity that is located between bottom-up and top-down explanations of nearly all behaviors and scientific phenomena. Biological systems theorists have called this region of complexity "the uncharted territory of ant country" after the phenomenon of ants using simple rules that lead to complex behavior (Stewart and Cohen, 1997). It is a bit like a chess game; at the beginning and end, the moves are all quite easy to understand, but in the middle, when you have a number of pieces on the board, even a chess master cannot work out your next move without knowing your overall plan.

Working upwards from intentions/decisions and other affective/cognitive factors, it is (just) possible to explain most behavior. However, the properties of affective/cognitive factors also need explanation, and these multiply upwards. In this sense, affect and cognitions, taken alone, cannot explain every behavior (or any of them!). On the other hand, simply moving to the ultimate levels and saying that nature or nurture explain everything is not very satisfying either (Institute of Medicine, 2006). Both extremes, by themselves, are almost useless as explanatory devices—we need to understand the influences on behavior (and our health) at both levels and the complexity of the linkages in between. The TTI is our attempt to understand "ant country"; to provide the linkages between the more traditional top-down and bottom-up approaches to understanding behavior.

Anyone in the business of HP must know two things: what causes HRBs, and how to effectively promote health-enhancing behaviors (like wearing seat belts) or deter health-compromising behaviors (like smoking cigarettes). This knowledge, however, has been evasive. We hope that those in the business of HP will benefit by pinning the TTI to their walls.

ACKNOWLEDGMENTS

We thank Alan Acock, Brad Corbett, Joseph Durlak, and Mary Jane Rotheram-Borus for very helpful comments on earlier drafts. Colored versions of the figures are available from the first author.

REFERENCES

Aarts, H. (2007). Health and goal-directed behavior: The conscious regulation and motivation of goals and their pursuit. *Health Psychology Review*, *1*(1), 53–82.

Aarts, H., and Dijksterhuis, A. (2000). Habits as knowledge structures: Automaticity in goal-directed behavior. *Journal of Personality and Social Psychology*, *78*(1), 53–63.

Abrams, D. (1999). Transdisciplinary paradigms for tobacco prevention research. *Nicotine and Tobacco Research*, *1*, S15–S23.

Adler, N. E., and Newman, K. (2002). Socioeconomic disparities in health: Pathways and policies. *Health Affairs*, *21*(2), 60.

Airhihenbuwa, C. O. (1995). *Health and culture: Beyond the Western paradigm*. Thousand Oaks, CA: Sage.

Ajzen, I. (1985). From decisions to actions: A theory of planned behavior. In J. Kuhl and J. Beckmann (eds.), *Action-control: From cognition to behavior* (pp. 11–39). Heidelberg: Springer.

Ajzen, I. (1988). *Attitudes, personality, and behavior*. Homewood, IL: Dorsey Press.

Ajzen, I. (1991). The theory of planned behavior. *Organizational Behavior and Human Decision Processes*, *50*(2), 179–211.

Akers, R. L. (1977). *Deviant behavior: A social learning approach* (2nd ed.). Belmont, CA: Wadsworth.

Akers, R. L., Krohn, M. D., Lanza-Kaduce, L., and Radosevich, M. (1979). Social learning and deviant behavior: A specific test of a general theory. *American Sociological Review*, *44*(4), 636–655.

Anderson, T. L. (1998). A cultural-identity theory of drug abuse. *Sociology of Crime, Law, and Deviance, 1*, 233–262.

Arnold, E. M., Rice, E., Flannery, D., and Rotheram-Borus, M. J. (2008). HIV disclosure among adults living with HIV. *AIDS Care*, 20(1), 80–92.

Atkinson, J. W. (1957). Motivational determinants of risk-taking behavior. *Psychological Review*, 64, Part 1(6), 359–372.

Bandura, A. (1977). *Social learning theory*. Oxford, England: Prentice-Hall.

Bandura, A. (1986). *Social foundations of thought and action: A social cognitive theory*. Englewood Cliffs, NJ: Prentice-Hall, In P. Norman (Ed.),

Bandura, A. (2000). Health promotion from the perspective of social cognitive theory. In P. Norman (Ed.), *Understanding and changing health behaviour: From health beliefs to self-regulation*, (pp. 299–337). Amsterdam: Harwood Academic.

Bandura, A. (2005). The primacy of self-regulation in health promotion. *Applied Psychology: An International Review*, *54*(2), 245–254.

Baranowski, T., Anderson, C., and Carmack, C. (1998). Mediating variable framework in physical activity interventions. How are we doing? How might we do better? *American Journal of Preventive Medicine*, *15*(4), 266–297.

Baron, R. M., and Kenny, D. A. (1986). The moderator-mediator variable distinction in social psychological research: Conceptual, strategic, and statistical considerations. *Journal of Personality and Social Psychology,* *51*(6), 1173–1182.

Bartholomew, L. K., Parcel, G. S., Kok, G., and Gottlieb, N. H. (2006). *Planning health promotion programs: An intervention mapping approach.* San Francisco: Jossey-Bass.

Bauman, K. E., Foshee, V. A., and Haley, N. J. (1992). The interaction of sociological and biological factors in adolescent cigarette smoking. *Addictive Behaviors, 17*(5), 459–467.

Baumrind, D. (1985). Familial antecedents of adolescent drug use: A developmental perspective. In C. L. Jones and R. J. Battjes (eds.), *Etiology of drug abuse: Implications for prevention* (pp. 13–44). Rockville, MD: National Institute on Drug Abuse.

Baxter, L. A., and Bullis, C. (1986). Turning points in developing romantic relationships. *Human Communication Research, 12*(4), 469–493.

Bearinger, L. H., and Resnick, M. D. (2003). Dual method use in adolescents: A review and framework for research on use of STD and pregnancy protection. *The Journal of Adolescent Health, 32*(5), 340–349.

Becker, M. H. (ed.). (1974). *The health belief model and personal health behavior.* Thorofare, NJ: Slack.

Beets, M. W., Flay, B. R., Vuchinich, S., Snyder, F. J., Acock, A., Li, K.-K., Burns, K. et al. (2009). Using a social and character development program to prevent substance use, violent behaviors, and sexual activity among elementary-school students in Hawai'i. *American Journal of Public Health,* 99(8), 1438-1445.

Bell, C. C., Bhana, A., McKay, M. M., and Petersen, I. (2007). A commentary on the triadic theory of influence as a guide for adapting HIV prevention programs for new contexts and populations: The CHAMP-South Africa story. *Social Work in Mental Health, 5*(3/4), 243–267.

Bell, C. C., Bhana, A., Petersen, I., McKay, M., Gibbons, R., Bannon, W., et al. (2008). Building Protective Factors to Offset Sexually Risky Behaviors Among Black Youths: A Randomized Control Trial. *Journal of the National Medical Association, 100*(8), 936–944.

Bell, C. C., and Fink, P. J. (2000). Prevention of violence. In *Psychiatric aspects of violence: Issues in prevention and treatment.* (pp. 37–47). San Francisco: Jossey-Bass.

Bell, C. C., Gamm, S., Vallas, P., and Jackson, P. (eds.). (2001). *Strategies for the prevention of youth violence in Chicago public schools.* Washington, DC: American Psychiatric Press.

Bell, C. C., and McKay, M. M. (2004). Constructing a children's mental health infrastructure using community psychiatry principles. *Journal of Legal Medicine, 25*(1), 5–22.

Bellack, A., Elkin, I., Flay, B. R., Fishbein, M., Gottman, J., Pequegnat, W., et al. (2001). *An integrated framework for preventive and treatment interventions.* Paper presented at the NIMH Intervention Workgroup meeting.

Berndt, T. J. (1979). Developmental changes in conformity to peers and parents. *Developmental Psychology, 15*(6), 608–616.

Bierman, K. L., Coie, J. D., Dodge, K. A., Foster, E. M., Greenberg, M. T., Lochman, J. E., et al. (2004). The effects of the Fast Track program on serious problem outcomes at the end of elementary school. *Journal of Clinical Child and Adolescent Psychology, 33*(4), 650–661.

Biglan, A. (1995). *Changing cultural practices: A contextualist framework for intervention research.* Reno, NV: Context Press.

Biglan, A. (2003). Selection by consequences: One unifying principle for a transdisciplinary science of prevention. *Prevention Science, 4*(4), 213–232.

Biglan, A. (2004). Contextualism and the development of effective prevention practices. *Prevention Science, 5*(1), 15–21.

Biglan, A., Brennan, P. A., Foster, S. L., and Holder, H. D. (2004). *Helping adolescents at risk: Prevention of multiple problem behaviors.* New York: Guilford.

Biglan, A., Mrazek, P. J., Carnine, D., and Flay, B. R. (2003). The integration of research and practice in the prevention of youth problem behaviors. *American Psychologist, 58*(6/7), 433.

Botvin, G. J., Griffin, K. W., and Nichols, T. D. (2006). Preventing youth violence and delinquency through a universal school-based prevention approach. *Prevention Science*, *7*, 403–408.

Brindis, C. D., and Lee, P. R. (1991). Adolescents conceptualization of illness. In R. M. Learner, A. C. Petersen and J. Brooks-Gunn (eds.), *Encyclopedia of adolescence* (pp. 534–540). New York: Garland.

Bronfrenbrenner, U. (1979). *The ecology of human development*. Cambridge, MA: Harvard University Press.

Bronfrenbrenner, U. (1986). Ecology of the family as a context for human development. *Developmental Psychology*, *22*, 723–742.

Bronfrenbrenner, U. (2005). *Making human beings human: Bioecological perspectives on human development*. Thousand Oaks, CA: Sage.

Brook, J. S., Brook, D. W., Gordon, A. S., and Whiteman, M. (1990). The psychosocial etiology of adolescent drug use: A family interactional approach. *Genetic, Social and General Psychology Monographs*, *116*, 111–267.

Brown, B. B., Clasen, D. R., and Eicher, S. A. (1986). Perceptions of peer pressure, peer conformity dispositions, and self-reported behavior among adolescents. *Developmental Psychology*, *22*(521–530).

Browne, D. C., Clubb, P. A., Aubrecht, A.M.B., and Jackson, M. (2001). Minority health risk behaviors: An introduction to research on sexually transmitted diseases, violence, pregnancy prevention and substance use. *Maternal and Child Health Journal*, *5*(4), 215.

Brug, J., de Vet, E., de Nooijer, J., and Verplanken, B. (2006). Predicting fruit consumption: cognitions, intention, and habits. *Journal of Nutrition Education and Behavior*, *38*(2), 73–81.

Brug, J., Oenema, A., and Campbell, M. (2003). Past, present, and future of computer-tailored nutrition education. *The American Journal of Clinical Nutrition*, *77*(4 Suppl), 1028S–1034S.

Brug, J., Oenema, A., and Ferreira, I. (2005). Theory, evidence and intervention mapping to improve behavior nutrition and physical activity interventions. *International Journal of Behavioral Nutrition and Physical Activity*, *2*(2).

Brug, J., van Lenthe, F. J., and Kremers, S.P.J. (2006). Revisiting Kurt Lewin: How to gain insight into environmental correlates of obesogenic behaviors. *American Journal of Preventive Medicine*, *31*(6), 525–529.

Busseri, M., Willoughby, T., Chalmers, H., and YLC-CURA. (2005, April). *Applying the theory of triadic influence to multiple adolescent health risk behaviors*. Paper presented at the Society for Research on Children Development, Atlanta, Georgia.

Carvajal, S. C., Evans, R. I., Nash, S. G., and Getz, J. G. (2002). Global positive expectancies of the self and adolescent substance use avoidance: Testing a social influence mediational model. *Journal of Personality*, *70*(3), 421–442.

Carvajal, S. C., and Granillo, T. M. (2006). A prospective test of distal and proximal determinants of smoking initiation in early adolescents. *Addictive Behaviors*, *31*(4), 649–660.

Carvajal, S. C., Hanson, C., Downing, R. A., Coyle, K. K., and Pederson, L. L. (2004). Theory-Based Determinants of Youth Smoking: A Multiple Influence Approach. *Journal of Applied Social Psychology*, *34*(1), 59–84.

Catalano, R. F., Berglund, M. L., Ryan, J.A.M., Lonczak, H. S., and Hawkins, J. D. (2004). Positive youth development in the United States: Research findings on evaluations of positive youth development programs. *The Annals of the American Academy of Political and Social Science*, *591*(1), 98.

Chalmers, H., and Willoughby, T. (2006). Do predictors of gambling involvement differ across male and female adolescents? *Journal of Gambling Studies*, *22*(4), 373–392.

Cloninger, C. R. (1987). Neurogenetic adaptive mechanisms in alcoholism. *Science*, *236*, 410–416.

Coburn, D. (2000). Income inequality, social cohesion and the health status of populations: The role of neo-liberalism. *Social Science and Medicine*, *51*(1), 135–146.

Coburn, D. (2004). Beyond the income inequality hypothesis: Class, neo-liberalism, and health inequalities. *Social Science and Medicine*, *58*(1), 41–56.

Comer, J. P. (1988). Educating poor minority children. *Scientific American, 259*(5), 42.

Commers, M. J., Gottlieb, N., and Kok, G. (2007). How to change environmental conditions for health. *Health Promotion International, 22*(1), 80–87.

Cosmides, L., and Tooby, J. (2003). *What is evolutionary psychology?: Explaining the new science of the mind.* New Haven, CT: Yale University Press.

Csikszentmihalyi, M., and Nakamura, J. (1999). Emerging goals and the self-regulation of behavior. *Perspectives on behavioral self-regulation, 12*, 107–118.

Dahl, R. E. (2001). Affect regulation, brain development, and behavioral/emotional health in adolescence. *CNS Spectrums, 6*(1), 60–72.

Dahl, R. E. (2004). Adolescent brain development: A period of vulnerabilities and opportunities. In *Adolescent brain development: Vulnerabilities and opportunities.* (Vol. 1021, pp. 1–22). New York: New York Academy of Sciences.

Dahlberg, L. L. (1998). Youth violence in the United States. Major trends, risk factors, and prevention approaches. *American Journal of Preventive Medicine, 14*(4), 259–272.

Damon, W. (1991). Adolescent self-concept. In R. M. Learner, A. C. Petersen and J. Brooks-Gunn (eds.), *Encyclopedia of adolescence* (pp. 987–991). New York: Garland.

de Bruijn, G. J., Kremers, S.P.J., Schaalma, H., van Mechelen, W., and Brug, J. (2005). Determinants of adolescent bicycle use for transportation and snacking behavior. *Preventive Medicine, 40*(6), 658–667.

de Bruijn, G. J., Kremers, S.P.J., van Mechelen, W., and Brug, J. (2005). Is personality related to fruit and vegetable intake and physical activity in adolescents? *Health Education Research, 20*(6), 635–644.

de Vries, H., and Lechner, L. (2000). Motives for protective behavior against carcinogenic substances in the workplace: A pilot study. *Journal of Occupational and Environmental Medicine, 42*(1), 88.

deBry, S. C., and Tiffany, S. T. (2008). Tobacco-induced neurotoxicity of adolescent cognitive development (TINACD): A proposed model for the development of impulsivity in nicotine dependence. *Nicotine and Tobacco Research, 10*(1), 11–25.

Deci, E. L., and Ryan, R. M. (1985). *Intrinsic motivation and self-determination in human behavior.* New York: Plenum.

Diamond, A., Barnett, W. S., Thomas, J., and Munro, S. (2007). The early years: Preschool program improves cognitive control. *Science, 318*(5855), 1387.

Diamond, A., and Kirkham, N. (2005). Parallels between cognition in childhood and adulthood. *Psychological Science, 16*(4), 291–297.

DiClemente, C. C., Marinilli, A. S., Singh, M., and Bellino, L. E. (2001). The Role of Feedback in the Process of Health Behavior Change. *American Journal of Health Behaviour, 25*(3), 217–227.

Digman, J. M. (1990). Personality structure: emergence of the five-factor model. *Annual Review of Psychology, 41*(417–440).

DiRocco, D. N., and Shadel, W. G. (2007). Gender differences in adolescents' responses to themes of relaxation in cigarette advertising: Relationship to intentions to smoke. *Addictive Behaviors, 32*(2), 205–213.

Dodge, K. A., and Pettit, G. S. (2003). A biopsychosocial model of the development of chronic conduct problems in adolescence. *Developmental Psychology, 39*(2), 349–371.

Drobes, D. J. (2002). Concurrent alcohol and tobacco dependence. *Alcohol Research and Health, 26*(2), 136–142.

DuBois, D. L., and Flay, B. R. (2004). The healthy pursuit of self-esteem: Comment on and alternative to the Crocker and Park (2004) formulation. *Psychological Bulletin, 130*(3), 415–420.

DuBois, D. L., Flay, B. R., and Fagen, M. C. (this volume). Self-esteem enhancement theory: Promoting health across the life-span. In R. J. DiClemente, M. C. Kegler and R. A. Crosby (eds.), *Emerging Theories in Health Promotion Practice and Research* (2nd ed.) San Francisco: Jossey-Bass.

Duncan, T. E., and McAuley, E. (1993). Social support and efficacy cognitions in exercise adherence: A latent growth curve analysis. *Journal of Behavioral Medicine, 16*, 199–218.

Dusenbury, L., and Botvin, G. J. (1990). Competence enhancement and the prevention of adolescent problem behavior. In K. Hurrelmann and F. Losel (eds.), *Health Hazards in Adolescence* (pp. 459–478). Germany: Berlin:/De Gruyter.

Eccles, J. S., Adler, T. F., Futterman, R., Goff, S. B., Kaczala, C. M., Meece, J. L., et al. (1983). Expectancies, values, and academic behaviors. In J. T. Spence (ed.), *Achievement and achievement motivation* (pp. 75–146). New York: W. H. Freeman.

Eells, E. (1991). *Probabilistic causality*. Cambridge: Cambridge University Press.

Elder, G. H., and Pellerin, L. A. (eds.). (1998). *Linking history and human lives*. Thousand Oaks, CA: Sage.

Elkind, D., and Bowen, R. (1979). Imaginary audience behavior in children and adolescents. *Developmental Psychology*, *15*, 33–44.

Elliott, D. S., Huizinga, D., and Ageton, S. S. (1985). *Explaining delinquency and drug use*. Beverly Hills: Sage.

Elliott, D. S., Huizinga, D., and Menard, S. (1989). *Multiple problem youth: Delinquency, substance use, and mental health problems*. New York: Springer-Verlag.

Ertas, N. (2007). Factors associated with stages of cigarette smoking among Turkish youth. *European Journal of Public Health*, *17*(2), 155–161.

Feather, N. T. (ed.). (1982). *Expectations and actions: Expectancy-value models in psychology*. Hillsdale, NJ: Erlbaum.

Ferreira, I., van der Horst, K., Wendel-Vos, W., Kremers, S., van Lenthe, F. J., and Brug, J. (2007). Environmental correlates of physical activity in youth—a review and update. *Obesity Reviews: An Official Journal of The International Association for The Study of Obesity*, *8*(2), 129–154.

Fishbein, M., and Ajzen, I. (1975). *Belief, attitude, intention and behavior: An introduction to theory and research*. Reading, MA: Addison-Wesley.

Flammer, A. (1991). Self-regulation. In R. M. Learner, A. C. Petersen and J. Brooks-Gunn (eds.), *Encyclopedia of adolescence* (pp. 1001–1003). New York: Garland.

Flay, B. R. (1993). Youth tobacco use: risk, patterns, and control. In C. T. Orleans and J. Slade (eds.), *Nicotine addictions: Principles and management*. New York: Oxford University Press.

Flay, B. R. (1999). Understanding environmental, situational and intrapersonal risk and protective factors for youth tobacco use: The theory of triadic influence. *Nicotine and Tobacco Research*, *1*, S111–S114.

Flay, B. R. (2000). Approaches to substance use prevention utilizing school curriculum plus social environment change. *Addictive Behaviors*, *25*(6), 861–885.

Flay, B. R. (2002). Positive youth development requires comprehensive health promotion programs. *American Journal of Health Behavior*, *26*(6), 407.

Flay, B. R., and Allred, C. G. (2003). Long-term effects of the Positive Action program. *American Journal of Health Behavior*, *27*, S6.

Flay, B. R., Allred, C. G., and Ordway, N. (2001). Effects of the Positive Action program on achievement and discipline: two matched-control comparisons. *Prevention Science*, *2*(2), 71–89.

Flay, B. R., and Collins, L. M. (2005). Historical review of school-based randomized trials for evaluating problem behavior prevention programs. *Annals of the American Academy of Political and Social Science*, *599*, 115–146.

Flay, B. R., Graumlich, S., Segawa, E., Burns, J. L., and Holliday, M. Y. (2004). Effects of two prevention programs on high-risk behaviors among African American youth: a randomized trial. *Archives of Pediatrics and Adolescent Medicine*, *158*(4), 377–384.

Flay, B. R., Hu, F. B., Siddiqui, O., Day, L. E., Hedeker, D., Petraitis, J., et al. (1994). Differential influence of parental smoking and friends' smoking on adolescent initiation and escalation of smoking. *Journal of Health and Social Behavior*, *35*(3), 248–265.

Flay, B. R., and Petraitis, J. (1991). Methodological issues in drug use prevention research: Theoretical foundations. *NIDA Research Monograph*, *107*, 81–109.

Flay, B. R., and Petraitis, J. (1994). The theory of triadic influence: A new theory of health behavior with implications for preventive interventions. *Advances in Medical Sociology, 4*, 19–44.

Flay, B. R., and Petraitis, J. (2003). Bridging the gap between substance use prevention theory and practice. In W. J. Bukoski and Z. Sloboda (eds.), *Handbook of drug abuse prevention theory, science, and practice* (pp. 289–305). New York: Kluwer Academic/Plenum Publishers.

Flay, B. R., Petraitis, J., and Hu, F. B. (1995). The theory of triadic influence: Preliminary evidence related to alcohol and tobacco use. In J. B. Fertig and J. P. Allen (eds.), *NIAAA Research Monograph- Alcohol and tobacco: From basic science to clinical practice* (pp. 37–57). Bethesda, MD: U.S. Government Printing Office.

Flay, B. R., Petraitis, J., and Hu, F. B. (1999). Psychosocial risk and protective factors for adolescent tobacco use. *Nicotine and Tobacco Research, 1*, S59–S65.

Fogg, B., and Borody, J. (September, 2001). *The impact of facility no smoking policies and the promotion of smoking cessation on alcohol and drug rehabilitation program outcomes*: Prepared for The Canadian Centre on Substance Abuse, Addictions Policy Working Group.

Foshee, V. A., Ennett, S. T., Bauman, K. E., Granger, D. A., Benefield, T., Suchindran, C., et al. (2007). A test of biosocial models of adolescent cigarette and alcohol involvement. *Journal of Early Adolescence, 27*(1), 4–39.

Foster-Clark, F. S., and Blyth, D. A. (1991). Peer relations and influences. In R. M. Learner, A. C. Petersen and J. Brooks-Gunn (eds.), *Encyclopedia of adolescence* (pp. 767–771). New York: Garland.

Frankenhaeuser, M. (1991). The psychophysiology of workload, stress, and health: Comparison between the sexes. *Annals of Behavioral Medicine, 13*(4), 197–204.

Freudenberg, N., Eng, E., Flay, B. R., Parcel, G., Rogers, T., and Wallerstein, N. (1995). Strengthening individual and community capacity to prevent disease and promote health: in search of relevant theories and principles. *Health Education Quarterly, 22*(3), 290–306.

Freudenberg, N., Silver, D., Carmona, J. M., Kass, D., Lancaster, B., and Speers, M. (2000). Health promotion in the city: A structured review of the literature on interventions to prevent heart disease, substance abuse, violence and HIV infection in U.S. metropolitan areas, 1980–1995. *Journal of Urban Health: Bulletin of the New York Academy of Medicine, 7*(3), 443–457.

Gallant, M. P. (2003). The influence of social support on chronic illness self-management: A review and directions for research. *Health Education and Behavior, 30*(2), 170.

Gell-Mann, M. (2003). *The quark and the jaguar: Adventures in the simple and the complex.* London: Abacus.

George, L. K. (ed.). (2004). *Life course research: Achievements and potential.* New York: Springer.

Gerrard, M., Gibbons, F. X., Houlihan, A. E., Stock, M. L., and Pomery, E. A. (2008). A dual-process approach to health risk decision making: The prototype willingness model. *Developmental Review, 28*(1), 29–61.

Giddens, A. (1987). Time and space in social theory. *Social Science, 72*(2–4), 99–103.

Glanz, K., Lewis, F. M., and Rimer, B. K. (2002). *Health behavior and health education: Theory, research, and practice* (3rd ed.). San Francisco: Jossey-Bass.

Glass, T. A., and McAtee, M. J. (2006). Behavioral science at the crossroads in public health: Extending horizons, envisioning the future. *Social Science and Medicine, 62*(7), 1650–1671.

Glenn, S. S. (1988). Contingencies and metacontingencies: Toward a synthesis of behavior analysis and cultural materialism. *Behavior Analyst, 11*, 161–179.

Goodstadt, M. S. (1978). Alcohol and drug education: Models and outcomes. *Health Education Monographs, 6*(3), 263–279.

Goodstadt, M. S. (1980). Drug education: A turn on or a turn off? *Journal of Drug Education, 10*, 89–99.

Gordon, R. (1983). An operational classification of disease prevention. *Public Health Reports, 98*, 107–109.

Gordon, R. (1987). An operational classification of disease prevention. In J. A. Steinberg and M. M. Silverman (eds.), *Preventing Mental Disorders* (pp. 20–26). Rockville, MD: Health and Human Services.

Graber, J. A., and Brooks-Gunn, J. (1996). Transitions and turning points: Navigating the passage from childhood through adolescence. *Developmental Psychology, 32*(4), 768–776.

Green, L. W. (1992). PATCH: CDC's planned approach to community health: An application of PRECEED and an inspiration for PROCEED. *Journal of Health Education, 23*(3), 140–147.

Green, L. W., and Kreuter, M. W. (2005). *Health program planning: An educational and ecological approach* (4th ed.). New York: McGraw-Hill.

Greenberg, M. T. (2004). Current and future challenges in school-based prevention: The researcher perspective. *Prevention Science, 5*(1), 5–13.

Gross, J. J. (2002). Emotion regulation: Affective, cognitive, and social consequences. *Psychophysiology, 39*(3), 281–291.

Hall, P. A., and Fong, G. T. (2007). Temporal self-regulation theory: A model for individual health behavior. *Health Psychology Review, 1*(1), 6–52.

Hansen, W. B., and Graham, J. W. (1991). Prevention of alcohol, marijuana, and cigarette use among adolescents: Peer pressure resistance skills versus establishing conservative norms. *Preventive Medicine, 20*, 414–430.

Hanson, S., and Hanson, P. (1993). The geography of everyday life. In T. Garling and R. G. Golledge (eds.), *Behavior and environment: Psychological and geographical approaches* (pp. 249–269): North-Holland.

Hart, B., and Risley, T. R. (1995). Meaningful differences in the everyday experience of young American children. Baltimore: Brookes Publishing Company.

Haug, M. (2001). *The use of formative research and persuasion theory in public communication campaigns: An anti-smoking campaign case study.* Paper presented at the Nordic Mass Communication Research Conference.

Hawkins, J. D., Catalano, R. F., and Miller, J. Y. (1992). Risk and protective factors for alcohol and other drug problems in adolescence and early adulthood: Implications for substance abuse prevention. *Psychological Bulletin, 112*(1), 64–105.

Hawkins, J. D., and Weis, J. G. (1985). The social development model: An integrated approach to delinquency prevention. *Journal of Primary Prevention, 6*(2), 73–97.

Hellerstedt, W. L., Rhodes, K. L., Peterson-Hickey, M., and Garwick, A. (2006). Environmental, social, and personal correlates of having ever had sexual intercourse among American Indian youths. *American Journal of Public Health, 96*(12), 2228–2234.

Herrenkohl, T. I., Maguin, E., Hill, K. G., Hawkins, J. D., Abbott, R. D., and Catalano, R. F. (2000). Developmental risk factors for youth violence. *The Journal of Adolescent Health, 26*(3), 176–186.

Higgins, E. T. (1987). Self-discrepancy: A theory relating self and affect. *Psychological Review, 94*, 319–340.

Hirschberger, G., Florian, V., Mikulincer, M., Goldenberg, J. L., and Pyszczynski, T. (2002). Gender differences in the willingness to engage in risky behavior: A terror management perspective. *Death Studies, 26*(2), 117–141.

Hirschi, T. (1969). *Causes of delinquency.* Berkeley: University of California Press.

Holder, H., Flay, B. R., Howard, J., Boyd, G., Voas, R., and Grossman, M. (1999). Phases of alcohol problem prevention research. *Alcoholism, Clinical And Experimental Research, 23*(1), 183–194.

House, J. S. (2002). Understanding social factors and inequalities in health: 20th century progress and 21st century prospects. *Journal of Health and Social Behavior, 43*(2), 125–142.

Hovell, M. B., Wahlgren, D. R., and Gehrman, C. A. (2002). The behavioral ecological model: Integrating public health and behavioral science. In R. J. DiClemete, R. A. Crosby and M. C. Kegler (eds.), *Emerging theories in health promotion practice and research: Strategies for improving public health* (pp. 347–385). San Francisco: Jossey-Bass.

Hover, A. R., Hover, B. A., and Young, J. C. (2000). Measuring the effectiveness of a community-sponsored DWI intervention for teens. *American Journal of Health Studies, 16*(4), 171.

Huba, G. J., and Bentler, P. M. (1982). A developmental theory of drug use: Derivations and assessment of a causal modeling approach. In P. B. Baltes and O. G. Brim (eds.), *Life span development and behavior* (Vol. 4, pp. 147–203). New York: Academic Press.

Hurdle, D. E. (2001). Social support: A critical factor in women's health and health promotion. *Health and Social Work, 26*(2), 72–79.

Ingram, B. L., Flannery, D., Elkavich, A., and Rotheram-Borus, M. J. (2008). Common processes in evidence-based adolescent HIV prevention programs. *AIDS Behavior, 12,* 374–383.

Institute of Medicine. (2006). *Genes, behavior, and the social environment: Moving beyond the nature/nurture debate.* Washington, DC: National Academy Press.

Jagers, R., Morgan-Lopez, H. T.-L., Browne, D., and Flay, B. R. (2007a). Mediators of the development and prevention of violent behavior. *Prevention Science, 8*(3), 171–179.

Jagers, R., Sydnor, K., Mouttapa, M., and Flay, B. R. (2007b). Protective factors associated with preadolescent violence: Preliminary work on a cultural model. *American Journal of Community Psychology, 40*(1/2), 138–145.

Janz, N. K., and Becker, M. H. (1984). The health belief model: A decade later. *Health Education Quarterly, 11,* 1–47.

Jessor, R., and Jessor, S. L. (1977). *Problem behavior and psychosocial development.* New York: Academic Press.

Jessor, R., Turbin, M. S., Costa, F. M., Dong, Q., Zhang, H., and Wang, C. (2003). Adolescent problem behavior in China and the United States: A cross-national study of psychosocial protective factors. *Journal of Research on Adolescence, 13*(3), 329–360.

Jessor, R., Van Den Bos, J., Vabderryn, J., Costa, F. M., and Turbin, M. S. (1995). Protective factors in adolescent problem behavior: Moderator effects and developmental change. *Developmental Psychology, 31*(6), 923–933.

Kamphuis, C.B.M., Giskes, K., de Bruijn, G. J., Wendel-Vos, W., Brug, J., and van Lenthe, F. J. (2006). Environmental determinants of fruit and vegetable consumption among adults: a systematic review. *The British Journal of Nutrition, 96*(4), 620–635.

Kandel, D. B., Wu, P., and Davies, M. (1994). Maternal smoking during pregnancy and smoking by adolescent daughters. *American Journal of Public Health, 83,* 851–855.

Kaplan, H. B. (1975). *Self-attitudes and deviant behavior.* Oxford, England: Goodyear.

Karlsson, P. (2006). *Margins of prevention: On older adolescents' positive and negative beliefs about illicit drug use.* Stockholm: Stockholm University.

Karoly, P. (1993). Mechanisms of self-regulation: A systems view. *Annual Review of Psychology, 44,* 23–52.

Kawachi, I., and Subramanian, S. V. (2007). Neighbourhood influences on health. *British Medical Journal, 61*(1), 3–4.

Kear, M. E. (2002). Psychosocial determinants of cigarette smoking among college students. *Journal of Community Health Nursing, 19*(4), 245–257.

Kearney, M. H., and O'Sullivan, J. (2003). Identity shifts as turning points in health behavior change. *Western Journal of Nursing Research, 25*(2), 134.

King, A. C., Stokols, D., Talen, E., Brassington, G. S., and Killingsworth, R. (2002). Theoretical approaches to the promotion of physical activity: Forging a transdisciplinary paradigm. *American Journal of Preventive Medicine, 23*(2S1), 15–25.

Kirby, D., Barth, R. P., Leland, N., and Fetro, J. V. (1991). Reducing the risk: Impact of a new curriculum on sexual risk-taking. *Family Planning Perspectives, 23*(6), 253–263.

Klepp, K. -I., Perez-Rodrigo, C., De Bourdeaudhuij, I., Due, P., Elmadfa, I., Haraldsdottir, J., et al. (2005). Promoting fruit and vegetable consumption among European schoolchildren: Rationale, conceptualization and design of the Pro Children project. *Annals of Nutrition and Metabolism, 49*(4), 212–220.

Kobus, K. (2003). Peers and adolescent smoking. *Addiction, 98,* 37–55.

Kocken, P., van Dorst, A., and Schaalma, H. (2006). The relevance of cultural factors in predicting condom-use intentions among immigrants from the Netherlands Antilles. *Health Education Research, 21*(2), 230–238.

Komro, K. A., Perry, C. L., Veblen-Mortenson, S., Bosma, L. M., Dudovitz, B. S., Williams, C. L., et al. (2004). Brief report: the adaptation of Project Northland for urban youth. *Journal of Pediatric Psychology, 29*(6), 457–466.

Komro, K. A., Perry, C. L., Veblen-Mortenson, S., Stigler, M. H., Bosma, L. M., Munson, K. A., et al. (2004). Violence-related outcomes of the D.A.R.E. plus project. *Health Education and Behavior*, *31*(3), 335–354.

Komro, K. A., and Toomey, T. L. (2002). Strategies to prevent underage drinking. *Alcohol Research and Health*, *26*(1), 5.

Konopka, G. (1991). Adolescence, concept of, and requirements for a healthy development. In R. M. Lerner, A. C. Petersen and J. Brooks-Gunn (eds.), *Encyclopedia of adolescence* (pp. 10–13). New York: Garland.

Kremers, S. P., Mesters, I., Pladdet, I. E., van den Borne, B., and Stockbrugger, R. W. (2000). Participation in a sigmoidoscopic colorectal cancer screening program: A pilot study. *Cancer Epidemiology, Biomarkers and Prevention*, *9*(10), 1127–1130.

Kremers, S. P. J., Visscher, T. L. S., Brug, J., Chin, A., Paw, M. J. M., Schouten, E. G., Schuit, A. J., et al. (2005). Netherlands Research programme weight gain prevention (NHF-NRG): Rationale, objectives and strategies. *European Journal of Clinical Nutrition*, *59*(4), 498–507.

Krieger, N. (1994). Epidemiology and the web of causation: has anyone seen the spider. *Soc Sci Med*, *39*(7), 887–903.

Krieger, N. (2007). Why epidemiologists cannot afford to ignore poverty. *Epidemiology*, *18*(6), 658–663.

Krieger, N. (2008). Proximal, distal, and the politics of causation: What's level got to do with it? *American Journal of Public Health*, *98*(2), 221.

Kugler, K. C., Komro, K. A., Stigler, M. H., Mnyika, K. S., Masatu, M., Aastrom, A. N., et al. (2007). The reliability and validity of self-report measures used to evaluate adolescent HIV/AIDS prevention programs in sub-Saharan Africa. *AIDS Education and Prevention*, *19*(5), 365–382.

Kuh, D., and Yoav, B.-S. (eds.). (2004). *A life course approach to chronic disease epidemiology* (2nd ed.). Oxford: Oxford University Press.

Kumar, R., O'Malley, P. M., Johnston, L. D., Schulenberg, J. E., and Bachman, J. G. (2002). Effects of school-level norms on student substance use. *Prevention Science*, *3*(2), 105–124.

Lambert, M. J., and Oglesk, B. M. (2004). The efficacy and effectiveness of psychotherapy. In M. J. Lambert (ed.), *Bergin and Garfield's handbook of psychotherapy and behavior change* (5th ed., pp. 139–193). Hoboken, NJ: Wiley.

Landsbaum, J., and Willis, R. (1971). Conformity in early and late adolescence. *Developmental Psychology*, *4*, 334–337.

Laub, J. H., and Sampson, R. J. (1993). Turning points in the life course: Why change matters to the study of crime. *Criminology*, *31*(3), 301–325.

Leatherdale, S. T., and Manske, S. (2005). The relationship between student smoking in the school environment and smoking onset in elementary school students. *Cancer Epidemiology, Biomarkers and Prevention*, *14*(7), 1762–1765.

Leatherdale, S. T., and Strath, J. M. (2007). Tobacco retailer density surrounding schools and cigarette access behaviors among underage smoking students. *Annals of Behavioral Medicine*, *33*(1), 105–111.

Lechner, L., De Nooijer, J., and De Vries, H. (2004). Breast self-examination: longitudinal predictors of intention and subsequent behaviour. *European Journal of Cancer Prevention*, *13*(5), 369–376.

Lechner, L., de Vries, H., and Offermans, N. (1997). Participation in a breast cancer screening program: influence of past behavior and determinants on future screening participation. *Preventive Medicine*, *26*(4), 473–482.

Lerner, R. M. (1978). Nature, nurture, and dynamic interactionism. *Human Development*, *21*, 1–20.

Lerner, R. M. (2006). Developmental science, developmental systems, and contemporary theories of human development. In *Handbook of child psychology (6th ed.): Vol 1, Theoretical models of human development*. (pp. 1–17). Hoboken, NJ: Wiley.

Lerner, R. M., Abo-Zena, M., Bebiroglu, N., Brittian, A., Lynch, A. D., and Issac, S. (eds.). (in press). *Positive youth development: Contemporary theoretical perspectives*. San Francisco: Jossey-Bass.

Lettieri, D. J., Sayers, M., and Pearson, H. W. (1980). *Theories on drug abuse—Selected contemporary perspectives: NIDA Research Monograph 30*. Washington, DC: U.S. Government Printing Office.

Levenson, P. M., Marrow, J. R., and Pfefferbaum, B. J. (1984). Attitudes toward health and illness: A comparison of adolescent, physician, teacher, and school nurse views. *Journal of Adolescent Health Care*, *5*, 254–262.

Lewin, K. (1951). *Field theory in social science: Selected theoretical papers*. Oxford, England: Harpers.

Li, K.-K. (2008). *Life course perspective: A journey of participation in physical activity*. Unpublished doctoral dissertation, Oregon State University.

Limbos, M. A., Chan, L. S., Warf, C., Schneir, A., Iverson, E., Shekelle, P., et al. (2007). Effectiveness of interventions to prevent youth violence: A systematic review. *American Journal of Preventive Medicine*, *33*(1), 65–74.

Link, B. G., and Phelan, J. (1995). Social conditions as fundamental causes of disease. *Journal of Health and Social Behavior*, *35*, 80–94.

Lowenthal, M., Thurner, M., and Chiriboga, D. (1975). *Four stages of life*. San Francisco: Jossey-Bass.

MacKinnon, D. P., Johnson, C. A., Pentz, M. A., Dwyer, J. H., Hansen, W. B., Flay, B. R., et al. (1991). Mediating mechanisms in a school-based drug prevention program: First-year effects of the Midwestern Prevention Project. *Health Psychology*, *10*(3), 164–172.

MacKinnon, D. P., and Lockwood, C. M. (2003). Advances in statistical methods for substance abuse prevention research. *Prevention Science*, *4*(3), 155–171.

MacKinnon, D. P., Taborga, M. P., and Morgan-Lopez, A. A. (2002). Mediation designs for tobacco prevention research. *Drug and Alcohol Dependence*, *68 Suppl 1*, S69–83.

Magnusson, D. (1981). *Toward a psychology of situations: An interactional perspective*. Hillsdale, NJ: Erlbaum.

Marmot, M. G. (2001). Inequalities in health. *New England Journal of Medicine*, *345*(2), 134.

Marmot, M. G., and Wilkinson, R. G. (2006). *Social determinants of health*, Oxford University Press.

McBride, C. M., Puleo, E., Pollak, K. I., Clipp, E. C., Woolford, S., and Emmons, K. M. (2008). Understanding the role of cancer worry in creating a "teachable moment" for multiple risk factor reduction. *Social Science and Medicine*, *66*(3), 790–800.

McCall, D., Doherty, M., Allison, K., Rootman, I., Plotnikoff, R., and Raine, K. (2005). *A school-based, school-linked ecological and systems-based research agenda on healthy eating*: School Health Research Network, Canada.

McKinlay, J. B., and Marceau, L. D. (2000). Public health matters. To boldly go. *American Journal of Public Health*, *90*(1), 25–33.

McLeroy, K. R., Bibeau, D., and Glanz, K. (1988). An ecological perspective on health promotion programs. *Health Education Quarterly*, *14*(4), 351–377.

Merton, R. K. (1938). Social structure and anomie. *American Sociological Review*, *3*(5), 672–682.

Merzenich, M. M. (2001). Cortical plasticity contributing to child development. *Mechanisms of cognitive development: Behavioral and neural perspectives*, 67–95. Mahway, New Jersy: Lawrence Erlbaum Associates, Inc., Publishers.

Michie, S., Johnston, M., Abraham, C., Lawton, R., Parker, D., and Walker, A. (2005). Making psychological theory useful for implementing evidence based practice: a consensus approach. *Quality and Safety in Health Care*, *14*(1), 26.

Midford, R., Wilkes, D.E.B., and Young, D. (2005). Evaluation of the in touch training program for the management of alcohol and other drug use issues in schools. *Journal of Drug Education*, *35*(1), 1–14.

Mills, B., Reyna, V. F., and Estrada, S. (2008). Explaining contradictory relations between risk perception and risk taking. *Psychological Science*, *19*(5), 429–433.

Millstein, S. G. (1991). Health beliefs. In R. M. Learner, A. C. Petersen and J. Brooks-Gunn (eds.), *Encyclopedia of adolescence* (pp. 445–448). New York: Garland.

Minkler, M., Wallace, S. P., and McDonald, M. (1995). The political economy of health: A useful theoretical tool for health education practice. *International Quarterly of Community Health Education*, *15*(2), 111–125.

Mohatt, G. V., Rasmus, S. M., Thomas, L., Allen, J., Hazel, K., and Hensel, C. (2004). "Tied together like a woven hat:" Protective pathways to Alaska native sobriety. *Harm Reduction Journal*, *1*(10).

Montemayor, R., and Flannery, D. J. (1991). Parent-adolescent relations in middle and late adolescence. In R. M. Learner, A. C. Petersen and J. Brooks-Gunn (eds.), *Encyclopedia of adolescence* (pp. 729–734). New York: Garland.

Morenoff, J. D., House, J. S., Hansen, B. B., Williams, D. R., Kaplan, G. A., and Hunte, H. E. (2007). Understanding social disparities in hypertension prevalence, awareness, treatment, and control: The role of neighborhood context. *Social Science and Medicine*, *65*(9), 1853–1866.

Mowrer, O. H. (1960). *Learning theory and behavior*. New York: Wiley.

Murnaghan, D. A., Sihvonen, M., Leatherdale, S. T., and Kekki, P. (2007). The relationship between school-based smoking policies and prevention programs on smoking behavior among grade 12 students in Prince Edward Island: A multilevel analysis. *Preventive Medicine*, *44*(4), 317–322.

Neal, D. T., Wood, W., and Quinn, J. M. (2006). Habits: A repeat performance. *Current Directions in Psychological Science*, *15*(4), 198–202.

Ngwe, J. E., Liu, L. C., Flay, B. R., Segawa, E., and Aban Aya Co-Investigators. (2004). Violence prevention among African American adolescent males. *American Journal of Health Behavior*, *28*, S24–37.

Nierkens, V., Stronks, K., and de Vries, H. (2006). Attitudes, social influences and self-efficacy expectations across different motivational stages among immigrant smokers: Replication of the Ø pattern. *Preventive Medicine*, *43*(4), 306–311.

Oetting, E. R., and Beauvais, F. (1986). Peer cluster theory: Drugs and the adolescent. *Journal of Counseling and Development*, *65*(1), 17.

Olds, D. L., Eckenrod, J., Henderson, C. R., Kitzman, H., Powers, J., Cole, R., et al. (1997). Long-term effects of home visitation on maternal life course and child abuse and neglect. Fifteen-year follow-up of a randomized trial. *Journal of the American Medical Association*, *278*(8), 63–643.

Orr, D. P., and Ingersoll, G. (1991). Cognition and health. In R. M. Learner, A. C. Petersen and J. Brooks-Gunn (eds.), *Encyclopedia of adolescence* (pp. 130–132). New York: Garland.

Ory, M. G., Jordan, P. J., and Bazzarre, T. (2002). The behavior change consortium: Setting the stage for a new century of health behavior-change research. *Health Education Research*, *17*(5), 500–511.

Ouellette, J. A., and Wood, W. (1998). Habit and intention in everyday life: The multiple processes by which past behavior predicts future behavior. *Psychological Bulletin*, *124*, 54–74.

Overton, W. F. (1973). On the assumptive base of the nature nurture controversy: Additive versus interactive conceptions. *Human Development*, *16*, 74–89.

Perry, C. L. (2004). Getting beyond technical rationality in developing health behavior programs with youth. *American Journal of Health Behavior*, *28*(6), 558–568.

Perry, C. L., Stigler, M. H., Arora, M., and Reddy, K. S. (2008). Prevention in translation: Tobacco use prevention in India. *Health Promotion Practice*, *9*(4), 378–386.

Perry, C. L., Williams, C. L., Komro, K. A., Veblen-Mortenson, S., Stigler, M. H., Munson, K. A., et al. (2002). Project Northland: long-term outcomes of community action to reduce adolescent alcohol use. *Health Education Research*, *17*(1), 117–132.

Petersen, I., Bhana, A., and McKay, M. (2005). Sexual violence and youth in South Africa: The need for community-based prevention interventions. *Child Abuse and Neglect*, *29*(11), 1233–1248.

Petraitis, J., Flay, B. R., and Miller, T. Q. (1995). Reviewing theories of adolescent substance use: Organizing pieces in the puzzle. *Psychological Bulletin*, *117*(1), 67.

Petraitis, J., Flay, B. R., Miller, T. Q., Torpy, E. J., and Greiner, B. (1998). Illicit substance use among adolescents: a matrix of prospective predictors. *Substance Use and Misuse*, *33*(13), 2561–2604.

Petraitis, J., Lampman, C., and Falconer, E. M. (2008). The evolution of risk-taking for mate attraction: Sex differences in attractiveness of hunter-gatherer and modern risks. *Manuscript in preparation*.

Phil, R. O., Peterson, J. B., and Finn, P. (1990). An heuristic model for the inherited predisposition to alcoholism. *Psychology of Addictive Behaviors*, *4*(1), 12–25.

Reiss, D., and Leve, L. D. (2007). Genetic expression outside the skin: Clues to mechanisms of Genotype x Environment interaction. *Development and Psychopathology*, *19*(04), 1005–1027.

Resnicow, K., and Vaughan, R. (2006). A chaotic view of behavior change: A quantum leap for health promotion. *International Journal of Behavioral Nutrition and Physical Activity, 3*(1), 25–31.

Reyna, V. F., and Farley, F. (2006a). Is the teen brain too rational? *Scientific American Mind, 17*(6), 58–65.

Reyna, V. F., and Farley, F. (2006b). Risk and rationality in adolescent decision making: Implications for theory, practice, and public policy. *Psychological Science in the Public Interest, 7*(1), 1–44.

Reyna, V. F., and Rivers, S. E. (2008). Current theories of risk and rational decision making. *Developmental Review, 28*(1), 1–11.

Richerson, P. J., and Boyd, R. (2005). *Not by genes alone: How culture transformed human evolution.* Chicago: University of Chicago Press.

Riggs, N. R., Greenberg, M. T., Kusché, C. A., and Pentz, M. A. (2006). The mediational role of neurocognition in the behavioral outcomes of a social-emotional prevention program in elementary school students: Effects of the PATHS curriculum. *Prevention Science, 7*(1), 91–102.

Rivers, S. E., Reyna, V. F., and Mills, B. (2008). Risk taking under the influence: A fuzzy-trace theory of emotion in adolescence. *Developmental Review.*

Roffman, J. L., Marci, C. D., Glick, D. M., Dougherty, D. D., and Rauch, S. L. (2005). Neuroimaging and the functional neuroanatomy of psychotherapy. *Psychological Medicine, 35*(10), 1385.

Rose, G. (1985). Sick individuals and sick populations. *International Journal of Epidemiology, 14*(1), 32–38.

Rosenberg, M. (1985). Self-concept and psychological well-being in adolescence. In R. Leahy (ed.), *The development of the self* (pp. 205–242). New York: Academic Press.

Rosenstock, I. (1974). The health belief model and preventive behavior. *Health Education Monographs, 2,* 354–386.

Rutter, M., and Garmezy, N. (1983). Developmental psychopathology. In P. H. Mussen (ed.), *Handbook of child psychology* (Vol. 4, Socialization, personality and social development, pp. 775–911). New York: Wiley.

Ryan, R. M., and Deci, E. L. (2000). Self-determination theory and the facilitation of intrinsic motivation, social development, and well-being. *American Psychologist, 55*(1), 68–78.

Sadava, S. W. (1987). Psychosocial interactionism and substance use. *Drugs and Society, 2*(1), 1–30.

Sandvik, C., De Bourdeaudhuij, I., Due, P., Brug, J., Wind, M., Bere, E., et al. (2005). Personal, social and environmental factors regarding fruit and vegetable intake among schoolchildren in nine European countries. *Annals of Nutrition and Metabolism, 49*(4), 255–266.

Scheier, L. M. (2001). Etiologic studies of adolescent drug use: A compendium of data resources and their implications for prevention. *Journal of Primary Prevention, 22*(2), 125–168.

Schofield, P. E., Pattison, P. E., Hill, D. J., and Borland, R. (2003). Youth culture and smoking: Integrating social group processes and individual cognitive processes in a model of health-related behaviours. *Journal of Health Psychology, 8*(3), 291.

Schols, A. M. W. J., and Brug, J. (2003). Efficacy of nutritional intervention in chronic obstructive pulmonary disease. In *Nutrition and metabolism in chronic respiratory disease* (Vol. 24, pp. 142–152).

Schulenberg, J. E., and Maggs, J. L. (2001). *A developmental perspective on alcohol and other drug use during adolescence and the transition to young adulthood.* Ann Arbor: Institute for Social Research, University of Michigan.

Segawa, E., Ngwe, J. E., Li, Y., and Flay, B. R. (2005). Evaluation of the effects of the Aban Aya Youth Project in reducing violence among African American adolescent males using latent class growth mixture modeling techniques. *Evaluation Review, 29*(2), 128–148.

Settersten, R. A., Jr. (2005). Toward a stronger partnership between life-course sociology and life-span psychology. *Research in Human Development, 21,* 25–41.

Shadel, W. G., Niaura, R., and Abrams, D. B. (2004a). Adolescents' responses to the gender valence of cigarette advertising imagery: The role of affect and the self-concept. *Addictive Behaviors, 29*(9), 1735–1744.

Shadel, W. G., Niaura, R., and Abrams, D. B. (2004b). Who am I? The role of self-conflict in adolescents' responses to cigarette advertising. *Journal of Behavioral Medicine, 27*(5), 463–475.

Sher, K. J. (1991). *Children of alcoholics: A critical appraisal of theory and research.* Chicago: University of Chicago Press.

Shonkoff, J. P., and Phillips, D. A. (2000). *From neurons to neighborhoods: The science of early childhood development.* Washington, DC: National Academy Press.

Sieving, R. E., Eisenberg, M. E., Pettingell, S., and Skay, C. (2006). Friends' influence on adolescents' first sexual intercourse. *Perspectives on Sexual and Reproductive Health, 38*(1), 13–19.

Sieving, R. E., Maruyama, G., Williams, C. L., and Perry, C. L. (2000a). Pathways to adolescent alcohol use: Potential mechanisms of parent influence. *Journal of Research on Adolescence, 10*(4), 489–514.

Sieving, R. E., McNeely, C. S., and Blum, R. W. (2000b). Maternal expectations, mother-child connectedness, and adolescent sexual debut. *Archives of Pediatrics and Adolescent Medicine, 154*(8), 809–816.

Snyder, C. R. (2002). Hope theory: Rainbows in the mind. *Psychological Inquiry, 13*(4), 249–275.

Snyder, C. R., Feldman, D. B., Taylor, J. D., Schroeder, L. L., and Adams, V. (2000). The roles of hopeful thinking in preventing problems and enhancing strengths. *Applied and Preventive Psychology, 15*, 262–295.

Sober, E., and Wilson, D. S. (1998). *Unto Others: The evolution and psychology of unselfish behavior.* Cambridge, MA: Harvard University Press.

Stanton, W. R., Moffatt, J., and Clavarino, A. (2005). Community perceptions of adequate levels and reasons for skin protection. *Behavioral Medicine, 31*(1), 5–15.

Steinberg, L. (1991). Parent-adolescent relations. In R. M. Learner, A. C. Petersen and J. Brooks-Gunn (eds.), *Encyclopedia of adolescence* (pp. 724–728). New York: Garland.

Steinberg, L. (2008). A social neuroscience perspective on adolescent risk-taking. *Developmental Review, 28*(1), 78–106.

Steinberg, L., Dahl, R. E., Keating, D., Kupfer, D. J., Masten, A. S., and Pine, D. (2004). The study of developmental psychopathology in adolescence: Integrating affective neuroscience with the study of context. In D. Cicchetti (ed.), *Handbook of developmental psychopathology.* New York: Wiley.

Stewart, I., and Cohen, J. (1997). *Figments of reality.* Cambridge, UK: Cambridge University Press.

Stigler, M. H., Perry, C. L., Komro, K. A., Cudeck, R., and Williams, C. L. (2006). Teasing apart a multiple component approach to adolescent alcohol prevention: What worked in Project Northland? *Prevention Science, 7*(3), 269–280.

Stokols, D. (1992). Establishing and maintaining health environments: Towards a social ecology of health promotion. *American Psychologist, 47*(1), 6–22.

Sunstein, C. R. (2008). Adolescent risk-taking and social meaning: A commentary. *Developmental Review, 28*(1), 145–152.

Suppes, P. (1970). *A probabilistic theory of causality.* Amsterdam: North-Holland.

Sussman, S., Dent, C. W., and Leu, L. (2000). The one-year prospective prediction of substance abuse and dependence among high-risk adolescents. *Journal of Substance Abuse, 12*(4), 373–386.

Tarter, R. E., Alterman, A. I., and Edwards, K. L. (1985). Vulnerability to alcoholism in men: A behavior-genetic perspective. *Journal of Studies on Alcohol, 46*(4), 329–356.

te Velde, S. J., Wind, M., van Lenthe, F. J., Klepp, K.-I., and Brug, J. (2006). Differences in fruit and vegetable intake and determinants of intakes between children of Dutch origin and non-Western ethnic minority children in the Netherlands—a cross sectional study. *The International Journal of Behavioral Nutrition and Physical Activity, 3*, 31–31.

Thorner, E. D., Jaszyna-Gasior, M., Epstein, D. H., and Moolchan, E. T. (2007). Progression to daily smoking: Is there a gender difference among cessation treatment seekers? *Substance Use and Misuse, 42*(5), 829–835.

Trochim, W. M., Cabrera, D. A., Milstein, B., Gallagher, R. S., and Leischow, S. J. (2006). Practical challenges of systems thinking and modeling in public health. *American Journal of Public Health, 96*(3), 538–546.

Turner, L., Mermelstein, R., and Flay, B. R. (2004). Individual and contextual influences on adolescent smoking. *Annals of The New York Academy of Sciences, 1021*, 175–197.

Twenge, J. M. (2006). *Generation me: Why today's young Americans are more confident, assertive, entitled— and more miserable than ever before.* New York: Free Press.

Verheijden, M. W., Bakx, J. C., Weel, C., Koelen, M. A., and Staveren, W. A. (2005). Role of social support in lifestyle-focused weight management interventions. *European Journal of Clinical Nutrition, 59*(Supplement 1), S179–S186.

Verplanken, B., and Aarts, H. (1999). Habit, attitude and planned behavior: Is habit an empty construct or an interesting case of goal-directed behavior? *European Review of Social Psychology, 10*, 101–134.

Victoir, A., Eertmans, A., Van den Bergh, O., and Van den Broucke, S. (2007). Association of substance-use behaviours and their social-cognitive determinants in secondary school students. *Health Education Research, 22*(1), 81–94.

Waldrop, M. M. (1992). *Complexity: The emerging science at the edge of order and chaos.* New York: Simon and Schuster.

Wang, Y., Tussing, L., Odoms-Young, A., Braunschweig, C., Flay, B. R., Hedeker, D., et al. (2006). Obesity prevention in low socioeconomic status urban African American adolescents: study design and preliminary findings of the HEALTH-KIDS Study. *European Journal of Clinical Nutrition, 60*(1), 92–103.

Weeks, K., Levy, S. R., Zhu, C., Perhats, C., Handler, A., and Blay, B. R. (1995). Impact of a school-based AIDS prevention program on young adolescents' self-efficacy skills. *Health Education Research, 10*(3), 329–344.

Werner, E. E., and Smith, R. S. (1992). *Overcoming the odds: High risk children from birth to adulthood.* Ithaca, NY: Cornell University Press.

Wheaton, B., and Gotlib, I. H. (eds.). (1997). *Trajectories and turning points over the life course: Concepts and themes.* New York, NY: Cambridge University Press.

White, F. J. (1997). Cocaine and the serotonin sage. *Nature, 393*, 118–119.

Wiefferink, C., Detmar, S., Coumans, B., Vogels, T., and Paulussen, T. (2008). Social psychological determinants of the use of performance-enhancing drugs by gym users. *Health Education Research, 23*(1), 70–80.

Wiefferink, C. H., Peters, L., Hoekstra, F., Dam, G. T., Buijs, G. J., and Paulussen, T.G.W. M. (2006). Clustering of health-related behaviors and their determinants: possible consequences for school health interventions. *Prevention Science, 7*(2), 127–149.

Williams, D. R., and Earl, T. R. (2007). Commentary: Race and mental health more questions than answers. *International Journal of Epidemiology, 36*(4), 758.

Willoughby, T., Chalmers, H., Busseri, M., Bosacki, S., Dupont, D., Marini, Z., et al. (2008). Testing an integrative model of adolescent risk behavior. *Manuscript in preparation.*

Wilson, D. M., Killen, J. D., Hayward, C., Robinson, T. N., Hammer, L. D., Kraemer, H. C., et al. (1994). Timing and rate of sexual maturation and the onset of cigarette and alcohol use among teenage girls. *Archives of Pediatrics and Adolescent Medicine, 14*(789–795).

Wilson, D. S. (2007). *Evolution for everyone: How Darwin's theory can change the way we think about our lives.* New York: Random House.

Wilson, D. S., and Csikszentmihalyi, M. (2008). Health and the ecology of altruism. In S. G. Post (ed.), *The science of altruism and health.* London: Oxford University Press.

Wind, M. (2006). *The development, implementation and evaluation of a school-based intervention to promote fruit and vegetable intake among 10–13-year-old European schoolchildren.* Erasmus Universiteit, Rotterdam.

Wind, M., deBourdeaudhuij, I. ., teVelde, S.J., Sandvik, C., Klepp, K. I., et al. (2006). Correlates of fruit and vegetable consumption among 11-year-old Belgian-Flemish and Dutch schoolchildren. *Journal of Nutrition Education and Behavior, 38*(4), 211–221.

Wolf, C. (2002). *Social impact assessment and policy.* Paper presented at the National Research and Development Centre for Welfare and Health, with the Ministry of Social Affairs and Health: Human Impact Assessment, Finland.

Wood, W., Quinn, J. M., and Kashy, D. A. (2002). Habits in everyday life: Thought, emotion, and action. *Journal of Personality and Social Psychology, 83*(6), 1281–1297.

Zimmerman, B. J. (2001). Theories of self-regulated learning and academic achievement: An overview and analysis. In B. J. Zimmerman and D. H. Schunk (eds.), *Self-regulated learning and academic achievement: Theoretical perspectives* (2nd ed., Vol. 2, pp. 1–38). Hillsdale, NJ: Erlbaum.

Zuckerman, M. (1971). Dimensions of sensation seeking. *Journal of Consulting and Clinical Psychology, 36*(1), 45–52.

Zuckerman, M., Ball, S., and Black, J. (1990). Influences of sensation seeking, gender, risk appraisal, and situational motivation on smoking. *Addictive Behaviors, 15*(3), 209–220.

THE INTERACTIVE DOMAIN MODEL APPROACH TO BEST PRACTICES IN HEALTH PROMOTION

Barbara Kahan
David Groulx
Josephine Pui-Hing Wong

A BEST PRACTICES MODEL FOR HEALTH PROMOTION

The Interactive Domain Model (IDM) is a comprehensive **best practices** approach to health promotion, adaptable to the local context. Individuals and organizations have used the IDM in a number of settings, for a variety of purposes, and with positive results. Although a number of evidence-based approaches exist (for example, Cameron, Walker, and Jolin 1998; Rychetnik and Frommer 2002), few match the holistic nature of the IDM, whose elements range from **values** and **theories** to understanding of the organizational and health-related environments.

RATIONALE FOR DEVELOPING THE IDM

Health promotion practitioners—program managers and implementers, researchers, and policy makers—intend to do the best they can to improve the health of individuals and communities. However, practitioners are overwhelmed with information, time demands, and competing perspectives; sorting out the best course of action to get the best possible results can seem like an impossible task. Difficulties compound when information conflicts, demands are unrealistic, and time and other resources are limited.

Given these circumstances it is not surprising that practitioners at the 1996 International Symposium on the Effectiveness of Health Promotion in Ottawa called for tools to guide their work. The Centre for Health Promotion, University of Toronto, took on this task and initiated a working group to explore possibilities. The Best Practices Work Group, composed of members of community health centers, public health units, government, and other groups with an interest in improving health promotion practice, was eventually joined by the Association of Ontario Health Centres, the Ontario Public Health Benchmarking Partnership, and the Health Promoting Hospital Network to form the Best Practices Partnership.

After an initial exploration stage, the Partnership conducted a survey of health promotion and best practices in Ontario. Although some survey participants expressed concern about the possibility of an imposed or "one size fits all" approach, survey results, overall, indicated strong support for developing and implementing a best practices approach to health promotion (Kahan, Goodstadt, and Rajkumar 1999). While the concept of best practices was becoming increasingly popular, no models to implement best practices in health promotion existed at that time. Further, no comprehensive models existed in any other related fields. (Most approaches at that time focused almost exclusively on evidence, as they do today, rather than on utilizing a broad range of key decision-making variables. A narrow evidence-based approach ignores, for example, the role of values in shaping research questions and methods and the impact of local conditions.)

The initial model, based on an extensive literature review, was refined through participation from the Centre for Health Promotion's Work Group and other Partnership members. The review identified existing approaches to practice, which contained one or more elements of the future IDM. No approach at that time contained all elements. The review drew on literature related to continuous quality improvement, evidence of effectiveness, role of theories, values and environment in practice, and health promotion in general (for example, Caplan 1993; Freudenberg, Eng, Flay, Parcel, Rogers, and Wallerstein 1995; Milburn 1996; Nutbeam and Harris 1998; Ovretveit 1996; Seedhouse 1997; Simnett 1995; Stokols 1996; for more references, see Kahan and Goodstadt, 1999 and 2001a).

Pilot testing results were positive. Information and encouragement from IDM pilot testing, workshops, reporting and discussion sessions, and Best Practices Partnership members provided the basis for continuing to improve the model and related resources.

Best practices in health promotion are those sets of processes and activities that are consistent with health promotion values, theories, evidence, and understanding of the environment, and that are most likely to achieve health promotion goals in a given situation.

—Kahan and Goodstadt, 2001a

According to the IDM, best practices and the best outcomes occur when processes and activities are consistent with health promotion underpinnings and understanding of the environment. There is no single best practice; best practices vary from situation to situation according to a number of variables ranging from values and underlying beliefs to current knowledge and available resources.

DESCRIPTION OF THE IDM

This section introduces the Interactive Domain Model, discusses the importance of consistency to the IDM, and provides an overview of the IDM Operational and Evidence Frameworks.

Introduction to the Model

According to the IDM, best practices and the best outcomes occur when processes and activities are consistent with health promotion underpinnings and understanding of the environment. There is no single best practice; best practices vary from situation to situation according to a number of variables ranging from values and underlying beliefs to current knowledge and available resources. In IDM workshops, when asked to identify factors that influence decisions, participants list the elements that constitute the model, that is, factors that fall into the following categories of domains:

- **Underpinnings:** values, **ethics** and goals; theories, concepts, and beliefs, **evidence**;

- **Understanding of the environment:** vision, an "idea perceived vividly in the imagination" (Barber 1998), which offers something to aspire to, and analysis of organizational and health-related environments

- **Practice:** processes and activities related to research (including evaluation), policy development, program design and implementation, and organizational development

These domains interact with each other in the context of the social, political, economic, psychological, and physical environments.

Several qualities embedded in the IDM and its definitions distinguish it from traditional best practice approaches. The IDM:

- Highlights the contribution to best practices decision-making of a comprehensive set of factors that includes, but is not limited to, evidence. In particular other models often omit the role of values;

FIGURE 17.1 *The Interactive Domain Model*

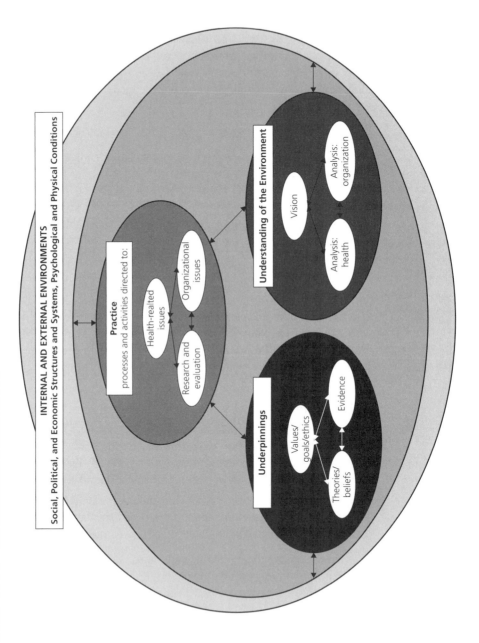

INTERNAL AND EXTERNAL ENVIRONMENTS
Social, Political, and Economic Structures and Systems, Psychological and Physical Conditions

Practice
processes and activities directed to:

Health-realted issues

Organizational issues

Research and evaluation

Understanding of the Environment

Vision

Analysis: organization

Analysis: health

Underpinnings

Values/ goals/ethics

Evidence

Theories/ beliefs

- Makes explicit the underlying values, beliefs and analyses held by key stakeholders on the one hand and embedded in practice processes and activities on the other hand, providing the opportunity to align thought and action;

- Encourages the integration of theory into practice, thereby increasing the possibilities for innovation, especially in the absence of definitive evidence;

- Emphasizes sensitivity to local conditions by working with the values, evidence, and understanding specific to the particular context;

- Increases awareness of broader society-wide environmental influences such as economic systems and power structures, rather than being restricted to the more readily discernible influences at the individual level;

- Emphasizes the importance of the organization in achieving best practices, rather than focusing exclusively on strategies directed to the health-related issue; and

- Focuses on processes as well as outcomes to build a strong foundation for optimizing the best outcomes possible.

Consequences of Consistency and Inconsistency

[The IDM] helps us evaluate things like values and beliefs—to see whether what we do is based on values, the values are not just on paper . . . It reduces the gap between the talk and the walk—it provides integrity . . .
—Hélène Roussel, quoted in Kahan et al., 2007

The domains included in underpinnings, understanding of the environment, and practice are interactive and mutually influencing. Thus, consistency among the domains is crucial to effective practice; best practices will not occur unless values, theories, evidence, and other domains are concretely translated into processes and activities.

Alignment among the domains increases the chances of achieving positive impacts, and misalignment increases the chances of negative impacts. For example, not translating values and concepts into analysis of the environment or practice will limit an organization's capacity to explore approaches that might result in better program outcomes. Without evidence or analysis, the organization will likely stagnate, with **beliefs,** processes, and activities remaining the same.

To illustrate the adverse effects of inconsistency between the domains using a real-life example, not integrating equity principles into practice has contributed to or perpetuated inequity of health outcomes. In general people with higher socio economic status are more likely to adopt health promotion information and programs than are people with lower socio-economic status. While over two decades of smoking cessation efforts have led to an overall decline in smoking among the general population, smoking continues to be a common practice among individuals and groups with low income and other social disadvantages (for example, see Chandola, Head, and Bartley, 2004). The association between smoking and chronic illnesses such as lung cancer has been well established over the last two decades. Unless health promotion strategies relevant to people with lower socioeconomic status are developed—in accordance with the value of health equity—disparity in health outcomes will persist.

Best practices will not occur unless values, theories, evidence and other domains are concretely translated into processes and activities.

TABLE 17.1 Addressing Equity in Health: a Hypothetical Example of Interactivity and Consistency Among the Domains.

Underpinnings	Understanding of the Environment	Practice
Values • One of the organization's stated **values** is EQUITY. • An all-stakeholder session is planned to identify the range of meanings for EQUITY and other **values** to see if a consensus is possible. **Evidence** • Evaluation and other **research** information has been collected to answer EQUITY-related questions. • **Evidence** about the link between income and program outcomes is unclear but will be pursued. **Theories/Concepts/Beliefs** • One of the organization's selected **concepts** to guide work is the social determinants of health, which include a society's degree of income EQUITY. This concept is supported by the current **evidence**. • One of the organization's **beliefs** is that income EQUITY is a prerequisite for social justice.	In the **environmental vision**, EQUITY exists in the workplace and community. The priority health-related issue is to increase the degree of income EQUITY in the community. **Research** shows that globalization, inadequate social safety nets, and racism contribute to lack of income EQUITY. **Environmental analysis** suggests higher welfare rates and minimum wage, a more progressive tax system, and community economic development and antiracism activities as methods to positively influence the local situation. A capacity to draw on is local leadership. A challenge to address is lack of political will to change the status quo. **Research** has provided data on the range of income levels in the community, and identified differences according to income level in: service access, participation in recreational activities, and health status. **Environmental analysis** identifies the priority organizational issue as an INEQUITABLE pay scale: staff at the lower end of the pay scale have difficulty making ends meet.	• An organizational policy is being developed to institute a more EQUITABLE staff pay scale. • An outreach program, which includes a van to give rides to people with low income, was implemented a month ago. • As a member of a community coalition the organization advocates for greater income EQUITY through higher welfare rates and minimum wage. • One staff member is working with a community group on a community economic development initiative. • Ongoing **research** is being conducted to provide more **evidence** regarding organizational and health-related issues. A number of EQUITY-related topics are being researched.

On the other hand, consistency among domains contributes to positive outcomes. Take for example, an organization that identifies "equity" as one of its values, as illustrated in Table 17.1. If domains align with this value, equity-related evidence, theories, and environmental analysis will provide the basis for practice-related decisions on equity-related issues, resulting in processes and activities designed to address equity-related organizational and health issues.

The IDM Frameworks

The IDM *Operational* Framework was designed to help practitioners integrate model concepts into practice. It contains four steps, each with its own set of questions, to apply to each of the IDM's domains:

- **Prepare a strong foundation for action.** What guides us? Where are we now? Where do we want to go?
- **Develop an action and evaluation plan.** How do we get to where we want to go: who does what, when, and how?
- **Implement, reflect and document.** What did we do? How did we do it? What were the results?
- **Revise.** What do we need to change?

As illustrated in Figure 17.2, Model domains are listed down the side of the Framework and Framework steps are listed across the top. The steps are similar to continuous quality improvement's Shewhart or Deming "plan-do-study-act" cycle (Levin 1994).

The Framework may look static on paper, but in practice the Framework has been used organically, depending on the purpose and situation (Kahan and Goodstadt, 2000, Kahan, et al. 2007). Groups' experiences with the IDM Framework have shown multiple ways of using the Framework, for example:

- Use a hopscotch approach or a set order;
- Work on one column or row at a time or work on several rows or columns at a time;
- Explore the domains briefly or explore them in-depth; and
- Focus on all or part of the IDM Framework.

Another organic dimension of the IDM Framework is its use as an ongoing process, with additions, deletions, and revisions to it as new information and insights arise.

The IDM *Evidence* Framework (Kahan and Goodstadt, 2005b), an elaboration of the IDM Operational Framework, was developed to assist groups whose main interest was identifying and using high-quality health promotion evidence. Like the Operational Framework, the Evidence Framework is based on the model's key concepts and relates evidence to underpinnings, the environment, and practice.

FIGURE 17.2 *The Evidence Framework for the IDM*

	Step 1: Prepare Foundation for Action Regarding Selected Issue			Step 2: Make Action and Evaluation Plan: *How do we get to where we want to go? who does what, when, and how?*				Step 3: Implement, Reflect, and Document		Step 4: Revise
	General guidelines: *What guides us?*	Current situation: *Where are we now?*	Picture of ideal situation: *Where do we want to go?*	Specific objectives to achieve ideal	Resources	Evaluation plan	Challenges	Activities and processes: *What did we do? How did we do it?*	Outcomes of activities and processes: *What were the results?*	Revisioins: *What do we need to change?*
UNDERPINNINGS										
Values										
Goals										
Ethics										
Theories										
Beliefs										
Evidence										
UNDERSTANDING OF THE ENVIRONMENT										
Organization vision										
Health vision										
Organization analysis										
Health analysis										
PRACTICE										
Address organization issues										
Address health issues										
Research/Evaluation										

APPLICATION

> Sometimes I wonder, do I use the IDM? Then I realize that I do, in the way I look at issues. Having worked to support the IDM and its Framework I now have a tendency in my work to look for what's behind things, what are the underlying assumptions, are we talking about the same things, do we have the same values. . . . The IDM pushes me to ask different questions of my colleagues—to know if we are using a common language, are we defining the research questions or issue statements the same way. It has forced me to have a systemic approach—having the IDM in mind helps me make the links. (Gagné 2005a and 2005b)

This section discusses who has used the IDM and how, and provides a case example of how to apply the IDM in practice.

Who Has Used the IDM and How

Individuals and groups who have used the IDM represent a variety of educational backgrounds, settings, languages, cultures, and countries. Participants in IDM processes have come from health promotion, clinical, and nonacademic backgrounds.

In addition to providing a planning structure, the IDM has guided evaluation and other research activities, built individual and organizational capacity, and provided conceptual foundations for other best practices tools and approaches. According to a 2007 follow-up of the IDM (Kahan et al., 2007), individuals and groups who have used the IDM represent a variety of educational backgrounds, settings, languages, cultures, and countries. Participants in IDM processes have come from health promotion, clinical, and nonacademic backgrounds.

Public health units, hospitals, academic institutions, community health centers, grassroots volunteer groups, and private business have used the IDM, as have consultants to governments and community agencies. These individuals and groups have applied the IDM to various issues, such as teen health, women's addictions, healthy child development, homelessness, diabetes, and partnerships.

Although the first language of most people using the IDM is English, at least one French-language group is actively using the IDM. IDM information is now available in English, French and Polish. The IDM has been used in the South Pacific islands, a very different culture to the one in which the IDM was conceived.

Examples of IDM application follow (from Kahan et al., 2007):

- **Planning and research.** A citywide plan to address housing and homelessness issues was developed using an IDM approach. L'Association des communautés francophone de l'Ontario-Toronto (L'ACFO-TO), a third of whose members are immigrants to Canada from a number of French-speaking countries in Africa, Europe, and the Caribbean, uses the IDM extensively for planning and evaluation. The IDM has shaped evaluations of a peer home visiting program for families with young children living in challenging circumstances, a community health center, and a collaboration of provincial, territorial, and federal health departments. The IDM was also used to

Applying the IDM in Different Cultural Contexts

One year we wanted to get into "how do we plan a project." We're talking about new immigrants, they're not concerned about planning, they're concerned about getting a job. The project was to plan the Francophone Community Builders program, but they skipped strategic thinking to go directly to concrete action without a sense of how the program would look at the end. After trying to do it for two or three Saturdays we were stuck, they didn't get the thinking process. So I said, "Let's choose a different example." I said to one participant, a traditional Algerian woman who wears a hijab, "We could plan your wedding—we'll use the MDI [French-language IDM] to do it." The need for strategic thinking became clearer because it was in their reality. Everyone knows someone who's gotten married.

Planning her wedding was wonderful, a beautiful example of inclusion and respect for culture. We had a Russian Francophile and people from France and Congolese—ten nations in all—focusing on this one wedding. Talk about inclusion, I had tears in my eyes every Saturday. It was a lot of fun. We looked at values: "What kind of values do you want in your wedding? Is there something that needs to be done in a specific way at the mosque?" We went into the evidence base, the theory part of the Muslim religion—what's the philosophy behind the rituals for the wedding. They learned that life is strategic. They were able with that easy example to put themselves into the process. It took a while— something like five or six Saturdays—at the end when we did the debriefing they said, "Wow, this is really amazing." They said, "This has taught me that I need to think about things in life. I can apply this in all areas." (Hélène Roussel, quoted in Kahan et al., 2007)

Having been convinced of the worth of the IDM, I added it to my resources and took it to the Pacific islands. I had been working with Pacific peoples in upgrading their health promotion skills for the past decade and had workshopped different aspects of these skills innumerable times over this period. Immediately that I started discussing the model with these Pacific peoples, I realized that if I were going to convince them of its merit, I had to take into account their traditional ways of teaching and learning, while being actively aware of their lower level of educational qualifications and their limited access to appropriate resources.

Thus the IDM has infiltrated our Pacific work, but it is not used as set out for Canadian or other resource-rich countries. Instead of a series of boxes and checks, we use story or narrative to draw attention to those issues we want covered. We make certain we include understanding of the environment; we always consider values and meanings in the under-pinnings. I know it has enhanced our Pacific work . . .

I will use a bit of story when I introduce different concepts, for example I will tell a story about a sea voyage before talking about the Ottawa Charter [for Health Promotion]. If I am wanting to learn about something I ask them to tell me their version, I phrase my question in such a way to allow them to give me their answer in a story format. They then might tell me, for example, about their uncle—the story is concrete, about a real body . . . Talking about things like "creating supportive environments" is so up in the air. Rather, I might talk about getting the village on-side, and choosing a night to meet when there's a full moon. The full moon is the spiritual piece, getting the village on-side is the social piece, the meeting place is the physical. (Ritchie, 2004) shape a Health Canada research project on effective primary prevention interventions for Type 2 diabetes.

- ■ **Conceptual foundations.** IDM concepts have influenced other models, tools, and individual understanding. The IDM forms the foundational underpinnings of the Toronto Public Health Practice Framework and has contributed to the development of the Nova Scotia Best Practices Framework, the European Quality Instrument for Health Promotion, and the Association of Ontario Health Centres bèst practices approach.

- ■ **Building organizational capacity.** The IDM has increased team and organizational cohesion through development of a common language and understanding around values and concepts, increased inclusion of key players previously not involved in many processes or activities, and placed the team's work in the context of the whole organization. It has increased identification, understanding, and addressing of organizational issues. It has also increased understanding of health-related issues leading to improved processes and activities to address these issues. In addition, IDM use has increased credibility for health promotion and research and increased consistency between practice, underpinnings, and understanding of the environment.

- ■ **Building individual capacity.** The IDM has been taught at the University of Toronto, Medical University of Warsaw, and the University of New South Wales. It has helped L'ACFO-TO volunteers increase their strategic thinking abilities. It has also increased individuals' understanding of health promotion and best practices, for example, to look for links and to take underpinnings and the environment into account.

Applying the IDM

The following case example, a composite of real life experiences (summarized from Kahan et al., 2007), illustrates the possible application of the IDM. All names and identifying characteristics are fictitious. It is important to remember that the only right way to apply the IDM is the way that works best for the individual or group.

The key task when using the IDM is to continually work to ensure consistency among the domains.

Karen P. is the manager of a "heart health" promotion program in a medium-sized public health department in a city with a high degree of poverty. After hearing about the IDM at a conference, she checked it out on the IDM Best Practices Web site at www.idmbestpractices.ca and read some of its supporting materials such as the *IDM Manual* (Kahan and Goodstadt, 2005b). Although interested, she was overwhelmed at the thought of integrating into practice not just values and evidence but also theories and beliefs, and vision and analyses of the various environments. After talking to someone familiar with the IDM she decided to start small, with the values piece of the IDM Framework.

It is important to remember that the only right way to apply the IDM is the way that works best for the individual or group.

She introduced the IDM to her team by using exercises from the *IDM Road Map for Coaches* (Kahan and Goodstadt, 2005a). At the end of the workshop the team agreed to try the IDM approach to best practices and a week later participated in a values clarification session. The only major disagreement occurred around the values of "individual autonomy" and "collective good": were they compatible or contradictory, and which was the closest to a health promotion value? The team decided to discuss these values later to avoid getting bogged down. Karen then introduced the one page values check-in from the *IDM Best Practices Check-In Forms* (Kahan and Goodstadt, 2004). The answers to the *Check-In* questions provided direction for future action to increase the reflection of values in practice.

After two months, Karen introduced the IDM to the community coalition of which the department was a member by conducting an exercise developed by L'ACFO-TO—using the IDM to plan a wedding. A few coalition members—community residents from the lower end of the income scale—responded to a request to join the heart health program's "best practices" committees.

At the four-month point, staff and volunteer committee members expressed dissatisfaction; for example, staff pointed to a low level of participation by volunteer members, and volunteers stated that they did not always understand staff member's comments. After some creative problemsolving the process was back on track.

At the six-month point, Karen and the team had completed an outline of the Framework and knew the areas in which they wanted to delve in more detail. They had a set of health promotion guidelines for underpinnings, understanding of the environment, and practice. For each of the domains they had brief notes, not always complete but enough to move forward with, on their current situation and their picture of the ideal. Team members Dana and Beckie, program participant Roger and community resident Estelle were working to refine the results into a usable action and evaluation plan, with concrete measurable objectives and indicators, and assigned responsibilities for implementing the tasks to achieve the objectives.

Documentation processes were in place and times scheduled to review what they had done so far and decide what to change in future. Despite some frustrations, all IDM participants, staff and volunteers, agreed that using the IDM was becoming easier over time and that they could see benefits already.

IDM IMPACTS

Three IDM reviews have identified a number of benefits resulting from its use. Over all, positive impacts included increases in:

- comprehensive/systematic planning
- consistency with principles/values
- health promotion and research knowledge/skills
- ability to address organizational-related issues
- group cohesion

Instances of no impact or negative impacts were observed only in the first pilot-testing phase and, in each case, positive impacts were also found. A description of the three reviews of the IDM and their results are summarized in Table 17.2.

TABLE 17.2 A Review of IDM Results.

	Review 1: pilot testing the IDM Operational Framework	Review 2: Pilot testing the IDM Evidence Framework learning module	Review 3: follow-up to IDM use and impacts
Authors	Kahan and Goodstadt, 2000	Kahan, 2007	Kahan, Groulx and Wong, 2007
Time period	Six months 1999–2000	Four months 2001–2002	2001–2007 (first and second pilot-testing periods omitted)
Cases	Three Ontario sites: public health department, hospital, community health center; individual participants included clinical and nonclinical staff and volunteers	six Ontario sites: public health departments, hospitals, community health centers; participants included clinical and nonclinical staff	Information from 26 individuals and 23 projects or organizations in North America, Europe and South Pacific islands; organizations included hospitals, public health departments, community health centers, community groups, academic institutions, private business; individuals included consultants, students, former pilot test participants and Best Practices Partnership members
IDM use	Planning	Research	Primarily planning, research, or building individual or organizational capacity
Health-related issues	Smoke-free cars, heart health, food security, and teen health	A variety of topics, from income as a barrier to health in the workplace to comprehensive school health	A variety of topics, from healthy child development to partnerships

(Continued)

TABLE 17.2 *(Continued)*

Research design	Observational case series based on: • participant feedback through informal conversation, feedback forms, workshop "check-ins," half-day mid-point review, half-day end-point evaluation session, two meetings with site contacts, end of project report from each site • facilitators' observations	Observational case series based on: • group evaluation interviews at the end of the project at five out of six sites • site reports on their experience with the project • facilitators' observations	Observational case series based on: • case studies • e-mail survey responses • semi-structured interviews • group discussion • author observations • other sources such as relevant documents and IDM Best Practices Web site profiles and reflections
Impacts	Impacts refer to one or more sites. Benefits at ***individual and team levels*** included increases in: • health promotion knowledge • group cohesion • ability to address issues within the team, organization and external environment • positive attitude to research Benefits regarding team's ***programs and activities*** included: • more comprehensive and systematic planning • greater clarity regarding issues • identification of actions and strategies to address issues • increased rigor, increased networking	Impacts refer to one or more sites. Benefits at ***individual and team levels*** included increases in: • understanding of health promotion and research • enthusiasm for research • group cohesion • systematic approach Benefits at the ***program level*** included: • increased understanding of issue • helped make time for research • varying degrees of progress towards implementing research plans	Benefits at ***individual and team levels*** included: • increased understanding of health promotion • change to practice approach that takes into account links between practice, underpinnings, and the environment, uses a broader range of information sources, and is more systematic or reflective Benefits at the ***program level*** included: • stronger relationships among staff and other stakeholders • increased use of evidence-based research • positive contribution to planning and research

Impacts (Continued)	At the **organizational** level, benefits included:	Benefits at **organizational level** included:	Benefits at the **organizational level** included:
	• greater awareness of best practices and health promotion issues, and greater credibility for health promotion • adoption of a best practices approach beyond the pilot site team Instances of **no** or **negative impact**: • may not have made a difference to planning at one site • one of several factors influencing volunteer disaffection at one site	• gave health-related issue more credibility • put organizational issues on the agenda • increased knowledge sharing • increased organizational cohesion • increased value placed on research No **negative impacts** from using the IDM Evidence Framework were identified.	• resurrection of an organization that was failing • increased cohesion • increased capacity • greater consistency between underpinnings, understanding of the environment, and practice **Other** benefits: • contributed to development of other tools and approaches • Impact on **outcomes for programs' priority populations:** No definitive conclusion about the IDM's contribution to outcomes for programs' priority populations is possible at this point but information collected to date is promising; for example, one organization which has used an IDM-like approach for thirty years has demonstrated very positive outcomes, with improvement in several developmental areas among children from challenging backgrounds.

(Continued)

TABLE 17.2 (Continued)

Impacts (Continued)

No **negative impacts** were identified during the Follow-up period.

Follow-up to the **pilot sites**:

A year after pilot testing the IDM Operational Framework all three sites reported ongoing benefits. One site responded to a follow-up request in 2004 with a positive report of IDM impacts. In 2007, two people who had participated at a second site responded to the Follow-up request: one reported knowledge of the IDM making no difference to quality or outcomes of that participant's work; the other reported a continued positive difference in personal understanding and approach.

In 2007, three of six sites who pilot tested the IDM Evidence Framework learning module provided an update. At one site two participants reported lasting personal benefits and two participants had no memory of having used the IDM. At the second site the IDM was in active use and achieving very positive results. At the third site IDM use was discontinued after a year and a half due to resource issues but the participant responding reported that benefits had resulted from its use. This site was considering resurrecting the IDM.

A description of impacts of IDM use follows in the context of six case studies of organizations that have used the IDM or an approach similar to the IDM. The information below is summarized from the 2007 IDM follow-up (Kahan et al., 2007).

L'Association des Communautés Francophone de l'Ontario-Toronto (L'ACFO-TO) L'ACFO-TO is a chapter of a provincial Franco-Ontarian grassroots volunteer-based organization. Its purpose is to assist Francophones to fully participate—on a daily basis in a large city where they are a minority—in various aspects of international "francophonie" such as socializing and doing business in the French language and enjoying French music, theater, and other arts. The degree of power and social inclusion experienced by individuals are strong social determinants of health; Francophones are marginalized in Toronto.

Since 2004 L'ACFO-TO has used the Modèle des Domaines Interactifs (MDI), the French-language version of the IDM, to plan and implement its activities. "We're really using the Model as a way to structure everything we do. . . . The Model will continue to remain the blueprint of where we are going." The organization also uses the MDI to teach strategic thinking to its volunteers and increase credibility with funders.

Using the MDI has resulted in a wide range of benefits for L'AFCO-TO, such as the development of a common language and understanding among its volunteer members increased planning skills, greater consistency between practice and values, the development of ethical principles, stronger vision, and more clearly defined objectives. "Because of the MDI we were able to take an organization that was on an artificial breathing system—it was about to die—and three years later have a complete 'building community' concept as a result of working on the foundations etc. The MDI has helped tremendously.

Brant Community HealthCare System (BCHS) The BCHS's association with the IDM started at the Willett Hospital, a small rural hospital in southern Ontario, during the pilot testing of the IDM Operational Framework. At that time the Willett was merging with a larger hospital in another location to become the BCHS. Initially volunteer members of the Willett's Community Well Being Team and hospital staff applied the IDM Framework to the topic of teen health. In addition to positive pilot testing impacts at the individual and program levels, such as skill enhancement, continued use of the IDM after the end of the pilot testing benefited BCHS as an organization in a number of ways. These benefits ranged from increased understanding and management of internal and external environmental factors to quality improvement and accreditation preparation. A key benefit was BCHS's adoption of a health promotion approach. "Our IDM work kick-started [BCHS's] new portfolio of Primary Healthcare Development. . . . What the portfolio would look like was completely open, so our work on the IDM Framework shaped it. The new portfolio was based on the Framework's underpinnings that we developed and resulted in business being done in a new way in a hospital setting. It helped us identify how the hospital could work with the community as a partner and how we could work as a system to address health issues. Health promotion became a part of the hospital's core business—that was a big deal.

Ceridian-Leade Health Leade Health Inc., formerly of Ann Arbor, Michigan and recently acquired by Ceridian Corporation of Minneapolis, Minnesota, focuses on health coaching in areas such as nutrition and physical activity, tobacco cessation, and stress management in order to facilitate overall health and well-being. Ceridian-Leade Health adopted the IDM in 2006, after researching different best practices models, in order to achieve the highest quality in coaching services and to establish a best practice model for the health coaching industry. The organization has used the IDM for program planning and evaluation, organizational change, evidence gathering, team building, values clarification, and as an everyday approach to work. It is still used since the acquisition by Ceridian to ensure consistency between all domains. "Using the IDM helped us fine-tune our designs, enhanced our coach training through developing competencies, brought us together. . . . We had a number of pieces we were working on and the IDM was the web that connected everything for us. When we talked about developing a practice we would look for our evidence, our experience, what else do we need. We were able to use what we learned from the IDM in decision making. The IDM gave us a framework to say 'is this part of our best practices, does it fit our focus' or 'that's not working, that doesn't fit'.

Regina Early Learning Centre The Regina Early Learning Centre (ELC), located in a Canadian prairie city of about 180,000 people, has worked for three decades to achieve healthy development for children in low-income families, primarily Aboriginal, through a range of programs for children and their parents. Using a home-grown approach to practice similar to the IDM, the ELC integrates into practice its values, evidence, and an understanding of the environment, and practices ongoing reflection and evaluation. According to an ELC outcome evaluation, between starting and finishing the ELC's preschool program the number of children with cognitive, language, and social-emotional delays decreased and a further number improved from a severe to a moderate delay. The changes observed were greater than would be expected due to maturation alone. According to the evaluation's key informant interviews, the ELC's impacts on the broader community ranged from "dissemination of knowledge and expertise" to "parents with increased skills who go on to participate in other organizations."

Womankind Addiction Service The mission of Womankind Addiction Service, part of St. Joseph's Health Care located in Hamilton, Canada, is to provide women with "effective and compassionate" withdrawal management and treatment. The IDM was used from the inception of Womankind to guide the development of this comprehensive women's addiction program. At the beginning of the merger between Women's Detox and the treatment-oriented Mary Ellis House, both sets of staff participated in the pilot testing of the IDM Evidence Framework learning module. In addition to unifying the two teams, IDM use resulted in Womankind's mission and values statements, which form the program's current guiding principles. The IDM continues to shape Womankind's strategic direction; it is also used as a filter to ensure its practices meet its stated values and mission. As a result of the IDM, "Womankind programming is based on current best practices, is flexible and poised to make changes based on emerging

FIGURE 17.3   *Toronto Public Health Practice Framework*

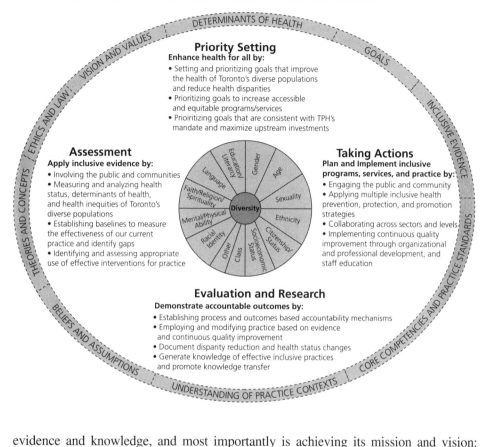

evidence and knowledge, and most importantly is achieving its mission and vision: helping women with addiction successfully journey towards recovery."

Toronto Public Health In 1997 Toronto amalgamated with five other municipalities to become a mega-city with a population of 2.5 million. Recognizing Toronto's increased cultural and linguistic diversity, growing social and economic disparities and the emergence of health needs related to globalization such as SARS, HIV/AIDS, and other communicable diseases, Toronto Public Health developed its practice framework in 2005 (Toronto Public Health, 2005) to guide its staff and members in integrating social justice, access, and equity principles into its programs and services. The Toronto Public Health Practice Framework has three core components: the diversity foundation that reflects Toronto's changing populations; Health Canada's Population Health Promotion Template that formulates the practice cycle; and the underpinnings of practice adopted from the IDM. (Figure 17.3.) The Practice Framework is being integrated into program/service development, implementation, and evaluation across all regions and programs. Preliminary feedback from health promotion staff working on a social marketing campaign suggests that the

> **Impact of IDM on an Individual**
>
> I think the IDM has influenced me in the kind of process that I take with the groups that I am working with. I work hard to get them to think about all the pieces that need to come together to make a best practice. I ask them to think about the values that they bring to their work and how that affects what outcomes they expect. I ask them to consider the theory and the evidence in literature when they are developing a practice.
>
> I think my involvement has been a factor in increasing my reflectiveness. I like to make sure that at some point in a project I take time to sit back and make sure that we haven't missed any steps, that everyone who needs to be involved has been and that where we are going is grounded in evidence. *(LS, quoted in Kahan et al., 2007)*

framework enhances staff reflexivity. "The Practice Framework enabled the staff to reflect on their work and identify the missing components that could make the campaign more effective and inclusive of the affected community, groups and individuals. As a result, Toronto Public Health staff working on the campaign had put 'community involvement' as one of the key priorities in the subsequent phases of the campaign."

STRENGTHS AND CHALLENGES

I think that probably the thing I valued most about [the IDM] was its comprehensiveness, how it takes into account all those different things (values, beliefs, theories, evidence, environment, practice, steps in the planning process, etc.), trying to link it all up into something coherent. What I understood as the most important messages of the IDM were the importance of considering all those things, (more or less) systematically, and to do it in a way that suits you and your context. (DJ, quoted in Kahan et al., 2007)

It is not an easy model to learn. . . . It doesn't happen over night. It is not a quick fix, it is a process. . . . In the end you need to consider other things besides what works—that's a hard lesson to learn. People want quick answers and this is a process-based model. . . . If a person is more focused on the product and the end point they wouldn't get a lot out of it. The challenge is to convert people if they're more product focused, get them to think in another dimension. (Jackie Kierulf, quoted in Kahan et al., 2007)

According to results from the recent IDM follow-up (Kahan et al., 2007), for many practitioners the IDM's key strength was the inclusion of values and other underpinnings, which function as a filter for health promotion practice. The inclusion of understanding of the environment assisted practitioners to address organizational issues that are often left on the back burner despite their importance to quality of practice.

For others, the IDM highlighted often concealed issues such as inequities. The IDM's emphasis on consistency between underpinnings, understanding of the environment, and

For many practitioners the IDM's key strength was the inclusion of values and other underpinnings, which function as a filter for health promotion practice. The inclusion of understanding of the environment assisted practitioners to address organizational issues that are often left on the back burner despite their importance to quality of practice.

practice was viewed by practitioners as promoting integrity or "walking the talk." The IDM was also evaluated positively for characteristics ranging from comprehensive to dynamic. Additionally, practitioners commented on the holistic nature of the IDM, that is, how it provides a "big picture" which makes visible the links between the different parts of the picture and incorporates all the elements essential to health promotion. Others commented on the IDM's adaptability to different situations.

Follow-up results show that one set of challenges to using the IDM is the circumstances of the organizational environment, in particular limited resources and conflicts between IDM and traditional approaches. For example, the IDM's comprehensive and critically reflective approach clashes with the more traditional approach of considering a limited range of factors and being oriented to quick action and easy solutions. In addition, while the IDM makes explicit the status of issues such as political commitment, resources and power equity, traditional approaches often ignore these topics because of their contentious nature.

Although no criticisms were made regarding the concepts underlying the Model or Framework, according to follow-up results one key challenge specific to the IDM is its complexity. A number of suggestions were made to simplify the IDM and its resources in order to make the IDM more usable and accessible. However, in general people found the benefits resulting from IDM use outweighed the challenges.

FUTURE DIRECTIONS

One of the key points is to demystify the idea that it's complicated, if our group has been using [the IDM] as a grassroots group, any group would be able to use it. . . . Although at first the model seems complicated, we have found it to be based on common sense. (Hélène Roussel, quoted in Kahan et al., 2007)

The concepts that shape the IDM have, to date, withstood the test of time: the IDM has been credited with contributing to many positive results in a number of different contexts, ranging from increased individual understanding of the connections between a number of decision-making factors to increased organizational capacity. At the same time, a number of unknowns are associated with it and room for growth and improvement exists in several areas.

Selective use of IDM elements may result in a narrow approach which ignores the political, economic, and social contexts of health promotion and perpetuates a disconnect between practice and other domains. Constant focus on one part of the Framework may result in lack of an ongoing process of implementation, reflection and revision.

One unknown relates to the IDM's impact on program outcomes for organizations' priority populations. Logically it makes sense that better outcomes will be achieved if practice matches evidence, values, theories, and understanding of the environment than if there is a mismatch. However, no full-scale study has examined results to see if real life fits the logic. Such a study, to follow outcomes from programs using the IDM over the course of a number of years, would contribute a great deal of knowledge about the IDM.

Another unknown relates to impacts of using parts of the Model or Framework as opposed to using it in its entirety. Selective use of IDM elements may result in a narrow approach which ignores the political, economic, and social contexts of health promotion and perpetuates a disconnect between practice and other domains. Constant focus on one part of the Framework may result in lack of an ongoing process of implementation, reflection and revision.

Room for growth involves exploring new IDM applications. For example, one practitioner suggested using the IDM as an advocacy tool: explicitly identifying underpinnings and understanding of the environment, and consciously measuring these against actual practice, provides the information required to push for greater consistency among all the domains. It is easier to maintain the status quo when assumptions are concealed, and more difficult to maintain the status quo when concrete evidence of inconsistencies between discourse, values, and practices are documented.

Room for growth also refers to the potential for more individuals and programs to actively use the IDM. Practitioners have suggested ways to increase dissemination and improve supporting resources, for example by establishing IDM coaches within organizations and by revising IDM materials to enhance ease of use.

Increased uptake further requires a fundamental change in attitude. Although a number of groups have reported using the IDM with desirable results, many practitioners may avoid it because of its apparent complexity. Ironically, the IDM has a very simple message—that what we do must match what we value, believe, and know if we are to achieve best practices and improved outcomes. However, its application is complex because health promotion practice exists in a world with many continually changing interactive elements, ranging from the nature of economic systems to power relationships, all of which differ according to factors such as geography, culture, and demographics. To use the IDM as a pathway through this complexity to reach our goals requires recognizing the importance of consistency between underpinnings, understanding of the environment and practice, and that the "best" is not always the easiest or quickest. Moreover, effective practice models must evolve over time to keep pace with changing realities.

> To use the IDM as a pathway through this complexity to reach our goals requires recognizing the importance of consistency between underpinnings, understanding of the environment and practice, and that the "best" is not always the easiest or quickest. Moreover, effective practice models must evolve over time to keep pace with changing realities

In the future, an IDM "vision" is a world where all practitioners—health promotion researchers, policy makers, and program managers and implementers—develop solid underpinnings and understanding of the environment and ensure practice is as consistent with these domains as possible through ongoing reflection and improvement. In this vision, reflecting on the integration of values, theories, evidence, and understanding of the environment into practice is second nature, coming as easily as riding a bicycle, with scraped knees from first attempts a distant memory. Work is very satisfying because it results in long-lasting benefits for the individuals and communities we work with. In this IDM vision, from morning to night our actions mirror what we value, believe, and know.

SUMMARY

The Interactive Domain Model (IDM), a best practices approach to health promotion, supports improved processes, activities, and outcomes by increasing consistency between what we value, believe, know, and do. (Kahan, B. and Goodstadt, M., 2001b).

Several qualities distinguish the IDM from traditional best practice approaches. The IDM situates evidence in relation to a comprehensive set of factors including values, supports innovation by recognizing the role of theory, emphasizes sensitivity to local conditions, encourages awareness of broader influences such as political and social environments, and highlights the importance of the organization.

The IDM Framework acts as an organizational and community change tool by leading participants through a practice cycle which involves building a strong foundation; making an action plan; implementing, reflecting, and documenting; and revising. IDM users, who represent a variety of backgrounds, have applied the IDM to a wide range of topics. Community groups, public health departments, hospitals, and other types of organizations have successfully used the IDM to plan, evaluate, clarify values, strengthen teams, and increase knowledge and skills.

REFERENCES

Barber, K. (Ed.) (1998). *The Canadian Oxford dictionary*. Toronto: Oxford University Press.

Cameron, R., Walker, R., and Jolin, M. A. (1998). *International best practices in heart health*. Toronto: Heart Health Resource Centre.

Caplan, R. (1993). The importance of social theory for health promotion: from description to reflexivity. *Health Promotion International*, 8(2), 147–157.

Chandola, T., Head, J. and Bartley, M. (2004). Socio-demographic predictors of quitting smoking: How important are household factors? *Addiction*, 99, 770–777.

Freudenberg, N., Eng, E., Flay, B., Parcel, G., Rogers, T., and Wallerstein, N. (1995). Strengthening individual and community capacity to prevent disease and promote health: In search of relevant theories and principles. *Health Education Quarterly*, 22(3), 290–306.

Gagné, Hélène. (April 2005a). *Profile of Hélène Gagné* (based on an interview with the Web site editor). IDM Best Practices Web site (www.idmbestpractices.ca).

Gagné, Hélène. (April 2005b). *Using the IDM in practice without naming it*. IDM Best Practices Web site (www .idmbestpractices.ca).

Kahan, B., and Goodstadt, M. (1999). Continuous quality improvement and health promotion. *Health Promotion International 14*(1), 83–91.

Kahan, B., Goodstadt, M., and Rajkumar, E. (1999). *Best practices in health promotion: A scan of needs and capacities in Ontario*. Toronto: Centre for Health Promotion, University of Toronto.

Kahan, B., and Goodstadt, M. (2000). *Pilot testing the Best Practices in Health Promotion Framework*. Toronto: Centre for Health Promotion, University of Toronto.

Kahan, B., and Goodstadt, M. (2001a). The Interactive Domain Model of Best Practices in Health Promotion: Developing and implementing a best practices approach to health promotion. *Health Promotion Practice*, 2(1), 43–67.

Kahan, B., and Goodstadt, M. (2001b). *The Interactive Domain Model computer program for Best Practices in Health Promotion, 2.12*. Centre for Health Promotion, University of Toronto.

Kahan, B., and Goodstadt, M. (2004). *Best practices check-in forms.*

Kahan, B., and Goodstadt, M. (2005a). *IDM best practices road map for coaches: a guide to using the Interactive Domain Model (IDM) for better health*, 2nd ed. Toronto: Centre for Health Promotion, University of Toronto.

Kahan, B., and Goodstadt, M. (2005b). *IDM manual*, 3rd ed. Toronto: Centre for Health Promotion, University of Toronto.

Kahan, B., Groulx, D., Wong, J. (2007). *Interactive Domain Model (IDM) best practices approach to better health: Follow-up to IDM use and impacts.* Toronto: Centre for Health Promotion, University of Toronto.

Kahan, B. (2007). *Pilot testing the IDM evidence framework learning module.* Toronto: Centre for Health Promotion, University of Toronto.

Levin, W. J. (1994). Using theory to improve population health: What health care can teach management. *Canadian Journal of Quality in Health Care, 11,* 4–15.

Milburn, K. (1996). The importance of lay theorizing for health promotion research and practice. *Health Promotion International, 11*(1), 41–46.

Nutbeam, D., and Harris, E. (1998). *Theory in a nutshell: A practitioner's guide to commonly used theories and models in health promotion.* Sydney, Australia: National Centre for Health Promotion, University of Sydney.

Ovretveit, J. (1996). Quality in health promotion. *Health Promotion International, 11*(1), 55–62.

Ritchie, Jan. (October 2004). *Profile of Jan Ritchie* (based on an interview with the Web site editor). IDM Best Practices Web site (www.idmbestpractices.ca).

Rychetnik L., Frommer M. A. (2002). *Schema for evaluating evidence on public health interventions* Version 4. Melbourne: National Public Health Partnership.

Seedhouse, D. (1997). *Health promotion: Philosophy, prejudice and practice.* Chichester, UK: Wiley.

Simnett, I. (1995). *Managing health promotion: Developing healthy organizations and communities.* Chichester, UK: Wiley.

Stokols, D. (1996). Translating social ecological theory into guidelines for community health promotion. *American Journal of Health Promotion, 10*(4), 282–298.

Toronto Public Health. (2005). *Toronto public health practice framework.* Toronto: Toronto Public Health.

CHAPTER

18

COMMUNICATION-FOR-BEHAVIORAL-IMPACT: AN INTEGRATED MODEL FOR HEALTH AND SOCIAL CHANGE

Everold Hosein
Will Parks
Renata Schiavo

MOBILIZING FOR HEALTH OUTCOMES AND SOCIAL CHANGE

The theory and practice of communicating about health and illness to mobilize individuals, families, communities, and societies toward health outcomes and social change has noticeably evolved over the past few decades. This evolution reflects emerging theories and empirical observations that point to the importance of an audience-centered, research-based, multidisciplinary, behavior-oriented, multifaceted, and strategic approach to communication interventions (Schiavo, 2007, p. 12; WHO, 2001 and 2003; Piotrow et al., 2003; Institute of Medicine, 2003; Bernhardt, 2004). There is broad agreement among theorists and practitioners alike that in order to "match how communication actually takes place" in people's everyday lives, an integrated blend of multiple action areas and channels is fundamental (Schiavo, 2007, p. 304; Exchange, 2006). Likewise, to improve, measure, and sustain impact, approaches should engage and mobilize all relevant participants in the health behavior and social change process (Parks et al., 2005).

In this context, Communication-for-Behavioral-Impact (COMBI) is a pioneering international model and planning framework for strategic communication and social mobilization that absorbs and applies lessons learned, good practices, and theoretical assumptions from a variety of disciplines to improve the reach and effectiveness of interventions that seek to promote health behavior and social change (WHO, 2003). COMBI's theoretical and practical foundation draws upon, among others, marketing, mass communications, information-education-communication, social mobilization, anthropology, and sociology (Renganathan et al., 2005).

Since 2000, the World Health Organization (WHO) and its partners have been applying COMBI in planning, initiating, and implementing strategic communications and social mobilization interventions in more than fifty countries in a variety of settings and disease areas that span from contributing to controlling and preventing outbreaks of infectious diseases (for example, by increasing public compliance to prevention measures for lymphatic filariasis or modifying behaviors to respond to early signs of dengue fever) to the reduction of maternal and infant mortality; HIV/AIDS programs; decreasing the incidence of household violence; and more recently promoting changes in diet and lifestyle.

To date, COMBI programs have reached a minimum of 100 million people worldwide and affected the health and/or social behavior of an average 60 percent of those individuals who have been reached by and engaged in COMBI interventions (Everold Hosein, personal data files, 2008). This chapter offers a synopsis of COMBI, outlining its theoretical foundations and public health applications.

WHAT IS COMBI?

COMBI is an integrated model and planning framework for social mobilization and strategic behavior communications interventions (Parks and Lloyd, 2004; Renganathan et al., 2005; Schiavo, 2007). Developed and tested over several years, COMBI incorporates the lessons learned from several disciplines and theoretical models and "draws substantially from the experience of private sector consumer communication" (Parks and Lloyd, 2004).

COMBI's theoretical foundation and ten-step planning methodology have progressively matured from work started in 1994 at New York University on *integrated marketing communication* (a planning concept "that recognizes the added value of a comprehensive plan that evaluates the strategic roles of a variety of communication disciplines and combines these disciplines to provide clarity, consistency, and maximum communications impact," Belch and Belch, 2004) applied to social development challenges. As a result, COMBI has its roots in the New York University's (NYU) annual summer institute on Integrated Marketing Communication for Behavioral Impact (IMC/COMBI) in Health and Social Development. Developed by the lead author (EH) with regular inputs from the United Nations Children's Fund (UNICEF), the United Nations Population Fund (UNFPA), NYU faculty, and originally, staff of Burson-Marsteller, Inc., the summer institute has been attracting professionals from the United States and international government agencies, multilateral organizations, and other leading public health institutions. In 2000, the institute became a training program conducted jointly in collaboration with the World Health Organization (WHO).

By incorporating principles and lessons learned from the private sector and more specifically IMC, COMBI reflects recent wisdom that recognizes the importance of transferring and integrating in public health and social development practice—and more generally in nonprofit practice—those skills and experiences that have proven to work in the private sector (Andresen, 2006; Curtis, Garbrah-Aidoo, and Scott, 2007). This trend has led to the flourishing of many global public-private partnerships where the private sector is sometimes charged with transferring knowledge and skills that may assist organizations in their health promotion and disease prevention efforts, and/ or help strengthen health systems (Curtis, Garbrah-Aidoo, and Scott, 2007).

To date, WHO and its partners have trained public health professionals and government agencies in COMBI from more than fifty countries in Africa, Asia, Eastern Europe, Latin America, the Caribbean, and North America. This training has increased local strategic communication capacity and resulted in the development and implementation of more than sixty COMBI programs worldwide (Hosein, 2008).

COMBI programs have been instrumental in mobilizing and communicating across cultural and geographical boundaries with a variety of audiences and levels of society, including the general public, policymakers, vulnerable populations, healthcare professionals, teachers, patients, parents, community development workers, spiritual pastors, local community leaders and groups, professional organizations, women, and many other communities and audiences (Renganathan et al., 2005). Although more evaluations are needed, COMBI's effectiveness has been already documented in many countries (Elder, 2005; WHO, 2005; Ramaiah et al., 2006; Bergada, 2006).

COMBI's Key Features and Other Theoretical Influences

Although the scope of this chapter does not include an in-depth description of COMBI's planning methodology, Box 18.1 features the HIC (inform and convince)-DARM (adopt and maintain behavior) model that informs COMBI's analytical planning (Hosein, 1979). This analytical frame of reference—a simplified version of the Transtheoretical Model—recognizes that behavior change often takes place in gradual and sequential steps and requires a sustained effort over a reasonable time period (Prokasha, Redding, and Evers, 1997).

In further refining COMBI, WHO and its partners also drew on the lessons learned and theoretical assumptions of several disciplines, including information-education-communication (IEC), social marketing, Integrated Marketing Communications (IMC) and social mobilization with the aim of providing an innovative framework for the planning, implementation, and evaluation of social mobilization and behavior communications programs (WHO, 2003; Renganathan et al., 2005). By incorporating good practices of these fields, COMBI has become a strategic framework with well-defined strengths and characteristics that include (Parks and Lloyd, 2004, Renganathan et al., 2005):

■ A strong emphasis on **behavioral impact** rather than awareness and knowledge-related results, which are important but insufficient steps to improving public health and social outcomes, as also prescribed by several authors (Andreasen, 1995; Schiavo, 2007).

■ Its focus on creating "**societal ownership**" through participatory research as well as planning, monitoring, and evaluation steps that aim collectively to engage and mobilize different social groups and communities, and to build national consensus on key issues and approaches.

■ The **cohesiveness of its steps** that address the model's primary concern, namely reducing disease burden.

■ Its reliance on the **integrated use of multiple communication action areas** and advances in communication technology and marketing.

■ The model's commitment to a **strong communication planning foundation** that relies on a comprehensive situation analysis and understanding of people's needs.

The importance of advanced planning and sound communication management—which are emphasized in COMBI—is well established (National Institute of Health and National Cancer Institute, 2002; WHO, 2003; Belch and Belch, 2004; Schiavo, 2007). Furthermore, measurable and well-defined behavioral results are increasingly recognized as the key planning objective of health communication programs and other interventions that seek to improve public health and social outcomes (Bertrand, 2005; Schiavo, 2007; WHO, 2003; Elder, 2005). Such behavioral results should be sought within the context of broader development initiatives that address multiple social, economic, organizational, legal, and cultural factors (WHO, 2001; Schiavo, 2007; Piotrow, 2003). The application of COMBI addresses the need for achieving these behavioral results through the integration of five mobilization and communication action areas (see Figure 18.1).

FIGURE 18.1 *The Five Integrated Communication Actions*

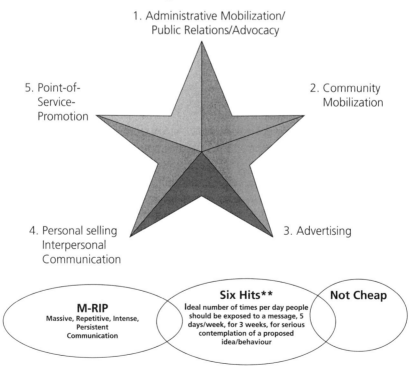

© Everold Hosein 1994. **Informal observation by Everold Hosein gathered from colleagues during work with Burston Marsteller, 1994–97.

The determination of precise behavioral results alongside the integrated blend of actions that are needed to achieve them is through a strategic and participatory approach to planning grounded in a comprehensive analysis of the health issue and situation. COMBI's key planning mantras are: "First: Do nothing—produce no T-shirt, no posters, no leaflets, no videos, until you have set out clear, precise, specific behavioral objectives." Second: "Do nothing—produce no T-shirts, no posters, no leaflets, no videos, until you have successfully undertaken a situational 'market' analysis in relation to preliminary behavioral objectives." The **situational market analysis** calls for "taking the recommended behavior back into the community and listening to its members to identify the 'communication keys' to help secure their involvement" (Schiavo, 2007, p. 51).

CASE APPLICATION: DENGUE FEVER PREVENTION AND CONTROL IN MALAYSIA

Dengue fever is the most important arbovirus infection in the world, as well as the most important infectious disease in the tropics after malaria (Gubler, 1998). Commonly transmitted by the mosquito species *Aedes aeygpti* (Linn.), dengue fever (DF) and its more severe form, dengue hemorrhagic fever/dengue shock syndrome (DHF/DSS), represent an increasing threat to global health (Gubler, 2002). More than a hundred countries are now affected in Africa, the Americas, the Eastern Mediterranean, Southeast Asia, and the Western Pacific.

Dengue outbreaks in urban areas infested with *Ae. aegypti* can be explosive, involving up to 70 to 80 percent of the population. Previously confined to urban centers, dengue is now spreading to rural areas wherever the vector is present. There are no cures for DF/DHF and until effective, safe, and affordable vaccines become available, the only existing prevention and control strategies are to reduce human-vector contact, using vector control and personal protection methods (Jacobs, 2000). Particular emphasis needs to be placed on the management or elimination of mosquito larval habitats in and around people's homes, work settings, municipal dumps, and in other less obvious places such as informal dump sites and playgrounds (WHO, 2001).

Key Issues in Dengue Fever Communications

For dengue programs to meet with success, a solid understanding of the local cultures and behaviors of affected populations including the general public, health care providers, politicians, policy makers, the media, and the private sector is needed (Gordon, Rojas, and Tidwell, 1990; Parks et al., 2000, 2005; Renganathan et al. 2004). Such a call reflects similar, long-standing recommendations made by social scientists working in other areas of public health (Manderson, 1998; Hahn, 1999; Farmer, 1999).

Until recently, however, public mobilization efforts related to dengue were generally based upon biomedical explanations of the disease and scientific observations of *Aedes* mosquitoes. Many of these efforts often took little account of local knowledge systems and practices (Gordon, 1998). For example, people in many diverse settings tend to associate mosquito breeding sites with public spaces such as drains, rubbish dumps, and areas of overgrown grass, or with even more distant sites such as swamps and rivers, not to everyday containers, packaging, and trash found around an individual's house (Ruiz and González-Téllez, 1992; Larson et al., 1997; Parks and Bera, 2001). Differences in the way people think about mosquitoes and the messages coming from dengue control programs may lead to people's apparent failure to act upon advice. A study in Mérida, Mexico, for example, revealed that many household members thought that mosquitoes found inside their homes were 'family' mosquitoes and did not cause illnesses. Disease-carrying mosquitoes, on the other hand, came from dirty standing water, overgrown vegetation, and garbage sites (Winch et al., 1991).

Dengue is often confused with other, less serious illnesses, and people may not believe dengue can be serious (Kendall et al., 1991). Such perceptions can influence the extent to which individuals protect themselves and their families from dengue, and the speed with which they respond to febrile illness during dengue outbreaks. Even at the height of dengue epidemics, people may fail to recognize disease symptoms. Delays in seeking medical attention as well as the frequency with which dengue is misdiagnosed or under-diagnosed can lead to the early stages of outbreaks (Kuno, 1995).

COMBI in Action in Malaysia

In January 2001, the Ministry of Health in Johor Bahru (MOHJB) decided to apply COMBI's integrated model to its strategic communication efforts with assistance from WHO. The trial followed COMBI's ten-step planning model (Figure 18.2) and consisted of twelve-week pilot project. Launched in August 2001 after a comprehensive situational market analysis, the project intended to affect behavioral change among residents of Johor Bahru City, the state's capital (approximately 1.2 million people).

Research data helped identify the following behavioral objectives:

1. To prompt family members in every home to conduct a weekly thirty-minute home inspection (both inside and outside) on Sundays to look for potential mosquito larval habitats and, if needed, take specific action to rid infested areas of these habitats.
2. To prompt the creation of a Dengue Volunteer Inspection Team (DeVIT) that would conduct a weekly larval site inspection of community surroundings (not within the definition of homes) and take specific action to rid the area of these habitats.
3. To prompt every individual with fever symptoms to suspect DF and go immediately (at least within one day) to the nearest health clinic for diagnosis and treatment.

FIGURE 18.2   Key Steps in Designing a COMBI Plan

WMC'S technical staff and consultants trained in COMBI planning apply a process in developing a COMBI plan. The building blocks of a COMBI plan are outlined below. It assumes a prior understanding of a few basic communication and marketing principles.

Identifying the behavioral objectives

1. The overall goal: a statement of the overall programme goal that COMBI will help achieve. For example... To contribute to the elimination of Lymphatic Filariasis in (location) by the year 2020.

2. The behavior objective/s: a statement of specific, measurable, appropriate and timebound behavioral objectives. For example... To prompt approximately 800,000 individuals (i.e. everyone other than pregnant women, new mothers of infants under a week old and children under 5 years of age) in (location) to accept the hand-delivered set of LF prevention pills (maximum 4) and to swallow these pills in the presence of a health worker/volunteer on October 27th, 2001.

3. The situational market analysis vis-a-vis the precise behavioral goal: a "consumer orientated" exploration of the factors influencing the attainment of the behavior objectives that will inform the strategy and the communication mix.

The situational market analysis

COMBI uses state-of-the-art participatory research techniques adapted from marketing, communications, anthropology, and sociology to identify behavioral issues amenable to communication solutions.

The situational market analysis involves listening to people and learning about their perceptions and grasp of the offered behavior(s) through tools such as TOMA (Top of the Mind Analysis), and DILO (Day in the Life Of). Their sense of the costs (time, effort, money) in relation to their perception of value of the behavior to their lives is explored through a Cost vs Value calculation.

Other tools such as the Force Field Analysis helps community members, field staff, local experts, and the COMBI specialist to analyse the social, political, ecological, moral, legal, and cultural factors that could constrain or facilitate adoption of the behavior.

The situational market analysis also examines where and from whom people seek information and advice on the particular health problem and why they use these information sources. The concept of positioning (used extensively in the advertising world), also helps the development of appropriate messages and communication approaches. Areas that require further investigation are also highlighted.

Finally, issues not substantially amenable to communication solutions, such as the ready availability of services, are documented so that appropriate organizational change or political action can be taken.

The communication strategy and mix

4. The overall strategy for achieving the stated behavioral result: a description of the general communication approach and actions which need to be taken to achieve the behavioral issues identified and presented as follows:
(a) Restate Behavioral Objective.
(b) Set out "Communication Objectives" which will need to be achieved in order to achieve behavioral result(s).
(c) Outline Communication Strategy: a broad outline of the proposed communication actions for achieving communication and behavioral results in terms of the five communication actions listed in #5.

5. The COMBI Plan of Action: a description of the integrated communication actions to be undertaken with specific communication details in relation (but not exclusive) to:

> **Public Relations/Public Advocacy/Administrative Mobilisation**
> **Community Mobilisation**
> **Personal Selling (Interpersonal Communication)**
> **Advertising**
> **Point-of-Service Promotion**

Implementation, monitoring and evaluation, budgeting

6. Management and implementation of COMBI: a description of how COMBI will be managed specifying the multidisciplinary planning team, including specific staff or collaborating agencies. (e.g., local advertising firms and research institutions), designated to coordinate communication actions and other activities such as monitoring. Also included are any technical advisory groups or government body from which the management team receives technical support or to whom it should report.

7. Monitoring implementation: a description of the process indicators to be used in tracking the reach and effect of the communication actions, including a description of how monitoring data will be gathered, shared and used.

8. Assessment of behavioral impact: details of the behavioral indicators to be used, methods for data collection, analysis and reporting.

9. Calendar/Time-line/Implementation Plan: a detailed workplan with time schedule for the preparation and implementation activities required to execute each communication action as described in #5.

10. The budget: A detailed listing of costs for the various activities described in #5, 6, 7 and 8.

For further information see the section on 'How can one find out more?'

The COMBI plan relied on the integration of its five action areas (Figure 18.1), and included:

- Advocacy and public relations activities to engage key local stakeholders, including politicians;

- The creation of social mobilization units such as (a) 48 Dengue Volunteer Inspection Teams (DeVITs), which included 615 volunteers and were instrumental in providing advice to 100,956 people, distributing 101,534 flyers and inspecting 1,440 vacant lots; and (b) bicycle riding teams (D'RIDERS), including local youth who were responsible for promoting the project and were accompanied by a van equipped with a Public Announcement system. At each location, local community leaders and residents greeted the team;

- A comprehensive advertising and public service announcement (PSA) strategy including two thousand vertical buntings posted along selected streets of Johor Bahru, a radio PSA in Malay and Chinese, a series of print ads that were carried by local newspapers and featured recommended behaviors;

- A school-based program that provided children and their parents with a single, two-sided self-instructional worksheet/checklist on how to deal with *Aedes* breeding sites at home was prepared in four major languages (Malay, Chinese, English, and Tamil);

- Radio talk shows hosted by local doctors to promote COMBI and provide listeners with information on dengue. Listeners were also encouraged to call in with questions; and

- Point-of-service promotion sites that were staffed by physicians and other health care providers to explain the behavioral goals of the project to every patient who attended the clinic for any given reason.

At the end of the twelve-week campaign, a post-intervention questionnaire survey was used to compare results against baseline data collected before the implementation of COMBI. Respondents were either household heads or anyone above the age of eighteen years. Out of 1,712 post-intervention respondents, 926 were considered "paired" respondents that is, they were the same respondents who had been interviewed during the baseline survey. [Almost all (99 percent) the respondents interviewed in the post-survey claimed that they had performed household inspections on Sundays compared to 71 percent in the pre-survey] ($p < 0.01$).

Short questionnaires were also developed to gather data on treatment-seeking behaviors among patients admitted and diagnosed with dengue in all government hospitals throughout Johore State. Patients admitted into Sultanah Aminah Hospital and Kulai Hospital (government hospitals serving Johor Bahru district) were considered as "cases," while those admitted in hospitals in other districts served as "controls." It was assumed that people who resided in other districts had not been exposed or involved in all the COMBI mobilization and communication activities. During the twelve-week study period, a total of 134 patients admitted into the two government hospitals in Johor Bahru district as well as 146 patients admitted into government hospitals in other districts participated in the study's interviews. Patients admitted into private hospitals were not interviewed. Results show that 59 percent of those admitted into Johor Bahru government hospitals sought treatment within twenty-four hours of the onset of the fever compared to 42 percent among those from control areas ($p < 0.01$). Apart from "exposure to COMBI," there were no associations between other variables and the time between the onset of fever and hospital admission. It was also noted that there was a slight decline in the number of cases in areas where DeVITs were established. No decline was measured in the non-DeVIT areas (Suhaili et al., 2004).

Conclusions

COMBI's application in dengue prevention and control has been successful in a variety of international settings (Parks and Lloyd, 2004; Elder, 2005). A key lesson learned from COMBI's application in dengue prevention and control is that intersectional coordination and active community involvement can be effectively stimulated but must be accompanied by improvements in the public health infrastructure, epidemiological and entomological surveillance, effective clinical management, emergency preparedness, and reinforcement of health policy and legislation (Parks et al., 2005).

THE ROLE OF COMBI IN PUBLIC HEALTH PROMOTION

As an applied profession with a strong behavioral and social science orientation, public health promotion heavily relies—or should rely heavily—on a research-based approach to design, implement, and evaluate programs that seek to improve public health and social outcomes. "Popular social-ecological models such as MATCH (Simons-Morton, Greene, and Gottlieb, 1996), Precede/Proceed (Green and Kreuter, 2002), and Intervention Mapping (Bartholomew, Parcel, Kok, and Gottlieb, 2001) emphasize the importance of multiple social levels of assessment and intervention" (Simons-Morton, 2006). This socioecological perspective has influenced recent trends and practices in health promotion and has lead to the current belief that behavioral change should be sought at community, policy, and social levels, as recognized by some key approaches and orientations in health promotion and in many other public health fields (Simon-Morton, 2006; Schiavo, 2007).

With its strong focus on social engagement and mobilization, COMBI is an essential tool and planning framework to promote health. Through its rigorous approach to researching situations, issues, and audiences, as well as its emphasis on mobilizing communities to achieve behavioral results that take into account the social, legal, and political environments in which such behaviors need to be adopted, implemented, and sustained, COMBI well reflects current and future directions in public health promotion. COMBI could be instrumental in implementing WHO's vision of health promotion "as a mediating strategy between people and their environments, synthesizing personal choice and social responsibility in health" (WHO, 1984). The key pillars of such a vision include yielding high levels of community and public participation; acting on what are recognized as key determinants or causes of health; and using a variety of approaches and interventions (WHO, 1984; Minkler, 1989). COMBI has proven to be effective in engaging public and community participation across health literacy and cultural boundaries in different ethnic groups and countries. Because of its widespread application in developing countries, COMBI has shown it is an effective planning framework to address the health and social issues of populations who may be the most vulnerable because of socioeconomic conditions, poor access to health care, low literacy levels, and other kinds of disadvantages (Renganathan et al., 2005).

WHAT COMBI CAN AND CANNOT DO

As previously mentioned, the rigorous application of COMBI to global public health communications and social mobilization interventions can move public health programs beyond "awareness raising" and toward the achievement of precise behavioral results. Increased awareness and knowledge about health behaviors have notoriously been insufficient bases for action, though they are essential steps in the process towards behavioral impact. COMBI makes a seamless connection between these steps and those needed for prompting desired behavioral responses. However, the following needs to be noted: COMBI makes behavioral promises with regard to the control of diseases. It promises to achieve the widespread practice of recommended health behaviors. COMBI programs work on the assumption that recommended behaviors have been selected to have an impact on the prevalence of a disease and are strictly related to its occurrence. If the "wrong" behavior is selected, a COMBI effort may very well be successful in getting the behavioral result but with little impact on the disease. Therefore, the early involvement of COMBI experts in identifying—together with the larger public health and disease management team—suitable behaviors that may have the most impact on disease incidence and prevalence may increase effectiveness of COMBI interventions in relation to potential reduction in disease burden. In general terms, involving communication experts at the early onset of strategic planning is a good practice in many different sectors.

COMBI adds the social mobilization element to marketing and behavioral sciences–based models ensuring that behaviors, products, concepts, or innovations will be widely diffused through various social channels. The demand stimulation brought about by social mobilization ensures an accelerated process of diffusion. At the same time, by adding the behavioral bite to the mobilization model, COMBI helps public health programs that usually have very small strategic communications budgets, to get value for their investment in terms of actual behavioral outcomes. COMBI's application can help program planners to allocate strategically their scarce resources.

As for the majority of global public health interventions and models, COMBI by itself cannot and does not always generate development. In fact, addressing issues of inequity, injustice, and poverty often requires the blending of different interventions, approaches, and professional competencies (Schiavo, 2007). Yet, COMBI's disease- or risk-focused approach as well as its initial application to communicable diseases and other so-called "diseases of poverty" could provide much-needed help to vulnerable populations, relieve them of a significant obstacle that keeps people in poverty, make progress against the most formidable childhood killers, and help strengthen health services. COMBI's application in Nepal, Vietnam, and Uganda has made significant strides in tackling specific diseases of poverty. To the extent that "development" is a process of individuals taking specific actions, the COMBI approach with its sharp behavioral focus may be of significant use.

COMBI programs often require substantial resources (depending on the magnitude and characteristics of the health or social issue being addressed). Therefore, COMBI programs cannot be easily implemented without advanced planning to secure adequate funds that would also consider the potential need for replication and scaling-up phases. However, regardless of the planning framework being used, this is a relatively common issue in communication interventions. Several authors have already argued that communication is often underfunded—even in areas such as immunization where its impact is well documented—and that the lack of adequate resources (including funds, human resources, and time) may have a negative impact on the effectiveness of communication efforts (Schiavo, 2007; Waisbord, 2005).

For communication to have long-lasting *behavioral* impact rather than just change knowledge or attitudes (which can usually be achieved at less cost), communication and mobilization activities must be (1) Massive, (2) Repetitive, (3) Intensive, and (4) Persistent (M-RIP). Ensuring M-RIP takes substantial resources. This initial investment, however, is always likely to save funds and other resources later on.

COMBI should not be promoted as having universal applicability in some fixed, rigid format. Countries and regions within countries vary greatly in terms of their social development experiences, political structures, literacy rates, settlement patterns, ethnic or tribal groupings, and so on. For example, the notion of participation and social mobilization may be perceived differently by various cultural and geographical groups (Schiavo, 2007). Therefore, the application of COMBI and all other planning frameworks and models should always take into account such differences. For example, in religiously conservative and male-dominated societies it may be difficult to encourage participation and create large alliances to advocate for women's health issues or other taboo topics such as family planning and AIDS education. COMBI programs may also be difficult to execute in those countries and situations where there are strict controls on the mass media and where governments may consider social programs their sole responsibility. In such countries, "mobilization" may remain coercive and communication channels strictly controlled. Nevertheless, COMBI programs can be designed within the framework of these restrictions, working within the reality of each "market" situation.

FUTURE DIRECTIONS

Although the application of COMBI has been mostly towards health outcomes, its key principles and methodologies are relevant to other areas. For example, COMBI has recently been used "as part of UNICEF's programs on child protection and juvenile justice in Moldova." (Schiavo, 2007, p. 51). Similar efforts are under way with UNICEF in Albania and Jordan. Moreover, COMBI has been used and has the potential to be used in combination with other strategic communication models (for example, CDCynergy, P-Process, CREATE! and ACADA) of other U.S. and international organizations for the development of tools and planning resources (John Hopkins University, 2005; UNICEF, 2006).

As for other public health models, COMBI continues to evolve and be integrated with emerging theoretical frameworks and approaches. Within WHO, COMBI is well positioned for use in combination with Healthy Settings, another health promotion framework that integrates health communication interventions with organizational change strategies. COMBI's emphasis on behavioral results may be also well suited to achieve organizational objectives. In fact, organizational change is "usually achieved as a result of the attainment of a series of behavioral objectives" (Schiavo, 2007, p. 223), which pertain to different organizational levels, senior officers, and staff members.

COMBI also continues to learn from other health promotion models. Future directions may include:

- Expanding on existing research efforts and steps to further *map the sociopolitical environment* into which and through which a newly devised COMBI program must be initiated and sustained. The sociopolitical environment can be defined as set of forces (demographic, economic, physical, technological, political/legal, and sociocultural) that are external to the COMBI program and are key to developing and maintaining successful influence on its intended audiences;

- Emphasizing the importance of *organizational change*, the "restructuring" of existing organizations to put in place the mechanisms needed to implement and manage COMBI programs and all related alliances and networks. Traditionally, COMBI programs have been managed within a broad and existing organization. Therefore, they often confront the issue of being integrated into that organization's structure as a legitimate philosophy and unit. Kotler and Anderson (1987) have argued that such integration evolves in three stages: an initial "resistance" stage, a growth stage and "acceptance" stage, and a mature or "established" stage. It is important that officials from local institutions are provided with adequate training and resources to integrate early on COMBI's activities with other more established activities within the organization.

Other future directions may emerge from the application of COMBI in additional settings and situations. In the meantime, COMBI has definitely contributed to revitalizing the field of global health communications and is now a mature approach that could serve as an essential part of the public health professional toolbox. As a model and planning framework for strategic communication for behavioral outcomes with a strong social mobilization component, COMBI is well positioned to result in an accelerated process of diffusion and acceptance of concepts, innovations, and behaviors in support of better public health and social outcomes.

SUMMARY

Applied in more than fifty countries, Communication-for-Behavioral Impact provides a strategic framework that has established efficacy in health promotion. The ten-step planning model used in COMBI has been carefully developed and its utility is well established. COMBI has been applied across a wide range of cultures, thereby demonstrating its adaptive capacity. The approach is based on prevailing theories in health promotion and is firmly grounded in the principles of community engagement. COMBI spans a wide range of intervention points, thereby optimizing its potential to create meaningful and lasting behavior change. The integration of five mobilization and communication action areas into the COMBI approach is vital to its success. Emphasis on social engagement and mobilization is a hallmark of COMBI, thereby making the method quite compatible with current thinking in public health practice.

ACKNOWLEDGMENTS

Everold Hosein and Will Parks wish to thank Renata Schiavo for joining them in writing and authoring this chapter, and for helping to position COMBI within the context of current theories and trends for the purpose of this publication. The authors gratefully acknowledge the efforts of national staff and partners in Malaysia's dengue program. The invaluable support of colleagues at WHO, UNICEF, UNFPA, NYU, and Burson-Marsteller, Inc., is greatly appreciated, especially Elil Renganathan and Asiya Odugleh-Kolev of WHO, Erma Manoncourt of UNICEF, and Jeff Carr of the Stern Business School at New York University. The credit for the ultimate success of any COMBI program is due to the individuals, families, and local communities who have embraced these activities and are dedicating time and effort to their implementation.

REFERENCES

Andreasen, A. R. (1995). *Marketing social change: Changing behavior to promote health, social development and the environment*. San Francisco: Jossey-Bass.

Andresen, K. (2006). *Robin Hood marketing: Stealing corporate savvy to sell just causes*. San Francisco: Jossey-Bass.

Bartholomew, L. K., Parcel, G. S., Kok, G., and Gottlieb, N. H. (2001). *Intervention mapping*. Mountain View, CA: Mayfield.

Belch, G. E. and Belch, M. A. (2004). *Advertising and promotion: An integrated marketing communications perspective*. (6th ed.). New York: McGraw-Hill.

Bergada, V. (2006). "National Communication Campaign promoting antenatal care—Pentru un Fat Frumos si Sanatos [For a Healthy and Beautiful Child]: The Moldova Experience" Presentation at 2006 UNICEF Middle East and North Africa (MENA) Region Workshop on Strategic Communication Planning. http://www.unicef.org.tn/html/pub_mena_wsc.htm. Retrieved May 2008.

Bernhardt, J. M. (2004). Communication at the core of effective public health. *American Journal of Public Health*, 2004, *94*(12), 2051–2053.

Curtis V. A., Garbrah-Aidoo, N. and Scott, B. (2007). Ethics in public health research: Masters of marketing: Bringing private sector skills to public health partnerships. *American Journal of Public Health 97*(4), 634–641.

Elder, J. (2005). Evaluation of Communication-for-Behavioral-Impact (COMBI): Efforts to control *Aedes aegypti* breeding sites in six countries. Tunis: WHO Mediterranean Centre for Vulnerability Reduction.

Farmer, P. (1999). *Infections and inequalities: The modern plagues.* Berkeley: University of California Press.

Gordon, A. J., Rojas, Z. and Tidwell, M. (1990). Cultural factors in *Aedes aegypti* and dengue control in Latin America: A case study from the Dominican Republic. *International Quarterly of Community Health Education, 3:* 193–211.

Gordon, A. J. (1988). Mixed strategies in health education and community participation: An evaluation of dengue control in the Dominican Republic. *Health and Education Research, 3,* 399–419.

Green, L. W., and Kreuter, M. W. (2002). *Health promotion planning: An educational and environmental approach.* Mountain View, CA: Mayfield.

Gubler, D. J. (1998). 'Dengue and dengue hemorrhagic fever.' *Clinical Microbiology Reviews, 11,* 480–496.

Gubler, D. J. (2002). Epidemic dengue/dengue hemorrhagic fever as a public health, social and economic problem in the 21st Century. *Trends in Microbiology 10,* 100–102.

Hahn, R. A. (1999). *Anthropology in public health: Bridging differences in culture and society.* Oxford: Oxford University Press.

Hosein, E. (1979). Communication training manual for IEC (Information-Education-Communication) officers of IPPF member affiliates in the Caribbean. Presentation at 1979 International Planned Parenthood Federation meeting, New York, NY.

Hosein, E. (2008) Communication for Behavioral Impact (COMBI): An overview of WHO's model for strategic social mobilization and communication. APHA 136th Annual Meeting, San Diego, CA, October 25–29, 2008.

Institute of Medicine. (2003) *Who will keep the public healthy?* Washington, DC: The National Academies Press.

Jacobs, M. (2000). Dengue: emergence as a global public health problem and prospects for control. *Transactions of the Royal Society of Tropical Medicine and Hygiene, 94,* 7–8.

John Hopkins University, Center for Communication Programs. (2005) 'Avian flu'. http://www.jhuccp.org/topics/avian_flu.shtml. Retrieved May 2008.

Kendall, C., Hudelson, P., Leontsini, E., Winch, P., Lloyd, L. and Cruz F. (1991). Urbanization, dengue and the health transition: Anthropological contributions to international health. *Medical Anthropology Quarterly, 5*(3), 257–268.

Kotler, P. and Andreasen, A.R. (1987). *Strategic marketing for nonprofit organizations.* 3rd ed. Englewood Cliffs, New Jersey: Prentice-Hall.

Kuno, G. (1995). Review of factors modulating dengue transmission. *Epidemiologic Reviews, 17*(2), 321–335.

Larson, A., Bryan, J. and Howard, P. (1997). Communities' roles in mosquito-borne disease control: Lessons from two Queensland studies. *Arbovirus Research in Australia, 7,* 141–146.

Manderson, L. (1998). Applying medical anthropology in the control of infectious disease. *Tropical Medicine and International Health, 3*(12), 1020–1027.

McKee, N. (1992). *Social mobilization and social marketing in developing countries: Lessons for communicators.* Penang: Southbound.

Minkler, M. (1989). Health Education, health promotion and the open society: A historical perspective. *Health Education and Behavior, 16,* 17–30.

Parks, W., et al. (2000). Campaigns that bite in strange places: social marketing and key containers in Fiji. Paper presented at the International Conference on Dengue and Dengue Haemorrhagic Fever, Chiang Mai, Thailand, 20–24, November.

Parks, W., and Bera, A. (2001). Linking social research, health communication and dengue control: An example from Fiji. *Arbovirus Research in Australia, 8,* 267–274.

Parks, P. and Lloyd, L. (2004) *Planning social mobilization and communication for dengue fever prevention and control: a step-by-step guide.* Geneva: World Health Organization.

Parks, W., et al. (2005). International experiences in social mobilization and communication for dengue prevention and control. *Dengue Bulletin,* Special Supplement, *28,* pp. 1–7.

Parks, W. with Grey-Felder, D., Hunt, J. and Byrne, A. (2005). *Who measures change? An introduction to participatory monitoring and evaluation of communication for social change*. South Orange: Communication for Social Change Consortium.

Piotrow, P. T., Rimon, J. G. II, Payne Merritt, A., and Saffitz, G. (2003). *Advancing health communication: The PCS experience in the field*. Baltimore, MD: Johns Hopkins Bloomberg School of Public Health, Center for Communication Programs.

Prokasha, J. O., Redding, C. A. and Evers, K. E. (1997). The Transtheoretical Model and stages of change. In Glanz, K., Lewis, F.M., Rimer, B.K. (eds) *Health Behavior and Health Education: Theory, Research, and Practice* (pp. 60–84). San Francisco: Jossey-Bass.

Ramaiah, K. D., et al. (2006). A campaign of "communication for behavioral impact" to improve mass drug administrations against lymphatic filariasis: Structure, implementation and impact on people's knowledge and treatment coverage. *Annals of Tropical Medicine and Parasitology*, *100*(4), June 2006, pp. 345–361.

Renganathan, E., et al. (2004). Towards Sustaining Behavioral Impact in Dengue Prevention and Control. *Dengue Bulletin*, *27*, pp. 6–12.

Renganathan, E., et al. (2005). Communication-for-Behavioral-Impact (COMBI): A Review of WHO's Experiences with Strategic Social Mobilization and Communication in the Prevention and Control of Communicable Diseases. In M. Haider (ed.), *Global public health communication: Challenges, perspectives, and strategies*. Sudbury, MA: Jones and Bartlett.

Ruiz, A. and González-Téllez, S. (1992). Community-based control of *Aedes aegypti* and dengue in Piritu, Syaye of Anzoategui, Venezuela. In Halstead, S.B. and Gómez-Dantés, H. (eds). *Dengue: A worldwide problem, a common strategy*. Mexico City: Ministry of Health.

Simons-Morton, B. (2007). Publication trends: A commentary on health education and health promotion publication trends. *Health Education and Behavior*. *34*, 26–31.

Simons-Morton, B. G., Greene, W. A. and Gottlieb, N. (1996). *Introduction to health ducation and health promotion*. Prospect Heights, IL: Waveland Press.

Schiavo R. (2007). *Health communication: From theory to practice*. San Francisco: Jossey-Bass.

Suhaili, M. R., Hosein, E., Mokhtar, Z., Ali, N., Palmer, K. and Isa, M. (2004). Applying Communication-for-Behavioural-Impact (COMBI) in the prevention and control of dengue in Johor Bahru, Johore, Malaysia. *Dengue Bulletin*, *28* Supplement, pp. 39–43.

UNICEF (2006). *Strategic communication for behaviour and social change in South Asia*. Nepal: Regional Office of South Asia.

Winch, P. J., et al. (1991). Beliefs about the prevention of dengue and other febrile illnesses in Mérida, Mexico. *Journal of Tropical Medicine and Hygiene*, *94*, 377–387.

World Health Organization, Regional Office for Africa. (2001a). *Health promotion: A strategy for the African region*. World Health Organization: AFR/RC51/12

World Health Organization (2001b). *Report of the consultation on: Key issues in Dengue Vector Control, toward the operationalization of a global strategy*. Geneva: WHO, CTD/FIL(DEN)/IC/96.1. http://www.who.int/emc-documents/dengue/docs/whocdsdenic20001.pdf.

World Health Organization. Mediterranean Centre for Vulnerability Reduction (2003). Mobilizing for action, Communication-for-Behavioral-Impact (COMBI). http://www.comminit.com/pdf/Combi4-pager_Nov_14.pdf. Retrieved Oct. 2005.

World Health Organization (2005). *Report of the scientific working group meeting on lymphatic filariasis*. Geneva, 10–12 May, 2005. Geneva: World Health Organization.

World Health Organization, Mediterranean Center for Vulnerability Reduction (2004). COMBI in action: Country highlights. http://wmc.who.int/pdf/COMBI_in_Action_04.pdf. Retrieved Nov. 2005.

19

ISSUES AND CHALLENGES IN APPLYING THEORY IN HEALTH PROMOTION PRACTICE AND RESEARCH: ADAPTATION, TRANSLATION, AND GLOBAL APPLICATION

Ralph J. DiClemente
Richard A. Crosby
Michelle C. Kegler

THE USE OF THEORY IN HEALTH PROMOTION

Social and behavioral science theory is integral to the design, implementation, and evaluation of health promotion interventions. Theory can be conceptualized as analogous to a roadmap. The "theory" roadmap guides the way for identifying and selecting which theoretical constructs to examine, for identifying targets of change, and for articulating the putative pathway through which these constructs interact to affect the likelihood of individuals engaging in specific health-protective or health-risk behaviors. By understanding the array of factors that affect people's health-risk and health-protective behaviors, and identifying mediating variables (proximal targets of change), the field can develop innovative and more effective strategies for changing health-risk behaviors (Glanz, Rimer, and Viswanath, 2008; Noar and Zimmerman, 2005).

Health educators, behavioral scientists, social scientists, and other professionals who design and implement health promotion programs generally possess competence pertaining to an extensive repertoire of behavioral theories. The theories described in this volume and elsewhere (Glanz, Rimer, and Viswanath, 2008) each have a unique set of tenets and propositions. This inherent integrity of theories is valuable to health promotion, as it creates a diverse range of "tools" that can be carefully selected and applied based on the need to either understand a given health behavior or foster conditions that will change a given health behavior. Indeed, there is nothing as practical as good theory. More precisely, we suggest that there is nothing as practical as finding the right theory that meets the specific prevention need.

Unfortunately, theory development to effectively serve health promotion practice is not yet a fully mature science. As editors of this volume, we have identified three priority areas for advancing theory that improves public health through health promotion programs that effectively avert disease. The first is that theory must be tested in practice-based contexts. Indeed, the epitome of theory development is that external validity that can best be established "beyond" efficacy trials. The challenge is to provide health promotion practitioners with user-friendly evaluation strategies that can be efficiently applied to theory-based programs. The second suggestion involves rectifying the lack of cross-cultural transfer regarding theories used in health promotion. Clearly, health promotion practice requires the ability to adapt theory-based prevention programs to local settings in any part of the global community. One challenge is to develop adaptation frameworks. Finally, we suggest that theory development should greatly expand the existing ecological models and be more inclusive of changes to the physical environment, as these changes may have substantial and sustainable effects on health behavior. A key challenge in this regard is to influence policy.

TEST THEORY IN PRACTICE-BASED SETTINGS

Health promotion practitioners and researchers use theories to understand why people behave the way they do, to identify mediating variables or proximal targets of change, and to suggest effective strategies for changing behavior (Glanz, Rimer, and Viswanath,

2008; Noar and Zimmerman, 2005). Given the significant potential of theory to improve health promotion practice, to what extent are theories actually used? In a recent review of the health behavior literature, Painter and colleagues (2008) assessed the use of theory in a sample of empirical articles from top-tier health promotion journals. They examined a continuum of use ranging from "informed by theory" to "creating or building" theory. They observed that 35.7 percent of the articles used theory, with articles describing intervention research more likely to mention a theory than articles describing nonintervention research. While the vast majority of theories were used to inform studies, there was minimal description of the theory or how it was used or measured in the article. More in-depth use of theory, in which a majority of constructs were applied or measured, was relatively rare. Rothman (2004) stated that some "lament the fact that too many interventions are not guided by a theoretical framework that specifies how they are supposed to elicit health behavior change."

The observation that theories are used most often in intervention research has interesting implications for the advancement of theory. Intervention research tends to emphasize efficacy trials and internal validity over effectiveness studies and external validity (Glasgow, Vogt, and Boles, 1999; Green and Glasgow, 2006). Efficacy trials use highly standardized protocols with well-trained staff often employed solely to deliver the intervention. They often take place in supportive organizational settings with motivated participants. Confounding variables are eliminated, minimized, or identified for later statistical control. The appeal of these rigorous designs is that the independent variable—the intervention—can be "proven" to cause the effect (that is, change in health behavior) with a fair degree of certainty. Alternative explanations for achieving the outcomes can be ruled out or minimized. The result can be a "program that works" if implemented with fidelity within a similar setting and for a similar population. The traditional research model argues that testing an intervention under ideal circumstances is a critical initial step. If it does not work in ideal circumstances, it is unlikely to work under less than ideal "real-world" circumstances. In this paradigm, intervention research should be followed by effectiveness and dissemination research.

The downside of this emphasis on internal validity over external validity is that interventions, often labeled evidence-based interventions, may have minimal relevance and applicability in the real-world practice environment (Green and Glasgow, 2006; Glasgow et al., 1999). To the extent that theory is tested through intervention research using this same model, the utility of theory in real-world contexts is also unknown (Suls and Rothman, 2004). Increased emphasis on external validity would provide valuable information on whether theories and interventions are effective in less ideal circumstances, such as when organizational settings are less enthusiastic, staff are stretched thin with multiple responsibilities, and participants are diverse along numerous dimensions, such as culture, race/ethnicity, education and health status (Glasgow et al., 1999). The cost of powering studies to test the applicability of theory across diverse settings and populations is prohibitive in any single study (Rothman, 2004). Replication or implementation research holds promise, but funding agencies tend to reward innovation over replication.

The applicability of theory across diverse contexts is of particular importance to advancing theory (Suls and Rothman, 2004). Learning the extent to which relationships between constructs hold across contexts would be invaluable in planning programs (Rothman, 2004). For example, can theories that explain cessation of a particular health behavior, for example, cigarette smoking, also explain maintenance of that behavior? While all health behaviors are complex, they vary substantively along a number of dimensions. One dimension, for example, is frequency (for example, annual mammograms versus maintaining a daily healthy diet). They can be tied to intentions or not. They can be addictive; they can be related to initiation or cessation. Unfortunately, insufficient work has been done to specify which theories fit best with which class of behaviors.

One partial solution to these dilemmas is for a more sophisticated exchange between theoreticians and applied researchers, particularly those conducting intervention research (Rothman, 2004). Researchers rarely suggest that a theory may not be applicable in a certain situation when hypothesized relationships are not confirmed (Noar and Zimmerman, 2005). Instead, measurement error, insufficient sample size, or weak intervention strategies are often blamed for lack of significant findings. With a few exceptions, there seems to be an aura of politeness about theories that keeps researchers from constructively criticizing each other's work. As a result, theories may not be evolving as quickly as possible and the field keeps using the same theories despite possible limited utility.

Branching out beyond intervention research to health promotion programs would also help to broaden our understanding of how well various theories function across contexts. Health promotion programs, some evaluated and some not, are designed to influence a range of behaviors from vaccinations to eating more fruits and vegetables. They are also designed for diverse populations ranging from Hmong women in Minnesota to African American men in the rural South. The primary purpose of health promotion programs, of course, is to improve a health outcome, not test theory. Nevertheless, these programs provide a great opportunity to learn about the utility of theories in a range of contexts. Thus, prevention research is not only a means of testing an intervention's effectiveness; it also can be used indirectly to test the theory on which the intervention is based.

Health promotion planning models, most notably PRECEDE-PROCEED and intervention mapping, begin with understanding a problem in a specific community or population (Green and Kreuter, 2005; Bartholomew et al., 2006). Starting with a problem rather than a theory does not lead naturally to testing a theory. The PRECEDE-PROCEED process identifies behaviors and environmental factors that cause the health problem, followed by identifying predisposing, enabling, and reinforcing factors that cause the behavior(s) of interest. Intervention mapping is also based on the identification of determinants, but is more explicit about using a social ecologic framework. This approach of starting with the theory of the problem encourages planners to pick and choose from various theories, since determinants are usually multilevel, and one theory is unlikely to address the full range of determinants.

This approach of starting with the theory of the problem encourages planners to pick and choose from various theories, since determinants are usually multilevel, and one theory is unlikely to address the full range of determinants.

Moreover, with the resurgence and the ascendancy of interest in ecological approaches, health behavior theories concentrated entirely at the individual and inter-personal levels may have limited relevance (Jeffery, 2004).

Despite different orientations to planning interventions, a more equitable exchange between practitioners and researchers in the production of knowledge about theory is an important next step. At present, theory development and testing seems to be the exclusive domain of researchers, with practitioners being interested bystanders, rele-gated to the sidelines, expected to simply learn and apply health behavior theories. A more balanced exchange could happen several ways. For instance, practitioners could be actively engaged in the design and implementation phases of research. This is hap-pening to some extent with the growth of community-based participatory research (Minkler, Wallerstein, and Hall, 2002; Israel, Eng, Schulz, and Parker, 2005).

A related strategy is to take advantage of opportunities within program evaluation to test theory and contribute to its development. Because evaluations are grounded in real-world contexts, they have the potential to inform the utility of theory in a range of settings. The design stage of program evaluation typically involves the development of logic models (CDC, 1999). Logic models are visual depictions of the logic underly-ing a program. By visually showing the connections between program activities and outcomes, a good logic model shows hypothesized relationships between constructs. These logic models, not surprisingly, often include constructs from health behavior the-ories with relationships between variables explicitly stated. For example, a logic model may posit that viewing a DVD that demonstrates healthy food preparation leads to increased self-efficacy for preparing healthy foods. Increased self-efficacy, in turn, leads to changes in food preparation behavior. Evaluation questions informed by logic models ask whether changes occurred as predicted. Mediation analysis can examine whether predicted relationships were supported, and if sample size is sufficient, longer causal chains can be examined through structural equation modeling. In addition, evaluations are usually prospective in nature, which enables examination of cause and effect rela-tionships between variables, unlike the cross-sectional studies often used to test theory. Even when evaluations do not meet certain standards of rigor due to funding or other practical constraints, they can provide valuable evidence that either supports or refutes health behavior theories or specific propositions within theories.

Testing theory is not the primary purpose of evaluation and could detract from its true purpose, which is to provide information to decision makers to improve or judge a program. Thus, evaluators and their clients would need to obtain a direct benefit to see the value in this form of collaboration. One approach would be to develop a repository of valid and reliable measures for common theoretical constructs tailored to specific behaviors. Common measurement across studies would greatly facilitate learning about the performance of theories across diverse situations, and the availabil-ity of good measurement tools would be useful to evaluators. Developing a way to share datasets and/or evaluation findings outside of the peer-reviewed literature would also be useful, given that evaluation reports are rarely published, thus inaccessible for many practitioners and researchers alike. This would allow for systematic comparison of selected theoretical propositions across studies (Rothman, 2004). Encouraging evaluators and practitioners to share their logic models would also facilitate this type of exchange, as would encouraging the publication of logic models and/or theoretical frameworks in peer-reviewed publications of intervention studies. Program evaluation can also help the field identify promising new approaches to health promotion, which can form the basis of new or expanded theoretical frameworks. By working collaboratively and by engaging more players in theory development, and the testing and refinement process, we will be able to improve our theories, and ultimately, have a greater impact on public health.

IMPROVING THE CULTURAL TRANSFER OF HEALTH PROMOTION THEORY

Health risk behaviors in developing countries continue to exact a substantial toll on the health and well-being of millions, causing considerable suffering, morbidity, and death. Many of these risk behaviors (for example, sexual risk behaviors, alcohol use, cigarette smoking) result in premature death from largely preventable diseases (such as HIV, cirrhosis, cancer, and heart disease) that exploit and amplify existing social and economic disparities, adversely affecting the labor force, placing additional fiscal stain on resource-constrained health care systems, and negatively impacting a country's national revenues. Increasing disease incidence, prolonged illness, and mortality incapacitates social systems, including governance. The net effect is reduced state capacity, creating an environment that further exacerbates the health crisis.

Although infectious diseases have historically accounted for much of the global disease burden, it is now apparent that chronic diseases are having a substantial impact on population-level health. Risk behaviors such as alcohol use and cigarette smoking affect the development of adverse health conditions associated with a significant and growing morbidity and mortality both directly and indirectly. Although health promotion interventions are urgently needed, developing programs through the design, implementation, and evaluation phase is a time- and cost-intensive process; often too costly and slow for resource-poor countries. Thus, the adaptation of existing programs is an attractive course of action. One strategy designed to promote the rapid dissemination of evidence-based health promotion interventions has been the cultural transfer of interventions, usually from United States and other Western countries to non-Western, developing countries.

With an upward spiraling of the global disease burden, addressing the myriad health threats in developing countries requires interventions designed to substantially reduce risk behaviors. To this end, there is growing recognition that theory-based health promotion interventions offer considerable promise as an efficacious strategy in modifying risk behaviors (that is, smoking) and, thus, reducing the burden of disease. As a consequence, there is a marked increase in the cultural transfer of theory-based interventions to developing countries.

Empirical investigation characterizing the relevance, applicability, and appropriateness of health promotion theories developed in one culture and transferred to another culture is lacking.

Empirical investigation characterizing the relevance, applicability, and appropriateness of health promotion theories developed in one culture and transferred to another culture is lacking. Indeed, theory is only indirectly assessed cross-culturally through the application and evaluation of theory-based interventions. The implicit assumption here is that if the intervention is effective (that is, if it modifies the targets of change, whether they be attitudes, beliefs, perceptions, behavioral intentions, or behaviors), then the underlying theory is ipso facto applicable to the culture. Because theory is usually assessed through this indirect approach, it is imperfectly assessed. Without increased attention to the cultural context of a new target population, interventions transferred from Western countries to non-Western countries may lack applicability, relevance, and acceptability for non-Western populations. This lack of cultural congruency may have adverse consequences, including lower acceptability of the intervention, lower intervention efficacy, and greater barriers to the broader dissemination of the intervention.

As the number of health promotion theories continues to grow, and theory is considered de rigueur in guiding their development, a key question arises; namely, what is the applicability of theory across diverse cultural contexts? Transferring theory-based interventions designed in the United States or other Western cultures to non-Western cultures (for example, Sub-Saharan Africa) has profound implications; both in terms of the appropriateness of the intervention for the new culture and the efficacy of the intervention.

The initial concern is the appropriateness of the theory for guiding the development and implementation of an intervention in a different culture. For example, some cultures are more collectivistic than others. Collectivism is a term used to describe any moral, political, or social outlook that stresses human interdependence and the importance of a collective, rather than the importance of separate individuals. The focus is on community and society, giving priority to group goals over individual goals. In some African countries, for example, "collectivism" is highly regarded and "individualism" disparaged. However, some health promotion theories have, as a fundamental tenet, a focus on changing individuals' attributes leading to their attainment of specified outcomes. These theories or their constructs may have less relevance and be less desired in collectivistic-oriented cultures. Thus, application of an intervention designed to promote individual gain or benefit may not be concordant with the cultural norms of the society and, thus, and likely to meet resistance.

Similarly, if the constructs articulated in Western theory that underlie interventions have less relevance to a particular culture or cultural group, then the intervention may be less effective in promoting behavior change. While we know of no study that specifically evaluates the applicability of health promotion theory, we are aware of studies that have assessed the applicability of health promotion intervention transfer to other cultures. Of course, though not isomorphic, evidence-based interventions are closely tied to and reflective of the underlying health promotion theory, mapping change strategies, methods, and activities on to constructs articulated within the theory.

Intrigued by the problem of the transfer of health promotion program between cultures, Sundberg and his colleagues (1995) developed an exploratory project that might later be useful for research and application. The purpose was to identify important questions and issues about transfer of programs to developing countries and to propose criteria or guidelines that might be used in considering possibilities for application of programs in other cultures. The methods for approaching this problem involved (1) the selection of a limited number of exemplary prevention programs, and (2) formulation of an interview guide based on preliminary hypotheses about issues and problems of program transfer to South and Southeast Asia and Latin America.

Their findings indicated that major cultural differences between developing countries and the United States exist; with all in-country community informants identifying significant differences. Frequently mentioned for all countries were strong family relationships and support in the developing countries, strong religious influences on daily life, and a more relaxed lifestyle in contrast with the competitive individualism in America. Teaching people to be self-directed and autonomous, as in some health promotion theories, not be seen as desirable in some other countries.

Comparing the different countries, some characteristics stood out as different from others; for instance, violence was mentioned as common in the Philippines and machismo as important in Mexico. Gender inequality and taboos on relations between the sexes are prominent in some countries. In India, for example, interviewees said that a girl getting pregnant before marriage would be ostracized by her family, even killed. Some respondents noted that the United States had a strong cultural and media influence, especially in Panama and Mexico. Informants noted the difficulty of disentangling cultural differences from socioeconomic status; poverty and low levels of education in other countries make for enormous contrasts with American lifestyles. Some respondents pointed out that there are two cultures within these countries: the rich, educated elites and the poor, more traditional majority, often living in rural settings, but also in urban slums. Overall, it was clear that a simple transfer of a health promotion program from the United States to a developing country in Asia or Latin America is nearly impossible.

While globalization, the view that the people and nations of the world should become more economically and politically integrated and unified, continues to escalate related to commerce, communication, and technology, a parallel, though not as rapid globalization is occurring in the field of health promotion. Many theory-based interventions are being exported, transferred, and translated for use in cultures where they were not developed. Indeed, it is reasonable to project an accelerating increase in the transfer of health promotion programs from the United States and other Western countries to developing countries. However, the empirical literature supporting this translation is equivocal. Clearly, there is a need to discuss strategies for enhancing the relevance, applicability, and acceptability of transferring theory to new cultures.

A key point in any discourse on theory and culture is that even in a single society, there is no homogeneous culture. Admittedly, one culture may predominate, but is not monolithic. Large societies often have subcultures, or groups of people with distinct sets of behavioral tendencies and beliefs that differentiate them from a larger culture of which they are a part. The subculture may be distinctive because of the age of its members, or by their race, ethnicity, class, or gender. The qualities that determine a

Health promotion theory should be assessed for relevance, applicability, and cultural appropriateness for within-country cultures to assure a goodness of fit.

subculture as distinct may be aesthetic, religious, occupational, political, sexual, or a combination of these factors. The United States, for example, is a rich mosaic of cultures reflecting diverse races, ethnicities, languages, age groups, gender, and regionalism. Thus, health promotion theory should be assessed for relevance, applicability, and cultural appropriateness for within-country cultures to assure a goodness of fit between the underlying behavioral and social science theory, the health promotion program, and the cultural context of the target population.

Culture as a concept has never been easy to articulate, describe, or define. Indeed, the diversity of definitions is staggering. For instance, in a thorough review of the literature, Lonner and Malpass (1994) identified over 175 definitions of culture. Today, most social scientists view culture as consisting primarily of the symbolic, ideational, and intangible aspects of human societies. The essence of a culture is not its artifacts, tools, or other tangible cultural elements but how the members of the group interpret, use, and perceive them. It is the values, symbols, interpretations, and perspectives that distinguish one people from another in modernized societies; it is not material objects and other tangible aspects of human societies (Banks, Banks, and McGee, 1989). People within a culture usually interpret the meaning of symbols, artifacts, and behaviors in the same or in similar ways. Thus, culture is a collective concept arising from conditions, shared experiences, and memories that are common to a group of people and transmitted intergenerationally. This definition may not be universal. Wilson and Miller (2003) have pointed out that in the field of HIV prevention, "culture" tends to be considered mainly in terms of oppressed racial or ethnic groups. However, across other disciplines, culture is generally defined as comprising widely shared sets of values, institutions, practices, and beliefs that (1) emerge as groups adapt to their environment and (2) are learned through social interactions that provide contexts for behavior and influence behavior (Brown, 1991; Scheer, 1994; Wilson and Miller, 2003). At the level of local community, over time these broad shared understandings give rise to a diverse combination of individual reactions, experiences, and identifications, such that the same cultural group living in different contexts may develop different cultural identities and behaviors (Birman, Trickett, and Buchanan, 2005).

Unfortunately, there has been insufficient research assessing the cultural relevance, appropriateness, and applicability of health promotion theories transferred to other cultures.

Understanding culture involves both a working knowledge of broad historical contexts and a local appreciation of individual and subgroup differences in the expression of culture. Characterizing the degree to which relationships between particular theoretical constructs are "stable" when applied in different cultural contexts can be invaluable in enhancing the efficiency and effectiveness of health promotion program planning (Rothman, 2004). For instance, consider theories that predict behavior. The behavior of condom use, for example, is not likely to be culturally comparable. Although all health behaviors are complex and vary substantively along a number of dimensions, understanding the cultural applicability of health promotion theories in a new cultural context would enhance their utility and, most importantly, may enhance the theory-based program's efficacy to promote the adoption and maintenance of health protective behaviors. Thus, defining the term culture in the context of the specific health promotion effort and identifying relevant cultural categories are therefore important steps in the process of considering the needs, assets, and preferences of a specific population. Unfortunately, there has been insufficient research assessing the cultural relevance, appropriateness, and applicability of health promotion theories transferred to other cultures.

There is no single approach to address the fundamental and complex issue of cross-cultural transfer of theory. One potential solution to address this gap in the literature on theory is to develop a continuum of research designed to understand the opportunities and challenges inherent in the cultural transfer of health promotion programs. Another potential solution would be to promote a more bountiful and efficient exchange of information between theoreticians and applied researchers (as suggested previously in this chapter). By enhancing the exchange between theory developers and theory users, we may be able to acquire another vantage point, one that offers a broader and culturally appropriate perspective for assessing the applicability of specific theories for particular cultures (Rothman, 2004). Indeed, when a culturally transferred theory is "unusable" in a new cultural context, namely, the hypothesized relationships between theoretical constructs (internally) and behavior (externally) are not observed, we as a field are quick to dismiss the findings. Indeed, we devalue our empirical evidence in favor of attributions that could logically and rationally account for the lack of observed significance between theory and its constructs and behavior. Often, we invoke methodological limitations as being responsible for the observed lack of associations or null findings. We assert that Type III implementation error, measurement error, insufficient sample size, or ineffectual intervention strategies are the methodological culprits, rather than the theory underlying the health promotion intervention may not be applicable to the cultural context (Noar and Zimmerman, 2005).

A third solution may be to test theory, and in doing so, contribute to its development as well as enhance our understanding of how well various theories function across cultural contexts by taking advantage of opportunities within program evaluation. Because evaluations are grounded in real-world contexts, they have the potential to inform the utility of theory in a range of settings. However, a caveat is warranted, as we noted in earlier sections of this chapter, this solution represents an indirect test of the cultural applicability of theory and, as such, is imperfect. For instance, it can be argued that it is not the theory per se that is poorly aligned with the culture, but rather the strategies, methods, and activities that are used to represent and articulate the constructs embedded within the theory that may not be culturally appropriate or relevant. However, rarely is theory testing a research activity. Though suffering from serious shortcomings, and notwithstanding the above noted limitations, the evaluation of health promotion programs does provide a rare "window of opportunity" to observe the applicability of theories across diverse cultural contexts (Cicchetti and Toth, 1992; Dishion and Patterson, 1999).

Key Principles

Over the past few years, a number of adaptation models have been developed, designed to provide a framework for adapting evidence-based HIV prevention interventions to other populations, venues, and cultures (Solomon et al., (2006); Bauman et al., (1991); McKleroy et al., (2006); Wingood and DiClemente, 2008). These frameworks provide a systematic approach for adapting evidence-based HIV interventions. Likewise, other evidence-based interventions have also been transferred cross-culturally. Unfortunately, while the adaptation and transfer of evidence-based health promotion interventions has gained increased traction in the field of health promotion, data describing the cross-cultural applicability of health promotion theory has not garnered the same degree of traction. Below we provide a brief, albeit less than comprehensive pragmatic set of strategies to consider when transferring health promotion theory to other cultures.

Strategy 1, *Assessment*, involves conducting focus groups, elicitation interviews, or other qualitative and quantitative assessments with the new population, applied researchers, and indigenous practitioners. Formative research is necessary to identify whether health promotion theory constructs can be located and interpreted in a new culture, and the culturally-appropriate language used to accurately describe these constructs. This assessment is fundamental to evaluating whether a particular health promotion theory will be applicable or relevant to the new culture. Focus groups or elicitation interviews should also be conducted with the proposed target population, with agency staff involved in implementing health promotion interventions, and other relevant stakeholders.

Strategy 2, *Decision*, involves (1) reviewing the empirical health promotion literature that uses the theory to guide research in this culture; (2) determining if the theory was appropriately applied, modified, or if particular constructs were deleted; and (3) deciding if the findings demonstrate that the theoretical constructs changed as a function of an intervention, according to the what the theory hypothesized. This step is critical to deciding if, indeed, the health behavior theory has accumulated empirical support within a particular cultural context.

Strategy 3, engage *Experts*. Experts need to be actively involved by (1) soliciting indigenous culturally competent researchers and practitioners as consultants to assess, prima facie, the cultural applicability of a particular health promotion theory; (2) asking cultural consultants to provide insight into the empirical literature that utilized the theory in terms of issues of program usability, perceived value, program implementation, other program evaluation measures (that is, attendance at group sessions); and (3) to assess whether the program has been disseminated and the level of program uptake by relevant stakeholders (that is, CBOs, clinics, schools, and so on).

Finally, it is obvious that the aforementioned strategies do not reflect a rigorous and validated approach to assessing the cultural applicability of health promotion theories. Unfortunately, more rigorous a priori theory testing is usually beyond the scope of researchers and practitioners given time and funding limitations. However, the strategies noted above do provide a systematic approach for collecting qualitative and quantitative data reflecting a range of metrics that could be valuable for assessing the cross-cultural applicability of health promotion theory.

DEVELOP ECOLOGICAL THEORIES AND FOCUS ON ENVIRONMENTAL CHANGE

This volume has presented theory in the context of three different paradigms: individual-level approaches, community-based approaches, and ecological approaches. Although the first and second paradigms are quite familiar in health promotion research and practice, the latter tends to be somewhat confusing and even elusive to many students and professionals. The confusion often arises from a simple misunderstanding of terms. To quickly rectify this, it is important to understand that an ecological approach is not synonymous with an approach that is strictly limited to changes in the physical environment. Unfortunately, this simple distinction has not always been clear in the literature.

In 1988, a seminal article pertaining to ecological approaches made it quite clear that the paradigm implied intervening at multiple levels of causation (McLeroy et al., 1988). Although various labels have been used over the years, these levels of causation can be loosely classified as intrapersonal (cognitive), interpersonal (relational), community, peers/social, cultural/societal, policy, and the physical environment. A true ecological approach can be viewed as one that draws on an "as needed" basis from each level of causation. Two well-known scholars in this area of investigation have defined ecological models of health behavior as: "Models proposing that behaviors are influenced by intrapersonal, sociocultural, policy, and physical-environmental factors; these variables are likely to interact, and multiple levels of environmental variables are described that are relevant for understanding and changing health behavior" (Sallis and Owen, 2002). The key phrase in this definition is "physical-environmental factors" as these variables make ecological approaches distinct from individual-level and community-based approaches. Clearly, it is important here to bear in mind that the primary goal is usually to effect change in individuals' health behaviors. Indeed, making changes to the physical environment can have strong and lasting influences on health behavior. The concept of "walkability" is an example of an increasingly popular and effective method of promoting physical activity (an otherwise difficult behavior to change). In addition to changing behaviors, changes to the physical environment can also have a direct effect on health (simple examples include the fortification of salt with iodine and adding fluoride to water supplies). An eloquent example of this direct effect can be traced back to the time of Sir Edwin Chadwick, who has been credited with providing sanitation services and clean drinking water to poverty stricken urban dwellers as a method of reducing infectious disease incidence in the mid-1800s (Duffy, 1990).

The international obesity epidemic serves to illustrate differences between a classic ecological approach and an approach based solely on physical-environmental factors. Swinburn and colleagues (1999) have used the term "obesogenic environments" to describe ways in which modern environments lead to physical inactivity and overeating. They have developed a framework for identification of key elements in obesogenic modern environments. Once identified, these key elements can become the target of change efforts. Clearly, using this approach, the key activity of health promotion is to change policy and perhaps pass legislation designed to favorably alter the identified elements that lead to obesity. In essence, changing the physical environment becomes the organizing goal of the health promotion effort. Indeed, the primary focal point of responding to the international obesity epidemic has increasingly become changing the physical environment (Brownson et al., 2001; Farley and Cohen, 2005). Alternatively, an ecological approach would encompass a broad-based view of "causes" concerning the obesity epidemic. Causes may include, or even emphasize, the physical environment (Trost et al., 2002) but cognitive and social variables may also be important, thereby becoming targets of health promotion efforts. The difference then hinges upon the degree of emphasis on changing the physical environment.

An important challenge for the future is to develop theory-based approaches to leveraging changes in the physical environment that can have truly profound influences on indicators of population-level health.

We suggest that health promotion theory is increasingly oriented toward an emphasis on changing physical environments to achieve favorable changes in health behavior. This phenomenon appears to be occurring in conjunction with the pubic health response to the international obesity epidemic and tobacco use; however, it is also becoming more common in other areas of health promotion, including the prevention of infectious disease. Unfortunately, theory development has focused primarily on the identification of physical-environmental structures that should be changed rather than how to actually achieve change in these structural elements. Thus, an important challenge for the future is to develop theory-based approaches to leveraging changes in the physical environment that can have truly profound influences on indicators of population-level health.

A second important challenge is to fortify the theoretical underpinnings of ecological approaches, thereby making the application of ecological theories in health promotion practice more efficient. This section of the chapter will address several issues that are relevant to meeting these two challenges.

First, it is important that ecological theories squarely address macro-level change. Macro-level change targets the superstructures of society, that is, influences that reach across populations and cultures. Because changing physical-environmental elements, identified as critical to achieving public health, may typically involve legislation, a key function of future theories will probably be centered upon changing how people who make laws and policies think and act regarding specified issues. The key role of these "intermediaries" has been described relative to physical activity (Stokols, 1996). Unfortunately, theory development has largely neglected this "how to" aspect of health-related changes to policy and law. Planning frameworks such as the PRECEDE-PROCEED model and MATCH have long recognized the value of efforts targeting policymakers and legislators. Thus, the next logical step in the progression is to develop and refine theory that can be used to address this neglected aspect of health promotion practice.

With increasing globalization, an important starting question becomes whether change efforts pertaining to policy and law are best made at the local level. In the United States, for example, tobacco-free workplaces and smoke-free communities have been created through the efforts of community coalitions and, until recently, change has usually taken the form of municipal legislation passed one city at a time. Clearly, local level change achieved through principles pertaining to building community organizational capacity is often the mainstay of community-based theories. Yet, for example, despite great success going "smoke free" in many U.S. communities, accelerated declines in tobacco consumption have yet to occur in recent years. Changes at more macro-level installations of policy and law may be far more difficult to achieve, but the corresponding gains in public health may also be far greater.

Changes in policy and law are only two examples of macro-level approaches. Macro-level approaches also apply to the distribution of health protective substances or products. In their work to eradicate onchocerciasis (river blindness) a drug (ivermectin) was distributed to people in endemic areas, but the distribution had to be "tightly controlled" because of its high value (Carter, 2007, p. 187). Of course, political support and assistance from law enforcement agencies are often required with respect to distributions efforts such as this one mounted by the Carter Center. Unfortunately, the great success of the Carter Center in disease eradication may be very difficult to replicate given that the stature of a former U.S. president undoubtedly provided great ease of access to heads of state, thereby facilitating the change process. Emerging theories will need to provide practitioners with a broader repertoire of methods that can be used to access key political figures.

As theory development proceeds, it is important to keep in mind that ecological theories must not create further health disparities. For example, the common tendency of persons lower in socioeconomic status to engage in relatively higher levels of health-risk behavior is well documented (Farley and Cohen, 2005). Although the question of "why" has not been adequately investigated, one contributing factor may be lack of access to services and education as they relate to health and health behavior. For example, an ecological approach to the promotion of vegetables and fruits that relies, in part, on Internet sites for message dissemination will largely "miss" an entire segment of the population who cannot afford Internet access. Naturally, such programs will neglect large segments of any population if provisions for affordable access to produce are not included in the ecological approach. Similarly, if the use of community infrastructure is one basis of leveraging change (in any behavior), those communities experiencing disintegration are likely to be left behind. By the same token, ecological approaches that capitalize on the use of media for health communication will neglect large segments of populations when uniform access to the selected media does not exist.

With increasing urbanization worldwide, disparities also exist for people in rural areas. Ecological approaches that are urban-centric will certainly exacerbate existing rural disparities.

> Ecological approaches that are urban-centric will certainly exacerbate existing rural disparities.

For example, the concept of *walkability* is certainly an excellent innovation for urban dwellers but a similar concept is unlikely to apply for rural residents. Rural residents in many countries (including the United States) lack access to high-speed Internet, thereby limiting the utility for this form of health communication. As the cost of transportation rises worldwide, rural residents are increasingly isolated from preventive services that are often focal points of health promotion efforts (for example, Pap testing, mammography, colorectal cancer screening). Rural residents are also less likely to live within the confines of geographically defined neighborhoods, thereby making some aspects of community-based intervention a less relevant portion of the ecological approach.

Yet another important consideration for further theory development is that ecological theories must be feasible for practitioners. Regardless of whether the intent is to change only the physical environment or to install a full-scale health promotion program using an ecological model, the theoretical underpinnings developed by researchers must be accessible to the practitioners using these principles. The development of complex logic models, for example, does little to assist the community-based practitioner in the process of gaining "buy in" from his or her community regarding a violence prevention program targeting high-risk teens. Practitioners deal with local realities, and often face challenges; they may or may not be interested in theory application as intended by researchers developing the approach or model.

Practitioners also lack the freedom to easily transcend their role as prescribed by their place of employment. This may be quite problematic when the use of an ecological model implies the ability to become a full-time administrator of the expansive health promotion efforts necessitated by leveraging change at multiple levels of causality. Indeed, ecological approaches are inherently demanding simply because they do involve a coordination of efforts across various domains of influence. Thus, unless funding is available to support at least one full-time, qualified practitioner (dedicated solely to the project), the orchestration of the ecological approach may well fail. In nations (including the United States) where medical paradigms greatly overshadow investment in prevention, the default position when funds are not available for full-time health promotion practitioners is to use existing staff to fill prevention functions. The result of the default position may be that a far less demanding approach be used, such as one that focuses exclusively on the individual level. In such circumstances, a preferable alternative may be to consider making changes only to the physical environment. While doing so is certainly very demanding in its own right, avoiding the complexities of also intervening at other levels of causality may be critical to making the single effort ultimately successful.

The relative emphasis on various components in any given model should be modifiable based on the behaviors being targeted for change. Finally, it is critical to note that ecological theories should have great flexibility. Ultimately, health promotion is not at all a monolithic activity. Models used successfully to promote the adoption of physical activity or improved dietary habits may look quite different from those used to prevent teens' abuse of substances or to avert incidence of infectious diseases. Thus, the relative emphasis on various components in any given model should be modifiable based on the behaviors being targeted for change.

For example, if the goal is to promote cancer screening, then the emphasis on changing the physical environment may be quite modest or even nonexistent, and the relative emphasis on patient-provider communication to modify people's decision-making may be greater. Conversely, if the goal is to promote HPV vaccine acceptance among young women in a medically underserved area, then the programmatic emphasis may be placed on advocacy for either publicly supported or corporate-supported vaccination programs. Although some level of health education may be important to promote HPV vaccine acceptance, this program component is unlikely to yield great return in the outcome behavior if women simply cannot afford the vaccine.

Further, the ability of models to provide tailored and targeted intervention programs is critical. Targeting, or audience segmentation, to use marketing terminology, is a concept that is critical to the resolution of health disparities. Models used successfully in one culture or even in one entire country may have little utility in other cultures or countries. If models are not capable of working across cultures and countries, the result will be a proliferation of models that will create a "communication divide" among professionals. The discipline of health promotion needs to be unified by theory rather than divided by theory.

Flexibility in the use of ecological models can also be thought of in terms of resources and personnel, with models being developed specifically for the constraints of low-resource environments. Indeed, models that stipulate changes in the physical environment need to be responsive to the larger concept of economic capacities. For example, making condoms easily accessible and available for free may be a key implication of an ecological model applied to HIV prevention in a developing country.

As a guide to action, a good ecological model should provide practitioners with practical methodologies for leveraging community and political resources necessary to marshal economic support for the vital program component of condom acquisition.

> As a guide to action, a good ecological model should provide practitioners with practical methodologies for leveraging community and political resources necessary to marshal economic support

A Paradigm with a Larger View

The development of highly flexible ecological models that are sensitive to health disparities emphasize macro-level change is a priority, as preventable disease continues to take a huge toll on the quality and quantity of human life. Yet, another paradigm may exist, one that has probably been overlooked for various reasons: the regulation of corporate efforts to promote unhealthy practices. The food industry, for example, has been tremendously successful in promoting high-calorie foods such as cheeseburgers, pizza, and fried chicken. Much like the tobacco industry, the food industry has fiscal resources that far outweigh those available in public health. Although health promotion programs may obtain resources to sponsor widespread media promotion of low-calorie foods, funding for such a campaign would be meager in contrast to the money spent by the fast food industry to promote high-calorie products. Other examples include policy changes such as federal subsidies for grocery stores to make fresh vegetables easily available to consumers (Kuchler, Abebayehu, and Harris, 2005) and laws that regulate the physical location of fast food restaurants (Ashe, Jernigan, Kline, and Galaz, 2003; Hayne, Moran, and Ford, 2004). Herein, then, lies the disadvantage of sole reliance on assorted ecological approaches: large-scale changes in cultural practices, policy, and law may be far less accessible to public health professionals than to corporate entities. Until prevention resources begin to resemble the finances allocated for medical treatment, public health professionals may be in a situation that requires advocacy for government regulation of health-damaging products (for example, tobacco, empty calorie foods, alcohol) as well as the often subtle corporate promotion of health-damaging practices (for example, use of firearms, riding all-terrain vehicles, and using over-the-counter drugs to regulate sleep cycles). Although this form of regulation may at first be threatening to the populace, the long-term national economic gains from medical savings may become a valued trade-off for the loss of corporate freedoms.

SUMMARY

Theories have been instrumental in underlying health promotion research. However, as the field of health promotion begins to globalize, we confront a number of challenges related to the relevance and cultural appropriateness of health promotion theory. The rapid globalization or translation of interventions from U.S. and Western countries to other developing nations, designed to reduce health-risk behaviors, necessitates a systematic assessment of cultural relevance and appropriateness if we are to maximize the potential of health promoton interventions and achieve the promise of health promotion on a global scale.

REFERENCES

Ashe, M., Jernigan, D., Kline, R., and Galaz, R. (2003). Land use planning and the control of alcohol, tobacco, firearms, and fast food restaurants. *American Journal of Public Health, 93*(9), 1404–1408.

Banks, J. A., Banks, and McGee, C. A. (1989). *Multicultural education*. Needham Heights, MA: Allyn and Bacon.

Bartholomew, L., Parcel, G., Kok, G., and Gottlieb, N. (2006). *Planning health promotion programs: An intervention mapping approach*. 2nd Edition. San Francisco: Jossey-Bass, 2006.

Bauman, L. J., Stein, R.E.K., and Ireys, H. T. (1991). Reinventing fidelity: The transfer of social technology among settings. *American Journal of Community Psychology, 19*(4), 619–639.

Birman, D., Trickett, E. and Buchanan, R. (2005). A tale of two cities: Replication of a study on the acculturation and adaptation of immigrant adolescents from the former Soviet Union in a different community context. *American Journal of Community Psychology, 35*(1–2), 87–101.

Brown, D. E. (1991). *Human universals*. Philadelphia: Temple University Press.

Brownson R. C., Baker E. A., Housemann, R. A., Brennan L. K., and Bacak L. J. (2001). Environmental and policy determinants of physical activity in the United States. *American Journal of Public Health, 81*, 1995–2003.

Carter, J. (2007). *Beyond the White House: Waging peace, fighting disease, building hope*. New York: Simon and Schuster.

Centers for Disease Control and Prevention. (1999). *Recommended framework for program evaluation in public health practice*. MMWR Recommendations and Reports, *48*(RR-11).

Cicchetti, D., and Toth, S.L. (1992). The role of developmental theory in prevention and intervention. *Development and Psychopathology, 4*, 489–493.

Dishion, T. J., and Patterson, G. R. (1999). Model building in developmental psychopathology: A pragmatic approach to understanding and intervention. *Journal of Clinical Child Psychology, 28*, 502–512.

Duffy, J. (1990). *The Sanitarians: A history of American public health*. Urbana and Chicago: University of Illinois Press.

Farely, T., and Cohen, D. A. (2005). *Prescription for a healthy nation: A new approach to improving our lives by fixing our everyday world*. Boston: Beacon Press.

Glasgow, R., Vogt, T., and Boles, S. (1999). Evaluating the public health impact of health promotion interventions: The RE-AIM framework. *American Journal of Public Health, 89*(9), 1322–1327.

Glanz, K., Rimer, R., and Viswanath, K. (2008). *Health behavior and health education*. 4th ed. San Francisco: Jossey-Bass.

Green, L., and Glasgow, R. (2006). Evaluating the relevance, generalization, and applicability of research: Issues in external validation and translation methodology. *Evaluation and the Health Professions*, *29*(1), 126–153.

Green, L., and Kreuter, M. (2005). *Health program planning: An educational and ecological approach*. 4th ed. New York: McGraw-Hill.

Israel, B., Eng., Schulz, A., and Parker, E. (Eds). (2005). *Methods in community-based participatory research for health*. San Francisco: Jossey-Bass.

Jeffery, R. (2004). How can health behavior theory be made more useful for intervention research? *International Journal of Nutrition and Physical Activity*, *1*:10, doi: 10.1186/1479–5868–1–10.

Kuchler, F., Abebayehu, T., and Harris, J. M. (2005). Taxing snack foods: Manipulating diet quality or financing information programs? *Review of Agricultural Economics*, *27*, 4–17.

Lonner, W., and Malpass, R. (1994). Where psychology and culture meet: An introduction to cross-cultural psychology, In W. Lonner and R. Malpass (eds.), *Psychology and Culture* (pp. 1–12). Boston: Allyn and Bacon.

McKleroy, V. S., Galbraith, J. S., Cummings, B. et al. (2006). Adapting evidence-based behavioral interventions for new settings and target populations. *AIDS Education and Prevention*, *18*, 59–74.

McLeroy, K. R., Bibeau, D., Steckler, A., and Glanz, K. (1988). An ecological perspective on health promotion programs. *Health Education Quarterly*, *15*, 351–378.

Minkler, M., and Wallerstein, N. (eds.). (2002). *Community-based participatory research for health*. San Francisco: Jossey-Bass.

Noar, S., and Zimmerman, R. (2005). Health behavior theory and cumulative knowledge regarding health behaviors: are we moving in the right direction? *Health Education Research*, *20*(3), 275–290.

Painter, J., Borba, C., Hynes, M., Mays, D., and Glanz, K. (2008). The use of theory in health behavior research from 2000 to 2005: A systematic review. *Annals of Behavioral Medicine*, *35*(3), 358–62

Sallis, J. F., and Owen, N. (2002). Ecological models of health behavior. In Glanz, K., Rimer, R., and Lewis, F. M. (2008). *Health Behavior and Health Education*. 3rd Edition. San Francisco, CA: Jossey-Bass.

Solomon, J., Card, J. J., and Malow, R. M. (2006). Adapting efficacious interventions: Advancing translational research in HIV prevention. *Evaluation and the Health Professions*, *29*(2), 162–94.

Stokols, D. (1996). Translating social ecological theory into guidelines for community health promotion. *American Journal of Health Promotion*, *10*, 282–298.

Suls, J., and Rothman, A. (2004). Evolution of the biopsychosocial model: Prospects and challenges for health psychology. *Health Psychology*, *23*(2), 119–125.

Swinburn, B., Egger, G., and Raza, F. (1999). Dissecting obesogenic environments: The development and application of a framework for identifying and prioritizing environmental interventions for obesity. *Preventive Medicine*, *29*, 563–570.

Trost, S. G., Owen, N., Bauman, A., Sallis, J. F., and Brown, W. (2002). Correlates of adults' participation in physical activity: Review and update. *Medicine and Science in Sports and Exercise*, *34*, 1996–2001.

Rothman, A. (2004). "Is there nothing more practical than a good theory?" Why innovations and advances in health behavior change will arise if interventions are used to test and refine theory. *International Journal of Nutrition and Physical Activity*, *1*:11, doi: 10.1186/1479–5868–1–11.

Scheer, J. (1994). Culture and disability: An anthropological point of view. In E. J. Trickett, R. J. Watts, and D. Birman (eds.), *Human diversity: Perspectives on people in context* (pp. 244–260). San Francisco: Jossey-Bass.

Sundberg, N. D., Hadiyono, J. P., Latkin, C. A., and Padilla, J. (1995). Cross-cultural prevention program transfer: Questions regarding developing countries. The *Journal of Primary Prevention*, *15*(4), 361–376.

Wilson, B. D. M., and Miller, R. L. (2003). On examining strategies for culturally grounded HIV prevention: A review. *AIDS Education and Prevention*, *15*(2), 184–202.

Wingood, G. M., and DiClemente, R. J. (2008). The ADAPT-ITT Model: A model for adapting evidence-based HIV interventions. *Journal of Acquired Immune Deficiency Syndromes*, *47*(Suppl), S40–S46.

INDEX